Traditional Institutions in Kembong (Cameroon)

BAESSLER-ARCHIV

Beiträge zur Ethnologie
Neue Folge Beiheft 11

Herausgegeben vom Ethnologischen Museum
Staatliche Museen zu Berlin – Stiftung Preußischer Kulturbesitz

von

Peter Junge und Viola König

Verlag von Dietrich Reimer Berlin

TRADITIONAL INSTITUTIONS IN KEMBONG (CAMEROON)

Hans-Joachim Koloss

with 261 colour photos

Verlag von Dietrich Reimer Berlin 2008

Alle Fotos vom Verfasser
Übersetzung: Dr. Emily Schalk
Grafik: Ulrich Gebauer

Bibliografische Information der deutschen Nationalbibliothek
Die Deutsche Nationalbibliothek verzeichnet diese Publikation in der Deutschen Nationalbibliografie; detaillierte bibliografische Daten sind im Internet über http://dnb.d-nb.de abrufbar.

Berliner Straße 53
D-10713 Berlin
www.reimer-verlag.de
und Staatliche Museen zu Berlin
Stiftung Preußischer Kulturbesitz

Layout und Satz: GrafikDesign M&S Hawemann, Berlin
Lithografien: Bild1Druck GmbH, Berlin
Druck und Verarbeitung: DZA Druckerei zu Altenburg GmbH, Altenburg
Gedruckt auf alterungsbeständigem Papier
Printed in Germany
ISBN 978-3-496-02811-6

Contents

Preface

We are particularly delighted to see that the research-work which Dr. Hans-Joachim Koloss started in Kembong in January 1980, has finally resulted in this book: "Traditional Institutions in Kembong (Cameroon)". The author, a German anthropologist, has documented in this book the history and cultural heritage of Kembong people. From the many beautiful and important photographs found in this book, we are pleasurably surprised to observe how much of our cultural past would have been lost forever, had the author not conducted his research-work in Kembong.

During his twenty-five years of contact with Kembong people and especially during the four intensive research-trips, which he made to Kembong in 2004/2005, the author has shown his profound understanding of the people's "way of life", their philosophy of existential reality and above all the people's fundamental belief pattern. In critically examining and analyzing the religious, social and political values, actions and institutions, the author rightly affirms that the ultimate and fundamental existential reality of Kembong people is, as everywhere in traditional Africa, "a community united in peace, harmony and co-operation". Though it has been impossible for mankind everywhere in the world to fulfil this ideal in the last consequence, the way of life shown by our forefathers was nevertheless directed toward achieving this objective: the maintenance of unity, peace, harmony, co-operation, morality and justice in the community.

Unquestionably, the work of Dr. Hans-Joachim Koloss in Kembong has benefited to a great extent from his research, which he had carried out in the Kingdom of Oku (North West Province of Cameroon) for many years – the findings are published in his outstanding work "World-View and Society in Oku (Cameroon)".

Impressive is his comparison of such distinctive political systems as the egalitarian society of the Ejagham with the monarchies of the Grasslands: The underlying principle is fundamentally the same in both traditions, the Chief or the King is dependent upon his people. It is the people who is the actual sovereign – Nelson Mandela was right when speaking of "democracy in its purest form".

There are several reasons for us to appreciate this book. For many centuries, our way of life has been exposed to aggressive foreign cultures. Ejagham people, like all Africans in recent decades, are faced with violent infiltration of western civilization in all of its facets and subtle ways – we are in greatest danger of losing our roots and becoming totally alienated. Dr. Hans-Joachim Koloss has dug deeply into the minds and memories – oral libraries – of our almost extinct wise men, the elderly and knowledgeable notables, and has stored in this book many vital aspects of our identity as a people.

In preserving our cherished past in word and picture, the author has given us the first critical and objective scientific research-document on our almost lost past. No doubt, this book has come to fill a vacuum in recording the authentic traditions not only of Kembong people but also of the Central Ejagham.

Ayukachale Peter Egbe
Hon. Rev. Dr.

Alfred Ayuk Ako
Chief of Kembong

Kembong (South West Province of Cameroon)
September 22, 2006

It is with the deepest regret that I must update the preface of the book "Traditional Institutions in Kembong (Cameroon)" with the sad news that His Royal Highness, Chief Alfred Ayuk Ako died on March 26, 2007 – he was the innocent victim in a street accident in Mamfe. There would have been no greater pleasure for him than to receive a copy of the published book, in which he and I wrote the original preface. Unfortunately, his tragic death preceded this publication.

The Kembong community in Cameroon and in the diaspora will perform the famous night dance during Easter 2008 to commemorate his illustrious life. This extremely rare sacred ceremony is reserved exclusively for men of highest honour and distinction among the Ejagham people. Chief Alfred Ayuk Ako will remain forever in the memory of our people.

Ayukachale Peter Egbe
Hon. Rev. Dr.
Kembong, (South West Province of Cameroon)
May 15, 2007

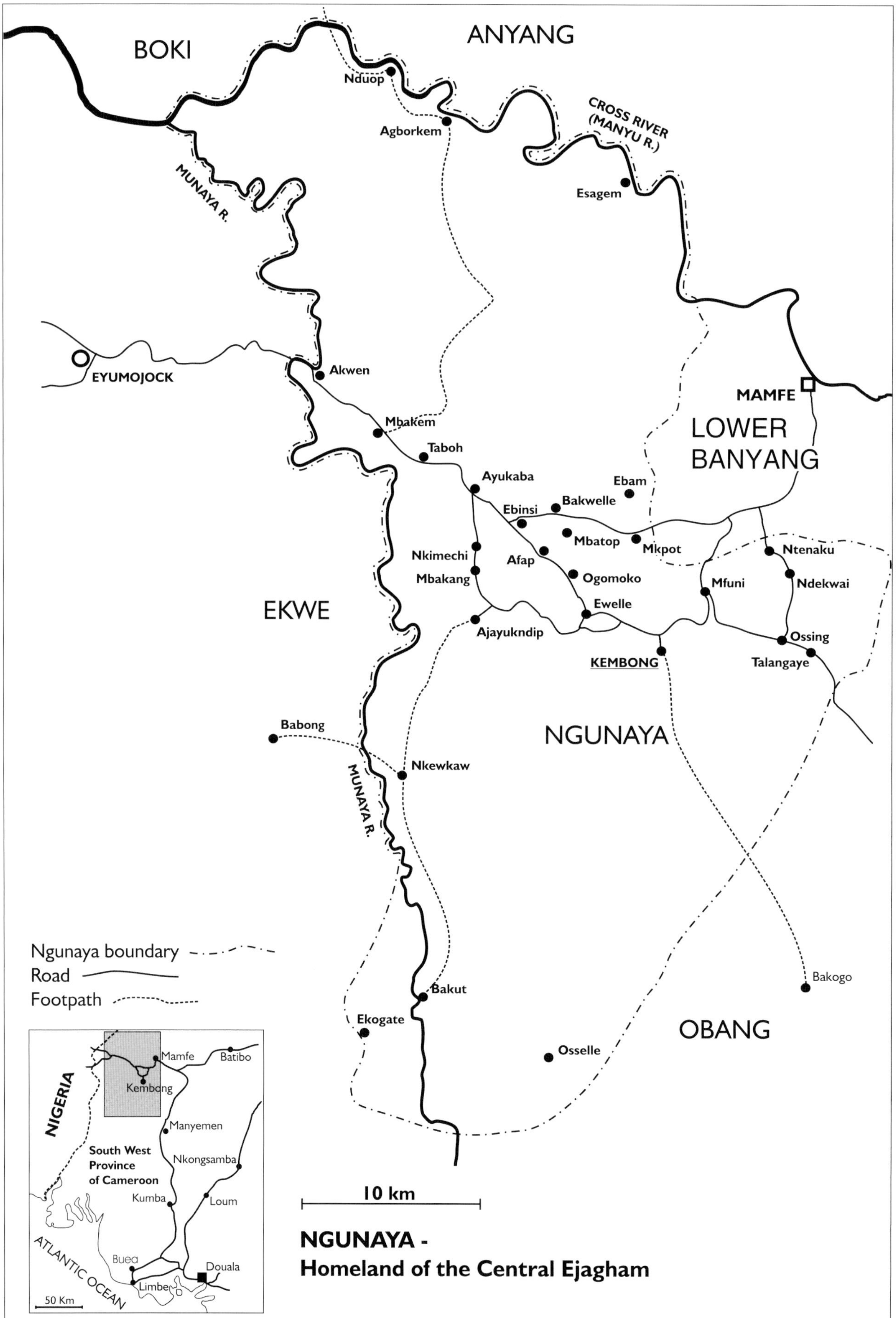

NGUNAYA -
Homeland of the Central Ejagham

1 Introduction: General information about Kembong and its history; the research project and its realisation

Kembong is the largest locality in the Ngunaya area of the Manyu Division, which belongs to the South West Province of Cameroon. In the census of 2005 the number of inhabitants in Kembong was 7,300.[1] The name "Ngunaya" can be translated as "mainland of the river", the "river" referred to being the Munaya ("small water"), which forms the western boundary of Ngunaya. In 2005, 28 localities with a total population of c. 28,000 people were accounted for in the Ngunaya area.[2] They belong to the Ejagham, whose settlement area encompasses the expansive forests of the Cross River region in southwestern Cameroon and southeastern Nigeria. Like numerous other peoples of Africa, the Ejagham were divided through the drawing of borders by the colonial powers, a demarcation that was mostly arbitrary, without any regard for the ethnic and historical background of the people affected.

The Ejagham have never represented a political unit; their unity is constituted instead by c. 150 localities or groups of peoples, who have always maintained their political independence as far as can be discerned. A certain affiliation among the Ejagham can be noted through their common language.[3] The religious and social traditions of the Ejagham are likewise similar to a great extent, and this applies to the economic, technical and political spheres as well. The Ejagham are basically an egalitarian society, who recognise neither kings nor chiefs, and in which all important decisions are made by the council of the respective community; this applies to all Ejagham groups in Cameroon as well. Apart from these, there are some groups in Nigeria with monarchical structures of government (cp. p. 50).

The settlements of the Ejagham are relatively small and, at least in Cameroon, the number of inhabitants in each is hardly more than 2,000. Now as in former times they are associated with their respective neighbours in various ways: through kinship, trade and membership in supra-regional societies. But these con-

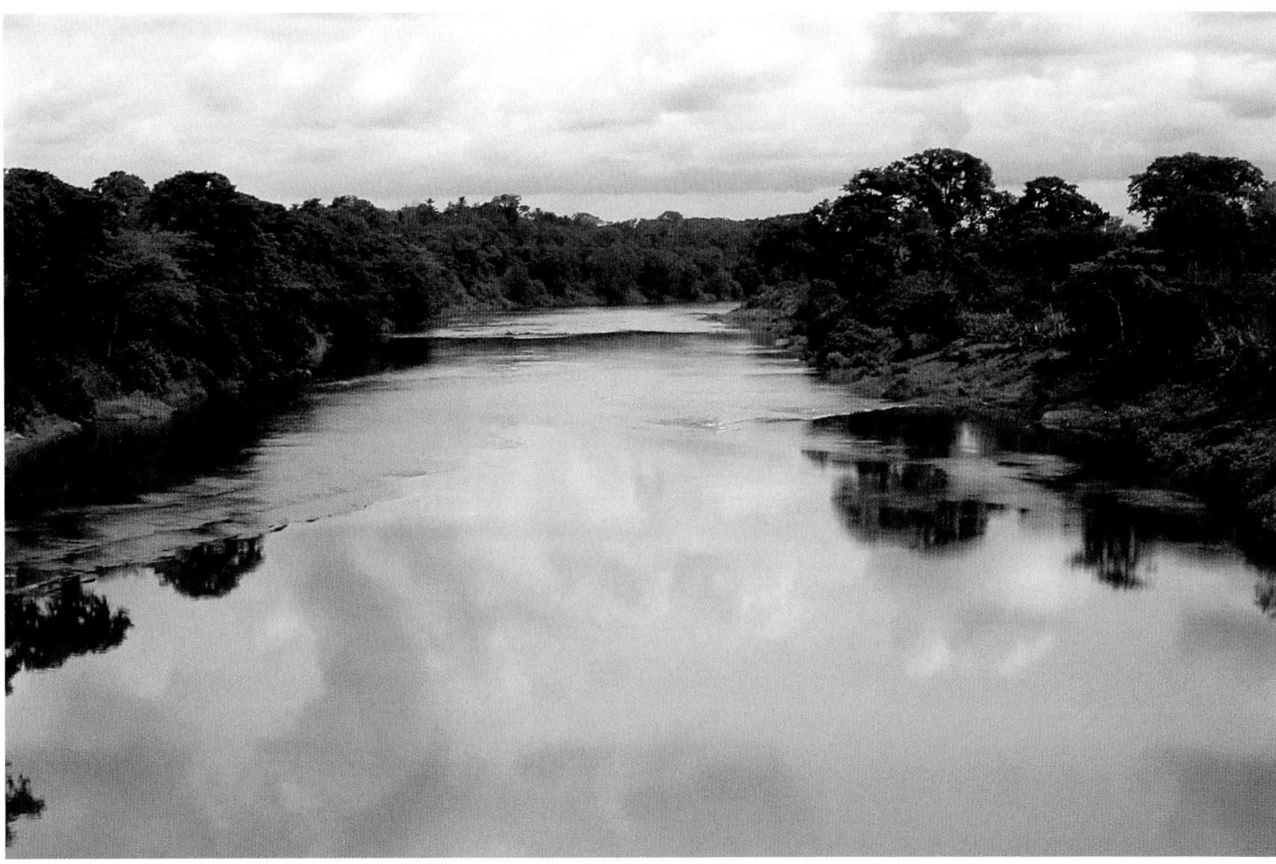

Fig. 1 The Cross River (Manyu River) near Mamfe (April 28, 2004).

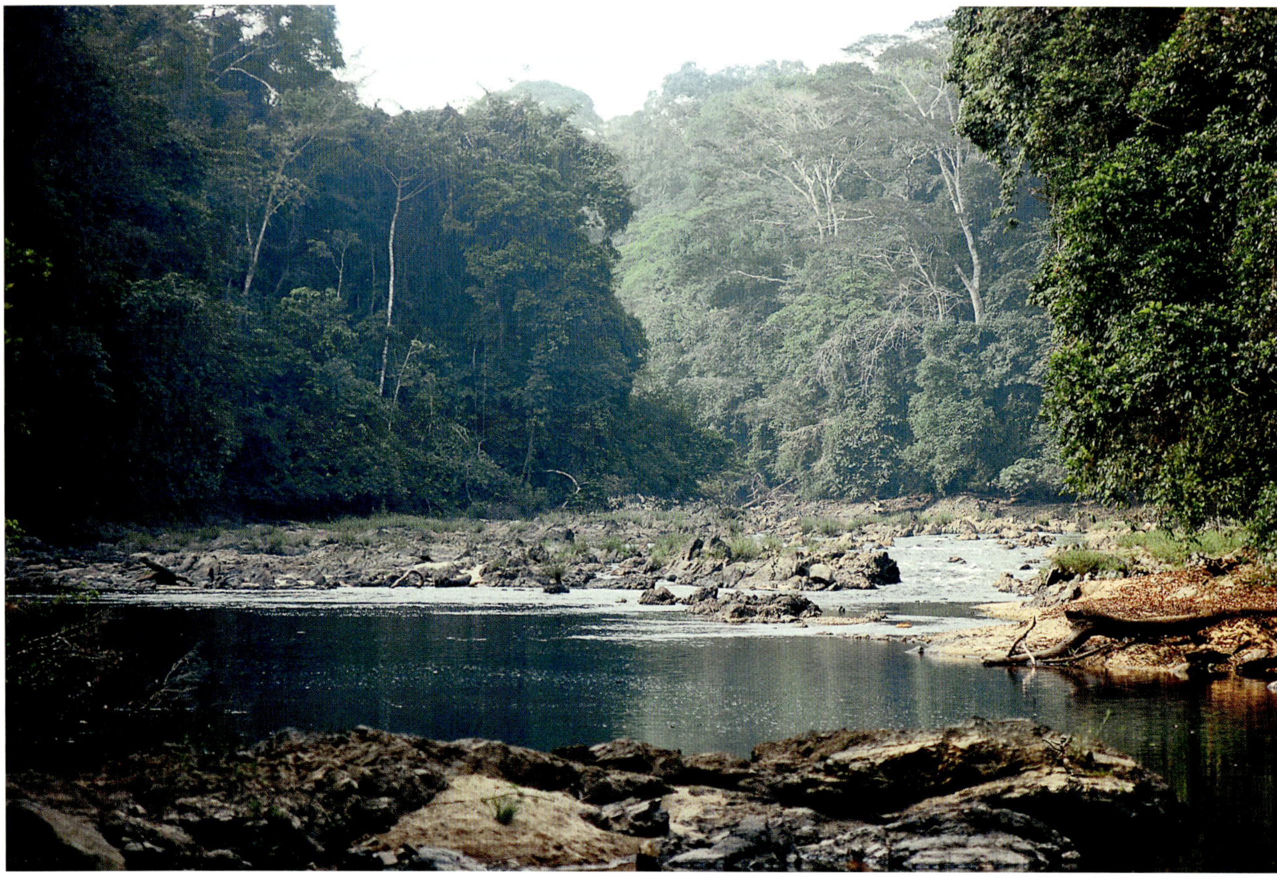

Fig. 2 The Munaya River to the east of Babong (February 19, 1980).

nections have been quite loose, and whoever left his own surroundings did so at a certain risk. There have always been occasional armed conflicts,[4] which usually occurred in the jungle regions in the form of attacks or "guerilla fighting".[5] Dr. Alfred Mansfeld (head of the District of Ossidinge – "Bezirksamtmann" – during the German era, 1904–1914) even reported actual head-hunting campaigns,[6] whereas corresponding references are absent in the writings of other authors. Yet the reaction to my inquiries in Kembong about head-hunting in pre-colonial times was surprise and irritation. None of the elders could remember ever having heard of such campaigns. I do not regard this information as a kind of answer in defence, for the same informants were not at all disinclined to report on human sacrifices at well-known "night dances", which from today's viewpoint are equally gruesome and offensive (cp. p. 112 ff.).

It seems that greater warlike campaigns seldom took place;[7] and when they were conducted, certain military alliances were involved. Nevertheless, they were not a matter-of-course. Referring to them, Mansfeld noted that during the revolt of 1904 in the Cross River region against the German colonial masters, which erupted after the murder of Count Pückler-Limburg, head of the district at that time, and five other Germans,[8] there could have been no common strategy among the revolting tribes. For, although "only fifteen minutes away from tribal brothers, with whom they were related tenfold through marriage, the parties were divided, among the Banjangs as well as the Keakas." While some groups resisted vigorously, others remained uninvolved; in fact they even supported the enemies by providing them with food.[9]

The various Ejagham groups use special designations for identifying themselves, and this also applies to the Ngunaya people, who call themselves the "Central Ejagham".[10] This designation did not appear until around 1930; in pre-colonial times mention was made only of "the Ejagham". In ethnographic literature the name "Keaka" mostly prevails,[11] which is the appellation of the Banyang, their eastern neighbours, for "Ejagham".[12] The name "Keaka" was adopted by the Germans from the Banyang, with whom they (the Germans) initially had contact in the Cross River region. The British, who administered the western part of the former German colony of Cameroon as a mandate after World War I, retained this designation.[13] However, the name "Keaka", although generally known,

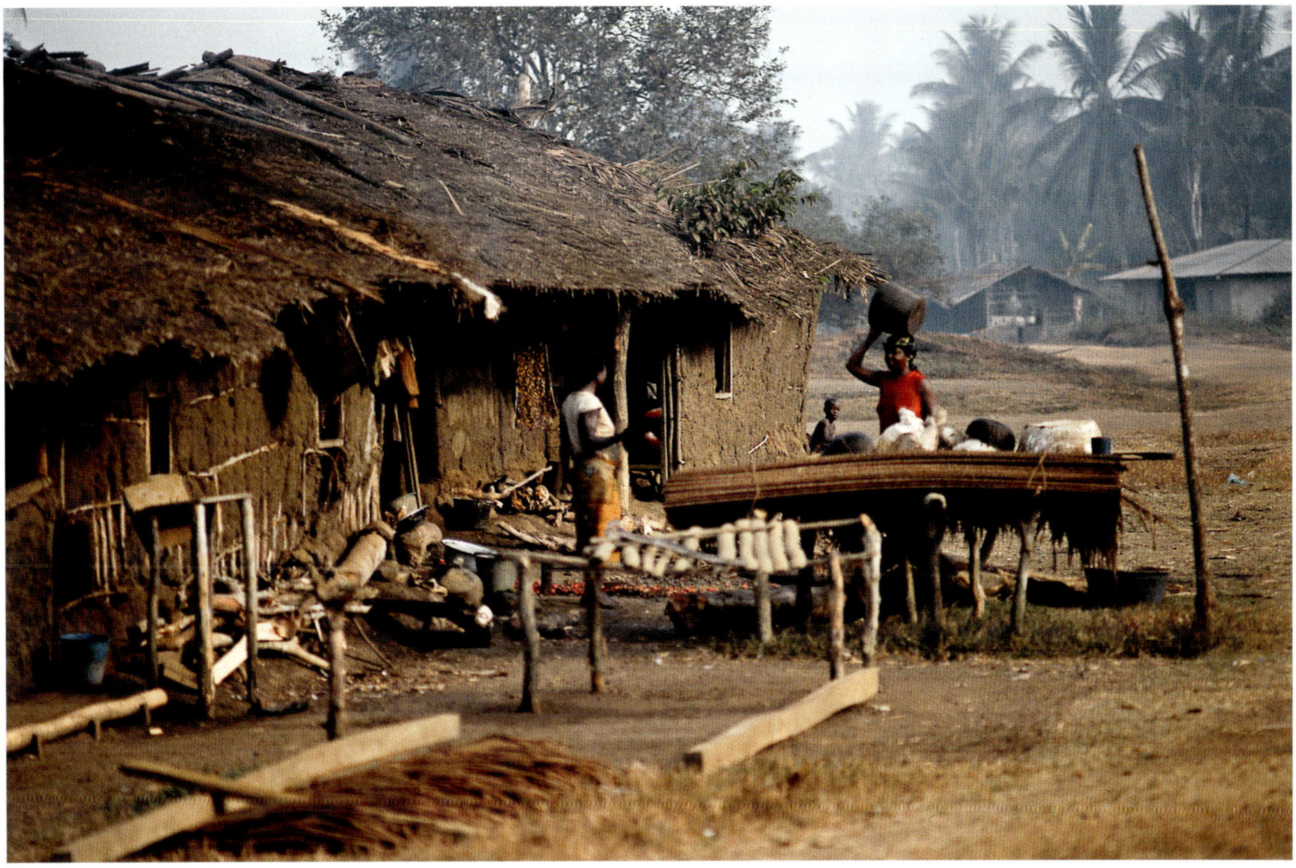

Fig. 3 Traditional 'mud houses' with a roof constructed from fronds of the raphia palm were still common in the Ngunaya area in the 1980s (Kembong, February 15, 1980).

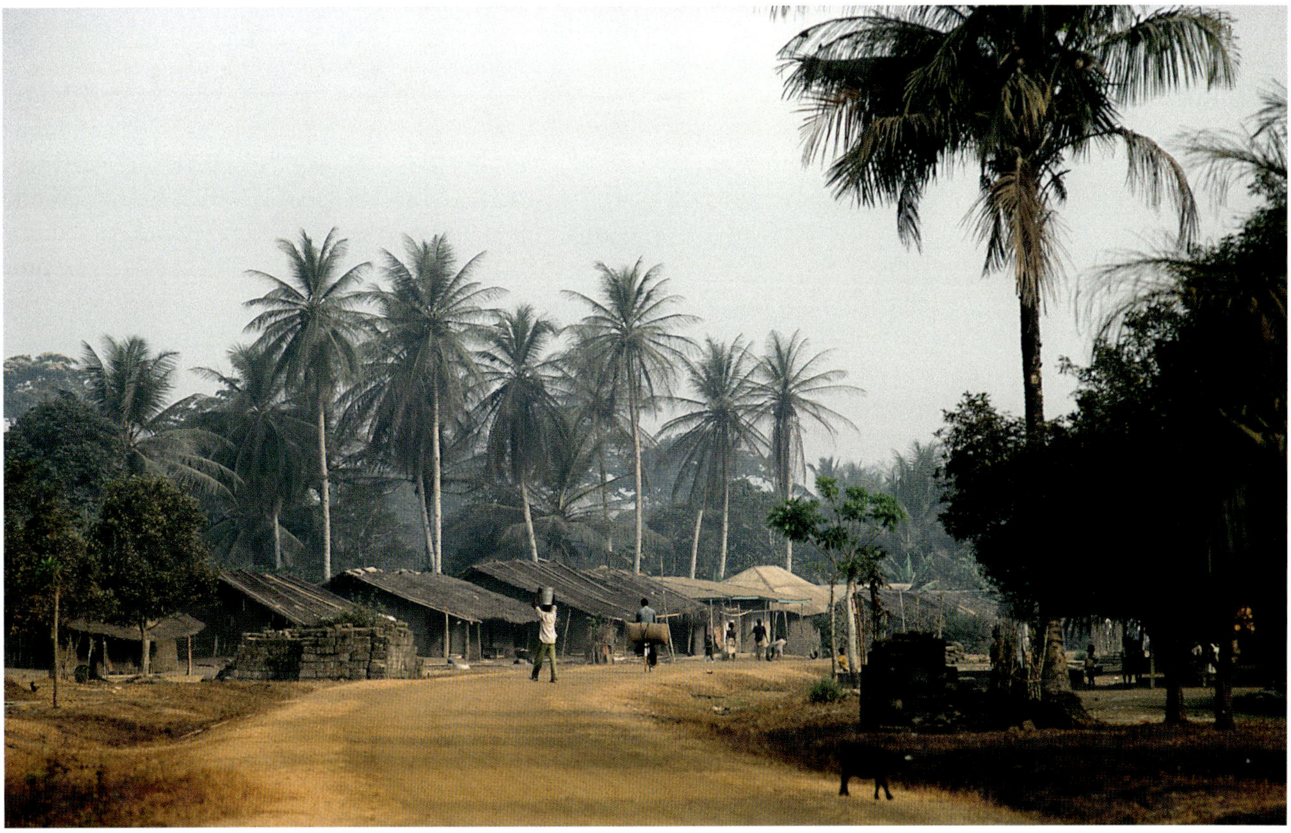

Fig. 4 Kembong's main street in 1980 (Kembong, February 15, 1980).

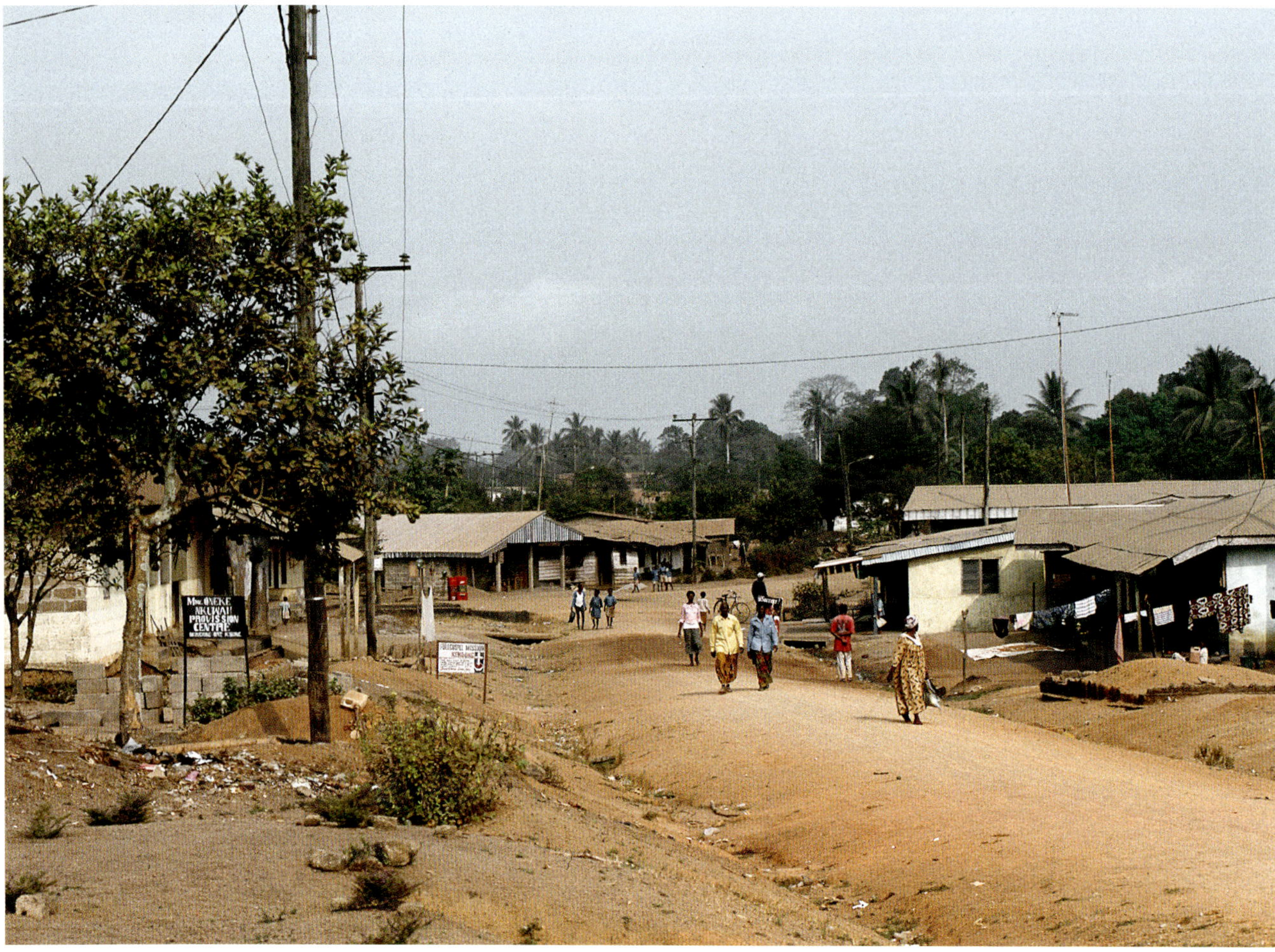

Fig. 5 Today modern houses built of brick with a corrugated metal roof dominate the scene. Electricity supply has become an important factor in the economic development (Kembong, January 21, 2004).

is not commonly used in the Ngunaya area, and, consequently, it will not be employed in this study. The Ngunaya people are proud of their membership in the great nation of the Ejagham,[14] although many possess only little knowledge about the Ejagham in Nigeria.

Delimited in the north by the Cross River,[15] the Ngunaya area borders there on the settlement area of the Boki and that of the Anyang; to the west it edges on the Njemaya area ("back of the river"), the land of the Ekwe, a people who likewise belongs to the Ejagham, just as the Obang, the neighbours of the Central Ejagham, who live to the south. The land of the Banyang lies to the east of the Ngunaya area. Thus, it was this central location of the Ngunaya area between the settlement areas of the Obang and Ekwe that led to the designation of its inhabitants as "Central Ejagham".[16]

With the penetration of western civilisation, "Old Africa" was subjected to change in almost every respect, and the Ngunaya area was no exception. The administration and jurisprudence in Cameroon had fallen into the hands of offices and courts long before, and the influence of schools and missions that were oriented towards European models had the same effect. They contributed profoundly towards undermining the prevailing traditional world-view in Africa: that the individual was no more than a part of society and that the present and the hereafter were inseparable, indeed, dependent upon one another. The monetary economy together with the penetration of western technology and the accompanying goods have had far-reaching economic and social effects in the Ngunaya area, too. Motorbikes, automobiles, radios and cameras have been familiar there for a long time, although most people cannot afford these items; the most recent consumer goods aspired for, televisions, computers and mobile telephones, are beyond the means of most people. In view of the few opportunities for earning money in the region, those goods remain unattainable for most of the population. They must be satisfied with the basic necessities. Especially due to the poor condition of roads, foremost during the long rainy season, the Manyu Division is difficult to reach, almost cut off from the rest of the world, and for this reason as well it is at a great economic disadvantage.

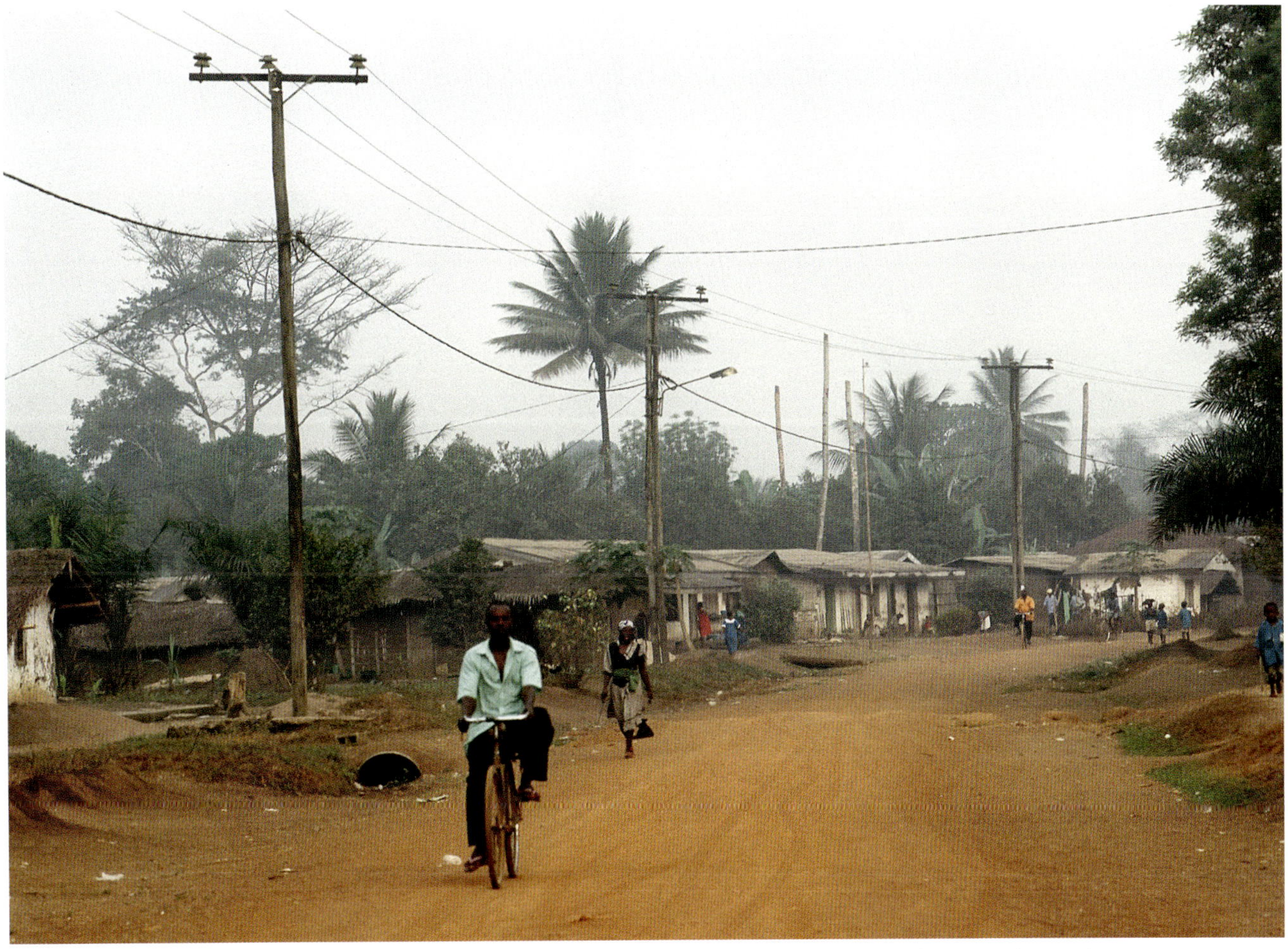

Fig. 6 Kembong's main street in 2004 (Kembong, January 28, 2004). Figures 4 and 6 were photographed from about the same location.

The most important economic basis in the Ngunaya area was and still is agriculture. This work is carried out mainly by women; men partake by clearing trees and underbrush. Mostly yams, cocoyams, plantains, cassava, maize, pineapple and beans are cultivated; cocoa and coffee are raised as cash crops. Benefit is also made of the fruits of many trees, such as the oil palm, papaya, mango, orange and avocado. Because of the fertile soil – at least in the area of Kembong – the farmlands can usually be cultivated for several years before they must lie fallow for the soil to regenerate. As the population density is relatively low, despite a considerable increase during the past decades, there is sufficient arable land available. In the past there were scarcely any problems due to land shortage. Whoever cleared a plot of forest that principally belonged to the whole community, could use it for cultivating plants and was considered its owner. If this person died without any heirs, ownership of the plot of land reverted to the community.

Likewise, animal husbandry plays a significant role in the economy, with goats, sheep, chickens, ducks and in recent years even large numbers of pigs being raised. Contrary to former times, when most men went hunting, today hunting is carried out primarily by a few professional hunters. With the many streams and runs, fishing is a prominent source of food and is mainly the task of women. The majority of the inhabitants of Kembong live from farming, but there are several men and women who have a store, a bar or a workshop for some kind of craft. Many men with the necessary training have a job in Mamfe, the main town of the Manyu Division, or in one of the other towns, usually on the coast. In many cases the men are able to visit their families in Kembong only sporadically. Indeed, finding ways to earn money in this remote region is not easy.

In the old days polygamy and patrilinear inheritance were commonplace. A man's wealth was measured foremost according to the number of wives, children as well as slaves that he possessed. Today, there are only few older men who have several wives; all of the others, particularly Christian men, are monogamous. Polygamous marriages are also disadvantageous for economic reasons; furthermore, many women are no longer willing to share their husband with other women. Never-

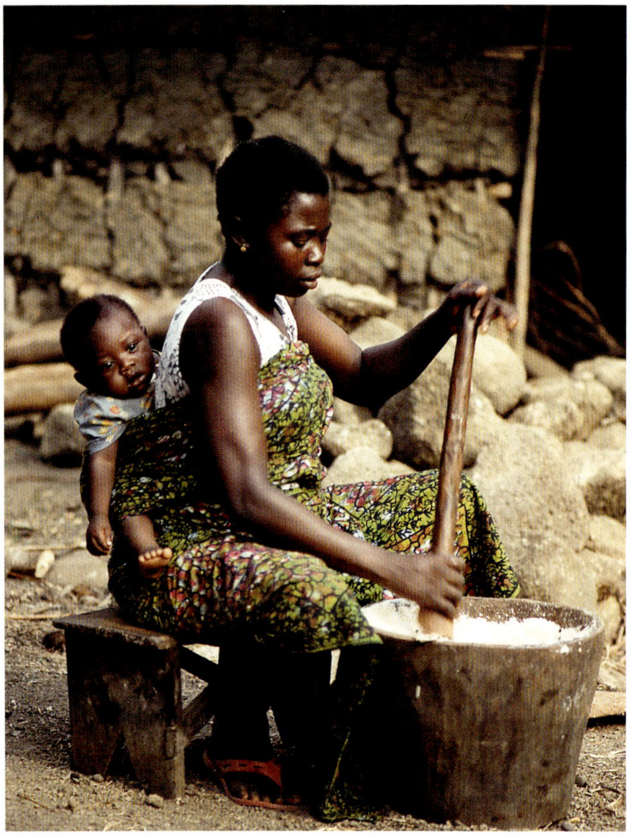

Fig. 7 This picture, taken in 1980 of a mother – her child on her back – at work with mortar and pestle, could just as well have been taken today (Kembong, February 18, 1980).

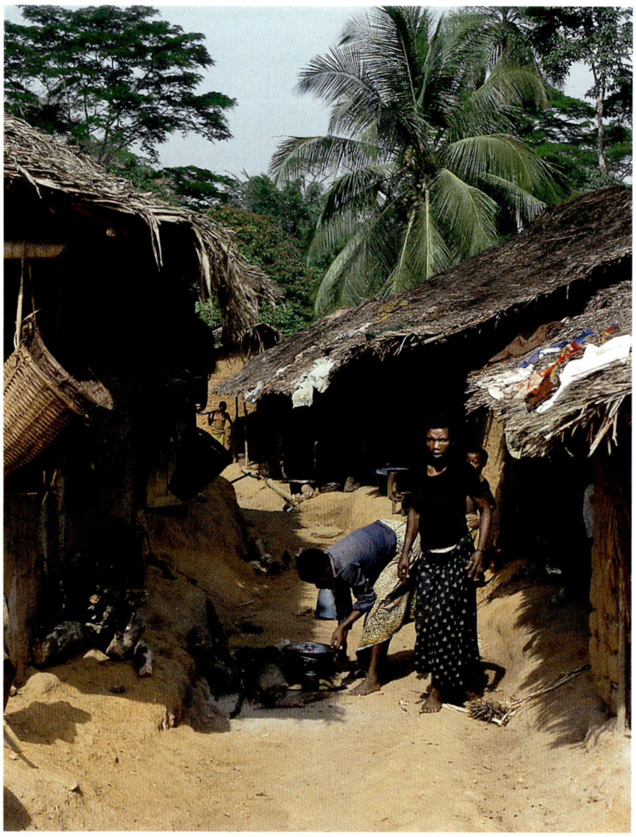

Fig. 8 A major part of the housework was carried out behind the individual houses (Babong, February 21, 1980).

theless, a family with many children is still the greatest wish of many households. Yet, children are a great financial burden for the family, although – in view of today's general social development – they are not necessarily a guarantee for reliable care and assistance to their parents in old age.

Mainly due to the monetary economy, in which it is possible for the individual to attain material security and thereby theoretically become independent of the old social bonds, extended families have greatly forfeited their former importance to smaller families. Nevertheless, extended families are still indispensable in ancestral and funeral ceremonies. Moreover, in former times there were even larger family units, so-called clans, which united the inhabitants of several localities. Their members could trace their origin from the same ancestors, whom they still invoked in prayer. But even then the clans were rather loosely bound units, which were usually called into action only in warlike confrontations and only then had one leader.[17]

The population in the surroundings of Kembong are members of the Nchemti clan, which was regarded as the most prominent and powerful clan of the Central Ejagham in earlier times. Nchemti was a legendary leader, who presumably came from Nyenya, today a quarter in Kembong. The dates of his life are not known. More is known about Mfontem, his successor. Mfontem was the leader of the troops of the Nchemti clan during the wars with the Kebus, who belong to the Mbo and live in the area around Nguti. They fought for the possession of the valuable salt resources in the area of Mbakang.[18] In the course of the conflicts, which began around 1870 and ended with the victory of Mfontem's troops in 1875, the magic medicines *Amok* and *Eyungi* were utilised, which had been acquired in Babong during these difficult times. It is said that a cannon, supposedly supplied by Elembe, chief of Ewelle, also played a role.[19] Furthermore, it was allegedly the sons of Mfontem, who expanded the influence of the Nchemti clan by founding a number of new localities: Ndekwai (near Ossing), Tale (Banyang), Fontem (Bangwa), Talangaye, Igbekaw (Ossing), Mbinjong (on the Mamfe-Kumba road) Osselle, Bakut as well as Bakogo and Nkogho in the Obang area.[20] Whenever a night dance took place in Kembong, the absolute peak in religious and social life, it was a tradition to invite the inhabitants of those localities, for they were considered relatives.

Even prior to colonial times the area around Kembong was an important trading centre, due to its location on several much-frequented trade routes that connected in particular the coastal region around Limbe (formerly Victoria) and Calabar and the area of Ikom with the Cameroon Grasslands. The exchange items included salt, domestic animals, tobacco, cotton, all kinds of European wares and – in earlier times – also slaves.[21] Kembong lost much of its prominence after the Germans enlarged Mamfe into an administrative centre in 1909 (it is still the main town of the Manyu Division). Kembong still holds regional importance as the location of the sole Customary Court, which is responsible for the entire Ngunaya region, besides the police station, which is entrusted with security and control of the surroundings. Represented in the Customary Court are the president and vice-president as well as one representative from each of the 28 localities in the Ngunaya area. The Court meets regularly and deals mainly with civil cases, such as conflicts concerning families, land and finances. Occasionally lesser offences such as insult and minor theft are tried as well. If a person does not accept the sentence of this court, whose sphere of jurisdiction extends to Manyemen, one of the main towns on the Mamfe-Kumba road, he has the chance of appealing to the next higher court in Mamfe.

The economic significance of Kembong is modest, and that applies to both its weekly market and the many small stores, whose merchandise scarcely extends beyond the needs of daily life. Kembong is known as a location of schools. Aside from a nursery school and three primary schools, particular mention must be made of the Government High School, which enjoys a good reputation. Its pupils come from nearby as well as from greater distances and then live in Kembong with guest families. The number of Christian churches in Kembong is remarkable. After the Basler Mission became active there in the 1920s, it was followed a short time later by the Catholic Mission. Over time several Christian churches became established in Kembong, including the Presbyterian Church, the Roman Catholic Church, the Baptist Church, the Apostolic Church, the Faith Revival Church, the Full Gospel Church, the Deeper Life Church and Jehova's Witnesses. Mention should also be made of the Health Centre, which is primarily responsible for ambulatory treatment in cases of illnesses. Patients with serious sicknesses or afflictions are sent to the hospital in Mamfe.

The real nucleus of the Manyu Division is Mamfe, the aforementioned administrative centre, with its 23,000 inhabitants (in 2005) and its economic and market position. Mamfe is the location not only of all important governmental offices and a judicial court, but also of a large number of stores selling an abundance of commodities, repair shops for vehicles, machines and all kinds of tools, in addition to a marketplace that is always open and of interest for many with its supply of agricultural products from the Grasslands, as well as banks, a state hospital and other smaller clinics. Mamfe, the "big city" with its bars, restaurants and cinemas, is easy to reach from Kembong by taxis, which are almost always available. A taxi-ride for a distance of 20 km takes about 30–40 minutes, depending upon the time of the year and whether or not the road can be used during the rainy season. The locality Eyumojock is also of importance for Kembong, as it is the location of the administration of the Sub-Division to which Kembong belongs. Yet, people usually travel to this town only when they have to visit an administrative office.

Yet, Kembong is not an old settlement, as one might surmise; it was not established until the German colonial period. Allegedly, around 1900 the Germans took over Ewelle after fierce fighting and then marched on to Okonyenge, today a quarter of Kembong, at that time an independent locality near Ewelle. In order to avoid further bloodshed, Tambe, the chief of Okonyenge, met the German forces and handed over an ivory tusk to them as a sign of submission. Later Tambe (whom Mansfeld erroneously designated as Chief of Kembong[22]) became involved in – in the eyes of Kembong's inhabitants – a condemnatory collaboration with the Germans, in that he showed them all of the small localities that were difficult to find in the dense forest. This action was considered as treason, for the Germans burned down the houses[23] and forced the inhabitants to resettle in the present area of Kembong. It was the plan of the Germans to consolidate small settlements and hamlets into larger localities for administrative as well as economic reasons.[24]

The new locality of present-day Kembong arose amidst the old hamlets Ebarensi, Okemebenem and Okemnjemeba, in which again thirteen nearby hamlets had been merged. Altogether, the three older hamlets mentioned first and the thirteen other hamlets constitute the sixteen quarters of Kembong, a row-village with houses aligned along the road for c. three kilometres in south-north direction. The southern area of the settlement borders on the rain forest and is called Upper Kembong; it encompasses the quarters: Ndengane, Takpang, Mbiofong, Nkonghobe, Ebarensi, Okune, Nchofang, Okemebenem and Nserong. The northern part is called Lower Kembong and includes the following quarters: Okemnjemeba, Abotabe, Okangku, Ayu-

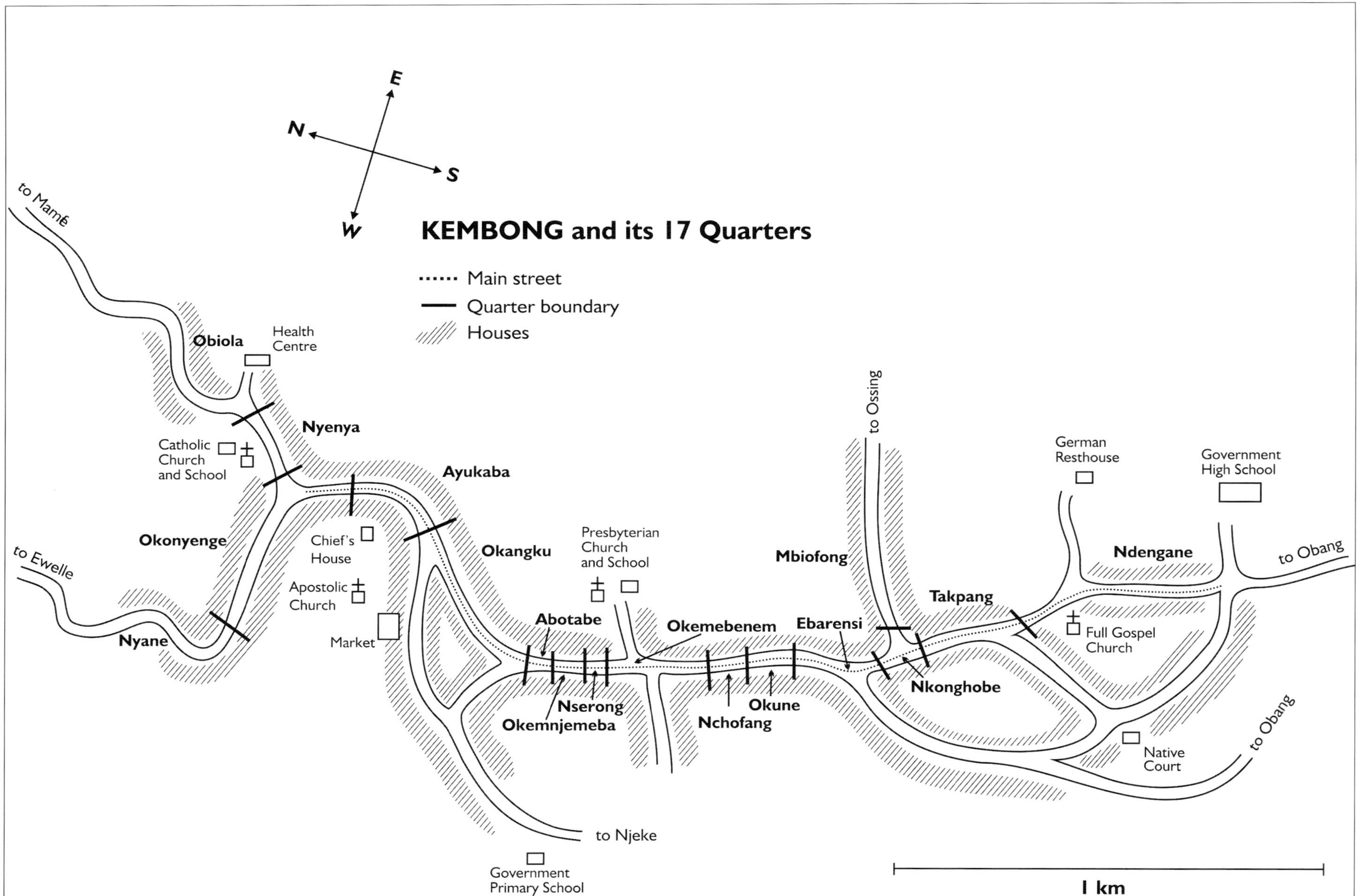
KEMBONG and its 17 Quarters
Main street
Quarter boundary
Houses
N
E
S
W
to Mamfe
to Ewelle
Obiola
Health Centre
Nyenya
Catholic Church and School
Okonyenge
Nyane
Ayukaba
Chief's House
Apostolic Church
Market
Okangku
Abotabe
Nserong
Okemnjemeba
Presbyterian Church and School
Okemebenem
Nchofang
Okune
Ebarensi
Mbiofong
to Ossing
Takpang
Nkonghobe
German Resthouse
Ndengane
Government High School
Full Gospel Church
Native Court
to Obang
to Obang
to Njeke
Government Primary School
1 km

kaba, Okonyenge, Nyane and Nyenya. Once completely independent, the hamlets enjoyed their independence as quarters of Kembong as well. All decisions that pertain to the community are – as ever – made by the council of the respective quarter (*Etek*). The secret society *Mgbe* sees that these decisions are enforced and that the laws are heeded. In 1984 an additional quarter, Obiola, which is located on the road to Mamfe, was added. The inhabitants of Obiola are descendants of slaves, most of whom lived in the Nyenya and Okonyenge quarters and who – according to the common opinion in Kembong – had been exploited, repressed and their human rights abused. So, the Kembong Traditional Council liberated them and gave them the status of a quarter like any other Kembong quarter.

Two stories, generally well-known today, relate the origin of the name Kembong during the German era. According to the first account, the Germans asked a man whom they thought to be indigenous as to the name of the settlement. The man, however, was a stranger to the area and could not supply any information and, thus, explained: "Nkebongho", which means, "I am wandering". But the Germans understood this answer to be the name of the settlement, and in this way the name "Kembong" emerged. The second account is likewise widespread knowledge in Kembong and was recorded by Mansfeld in 1908: "Forty years ago the village's name was Fontem, and it was governed by the chief Abandep. His son Atakam left the village and restlessly roamed the countryside for months; people therefore called him: 'a fool' = *mbung*, and the place that he finally chose was called 'place of fools'."[25]

I first became acquainted with the Cross River region in March 14–21, 1975, during a study trip throughout western Cameroon. At that time I stayed with two acquaintances, mostly in Mamfe and surroundings as well as in Ashum in the southern Banyang area. While in the latter place, I was able to witness a performance of *Obasinjom*, one of the most important masks of the whole forest region. Equally impressive for me were the large figures modelled in cement and commemorating the deceased *agbokarem*, those women who once formed an elite level in society and were members of the special society *Ndem*. The mask *Obasinjom* as well as the *agbokarem* with their commemorative figures, which at that time could still be found throughout this region, were to become two of the most important themes in my later research in Kembong.

My first longer research sojourn in the Cross River region was five years later, from January 21 to February 28, 1980. This stay was related to ethnological field work, which I had conducted since 1975 in the kingdom of Oku in the Cameroon Grasslands of the North West Province.[26] At that time I had concentrated extensively upon the masks and magic medicine in Oku, for which the kingdom was and still is renowned today. However, the field work was difficult, on the one hand due to the insufficient state of research, for there were hardly any publications on this theme. On the other, it was not easy to gain access to the secret societies. Even today these societies keep strict guard on all secrets pertaining to *jujus* against outsiders.

In the course of time I was able to accumulate and document the most important contexts and relevant material in my area of research. Yet, I was nevertheless convinced that it would be useful and recommendable, indeed absolutely necessary, to become acquainted with other parts of Africa besides the kingdoms in the Cameroon Grasslands. I was convinced that the observation of masks and magic medicines in completely different societies would further my studies in Oku and so supply additional possibilities for comparisons.

At that time it seemed reasonable to go to the Cross River region, which although it borders on the Grasslands to the west, belongs to an entirely different world in cultural respect. Whereas the Grasslands are a highland with savanna-like flora and a climate that is pleasant for Europeans, the Cross River region encompasses a vast rain forest with a hot and humid climate that stretches to the west and south. The borderline is just as distinct in a cultural-historical respect. While the Grassland kingdoms are characterised, among other things, by their magnificent and imposing palaces, the rain forest societies are with few exceptions small egalitarian societies with only loosely structured chiefdoms. Due to the proximity to Calabar, which from the 15th century onwards developed into an important trading centre for European merchants, European influence was felt in the rain-forest area at an early time. Tribes from the Grasslands, by contrast, presumably penetrated into that area from the east and settled there only as late as c. 300 years ago. Cultural exchange between these two large cultural regions – the rain forest and the Grasslands – was apparently none too extensive in pre-colonial times, with the exception of crossing points such as Bangwa and Widekum, yet there were more or less well-established trade networks, above all the slave trade.

Corresponding with my research program in Oku, during my first research trip to Kembong I concentrated mainly on magic medicines (*ajom*), to which one particular mask belonged that was of special interest to

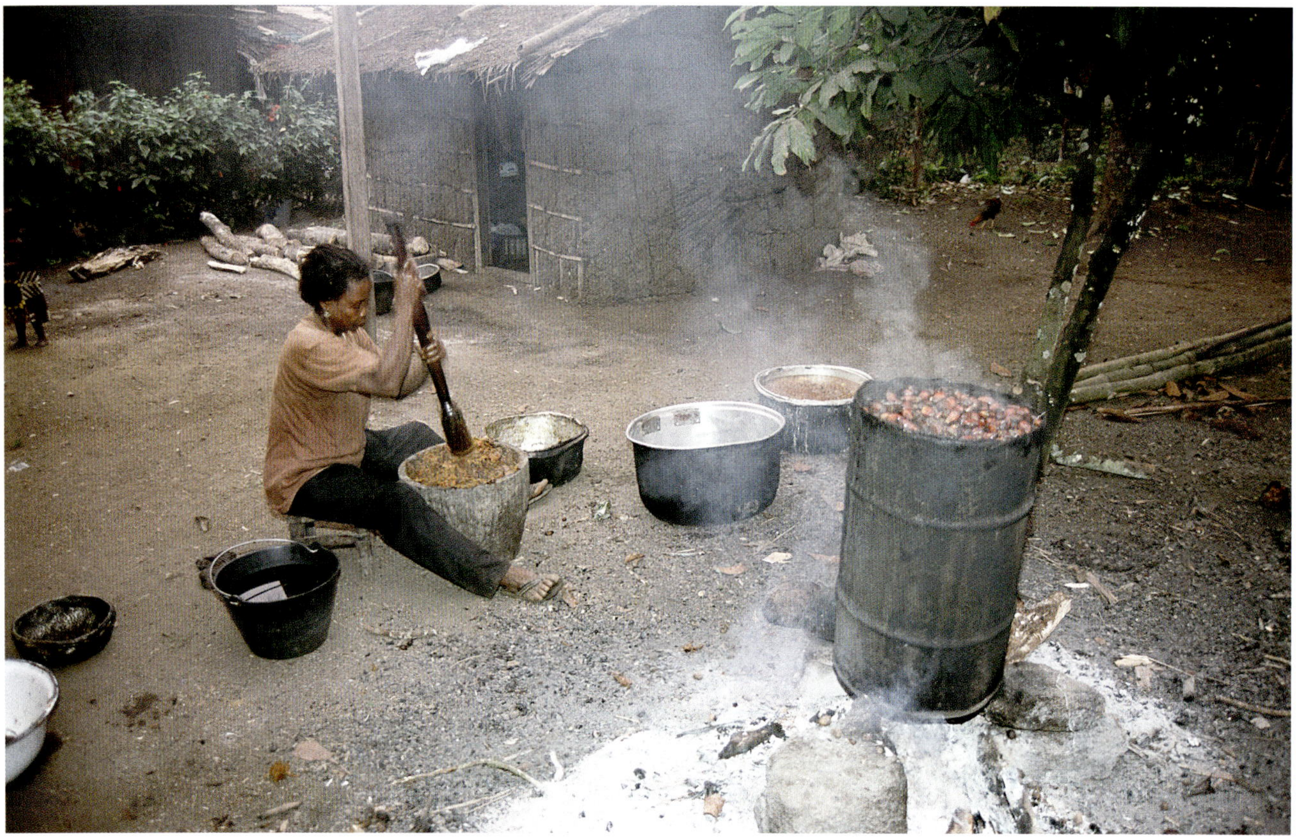

Fig. 9 Obtaining palm oil. The ripe fruits are first boiled in water (right) and then pounded in a mortar with a pestle (left) (Kembong, January 20, 2004).

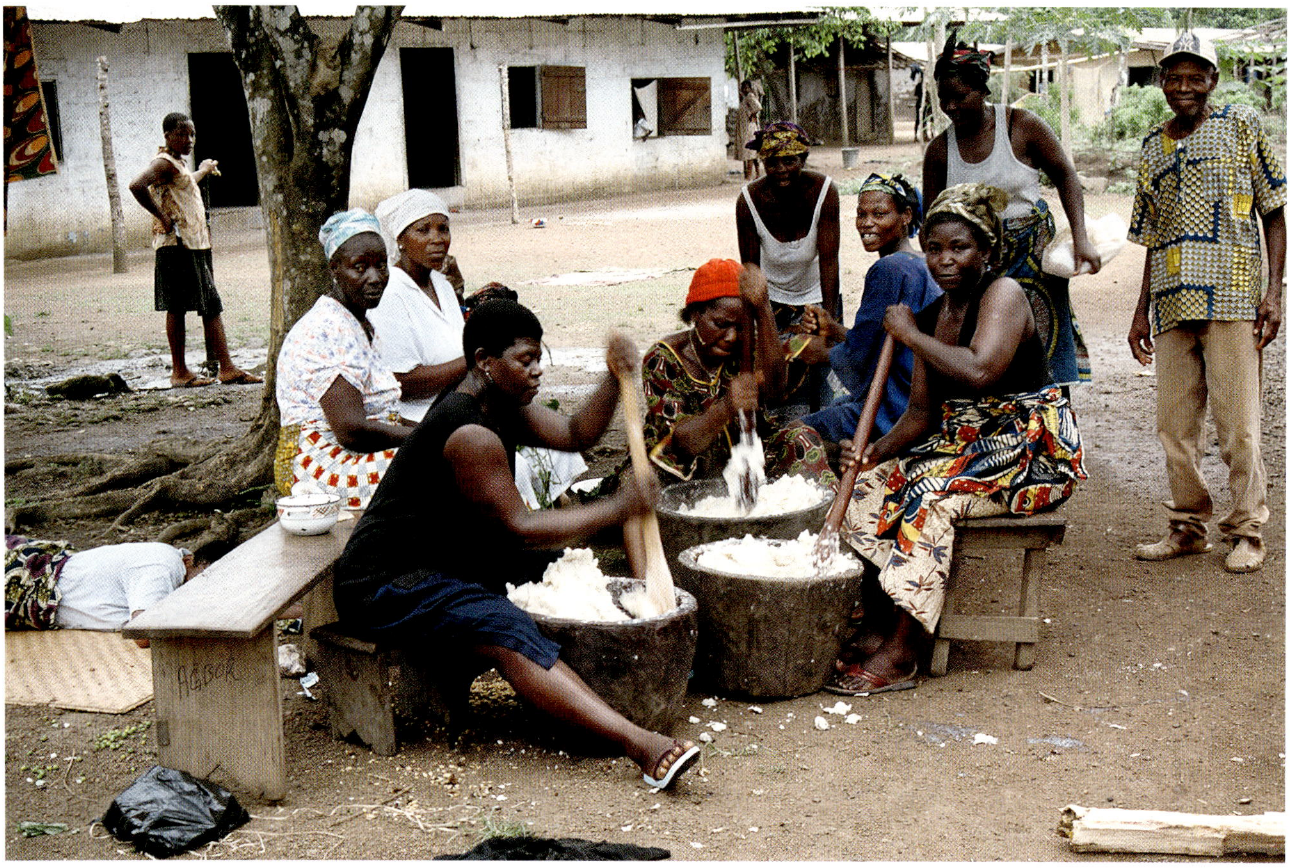

Fig. 10 Women preparing food for a death celebration (*aboku*), using mortars and pestles (Kembong, April 20, 2004).

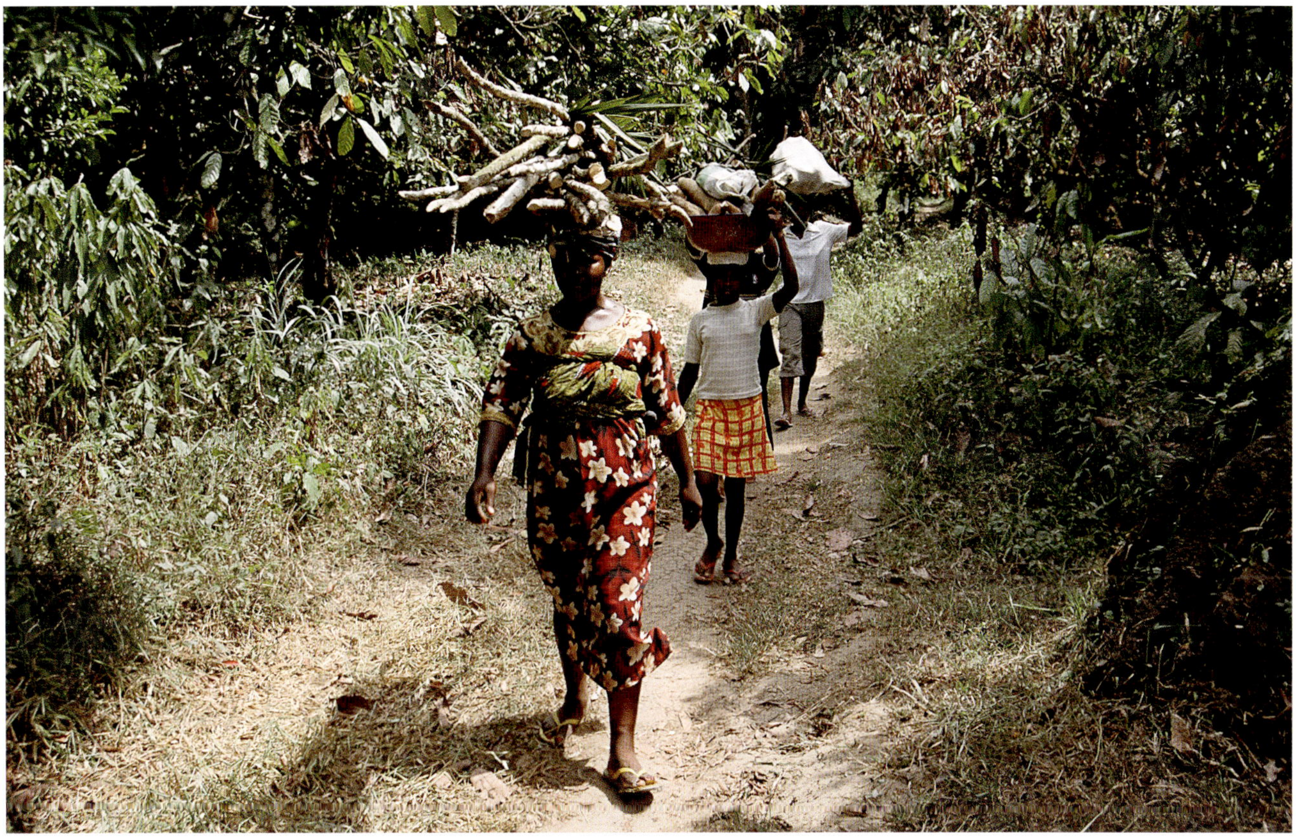

Fig. 11 Women returning from work on the farmland, carrying crops and fire wood (Kembong, January 29, 2004).

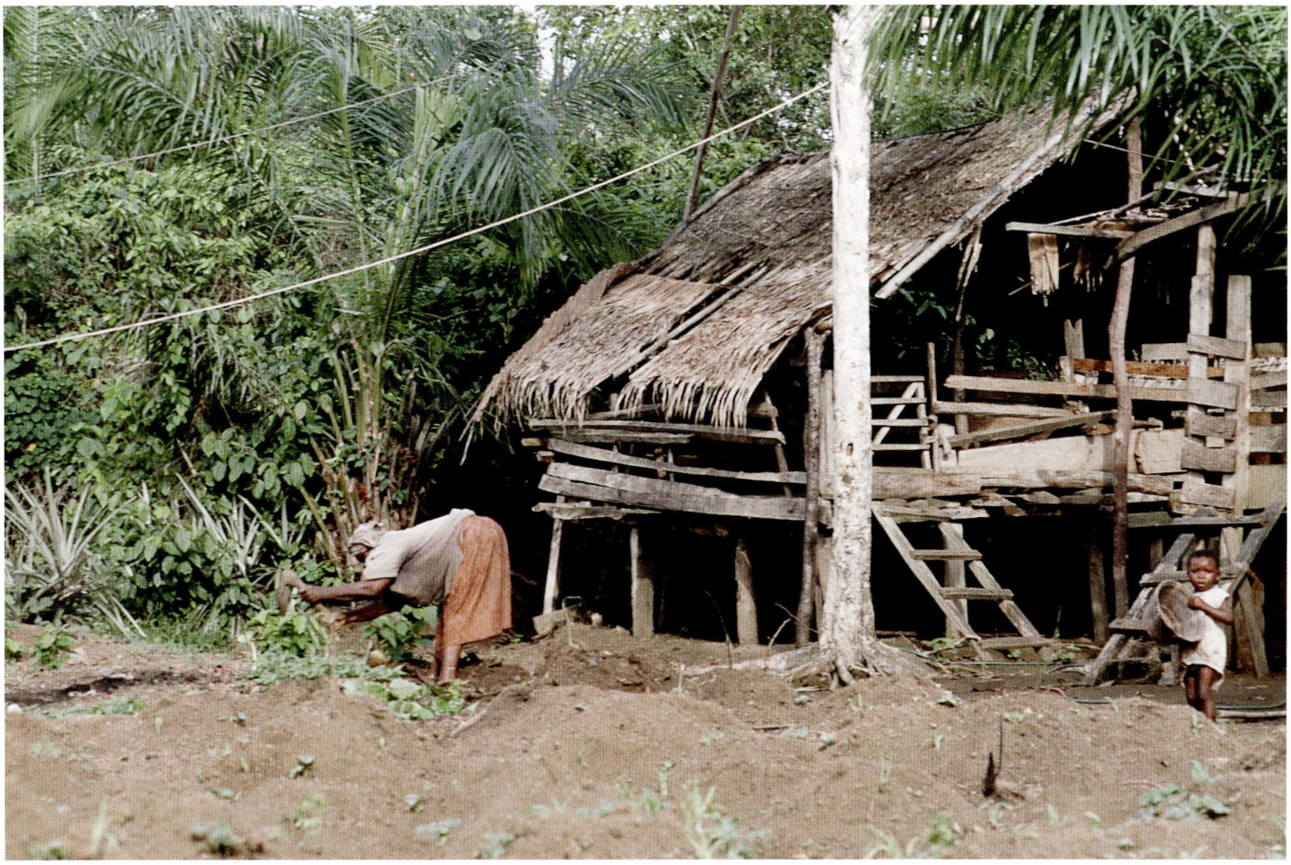

Fig. 12 A woman working the soil in her garden with a hoe. On the right, a present-day pigsty elevated upon posts (Kembong, April 17, 2004).

me, *Obasinjom*. Aside from the direct correlation between magic medicines and masks, which I was able to study intensively in the Grasslands and which I also found present in the forests, the "swearing of medicine" was of particular note to me. For in this medicine ritual, in which magic medicine is activated against witches, thieves, adulterers and other offenders, a character is clearly expressed which is both person- and robot-like and unpredictable. Widespread in the rain forests, the "swearing of medicine" is also known in the Grasslands, but there it is illegal and was seldom practised, at least during the first years of my work in Oku. Therefore, it was difficult to obtain sufficient information about this method of using medicine. In Kembong, on the contrary, the employment of magic medicines (*ajom*) was well-known, especially to ward off the much feared witches. I soon realised that the magic medicines were entities with their own supernatural facilities and powers, but not connected with so-called wild spirits, as is so often maintained in ethnological literature. I was able to discover correlations in Oku at a later time and after a longer stay, in which medicines and masks still number among the greatest secrets.

Upon completion of my research project in Oku in 2000 with the publication "World-View and Society in Oku (Cameroon)", I decided to continue the studies once begun in Kembong. Although magic medicines and masks were, as ever, my foremost interest, I hoped to gain a general overview of traditional life of this acephalous society. The question was whether or not it was sensible to conduct a research project such as this today, that is, at a time in which the way of life and living conditions in all of Africa have changed fundamentally through globalisation.

As in many other regions of Africa, in Kembong certain forms of belief have been maintained to this day, despite western influence. For many people in Kembong prayers and offerings to the ancestors are still customary, and funeral rituals are often performed in the old traditional way. Little doubt exists about the reality and might of witches, those persons who are said to possess supernatural facilities, to become invisible and to transform themselves into animals in order to follow their malevolent nature. In Cameroon as in numerous other African states, witchcraft has even been acknowledged to the extent that it is dealt with as a normal offence and correspondingly tried in public courts. By contrast, this has seldom occurred in the Ngunaya area. There the problems with witchcraft were solved by traditional methods in the past and to some extent still today. Rituals and ceremonies, which were in association with ancestral cult and with the pursuit and punishment of witches, were considered an absolute necessity in Kembong well into recent times. Secret societies also played an important role in this sphere of life and for that and other reasons most of them are still active today.

In general, little has survived of older forms of handicrafts and their techniques. Carving and weaving are rarely practised in Kembong.[27] Although the majority of houses today are built of brick with metal corrugated roofs (figs. 5, 6), it is noteworthy that the traditional house construction has prevailed. It is probably due to the difficult economic situation that notably many traditional "mud houses" are still in use and even new ones are built in the old tradition (figs. 23–26). They are well suited for the hot, humid climate, especially the roof made of fronds of raphia palm, which allow an optimal air circulation while resisting the strongest downpours of rain. And as the people proudly noted, even bullets from a rifle could not penetrate these walls made of mud. Furthermore, these houses are relatively simple, economical and quick to construct. At least in Kembong earth can be utilised as a building material without any additional substances; it just must be mixed with sufficient water. Moreover, there is no need for specialised craftsmen to build a house. It is usually erected by members of the respective family. It is the task of the men to build the framework and to cover the roof, the task of the women to construct the walls.[28]

Although numerous elements of the traditional way of life can still be observed, the present context within which they function is no longer the same as before. Disregarding all of the changes that modern times have brought about, specific institutions and activities that once essentially determined daily life do not exist at all or they are hardly possible today, such as polygamy, tribal wars, slavery and slave trade, human sacrifice, autopsy of corpses, circumcision and long-term initiation of women etc. In addition, one cannot expect to observe "completely authentic" ways of life, as Kembong is not an old settlement, but a product of the colonial era. Yet, despite all of the influences that have resulted from the onslaught of western civilisation, some important spheres of the older life have still been maintained in Kembong: the activities of extended families, the village community, secret societies, ancestral worship, cult of the dead, witchcraft and magic medicine. They constitute the theme of the present study and, moreover, their existence justifies the "ethnographic present".[29] In order to delineate the institutions and material under study more exactly, they should be discussed and presented in accordance with comparative research on corresponding contexts

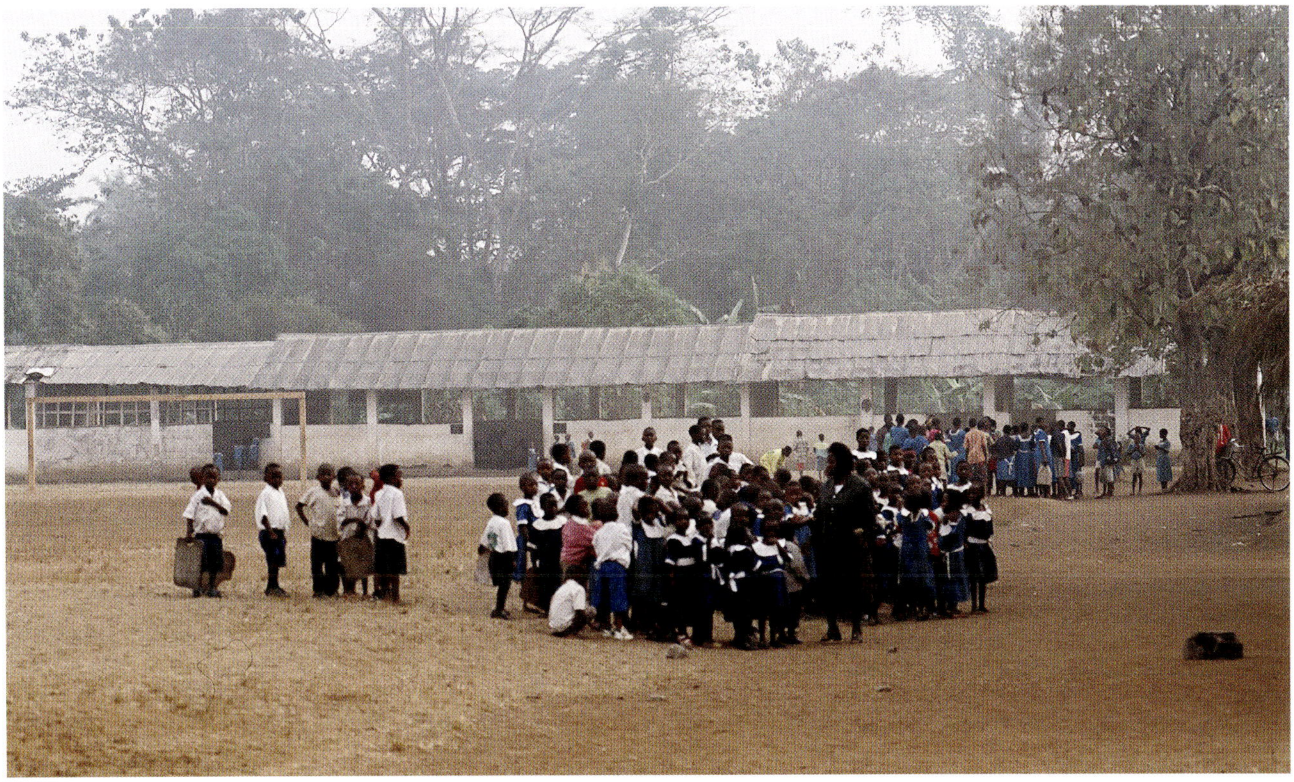

Fig. 13 The Primary School of the Presbyterian Church (Kembong, January 28, 2004).

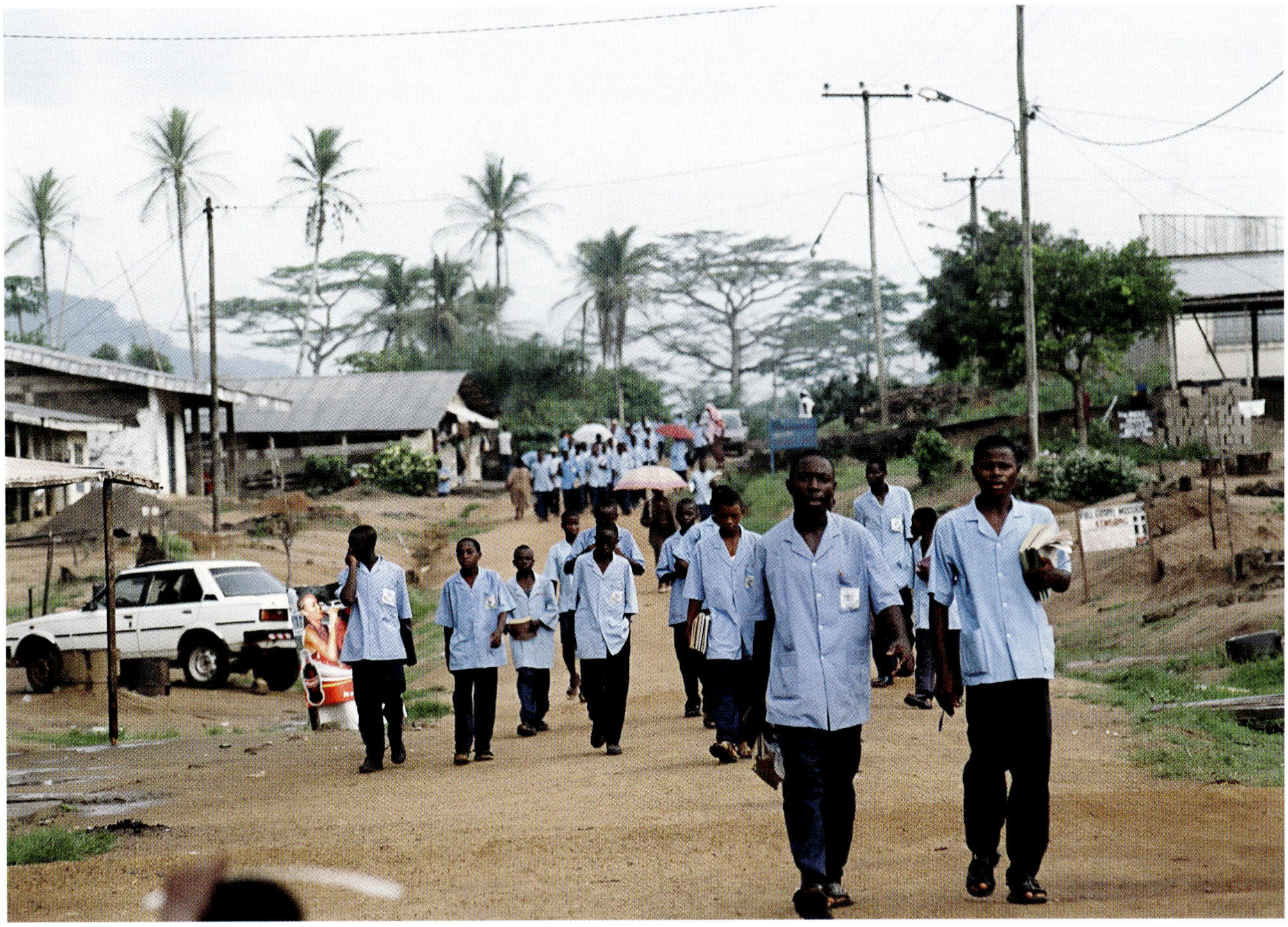

Fig. 14 High school students in their uniforms on Kembong's main street (Kembong, April 26, 2004).

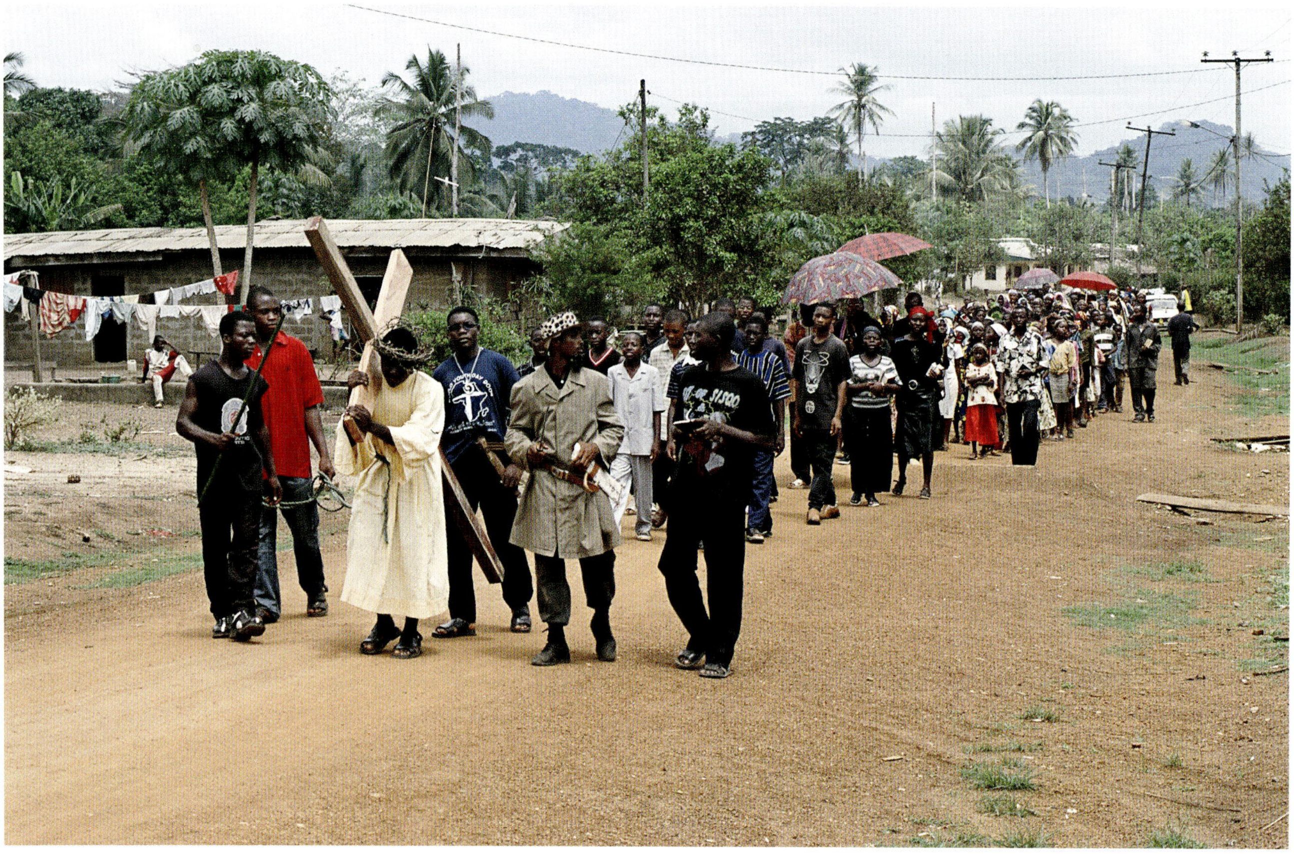

Fig. 15 Procession of the Catholic Church in Kembong on Good Friday. A parishioner represents Jesus Christ with a crown of thorns carrying the cross (Kembong, April 9, 2004).

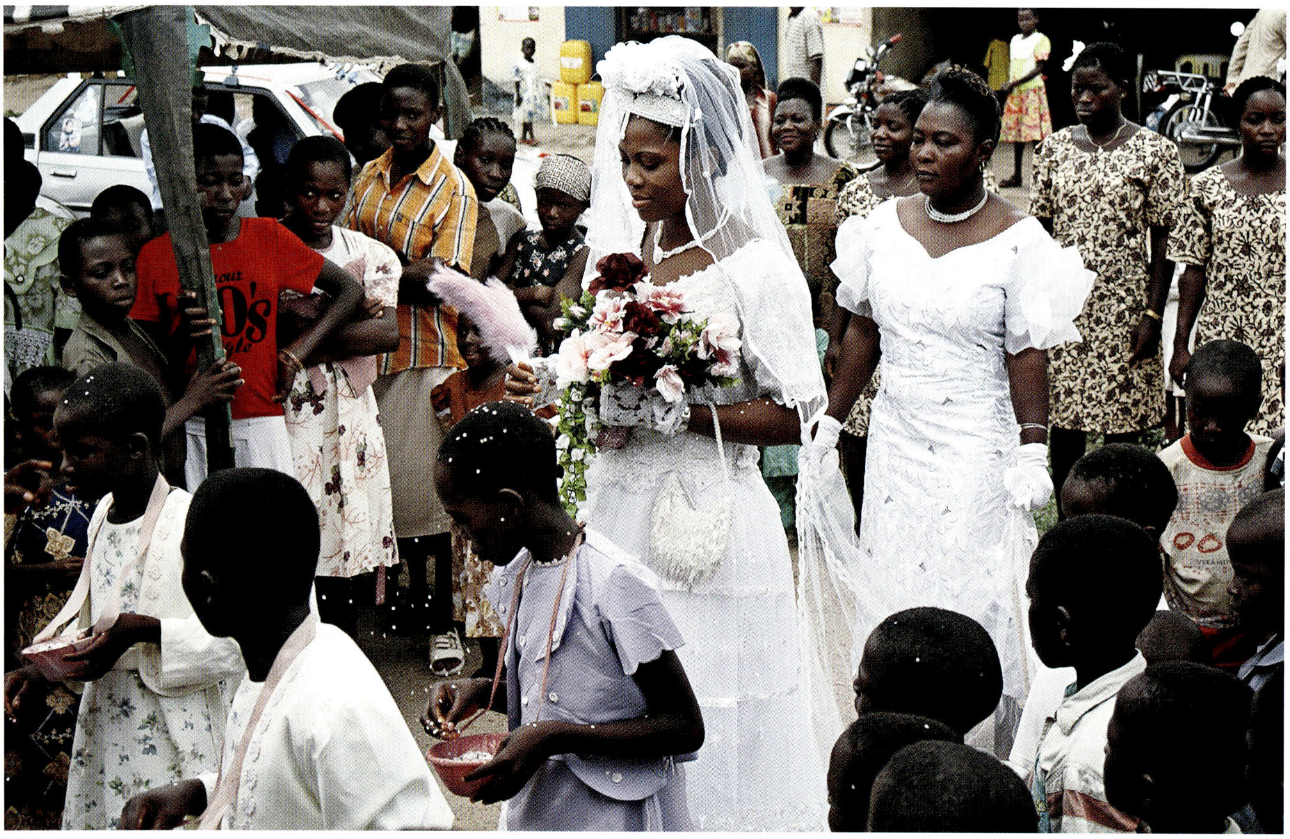

Fig. 16 A Christian wedding, with the bride dressed in an elegant bridal gown, accompanied by her attendants in festive attire (Kembong, April 3, 2005).

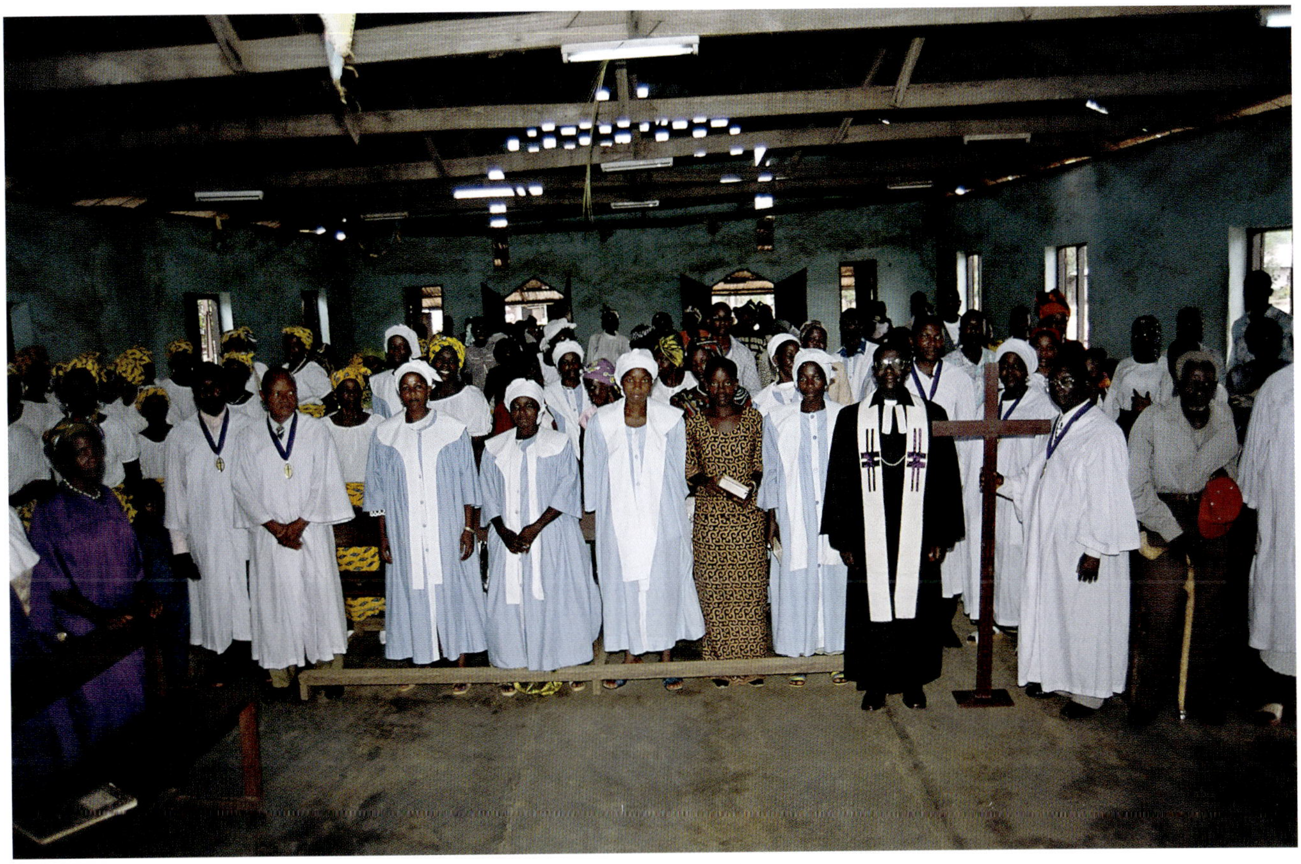

Fig. 17 Easter Sunday service in the Presbyterian Church (Kembong, April 11, 2004).

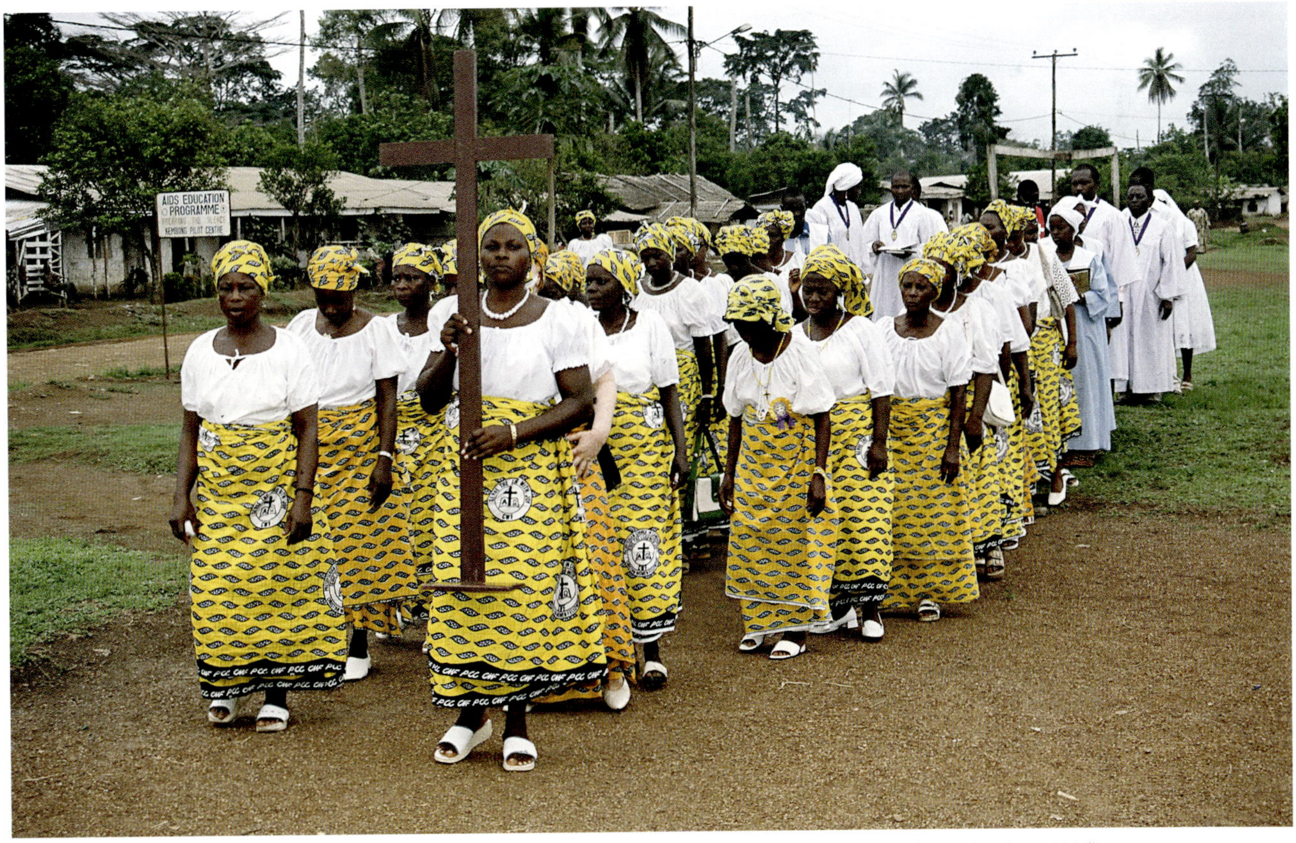

Fig. 18 Christian Women Fellowship of the Presbyterian Church, in a procession on Easter Sunday (Kembong, April 11, 2004).

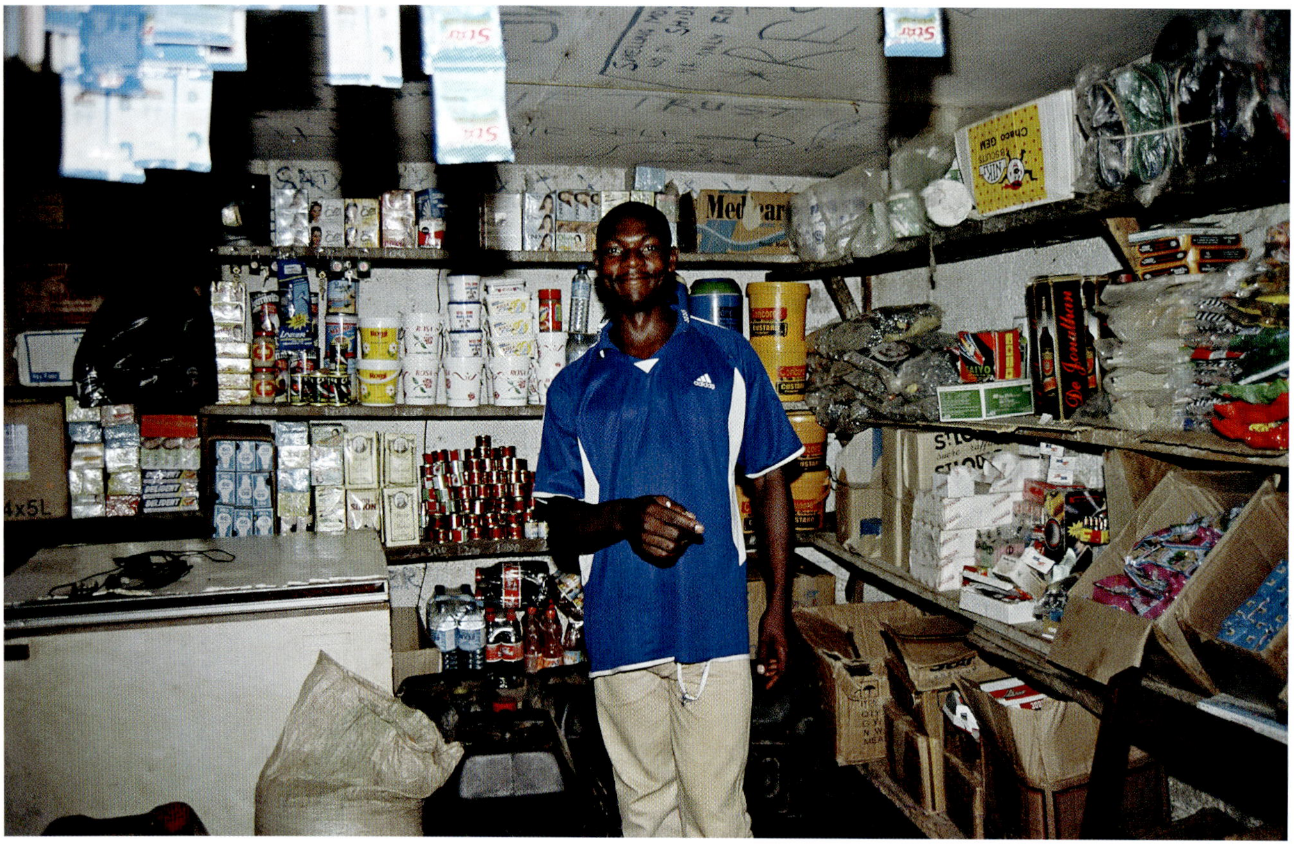

Fig. 19 One of the many small stores with the basic necessities for daily life. On the left, a freezer for the ever-present seafood (Kembong, April 3, 2005).

in the Cameroon Grasslands. For it is precisely the comparison between these basically very different cultural areas – the forest with the Ejagham, on one side, and the Grasslands, on the other – through which the various traditions can be grasped or at least more clearly determined – and this applies to the same extent to both regions.

During the years 2004 and 2005 I was able to undertake four research trips to the Ngunaya area: in specific, January 14 – February 4, 2004, April 7 – May 4, 2004, March 20 – April 10, 2005, and November 16 – December 8, 2005. During this time I concentrated from the very beginning on Kembong, the largest community in the region. Not only were most of the secret societies at home there, they were – and this was the crucial factor – still active. Nevertheless, I endeavoured to obtain information about these societies in other localities. Aside from a short side trip to Babong in 1980, which belongs to the Ekwe people, I had various contacts with informants in the villages of Ewelle, Ogomoko, Afap, Ayukaba, Mbakang, Ajayukndip and Nkewkaw. It was of essential value for my research that during the time of my sojourn an unusually large number of ceremonies and other important events took place, in which I was able to participate with hardly any limitations. Whereas I often had the opportunity to partake in the manifold funeral ceremonies for deceased big men of the *Mgbe* society, the night dance on March 26, 2005 in Kembong was the absolute zenith of my experiences. Night dances, which are held solely for the most prominent and important men, take place very rarely. And it is precisely only these night dances in which the skin-covered masks, for which the region is renowned, appear. I also viewed other masks of this region several times in their performances. Aside from the medicine men and diviners, whom I often met, the encounter with the last living *mgbokandem* made a lasting impression upon me. The *agbokarem* once formed an elite and esteemed society for women, and thus it is understandable that after the death of a member an imposing life-sized commemorative figure was dedicated to the person and placed in public view. These figures could still be seen everywhere in the Ngunaya area in the 1980s.

In all ceremonies, rituals and other events which I experienced, I always had the opportunity to take photographs and to make sound recordings, which I contributed to the Department of Ethnomusicology in the Ethnological Museum in Berlin. As in my work on the Cameroon Grasslands, I paid special attention to docu-

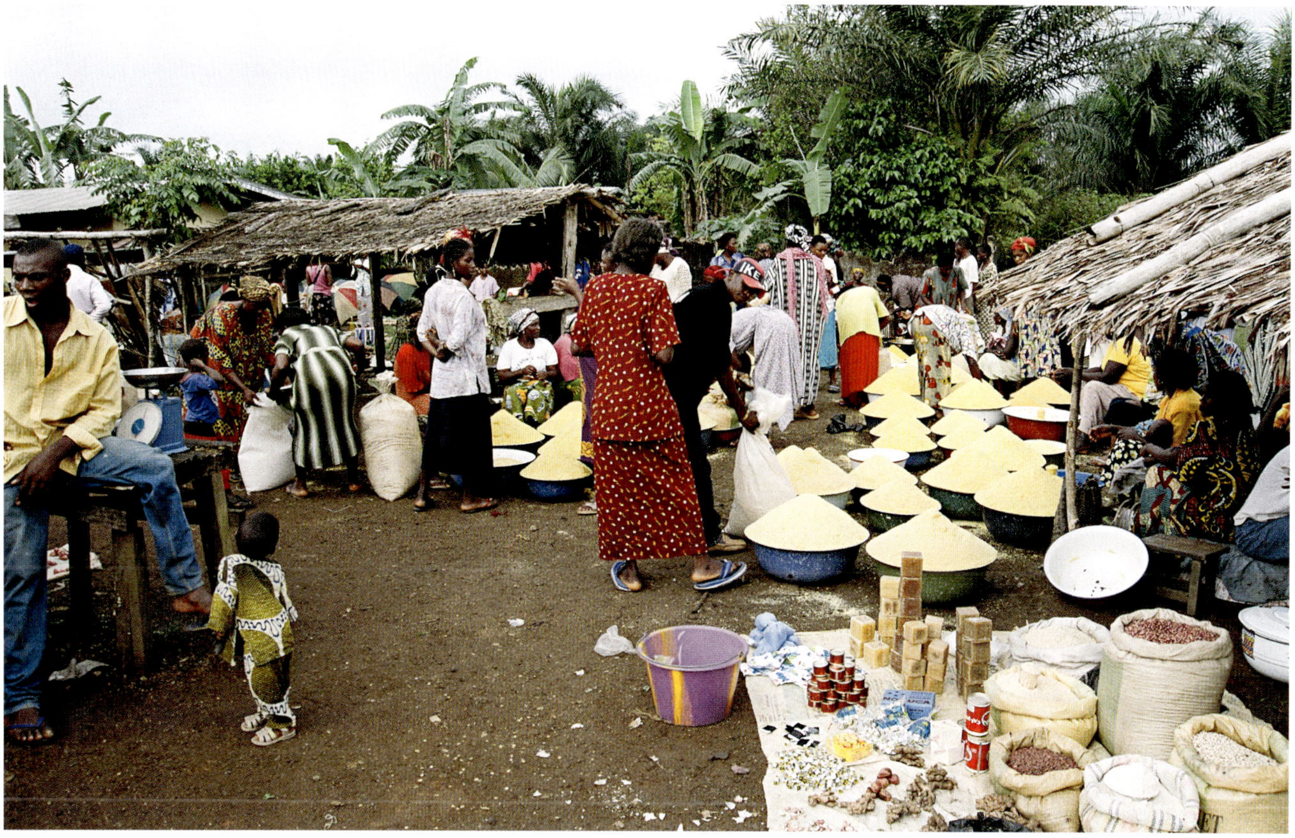

Fig. 20 The weekly market in Kembong takes place every Tuesday. Mainly local produce is on offer (Kembong, April 27, 2004).

menting prayers and other verbal expressions, in specific: as they were actually spoken or the way in which they might have been spoken in certain situations.

It was above all the big men in these societies who not only allowed me to partake in the respective events, but who were also my most important informants. Just as the dignitaries in Oku, who were decisive authorities for my research there, these big men belonged to those "old wise men" of Africa, who were highly esteemed in their community and whose dignity and intelligence left a great impression, upon Europeans as well.

My main informants in 1980 were *Ata* Tanyiashuh and *Ata* John Etchu, the big men of *Obasinjom*. *Ata* John Etchu was also a *seseku*, that is, chief of a *Mgbe* lodge. Both men had a comprehensive knowledge of their culture and knew many details about the colonial period. *Ata* Tanyiashuh had once met Mansfeld. He described Mansfeld as a small man with straight hair and glasses.[30] I saw *Ata* Tanyiashuh and *Ata* John Etchu almost daily during that time; their support for my work remains unforgettable.

In addition to the big men of the medicine societies (*ajom*) – Ayuk Tambla of *Enok Ateng* (from the locality of Afap), Hollford Ndip of *Mfam*, Moses Ojong of *Amok* and Agbor Enow of *Okeboho* –, further important authorities for me were the last but still living *agbokarem*, in particular Ebob Arrey. When I returned to Kembong after almost a quarter of a century, these informants were no longer alive, with the exception of Ayuk Tambla. Their generation, which had experienced the "olden days", is more or less extinct.

In 2004–2005 my prime areas of research were *Obasinjom* and *Mgbe*, and their chiefs as well as other high-ranking members were my major informants. They included in *Obasinjom*: Adolf Ojong Agbor (Okune) and other medicine men from Upper Kembong; in *Mgbe*, besides many, mostly older members, a number of *boseseku*: Ayuk Sampson Eno (Okemebenem), James Awoh (Okangku), Ateke Johnson (Takpang), Akobenem Sampson (Mbiofong), Ojong Samuel Ebot (Okune) and Elias Tanyi (Okonyenge). Further contact persons were Agbor George (Okangku) of *Angbu*, Samuel Tanyi Tambe (Okonynenge) of *Nkanda*, *Nchebe* and *Obasinjom*, and Alice Manchang and Batemanyo Pauline of *Mawu*. Information about *Ndem* from Bessem Bate (Ewelle), the last living *mgbokandem* in the entire region, was, needless to say, of paramount importance. Here I extend my most sincere thanks to all of these persons,

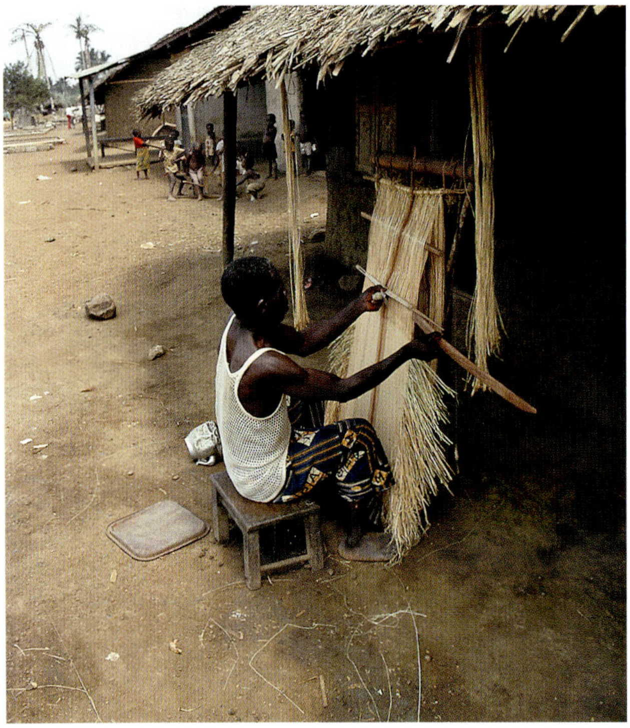

Fig. 21 A man weaving on a simple loom frame. Mostly large handbags were woven out of raphia fibres. Today this time-consuming work is rarely carried out; traditional handmade products have been replaced by cheap industrial goods (Kembong, January 23, 1980).

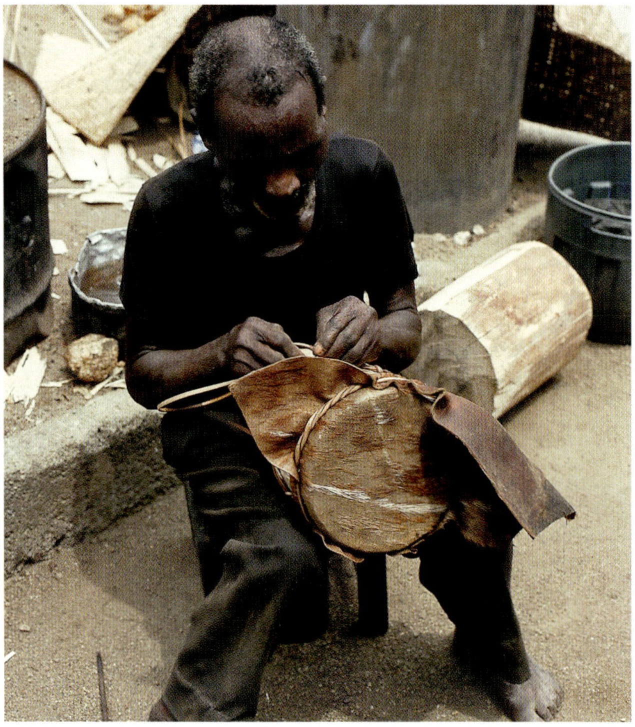

Fig. 22 A man stretching the hide of an antelope over the drum (Kembong, February 13, 1980).

and to Mr. Arreybesong Ashu Samuel, who accompanied me as translator during my research trips in 2004.

The gratitude which I wish to express to Hon. Rev. Dr. Ayukachale Peter Egbe (born in 1946) must be of another dimension. As far back as in 1980 my work profited decisively from his earnest participation, together with his great interest in the culture and history of his own community. In 2004 I met him again in Kembong; he had attained a doctoral degree in the meantime and had been a Member of Parliament in Yaoundé (1997–2002). During my research sojourns in 2004 and 2005 he not only showed me generous hospitality, but also supported my work in every way imaginable. It was he who set up my contact with the numerous secret societies, who knew the most important informants, and was ultimately the authority on almost all questions that arose in the course of research. His father, Ayukachale Daniel, was once a *seseku*, his mother Clara Oneke a *mgbokandem*. Both parents died in 1974. His support, which included reading the manuscript and transcribing words from Ejagham into English, was indispensable – I am very indebted with gratitude to Dr. Ayukachale. Finally, my thanks are extended to the Chief of Kembong, Mr. Alfred Ayuk Ako, for his great support, which was always of benefit to me, as well as for his information, particularly about the events and developments in Kembong during the past decades.

This research on the Central Ejagham was made possible by the Ministry of Scientific and Technical Research in Yaoundé (Cameroon), to whom I am indebted for its generous support for my work. The studies in Kembong could be carried out by means of the Deutsche Forschungsgemeinschaft (German Research Foundation) in Bonn; the publication of this work was realised with the funding of the Staatliche Museen zu Berlin – Preussischer Kulturbesitz (National Museums in Berlin). I should like to express my gratitude to both great institutions for the support that they have provided for this publication.

Several persons have been of great assistance to me in this work: My sincere thanks go to Ulrich Gebauer, Ethnological Museum Berlin, for his precise drawing of the maps. Sincere thanks are extended to my friend Klaus Klimmek (Bielefeld) for the many motivating discussions and proposals. I am very much obliged to Dr. Emily Schalk for taking on the task once again of translating these results of my work. Finally, I wish to express my special thanks to my wife Margarete. Not only did she accompany and support me on both of my past research trips to Kembong, but over and above she undertook the extensive work of preparing the manuscript for publication. I am very indebted to her for her contemplative and engaged participation in all aspects of this research project.

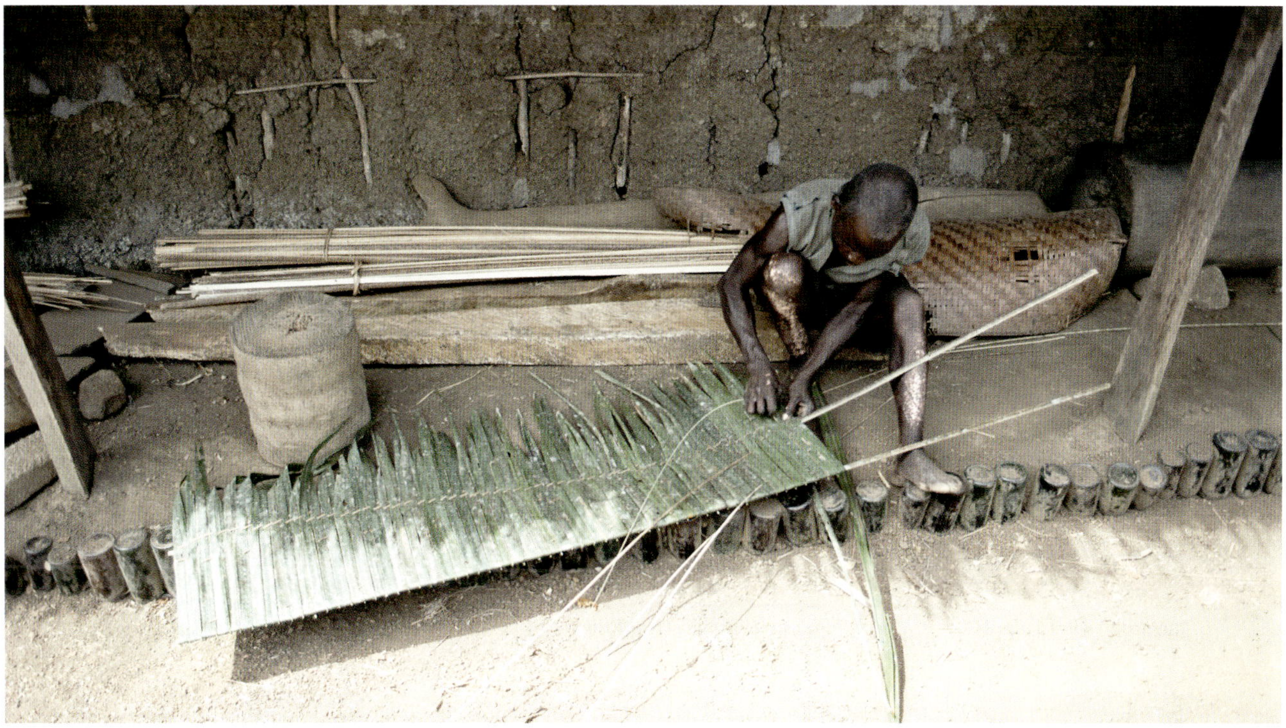

Fig. 23 Roof elements are made of fronds of the raphia palm (Kembong, January 30, 1980).

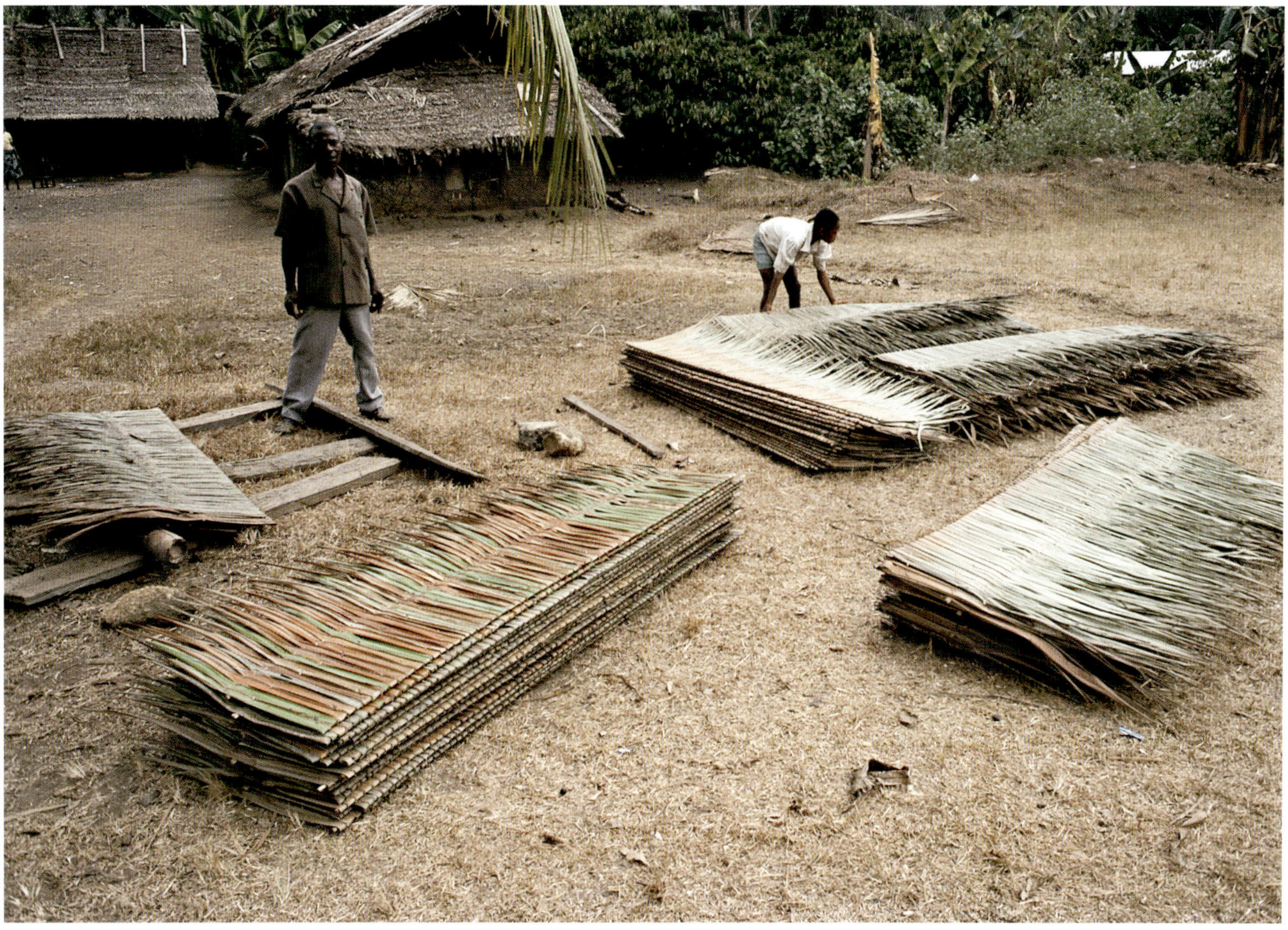

Fig. 24 Roof elements for a new mud house (Kembong, February 4, 1980).

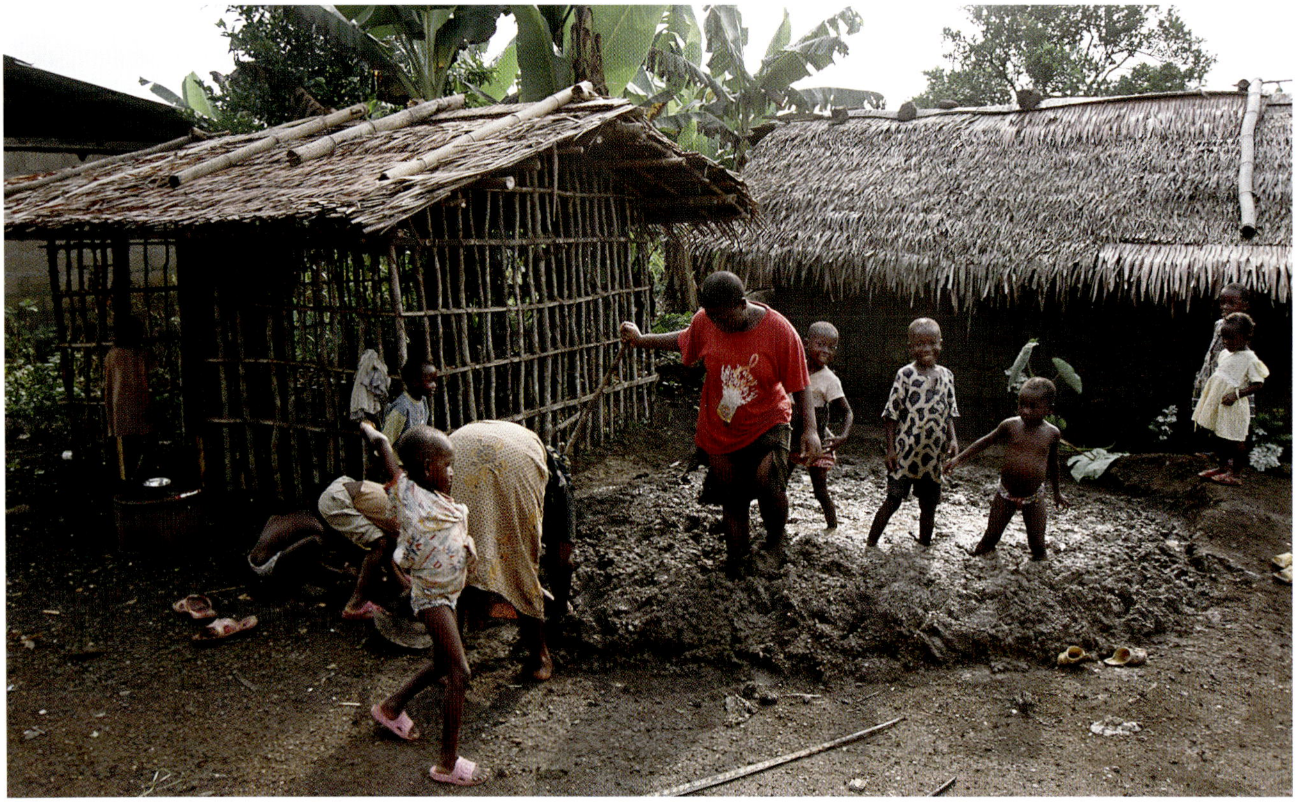

Fig. 25 Building a house. Women and children stamp the mud mixed with water. To the left, the framework of the house (Kembong, November 25, 2005).

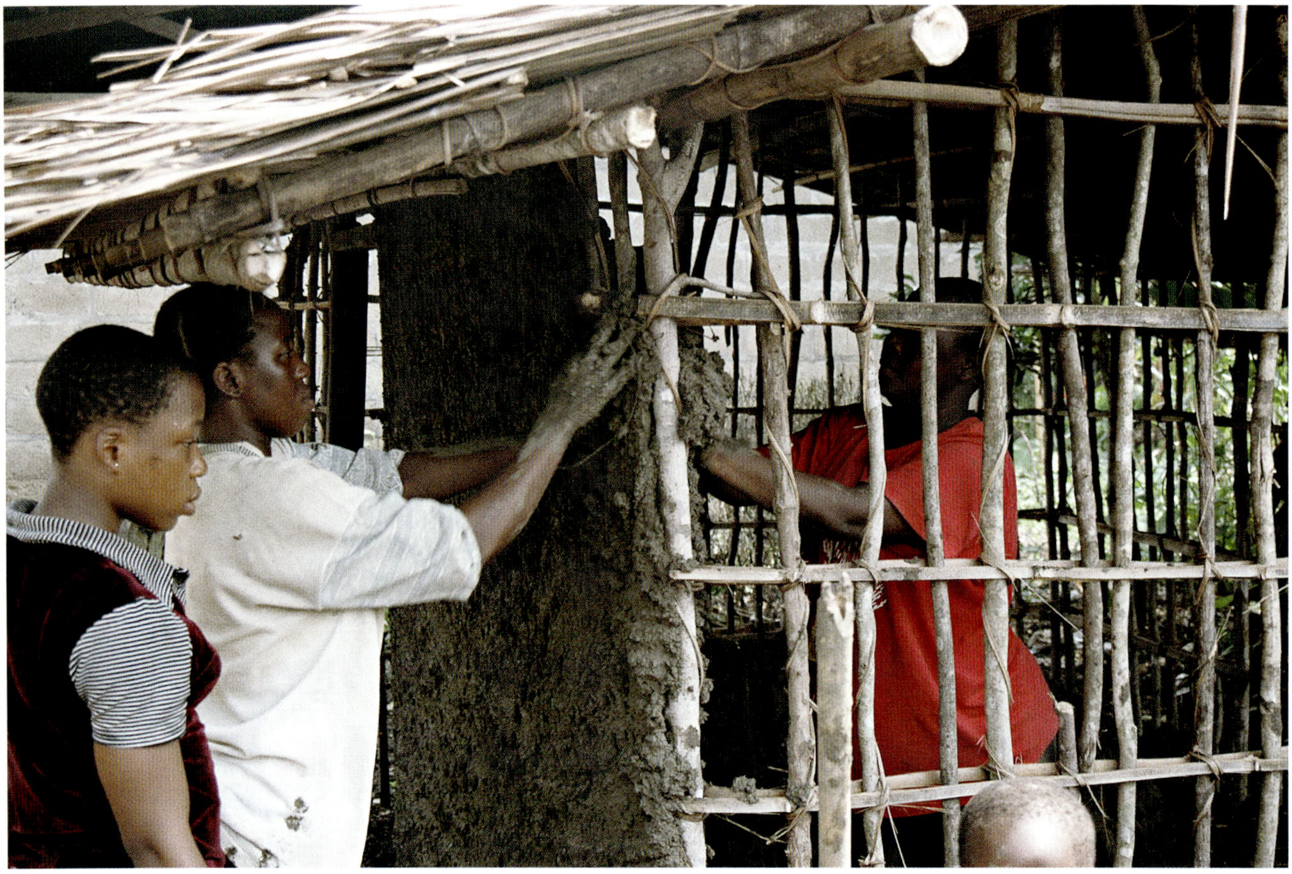

Fig. 26 From both sides women fill the frame walls with the stamped mud (Kembong, November 26, 2005).

Footnotes

1 According to an intelligence report of 1937 on the Kembong area, there were 1,324 inhabitants in Kembong at that time (Ruel 1969:5).

2 According to census figures for the Central Ejagham of former times the following data are available: Mansfeld 1908:8 (4,535); Talbot 1926:II:6 (7,542); Rutherfoord 1926:§ 6 (8,907); E. and S. Ardener 1960:406 (9,098, according to the census of 1953); Ruel 1969:5 (7,826).

3 For the linguistic material and corresponding linguistic assignment see De Wolff 1981:57 ff.; Röschenthaler 1993:19 f.; Onor 1994:24 ff.

4 For a list of the "short wars" that occurred in various localities during the last 30 years, that is before 1908, see Mansfeld 1908: 16 f.; see also Ruel 1969:181 f.

5 Ruel 1969:184.

6 Mansfeld 1908:158. Head-hunting was widespread in south-eastern Nigeria (cp. e.g. Talbot 1912:271 ff. and Horton 1971: 44 f.).

7 Mansfeld 1908:16; Ruel 1969:182.

8 Müller 1904; Mansfeld 1908:18; see also Agbor 2001:16 ff.

9 Mansfeld 1908:159; Ruel 1969:182.

10 Mansfeld 1908:12; Röschenthaler 1993:20; Agbor 2001:3.

11 Cp. for example Fagg 1964:52; Olderogge 1969:37 ff.; Schädler 1975: 162 ff.; Campbell 1983:34; Röschenthaler 1993:20 ff.

12 Mansfeld 1908:12 f.; Ruel 1969:2 ff.; Röschenthaler 1993:20.

13 Rutherfoord 1926.

14 Cp. Onor 1994.

15 In the language of the Ejagham the river's name is *Manyu*. The region, correspondingly, is called Manyu Division.

16 Ruel (1969:2 ff.) just as Nicklin (1979) named the Ngunaya people "eastern Ejagham".

17 For details about the clans of the region, see Rutherfoord (1926:§§ 2–5, 27–75) and Agbor 2001:4 f.
Among the neighbouring Banyang "Nchemti" designates a meeting, gathering, union, association or federation, and is also the name for new political bodies such as community groupings, clan unions and chiefs' councils (Ruel 1969:118, 205, 263). I was unable to ascertain whether or not this term stands in any kind of association with the name of the clan-founder of the Central Ejagham.

18 For further information about the salt resources in this region, see Mansfeld 1908:4 and Agbor 2001:6.

19 Rutherfoord 1926:§§ 12–14, 27–31; Agbor 2001:4 ff.; Ruel 1969:183.

20 See also Röschenthaler 2000:197.

21 According to Rutherfoord (1926:§ 306) "Kembong was, in pre-European days, a centre of the slave trade and a regular market. Slaves came chiefly from Bangwa country and were obtained very easily, the system being that 25–30 pieces of cloth and one gun were passed from village to village to Bangwa and Bali and a slave was passed down in return. Debtors were sold out of the villages as slaves, and a murderer compensated the bereaved family by giving one of his family as a slave. Slaves lived in a separate quarter known as the "Asunk Quarter". During the German era slavery was suppressed, but it appears that at Kembong slaves were still sold secretly and in small numbers to avoid attracting attention. The present chief of Kembong has served a sentence in prison for slave-dealing. There has been no attempt to revive slavery in recent times and it now appears to have been completely abolished". Cp. also Mansfeld (1908:167), where he reports that in the Ossidinge District "Slave trade … still continued until about fifteen years ago (that is, until c. 1890, H.-J. K.), individual slaves are still sold today and household slaves are present everywhere." For more on slave trade in this region, see Chem-Langhëë and Fomin 1995. According to these authors Kembong – or more likely the environs of present-day Kembong, for this locality only emerged in the German colonial era – was a centre of slave trade.

22 Mansfeld 1908:265.

23 Agbor 2001:17.

24 Cp. Röschenthaler 2000:192. Measures of forced resettlement such as this were also carried out by the German colonial administration with the Banyang (Ruel 1962:100; 1969:26 f., 33 ff.).

25 Mansfeld 1908:15.

26 Koloss 1984:71.

27 Men were the ones who used to do the weaving, above all bags. They utilised a type of loom that is widespread in western Africa and the fibres of the raphia palm as material. (Mansfeld 1908:110 ff. and Talbot 1912:270; cp. Nicklin 1980 (raphia weaving among the Annang Ibibio)).

28 Mansfeld supplied unusually detailed descriptions with sketches and photographs of house construction (Mansfeld 1908:22 ff., 1924:48, 89 ff.; cp. Talbot 1912:270).

29 The state of research in ethnology regarding the Cross River region in Cameroon is not at all favourable. A significant older source of information together with valuable photographs and sketches are the "Urwald-Dokumente" by A. Mansfeld (1908), who was the head of the District of Ossidinge in the former German colony Cameroon from 1904 to 1914. The work by F. Staschewski on the Banyang also stems from that time (1917). A further important document is the "Assessment-Report" of 1926 by the British District Officer of the former Mamfe Divison, I. W. C. Rutherfoord. The document contains comprehensive material on the history and sociology of the Central Ejagham. Sixty years elapsed after Mansfeld's publication of the "Urwald-Dokumente" before another outstanding work about the region appeared, namely M. Ruel's "Leopard and Leaders", with a convincing detailed analysis of the political system of the Banyang. As close cultural relations exist between the Banyang and the Central Ejagham, this work is also valuable with reference to the Ngunaya area. Aside from a few shorter studies in the 1970s and 1980s (R. F. Thompson, K. Nicklin, E. Leib and R. Romano), particular mention should be made of the publications of U. Röschenthaler, with contributions on cultural aspects of the women (since the 1990s). Further reference is made here to the unfortunately unpublished work about the Central Ejagham (2001) by A. W. Agbor, who is from Kembong. This study throws light on many ethnologically relevant conditions. The number of publications about the Ejagham and their neighbouring tribes in Nigeria is, by contrast, abundant, and cannot be listed here in detail. Yet, there the special topics of masks and magic medicine are given little attention. Finally, the comprehensive and knowledgeable works of P. A. Talbot, written during the first third of the 20th century, are still a "must" for all ethnological research on the area of western Cameroon and eastern Nigeria. S. O. Onor's "The Ejagham Nation" (1994) offers an interesting and informative overview of the culture and history of the Ejagham in Nigeria.

30 Though difficult to identify, Mansfeld is pictured in a photograph in Talbot 1912:154.

2 Elements of religious world-view

2.1 God and the ancestors

Among the Ejagham the belief prevails – as generally in Africa – in one god of creation, who created the world and all life upon it, including mankind. In our case the god of the Ejagham is a twofold figure, who embodies *Ata Obasi*, that is, Father God, and *Mma Obasi*, Mother God. *Ata Obasi* is the celestial god, and *Mma Obasi* as *Obasi Nsi*, the earth goddess.[1] Thus the characteristic traits of each are therefore quite different, as described by S. O. Onor: "The former (*Ata Obasi*) was thought to be very fierce and vindictive while the latter (*Mma Obasi*) was conceived as caring, forgiving and magnanimous. However, both were regarded with high esteem and treated as such in the belief and understanding that both of them required utmost attention and reverence if a man was to lead a successful life on earth."[2] Although perceived among the Central Ejagham as being two different deities, they nevertheless form an indivisible unit and are always invoked together in prayer. Indeed, they represent one single god, who has both male and female characteristics.

Contrary to other African creator gods, who having created the earth retreated and are no longer concerned with the fate of mankind, *Ata Obasi* and *Mma Obasi* exert a profound influence upon human life. Indeed, every living being and every action is dependent upon God, and it is a known fact that no undertaking can succeed without His assistance. He can inflict mankind with sickness (*emangha Obasi*, "illness from God") and even cause death.

The Ejagham have no visual concept of the external form of God, which is altogether typical of old traditional Africa. No one knows whether to picture Him in the form of a human being or to conceive of Him as a spiritual power. Aside from the belief that God has unlimited omnipotence, there is no conception of His origin and existence. Indeed, it is said that all living beings and inanimate things as well owe their very existence to their apportionment from the power of God. P. A. Talbot already pointed out this conception, which elucidates the pantheistic character of the religious concept among the Ejagham: "All these powers, from the great gods down to the smallest things on earth, exist by virtue of emanations from the supreme deity; the greatest, such as the Earth Goddess, possessing infinitely more of the essence of divinity than, for instance, an animal or stone."[3] God is omnipresent, the holder over all forms of being, and, consequently, there are no special sacred places in which He abides nor are there any "priests" for Him. Although God does not need offerings, all things offered, especially to the ancestors, are ultimately meant for Him.

Even today a remarkable lot of men and women in Kembong still invoke after the morning bath God and the ancestors. With a bowl full of water in both hands they pray for their support and promise to lead a righteous life: "*Ata Obasi, Mma Obasi*, I am praying that if I intend evil things against anybody, you two should punish me. But if I have a pure heart and if anybody intends evil things against me and my family members, do not allow such actions." A further example of these morning prayers is: "*Ata Obasi ka oso, Akeku ka Nsi*, I am washing my face this morning. As the day will go, let me meet only with weak animals and not with powerful and dangerous ones. A person with problems should be distant from me. I should always meet with food and not with problems." Then the water is poured upon the earth in offering. If a hissing noise occurs, it is the sign that the offer has been accepted – and the joy is correspondingly great.[4]

Ake kale eri mba Obasi ("giving food to God") is a ceremony of offering made directly to God without expressly including the ancestors. It is conducted at the beginning of the planting season after several bad harvests in the past and is the duty of the eldest man in a community. Women hand him fruit from all of the plants that are to be cultivated, which he places in a basket. Then he commences his prayer: "*Ata Obasi, Mma Obasi*, we have brought food for you. As we start our planting season this year, we are begging you to bless our crops, so that we will have a good yield this time." In this manner all of the plants are offered to God, and the basket is hung from a frame consisting of two vertical posts secured in the earth and a cross timber. A chicken is brought as a further offering; it is tied to a long pole that is then leaned against the basket. I was told that this ceremony was last conducted in Kembong about 2000.

In Ejagham, as in almost all of Africa, the ancestors as mediators to God exercise constant influence upon people's life. They can almost be reckoned as part of the community of the living. In contrast to God who lives in heaven, the ancestors' sphere is in the earth.[5] The ancestors bestow the people with blessings, and they punish them if they offend the laws that have always enabled them to live together. This applies not only to simple theft, adultery, armed robbery, murder and other condemnatory crimes, but also to seemingly less serious offences. For example, a person who does not carry sufficient responsibility for the parents-in-law and thus brings shame to the ancestors must reckon with sanctions.

The social values and institutions of the Ejagham, which are the consequence and expression of their religions laws, likewise correspond broadly with those of most other African peoples. Their fundamental principle is that a society united in peace, harmony and cooperation and in which the ancestors hold a central and respected position, represents the highest social value and can be understood as one of the essential elements of African philosophy.[6] The profound responsibility of the living for the ancestors demands that they must never forget their forebears. Thus, it is a matter of fact that the names of the deceased are retained in the family by passing them on to new-born children. The ancestors also expect – as mentioned above – that one address them in the daily morning prayers and that they receive their portion of drink at feasts in the form of libations.

For the Ejagham the veneration of the ancestors has its most prominent place within the family. It is, however, also the duty of other social organisations – secret societies, quarters, localities[7] – not only to give their deceased members a proper burial, so that they can enter into eternal peace, but also to show them their due honour as ancestors and never forget them. Indeed, the communities are also dependent upon the blessings of the ancestors. The fact that the individual is not only inseparable from his family, but also from the societies in which he is a member becomes impressively apparent at the moment of his death. For then not only is his family responsible for the necessary funeral rituals, but also the respective secret societies.

Everyone, men as well as women, can invoke the ancestors of his or her family through prayer. It is only important that at the same time God be addressed, for it is in His power that the fate of mankind lies, and He is the one who bestows mankind with blessings and help – or not. Therefore, *Ata Obasi* and *Mma Obasi* are always named first in prayers to the ancestors. When a man or a woman prays, only the names of good ancestors are called. A relative who lived a wicked life before his/her death is never used as a mediator between the living and God. Wicked people should be forgotten as soon as possible; no one should remember such a person. In praying, the names of deceased relatives are named from the most recently deceased to the final person to be remembered in the family line. In the prayers those ancestors are called expressly, whom the living no longer remember. The Ejagham can only turn to the ancestors of their own family in their prayers, never to those of other people – even if they were good people during their lifetime. Whereas within the sphere of the families, all the dead are reckoned as ancestors provided they led a blameless life, in the ceremonies of secret societies, e.g. *Mgbe* or *Obasinjom,* only the former chiefs are invoked.

When a person suffers from a severe illness, he or she may pray to his or her ancestors for help. In serious cases or when a diviner has traced the cause of the illness to the ancestors, a particular sacrifice has to be made, which is often prescribed in detail by the ancestors. Such sacrifices have several names: *akeku efohe* ("fanning the ancestors"), *akeku efoko* ("appeasing the ancestors"), *akeku ejoho* ("placation of the ancestors") and *akeku akale* ("gift for the ancestors"). In contrast to the Cameroon Grasslands, where sacrifices are made by men only, among the Ejagham women may carry out this function, too. Such sacrifices are often associated with severe illness, but in principle they may be conducted at any time in order to commemorate the ancestors and to ensure their beneficence.

The ritual procedure involved in an offering to the ancestors is remarkably modest and simple. The offering itself consists of roasted grains of maize mixed with oil and of water and palm wine (figs. 27–32, 65, 66, 74, 78, 125–128, 137, 252). Although modest in amount the substances are of symbolic significance. They are held first in the left hand and then placed in the right hand, while more or less common prayers are spoken. The offering made with the left hand is intended for the ancestors, while that with the right hand is for the living.[8] On important occasions the sacrifice of an animal is required. In former times the sacrifice of a slave was mandatory at the night dance.

Chickens, particularly cocks, are by far the most important sacrificial animals for the Ejagham, who regard them as being pure and having but little blood. It is said that chickens are close to the ancestors: When they stand motionless on one leg, they are thought to be communing with them. After each sacrifice, the testicles of the cock are examined. If they are white, the

Offering of food to the ancestors at the end of a death celebration (*aboku*) (Kembong, January 20, 2004) (fig. 27–32).

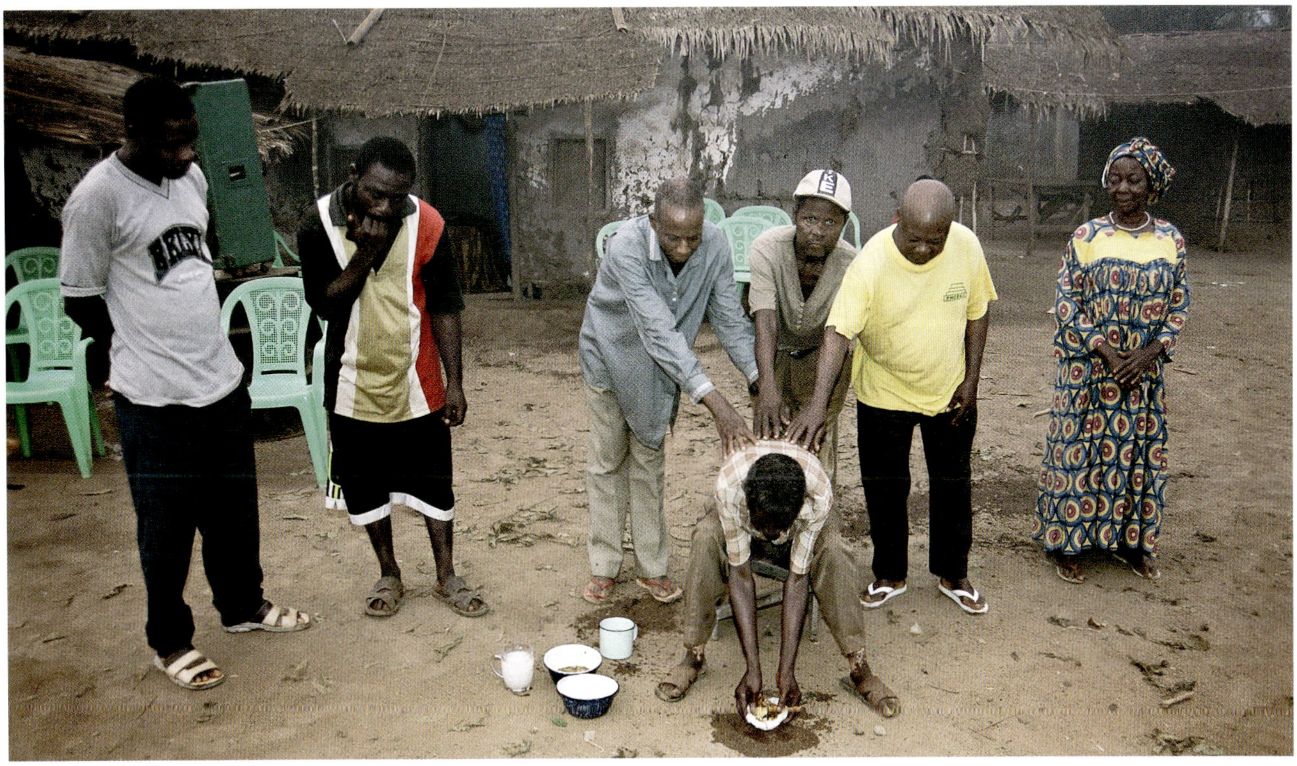

Fig. 27 A death celebration (*aboku*) closes with an offering of food to the ancestors (*etaah nji eyatek*). Members of the family place their hands upon the back of the head of the family as a sign of their solidarity and togetherness (Kembong, January 20, 2004).

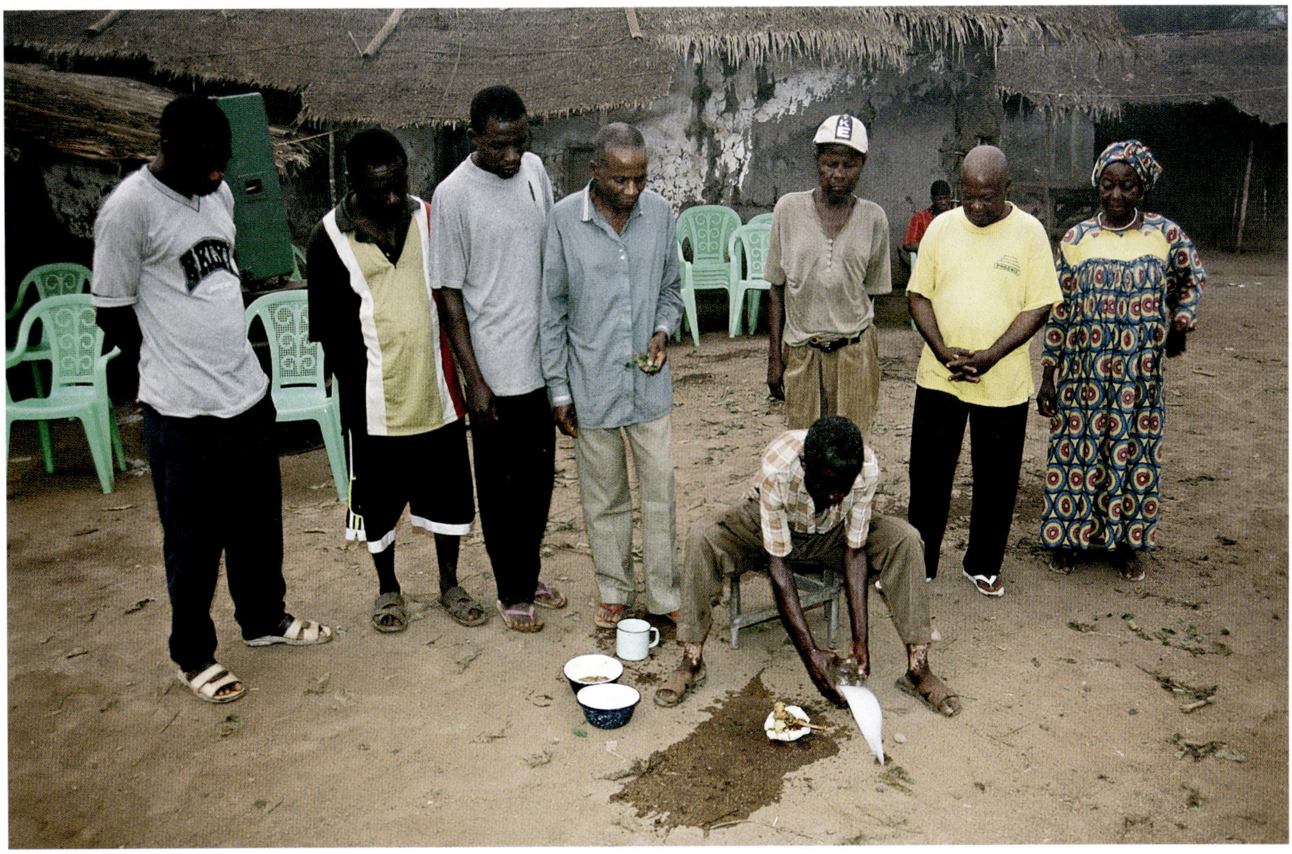

Fig. 28 The head of the family now makes an offering of palm wine to the ancestors (Kembong, January 20, 2004).

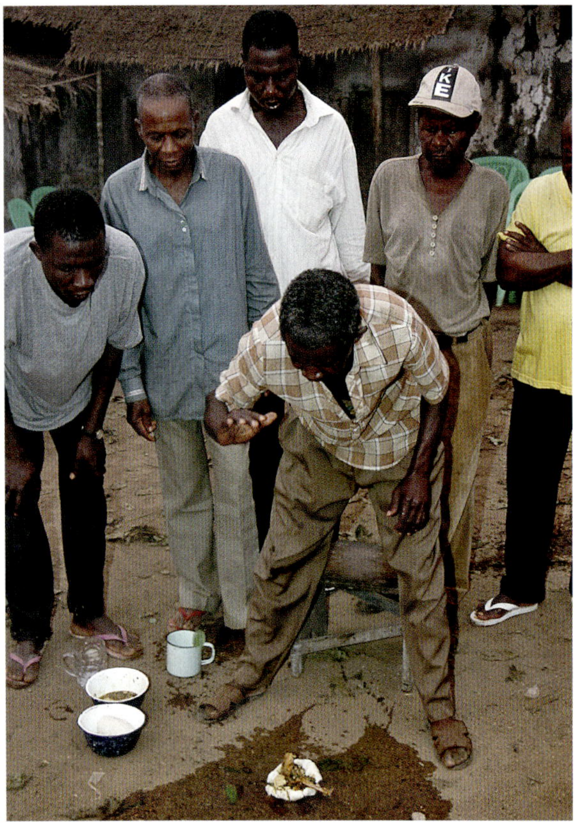

Fig. 29 The family watches the oracle with two leaves (*ebanghaah*) in great suspense. The result shows that the ancestors have accepted the offering and are satisfied (Kembong, January 20, 2004).

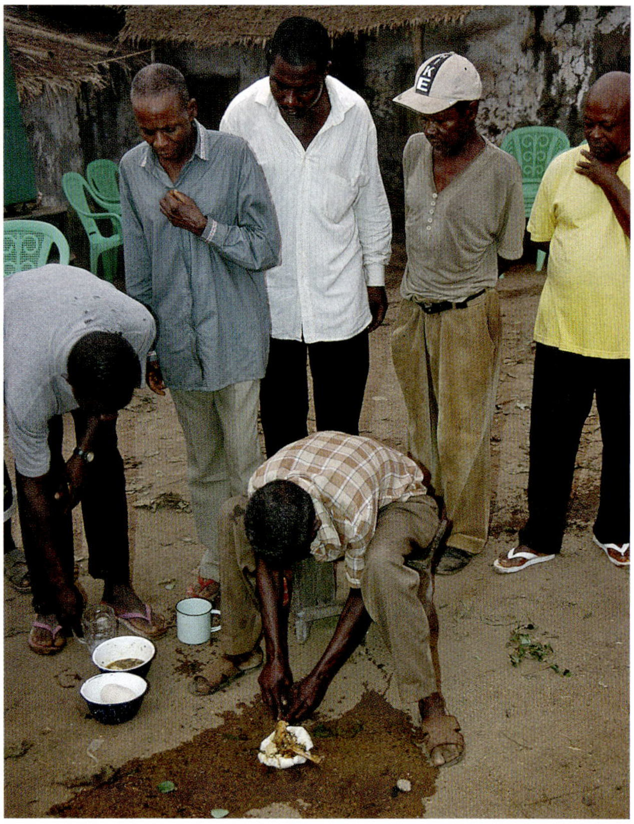

Fig. 30 The family head mixes the offering food and a leaf (*oyotnsi)* with his forefingers and adds his saliva to the mixture (Kembong, January 20, 2004).

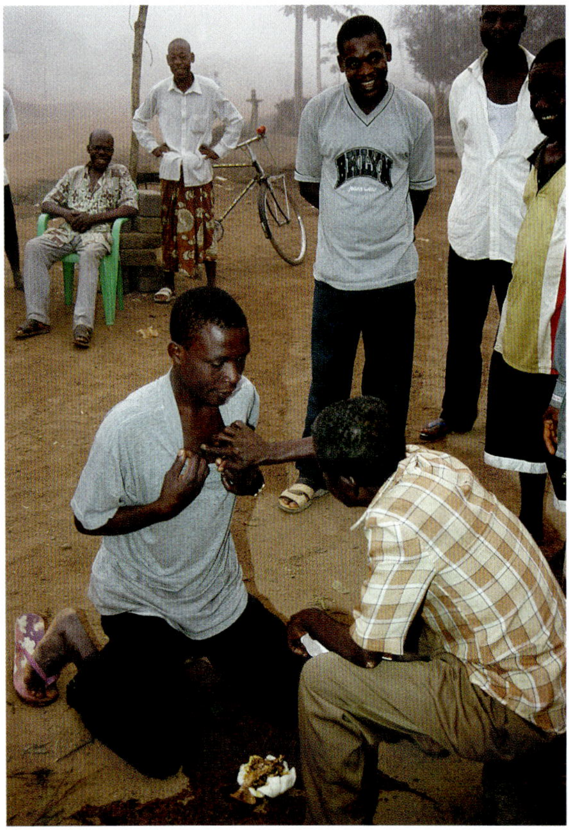

Fig. 31 With his finger he rubs part of the mixture on the breastbone of a family member (Kembong, January 20, 2004).

sacrifice has been accepted; otherwise it must be repeated.[9] In Oku the chicken is also the sacrificial animal, but for another reason. It is said to be "devilish", because it can recognise danger. Even shut up in a completely dark coop, a chicken will cackle if a bird of prey circles above the compound. Thus, its blood is considered to be particularly potent and must flow over a newly made medicine.[10]

Whereas the course of the offering is usually rather systematic and stiff, the concluding oracle with the throwing of two leaves (*ebanghaah*) is of great interest. The upward or downward position of the top and bottom side of the leaves on the ground is decisive (figs. 29, 67, 253). If one leaf lies upwards and the other downwards, this means that the offering has been accepted. Should both leaves fall with the upper side upwards, it is said that the ancestors are laughing. But the ancestors' complete rejection of the offering is shown when both leaves lie with the underside facing upwards. The oracle is repeated until the ideal position is attained, that is, one leaf upwards and the other downwards. If the ideal result is reached with the first throw, this means unlimited acceptance by the ancestors, and the persons present applaud. If the positive result occurs after three throws, everyone is more or less satisfied. But

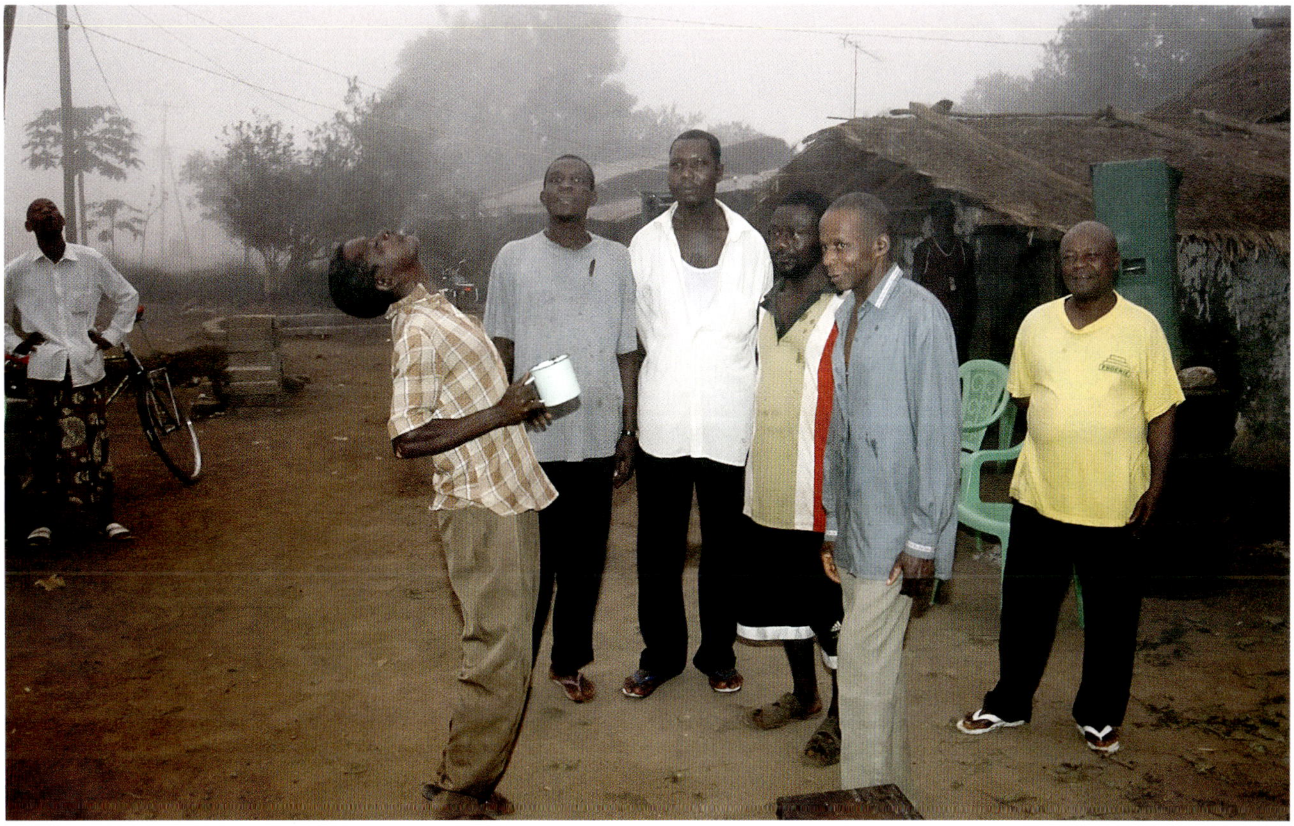

Fig. 32 In concluding the ritual, the family head blows water into the air; the falling droplets are considered to be a blessing (*oyotnsi*) (Kembong, January 20, 2004).

if five throws are necessary, one is very sceptical, for there may be problems looming somewhere. And if even more throws are necessary, a diviner must be consulted.[11]

Many ceremonies of offering are conducted in this manner, yet they can occur in diverse social groups and for very different reasons. *Akeku efoko* refers to the ceremony performed by a male or female family head to appease the ancestors. *Ajom Mgbe* designates the ritual performed by a *seseku*, the leader of a lodge of *Mgbe* (cp. p. 85 ff.). *Ajom Etek* refers to the ritual performed by the eldest member at a village meeting after having drunk palm wine (cp. p. 53). *Ajom Ndem* was the name of the ritual performed by *agbokarem* in former times (cp. p. 208).

Oyotnsi (pl. *ayotnsi*) is another ritual for ancestors, a form of blessing upon an individual by members of his or her family. The ceremony is meant to foster the general well-being and often conducted prior to difficult undertakings, such as a long journey, but in particular before a girl leaves her parents' compound to marry into another family. Sometimes *oyotnsi* is performed to encourage the quick convalescence of a sick person. The family members gather at the home of the family head. After consuming food and drink, a small hole is dug in the ground in front of the family head. Every member present says a wish in the form of a prayer for the one to receive the *oyotnsi*. At the end of the prayers, the members spit one by one into the hole. When everyone has taken his/her turn, the receiver kneels in front of the eldest person, who mixes the substance in the hole with his/her two forefingers. While the mixture is being rubbed upon the chest of the receiver and usually also of other persons, the prayers of the family members are repeated slowly. At the end of the ritual the family head takes a sip of water and blows it into the air. The drops of water that fall upon all persons present are considered a blessing. Those thus blessed go away with encouragement, knowing that they received the blessings of their family members and also from their protecting and guiding ancestors (figs. 30–32).

The presence of ancestors is greater among the Ejagham than is the case in the Cameroon Grasslands, where they are mostly invoked only in times of trouble. The Ejagham, by contrast, make mention of the ancestors even in daily meals and when drinking palm wine, leaving a small portion as a symbol of their partaking of the meal or drink. Thus, A.W. Agbor writes: "Most people as such have it as regular habit that they never drink or eat without throwing some portion of the food or drink on the ground to the ancestors."[12] In the Grasslands, contrarily, the ancestors are offered food and palm wine only in association with official ancestral ceremonies, which do not often take place.[13]

Ritual drinking is an important event in all social spheres and takes place relatively frequently, often in connection with councils and discussions. In correspondence with the official and ritual character of these gatherings, proper behaviour is expected of the participants, for example, the seating order is regulated, with the bench for the big men at the head of the room, as well as the order in which those present take the single drinking vessel, one after the other. Only the elders, who have their place on the bench, remain seated while drinking; the others must stand. Communal drinking, always out of one glass, is a special sign of congeniality and solidarity: "Only friends drink from the same cup". At the same time it joins the living with the dead (figs. 70, 94, 136, 147).[14]

2.2 Spirits

The belief in so-called spirits of nature is typical of the inhabitants of the forest area in southwestern Cameroon and southeastern Nigeria. They are encountered in conspicuous natural formations, such as rocky cliffs, rivers, waterfalls, springs, large trees etc. These spirits are omnipresent and omnipotent in their sphere and bestow fortune and prosperity upon those who follow their dictums and taboos. Otherwise they can cause a person the most diverse problems and afflict him with misfortune and failure. Although there are certain regional differences in the significance of these spirits for man as well as in the cult that is associated with them, there are recognisable common features that render a marked specificity to this form of belief. Among the Ejagham these spirits are called *arem* (sg. *ndem* or *nimm*). In general the *arem* are considered female, and it is mostly women whom they draw into dependency through trance.[15] The spirits expect relatively regular offerings from these "priestesses", but they reward the priestesses with generous gifts: wealth, beauty, fortune and usually the capabilities of prophecy and healing.[16]

In the coastal area the spirits are more associated with everything that has to do with water and accordingly are conceived as being water spirits. For the coastal Efik *ndem* is a water spirit and it is the king, who functions as the highest priest.[17] The concept of water spirits in the form of a water nymph, half human and half fish, is widespread along the west African coast. In this cult, too, the female element predominates: The water spirits are generally regarded as female, and their "priestesses" are mostly women, who are likewise drawn into dependency through trance. These water nymphs, known everywhere along the coast as *mammy wata*, have a rather European or Indian appearance due to their long, smooth hair.[18] The possibility cannot be excluded that this cult derived from European influences, which have been in effect there since the 15th century. On the other hand, it is noteworthy that members of the cult should avoid contact with objects of European provenience, such as lacquer paints. In fact, J. Ittmann reported[19] that on the Cameroon coast foreign materials such as books or even a simple piece of paper, that is "strong means", were used to scare away the spirits, the *mengú*. The spirits could not withstand European articles. In the meantime the *mammy wata* cult has spread inwards over large parts of the hinterland[20] and has also reached Kembong, as will be shown in the following.

The Ejagham believe that the *arem*, who are invisible to normal humans, can be encountered everywhere. Their contact persons are special priestesses, who also act as diviners and healers with the aid of the *arem* and, thus, are of great service for the community. These so-called priestesses, *abu arem* (sg. *mbu arem*), are predominantly women; men seldom act as priests. The priestesses are mostly sought out by the *arem* and are bestowed with supernatural capabilities and powers. Yet occasionally "ordinary" women can attain similar knowledge and abilities by attending instruction from an active *mbu arem*; thereafter they can seek contact with the *arem*. The state of trance plays a special role in the calling of the *abu arem* and later in their contact with the *arem*. The encounter with the spirits usually takes place at a special shrine, where more or less regular offerings are made.

During my stay in Kembong in 2004, I had the opportunity of making the acquaintance of a *mbu arem*. Hanna Agbor was born in 1963. She was normal at birth, but later experienced frequent and intense dreams. Europeans often appeared in her dreams, with whom she played, ate and drank. Much of the actions in the dreams took place in water. As a young girl Hanna Agbor fell sick and suffered from psychic problems. Once for no reason she ran into the forest alone and was found there later by her family and neighbours. The dreams continued as Hanna Agbor became older; she usually dreamt that she was in water. In one of her most peculiar dreams she held a clay pot filled with water in her hands and gave it to many people who wore red caps, who had waited for her on the river bank to drink the water. She took the last sip herself

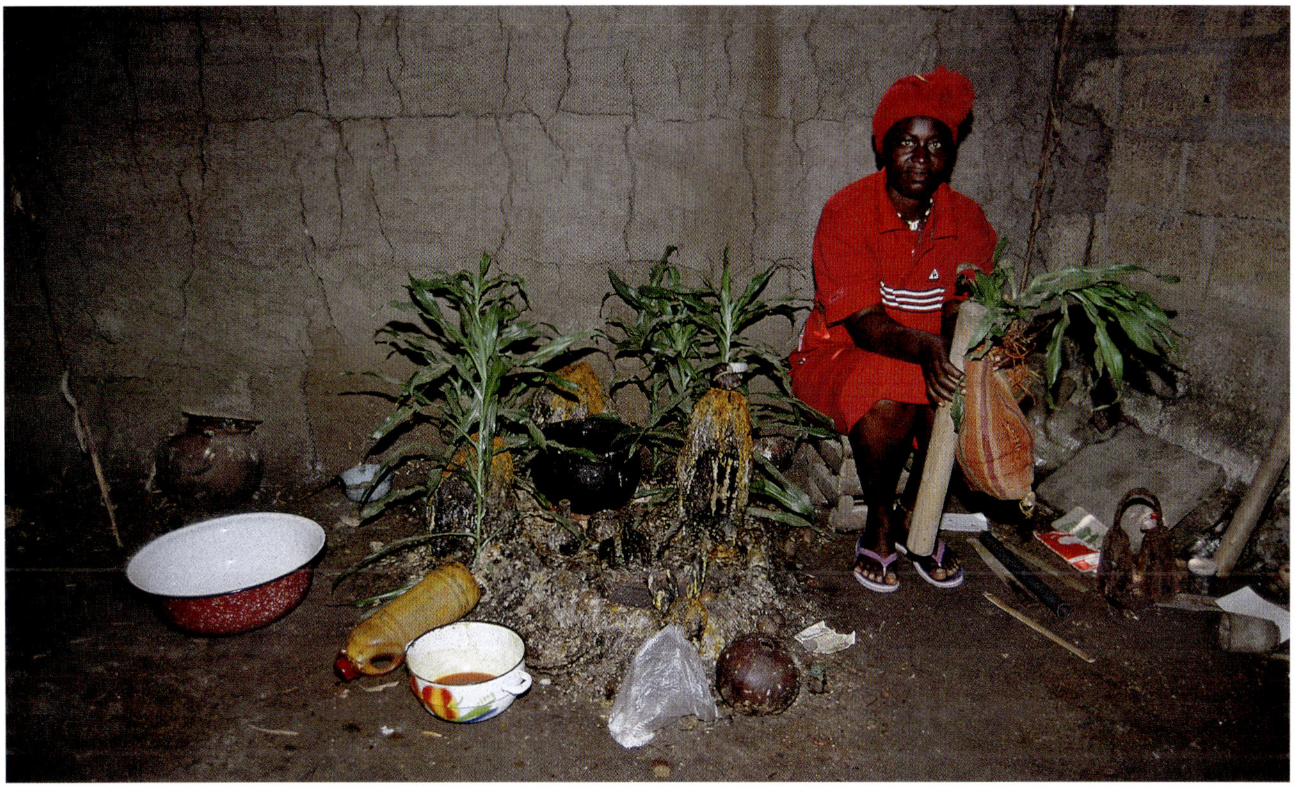

Fig. 33 Hanna Agbor, a priestess of the spirits (*mbu arem*), sitting next to the altar for the spirits (*arem*). She holds a bamboo blowpipe; to her left is a double bell. A black vessel, medicine plants and remains of offerings, among other things, can be seen at the altar (Kembong, January 24, 2004).

and blew it into the air; the drops that fell upon those present were considered – as in the ancestral ceremonies (cp. fig. 32) – to be blessings. Through this dream Hanna Agbor realised that she was destined to be a healer. She became seriously ill and once again had psychic problems. One night she saw the spirits for the first time in a dream. They commanded her to go to a certain person, who would be able to heal her. At first Hanna Agbor defied this command. Only after further warnings did she follow the order, although the man recommended to her (his name was Peter) had died in the meantime. In his place a woman and the son of the deceased made an offering in the bedroom of the deceased. Immediately thereafter Hanna Agbor was healed. These happenings occurred in 1989.

Since that time Hanna Agbor has been in constant contact with the *arem*, that is, with the spirits that look like humans; among these are also Europeans. As mentioned above, the spirits are present everywhere, in the air, upon the earth, but above all in water, meaning the ocean, sea, lakes, rivers and streams. Hanna Agbor designated the spirits of all the waters as *mammy wata*. Quick and direct communication with the spirits is achieved by playing musical instruments. With a wind instrument made of Indian bamboo the spirits can be contacted who are in the countryside, the spirits in

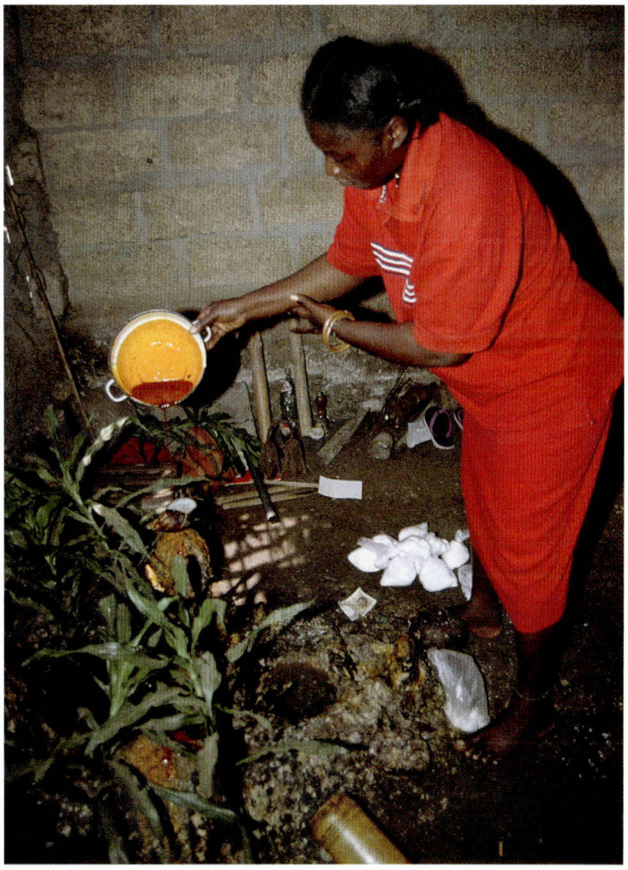

Fig. 34 Hanna Agbor makes an offering of palm oil to the spirits by pouring the oil over the altar (Kembong, January 24, 2004).

water are called with an iron bell, and a double bell made of iron calls the ancestors in the whole world. These musical instruments are taboo for non-initiated persons. Whoever uses them without permission can be killed immediately by the spirits. Communication with the *arem* is established in a special location, in Hanna Agbor's case in her "temple" for the *arem*, which comprises a room with an altar in her house. The altar consists of a pedestal upon which stands a clay vessel with water; it is framed by two green medicine plants (*Dracena* sp.), called "life-plant" in the Grasslands and indispensable in many religious practices there.[21] The offerings – usually palm oil and salt – are made upon the altar, and therefore the whole area is covered with their remains (figs. 33, 34).

Hanna Agbor became a diviner, who – as she herself assured me – knows all, who can explain every secret, and who can heal illness. She touches the sick person with her hands, and through her powers the malady is alleviated and soon heals. In every treatment patients are given water from the altar vessel to drink; it is full of blessings and accelerates the healing process. Through her communication with the spirits Hanna Agbor knows that she originates from the Arctic Ocean, specifically from Greenland. She assured me that she has never been in Nigeria, where the cult of *mammy wata* has long been known and practised intensively. Hanna Agbor is married and has children, which is rather uncommon among priestesses. She has resettled in Kumba, one of the larger towns in the South West Province, where she is esteemed and much sought after as a diviner and healer.

The *arem* carry special significance among the Ejagham, insofar as only with their assistance can children be conceived and born.[22] According to tradition the conception of a child is achieved not only through the sexual union of man and woman, but also requires the presence of a *ndem*, who first enters the womb of the woman. Only when this has been accomplished, can the woman become pregnant. In this way every child is a manifestation of an invisible *ndem*. The *ndem* takes on human form at the birth of the child, but remains in contact with the realm of the *arem*. When the child laughs, one knows that the *arem* are playing with it. When it cries, the *arem* have frightened or scolded it. The bond of children with the *arem* remains firm as long as the children are innocent. Once they have committed sin, the tie is forever terminated. Thus, the participation of "innocent" children between the ages of four and ten is almost indispensable at the death celebrations of *aboku*, at which they are the first to receive a portion of the festive meal following the performance of their mask *Nchockandah*. At the same time they must pass judgement as to whether the meal is good and sufficient. If this is not the case, the *aboku* cannot take place. At this moment the children are said to be the visible presence of the invisible *arem* (cp. p. 93 and figs. 100, 101).[23]

If a woman has difficulties in becoming pregnant, she can pray to the *arem* for help. She can make an offering of an egg, placing it upon a small round pebble.[24] She can also consult a priestess, who then makes the offering for her. Childlessness is not seen as punishment for immoral behaviour, but it is still said that "bad" women have more difficulties in conceiving than those women who lead a proper life.

2.3 Witches and magic medicines

People of traditional Africa are quite aware that peace and unity in the community are more of an ideal and a wish than a reality. Yet in Kembong not only are the tensions and conflicts reckoned with, which are indeed part of daily life in the whole world, but also the dangerous powers of witches who are believed to be present nearly everywhere in Africa. It is common knowledge that the principal aim of witches is to destroy peace in society, and that witchcraft is the cause of all things wicked and criminal. In fact, the Ejagham say that witches are willed by the gods and that they make the witches bring malady and death to people. Without witches everything would be good.

Witches (*aje,* sg. *nje)* are persons who can make themselves invisible or turn themselves into animals in order to commit serious crimes, most notably murder. The belief in their effectiveness is an important fact of daily life in the Cross River region, as evidenced by the number of socio-political institutions and magic rites and practices that exist to fight against them. It is said that witches do not only appear individually, but also form societies much like regular societies in which members are required to pay dues. In their case, however, these dues are not paid with domestic animals (for example, chickens and goats) but with members of the witches' families: they are forced to give their own blood, so to speak. The society "eats" the victim, or rather his vital force, which is gradually drained out of him until he dies. The soul of the witch leaves her sleeping body at night to carry out the task, perhaps transforming itself into an animal, and returns at dawn.[25]

Witches are said to be constantly on the lookout for new ways of destroying their victims. They turn themselves into owls, using their tongues to penetrate walls and draw blood from sleeping people. They carry them off in the guise of huge birds. As pythons, they poison victims by spitting on them, and they murder in the form of leopards, elephants and other dangerous animals. In invisible form witches might beat their victims with clubs or cutlasses, pull them from their boats into the water to drown or rob them of their hearts. Attacks in dreams are especially common. Witches even have ways of forcing people to commit suicide. However, the study of witchcraft implies special problems. Since the malevolent activities of witches are always invisible and done in utter secrecy, ordinary humans can have only incomplete knowledge of them. In fact, one would run the risk of being suspected as a witch, if one exhibited too much knowledge about them.

In earlier times the fear of witches used to be so intense that people would not leave their houses after dark. This fear remains even today, not only in isolated rural areas, but also in cities. Witches are blamed for most accidents, serious illnesses and deaths. The Ejagham say: "Nobody dies without a cause", the only natural deaths being those of the elderly. Because witches are the powers of invisibility, of darkness and of the night, their society is called *ekume atu* ("sitting in the night") or *echem atu* ("meeting in the night").

Although a witch can be male or female, women are said to have a greater affinity for witchcraft.[26] Their supposedly greater supernatural powers indicate the presence of sexual antagonisms within traditional Ejagham society. Supernatural powers are considered hereditary and manifested in certain physical characteristics. The stomach of a witch is thought to contain miniatures of those animals into which she transforms herself. A concentration of these on the left side of the stomach indicates that the predisposition was inherited from mother, from father if on the right. Victims of witches also reveal a sign: Small pieces of meat are found in their hearts. This explains why autopsies used to be performed – and occasionally are still today – on all corpses by the men "with four eyes" (that is those who have extraordinary powers of seeing, similar to the diviners).[27] These men also possess some supernatural abilities and use them only for the good of society. They can determine whether the deceased was a victim of witchcraft or a witch herself. If medicine has killed a witch, her blood will turn to water. Her corpse will then be treated with medicine to destroy her dangerous soul.[28]

It is necessary to remember that in Africa all calamities are blamed on social problems and conflicts, and witches more or less fulfil the role of scapegoats. Public pressure often leaves an accused person, even if innocent, no choice but to admit a crime of witchcraft. Among some peoples it is believed that a person can subconsciously act as a witch. Under these conditions, everyone runs the risk of being accused as such. These subconscious aspects of witchcraft have not yet been studied in depth, and therefore R. F. Thompson's findings in this regard are all the more valuable, especially since they also concern the Cross River region. According to Thompson some women accused of being witches were questioned by the mask-medicine *Obasinjom*: "'Have you done this?' They answered, 'Yes'. He asked again, 'were you at a certain place?' They answered, 'Yes'. He asked again: 'Were you at a certain place?' Again they answered, 'Yes'. They apologised and said they did not know that their powers had been so destructive. They begged forgiveness. They offered material amends and these were accepted."[29]

In association with witches are also those spirits of the dead, who allegedly return to earth as wandering souls, in whatever figure and for whatever motive – to seek out their survivors and torture and tyrannise them in every way imaginable. This belief is found among the Ejagham as well as many other peoples in Africa. It is said that there are also "devils" (*akepansi*, sg. *nkepansi*) among these returned dead souls, who behave properly. They have left their homeland – a relief for all – and settled in a foreign unknown land, from where they continually support their family relatives financially.

It is said that a person can be born as a "devil" and that the corresponding dispositions are inheritable. Moreover, it is assumed that those persons who have always been in contact with dangerous medicines during their lifetime can after their death become a threat for the living, due to their special powers. If it is suspected that the deceased might return as a wandering soul, preventative measures are made to hinder this by treating the corpse with certain medicines.[30] If the wandering soul turns against its relative despite this treatment, the ultimate measures must be taken: It is usually the mask *Angbu* that then goes into action and destroys the returned soul (cp. p. 125 ff.).[31] It is a matter of course that in all cases of death special attention is paid that the rituals of death are conducted, so that the deceased, as mentioned above, can enter the land of the dead and find his or her peace there as well as bestow his or her family with blessings and fortune.

The psychological and social aspects of witchcraft in the Cross River region are also more or less typical of witchcraft in the kingdom of Oku in the Grasslands, although there are important differences. In Oku, women are not believed to have greater supernatural powers than men, nor are these powers considered hereditary or accompanied by physical signs. Consequently, autopsies are relatively unknown. One has the impression that witchcraft in Oku, as compared to that among the Ejagham in Cameroon, is more abstract in the sense that accidents and all evil are usually blamed on rather obscure causes and "ghosts". In fact, all thoughts and actions that threaten the social order are considered witchery. With the help of medicines, attempts are made to ward off these anonymous and dangerous powers. Should, however, criminals or witches be detected by a diviner, it is the duty of the much feared secret society called *Kwifon* to punish them.[32]

Bad things propagate bad things, and therefore witches and other anti-social and offensive persons should be forgotten as soon as possible after their death – only good persons are a possilibilty as ancestors. Certain actions are considered dangerous and unclean, such as killing people, but there are also places and villages that are accursed, and it is better to avoid them. This applies to a "bad death", to which all cases of death are reckoned that are out of the ordinary, such as suicide, the death of a pregnant woman, drowning and cases of death following a severe and loathsome illness, lightning, falling branches and trees and – in recent times – automobile accidents and plane crashes. There are remarkably many institutions among the Ejagham, for example, *Angbu* (cp. p. 125 ff.), *Nsibiri* (in former times) and certain medicine men who specialise in removing or ritually cleansing dangerous things or persons who are marked by fault.

A natural and logical antidote against witches which is used in almost all of Africa is medicine, the prime remedy that secures mankind's good fortune and well-being in general. It is natural and logical, because it consists of substances from animals, but above all of grasses, leaves and tree bark. On the one hand, these substances are considered devilish and dangerous, while, on the other, they possess beneficial properties. The production of medicine is not simply a technical procedure that follows a certain recipe; on the contrary, it demands the observation of a complicated ritual, in which diverse religious and social convictions are effective. For the Ejagham, among other peoples, a life without medicine is unimaginable. As medicines stem from the ancestors and as their production as well as their use represent fundamental parts of cultic life, the most important aspects of medicines should be dealt with here.

The production and use of medicines are by no means the same in the various regions of Africa; quite the opposite, the differences are manifold. In general the vegetal components and the other ingredients of medicines are pounded, rubbed or roasted over fire and then made a powder or paste with the addition of further substances. "Good" medicines that bestow blessings are used to prevent or heal sickness and are usually consumed. Many Africans use medicines daily: against illness and misfortune of any kind, as a protection against inimical forces, for a successful completion of projects and undertakings, and for many other purposes. Medicines of this kind are well-known among the Ejagham; yet they do not have the same importance there as, for example, in the Cameroon Grasslands. For the Ejagham it is foremost the ancestors who guide the fate of mankind and in whom people entrust their daily life to a far greater extent than those people living in the Cameroon Grasslands. The latter depend more upon the efficacy of medicines, which are ultimately derived from the ancestors, too.

Great fear exists of "bad" medicines, which are employed against witches and other destructive forces. According to the correct use of the respective medicine and the particular circumstances, bad medicines are deposited, buried and sometimes even burned at special "places of offering", such as crossroads and other conspicuous locations. In the Cameroon Grasslands bad medicines are the most prominent possession of secret societies and likewise represent the greatest secrets. The masks draw their strength from these medicines, and, furthermore, it is the medicines that shield and safeguard the secret societies against outsiders, above all against women. Whoever should see something forbidden or offend the laws of the secret society in some way, will be pursued by the medicine and punished. This kind of "preventive" medicine is not common among the Ejagham, particularly not among the secret societies. Bad medicines are greatly feared and are only utilised, when criminal acts have already taken place. The frightening aspect is the mere threat of bad medicines and not their immediate use from the very start. Like the succinct saying of the Central Ejagham: "One does not play with medicines."

A widespread method applied in Africa is to transfer bad medicine upon some kind of carrier and with that to empower the carrier or "fetish", which can be activated against dangerous forces and offenders.[33] As initially mentioned, it is precisely these magic medicines that hold great significance for the Ejagham and are widely used by them. Medicines for healing illnesses are called *abla* (sg. *ebla*), whereas bad medicines are designated *ajom* (sg. *njom*). The latter are also known as *juju*, from Pidgin-English, among the Ejagham, a designation that is commonly used for secret and dangerous magic medicines in many regions of Africa.[34]

The Ejagham as well as peoples in the Grasslands believe that once set into life, magic medicines are unpredictable beings and powers that fight not only against enemies, but at times against their owner as well, especially if the owners have neglected to conduct rituals of medicine and the *juju* feels forgotten. Moreover, as the *jujus* have their own names with which they are addressed, it seems logical to view such medicines as autonomous beings, that is, as spirits, demons and other transcendental powers.

The actual circumstances surrounding the medicines emerge from the prayers, which are spoken during the various rituals of medicine. They are – again in both cultural regions – directed entirely towards God and the ancestors. God and the ancestors are thanked for having created medicine, and they are entreated for their aid in the respective circumstances. Although the medicines are considered to be self-willed, quite mysterious and unpredictable beings, it is also general knowledge that they do not exercise their own power, but are ultimately directed by God and the ancestors.[35]

Therefore, contrary to other ethnological studies, in my work medicines are not understood as autonomous ghosts, demons or minor deities, who merit a cult of their own, nor as impersonal powers that magicians can use in destructive, secret and illegal ways. Instead, medicine is God's gift to mankind – their only means to send off all kind of hostile and dangerous forces. For the ancestors can only be begged to bestow blessings and protection, but not to punish wrongdoers and criminals. The following story of the uses and origin of medicine summarises my study. Only few Ejagham know it today:

At first God and man lived together in peace and mutual trust. One day this harmony was disrupted when a well-to-do man was attacked, his wives and animals killed, and his children bewitched by a less successful, greedy man. The victim appealed to help to God, who showed him herbs with which to protect himself. "I will give you these medicines, which will fight evil powers. From the leaves you can form medicines: *Mfam, Amok* and *Okeboho.*" The man then went into the bush, collected the herbs God had named, prepared the medicines and was able now to crush the witch and her companions. In addition, God taught man the art of divination, enabling him not only to discover witches before they could do any harm, but also to find truth and righteousness in all walks of life. After God had revealed these secrets to his people, he closed the door. God and man were separated and apart.

2.4 Divination

Widespread in traditional Africa, this complicated religious system functions only through the institution of a diviner (*mbuebu*, pl. *abuebu*). It is the diviner who mediates between the supernatural sphere and the living of this world by naming the reasons for suffering and misfortune and by advising how to rid oneself of them. If the calamities stem from God and the ancestors, the diviner can determine the cause of their displeasure and recommend the necessary ceremony of offerings in order to appease them. If, however, he sees witches or other sinister forces as the cause of misfortune, the only possibility that remains for the victim is to turn to the medicine societies (*ajom*) for help. For it is these societies who have the means to drive out dangerous powers. Diviners of the Ejagham can also aid in clearing up crimes, and they offer advice about planned trips and other undertakings. However, their real sphere of work is the confrontation with ancestors and witches.

When I was among the Ejagham for the first time in 1980, there were only a few diviners still present. Andreas Tanyi was the sole active diviner in Kembong (fig. 35); he died in the 1980s and, as far as I know, had no successor. When I arrived in Kembong in 2004, not a single diviner resided there. People with a 'problem normally went to Kofi Otang in the village of Njeke (fig. 36). I was able to make Kofi Otang's acquaintance at that time. He was over 90 years of age and passed away on April 17, 2004, during my research visit in Kembong. At present the last and sole diviner of the region is Agbor Cyprin Ashu in Ajayukndip; he is 39 years old (fig. 37).

I have to thank these three diviners or *abuebu* for information pertaining to the following descriptions. The artefacts that they once used or still use in their work were largely the same. Similarly, there were no great variances in their information about the theoretical background, that is, their dependency in their work upon the ancestors. Indeed, their information corresponded largely with the reports of Mansfeld and Talbot from the early 20th century.[36]

A person can become a diviner only if he is chosen by God and, thus, is endowed with a special faculty. Only those, the "people with four eyes", are able to interpret

Three diviners (*abuebu*) seated upon a traditional mat and hold their oracle artefacts (figs. 35–37).

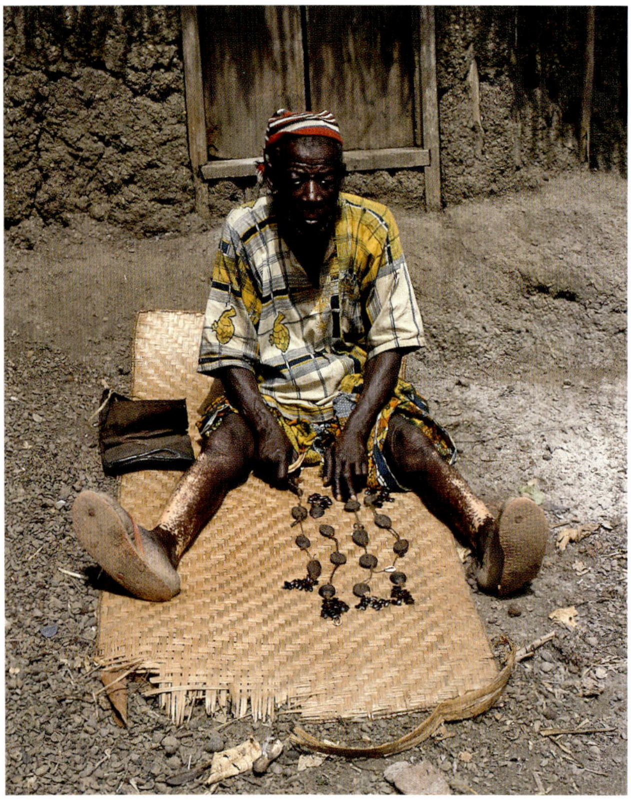

Fig. 35 Andreas Tanyi from Kembong (February 17, 1980).

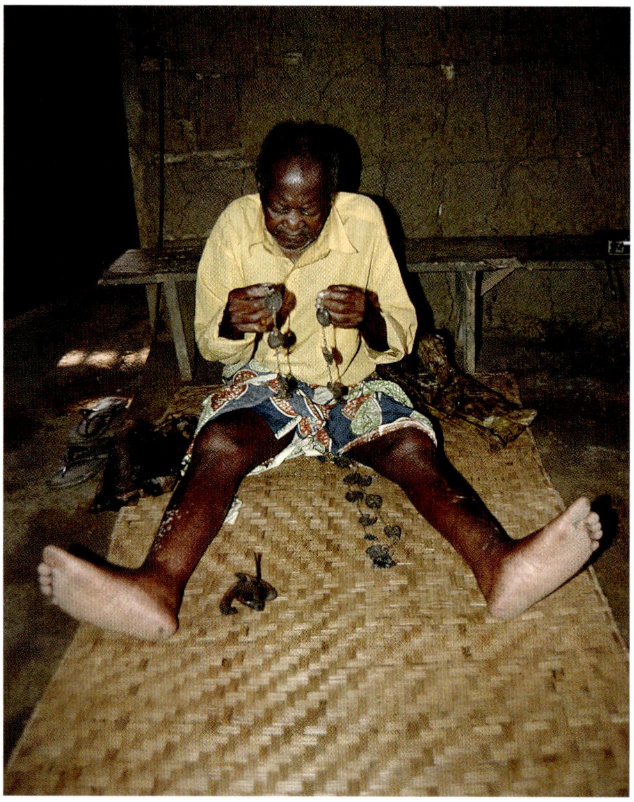

Fig. 36 Kofi Otang from Njeke (January 29, 2004).

the signs and tidings from God and the ancestors correctly and to recognise things in their context that are invisible to ordinary humans.[37] Diviners are not necessarily healers, although they often act as such. They do not have a special relationship with the ancestors; they encounter the ancestors in the same way as ordinary people – only in dreams. The faculty as a *mbuebu* must be inherited, and this means that the corresponding education is usually provided by the father. This was the case with the diviners whom I met. Besides, it is said that persons not related to the family are unable to pay the high costs of this education. In Agbor Cyprin Ashu's case, a ritual was conducted at the end of his schooling, in which his father rubbed his face with a medicine to equip him with additional strength. Sometimes parents are not agreed, when a son with the accordant abilities expresses the desire to become a diviner. In such cases these abilities or talents can be eliminated in a medicine ritual, during which the person's face is likewise rubbed with medicine. It should also be mentioned that among the Ejagham twins are not predestined to be diviners, as is the case in the Cameroon Grasslands.[38]

The typical oracle artefact (*ebu*, pl. *bebu*) of the Ejagham consists of four ropes (*areck ebu*, sg. *ndeck*

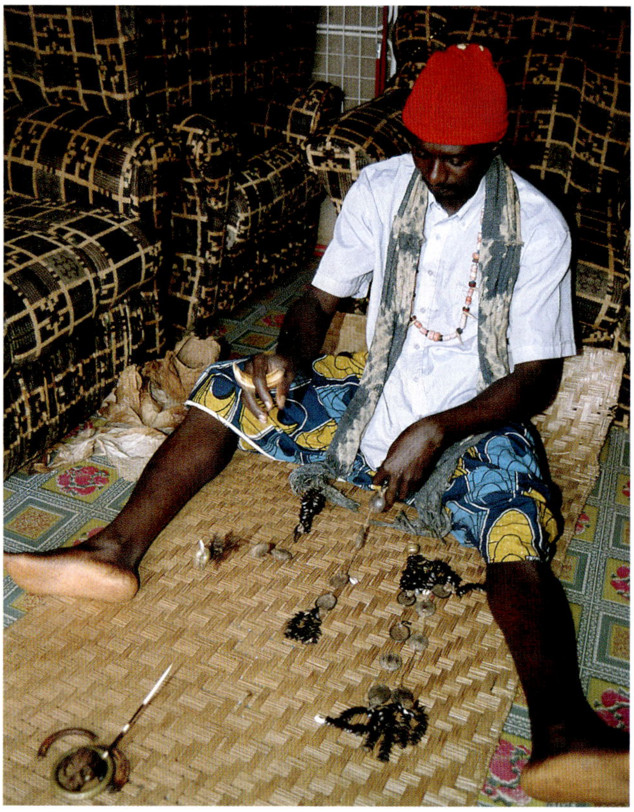

Fig. 37 Agbor Cyprin Ashu from Ajayukndip. In the foreground on the left are other artefacts for the oracle: the skull of a bush-baby, two teeth of a bush-pig, a brass arm ring and a porcupine quill (April 19, 2004).

ebu), to which four halves of the nut of a young mango fruit are fastened. In addition there are things such as cowrie shells, small brass bells, shells of fruit etc., which are supposed to further the search for truth. Still other things belong to the diviner's equipment, which lie in front of him when he sits on a mat with outstretched legs and inquires the *ebu*. In the case of Agbor Cyprin Ashu there was the skull of a bush-baby (*efi nyam*), which is a small animal of prey that holds its catch in its teeth and never lets it loose (fig. 37). The diviner was to proceed in an equally consistent and goal-oriented manner with his activities. Two teeth of a bush-pig, a brass arm ring and a porcupine quill served to ward off inimical influences. The diviner held another tooth of the bush-pig in his hand. With this tooth he could touch the mango kernels and awaken them – they were expected to say something.

At the consultation of the oracle two ropes, each are thrown upon the ground. Then the answer is seen in the position of the mango kernels: whether the upper or lower side faces upwards. However, there are substantial differences among diviners in the interpretation of the signs. Accordingly, the ropes held in Kofi Otang's left hand sent the message of his maternal ancestors; those in his right hand, of the paternal ancestors of the family. On the opposite, in Agbor Cyprin Ashu's case, the information for the ropes in his left hand came from those ancestors who had died at a very old age. The ropes in his right hand were the matter of ancestors who died at an early age. Evidently every diviner has his own system, about which he dislikes giving any information.

The oracle artefact is, nevertheless, not a dead or lifeless object, like dice in Europe whose result follows a principle of chance. Far more than that, *ebu* serves God and the ancestors as a mediator for their tidings to mankind, and correspondingly they exert an influence upon *ebu's* statements. In addition, an *ebu* must be treated with medicine regularly once a year, in order that it receive new powers to see and hear. This is perceptible in a prayer once spoken by Andreas Tanyi: "I want to empower you, as you have been dead. And now I awake you to see and to talk as a new person. Forget the old talks and from now see and talk as a new person."

Like the magic medicines (*ajom*), *bebu* also exhibit human-like traits. Their owners invoke them in prayer, each *ebu* with its own name. The *ebu* of Agbor Cyprin Ashu is named *aye nne amenge ejun* ("making a person know something"), that of Kofi Otang had the name of one of his ancestors, Achalle Moli. Nevertheless, it is clear that the existence and effectiveness of the *bebu* as well as the *ajom* stem from God and the ancestors. Yet, the *bebu* do not belong to *ajom*. An *ebu* serves the search for truth alone; its powers cannot be directed against human beings. If a diviner sees the approach of danger or misfortune, he will turn to the owner of a magic medicine (*njom*) with the request that it – in this case it was *Amok* – be activated. "*Amok,* anyone who wants to bring trouble into the village – if he succeeds bringing the trouble, go to war against him. But if he withdraws, as this *njom* is sworn, let him free."

Diviners have no taboos to observe in association with their work. That being said, they must not consult the oracle every day. Agbor Cyprin Ashu, for example, does not receive any clients on Sundays, for Sundays are the market day in Ajayukndip and there is much restless activity and noise, especially since people go to church. A *mbuebu* needs peace for his work, otherwise he cannot concentrate. Agbor Cyprin Ashu begins his work only after eight o'clock in the morning, when the clouds and the fog have cleared, and the "sight" is clear and wide. If there is a case of death in his locality, he does not give any advice until the body is buried. Otherwise the *ebu* would be concerned only with the deceased.

At work the diviner sits upon a mat of local make – "that was always so." In this way he is close to the ancestors, whose sphere is the earth. Accordingly, those seeking advice must take off their shoes, or else the diviner would not be able to see and speak well. In order to protect himself from invisible hostile powers, Agbor Cyprin Ashu wears a special red wool cap applied with a few cowry shells and a bead necklace. Before he consults *ebu*, he draws the aforementioned porcupine quill across his eyes, which is supposed to enhance foresight.

The *bebu* are activated in the same manner as *ajom*, that is, the diviners spit alligator pepper[39] upon them, sometimes even medicines, and assure themselves of the ancestors' support through prayers. Thus, Agbor Cyprin Ashu went about as follows: After spitting medicine upon the oracle ropes, he addressed his *ebu*: "*Aye nne amenge ejun*, this is your food. Wake up and see places." Then he poured some of the whisky that was always among the fees of the clients over it, saying, "This is your wine, wake up and start work." The ancestors received their whisky in front of the door to the house. "This is your wine. Take it and drink it and let the work go ahead."

Both of the other *abuebu* began their work in a similar manner. Andreas Tanyi first addressed his deceased father. "My father, if you did not teach me this profession, then when I perform this sorcery, let me not be successful. But if you taught me, let what I say be true." After this he turned to the *ebu* itself and spoke, "This question, which the man will bring. If you have the answer, tell me. But if you don't have the answer, be quiet, even if I ask you 15 or 20 times – be quiet." Kofi Otang also sought the support of God and the ancestors, after he had spit alligator pepper upon the oracle ropes. "*Ata Obasi* and the ancestors, I have now put down my equipment for divination. May you open my eyes to understand the signs well in order to save lives."

A diviner usually needs very little information from their clients; he receives it primarily from the *ebu*. The diviner does not question the *ebu* aloud, but confers with it in thought. The most frequent problems with which the diviner is confronted are illnesses, which can have the most diverse causes. It is expected of the *abuebu* that the diviner not only find the reason for illness, but also be able to advise clients how to overcome the malady. If the illness is associated with punishment from God and the ancestors, certain offerings must be made to appease them. If the illness was caused by a witch, she must be found with the aid of magic medicine (*njom*) and forced to leave her victim. If an illness is the result of an attack by magic medicine, the respective *njom* must be appeased in a special ritual. In all cases in which illness is traced back to an external power, the respective problem must be solved before the process of healing can begin.

Diviners offer only general advice for problems concerning daily life. In the case of thievery, for example, they can determine whether the thief comes from the family itself or from the neighbourhood, or whether he is a stranger. If someone is suspected of wrongdoing, diviners can determine whether or not the suspicion is justified. Many clients wish to know whether a planned undertaking will be successful. And there are numerous other questions pertaining to the future, to which the diviner is expected to find an answer, even preceding the birth of a child, whether it will be a boy or a girl.

The payment that Agbor Cyprin Ashu asked for in 2005 for his information was an average of 3,000 Francs CFA (about 5 Euro). The question as to the honesty of a diviner is seldom raised. No one would ever suspect lies or unfounded statements from a diviner. For in such a case, the diviner would be subject to the wrath of his ancestors, and there would also be the danger that the deceived clients could swear medicine against him.

Footnotes

1 Cp. Talbot 1912:13, 16 f., 66, 70; 1926:II: 66 f.; Nicklin 1983:66; Agbor 2001:12.
2 Onor 1994:106.
3 Talbot 1926:II:78 f. We can be thankful for his insight, which Evans-Pritchard also gained later during his research on the Nuer and which he summarised in his renowned theory of "the one and the many": "These spirits may be regarded as hypostases, representations, or refractions of God" (Evans-Pritchard 1977:93, 195, 200, 284, 319). The theory of "the one and the many" played a special role in the works of R. Horton about the Kalabari (1993:211 f.). Cp. corresponding references pertaining to the concepts of God (Koloss 2000:211 f.).
All life force ultimately derives from the creators *Ata Obasi* and *Mma Obasi*, upon which humans and other living beings are dependent. However, the Ejagham do not believe that this force is only bestowed if a person leads a moral and faithful life that is pleasing to God. By contrast, this particular belief exists among numerous other tribes and in Oku as well (cp. Koloss 2000:57, 445 ff.). There the magnitude of life force from God can even serve as a measure for the moral behaviour of an individual. In Oku life force is thus one of the central elements of religious world-view; for the Ejagham, by contrast, it does not carry this significance, in fact there is no specific term for "life force".
4 Talbot was among the first to mention the morning prayers of the Ejagham (1912:21 f.; 1926:II:68); cp. Agbor 2001:12.
5 There are tribes in the Grasslands, according to whose religious traditions the sphere of the ancestors is also in the earth. Yet this does not apply to all Grassland peoples. In Oku, for example, the ancestors "are present everywhere and are always near to mankind" (Koloss 2000: 400).
6 Cp. Koloss 2000:58, 446 f.
7 Talbot already made reference to this (1926:II:301).
8 This kind of ceremony of offering is already described by Mansfeld (1908:240 f.) and Talbot (1912:21 f., 39 f., 53 f., 66 f.; cp. Ruel 1969:314 f. and Röschenthaler 1993:236).
9 Mansfeld mentions this oracle as well (1908:176).
10 Koloss 2000:98.
11 Cp. Talbot's mention of this oracle (1912:53 f., 66 f.); cp. also Röschenthaler (1993:236).
12 Agbor 2001:13.
13 Koloss 2000:401.
14 In the Cameroon Grasslands each participant uses his own cup for drinking palm wine at official meetings, ceremonies etc. But in general, drinking and eating together are seen as especially characteristic of close friendship and harmony, and, hence, this is only allowed among friends, never enemies (cp. Koloss 2000:58, 452). Likewise Balz (1984:340) notes that among the Bakossi, "...eating and drinking together strengthens the community ties." Similar to the Ejagham, the Bakossi are a people who in former times were characterised by an egalitarian social structure. They inhabit the area north of Kumba, about 90 km southeast of Kembong.
15 Being in trance does not play an insignificant role in the Cameroon Grasslands (Koloss 2000:57).
16 Talbot 1912:94 ff.; 1926:II:130 ff.; Anonymous 1957:166; Hackett 1989:28 ff.; Röschenthaler 1993:64 ff; Onor 1994:23 f.
17 Latham 1973:35.
18 Ittmann 1957; Salmons 1977.
19 Ittmann 1957:143, 151; cp. Salmons 1977:11 and Röschenthaler 1993:70 f.

20 Ittmann 1957:136; Salmons 1977:14.
21 Koloss 2000:59.
22 The Banyang use *ndem* (pl. *arem*) to designate the "dead" or "spirit of the dead", "corpse" but also "foetus" (Ruel 1969:63, 203).
23 A similar view concerning the special relationship of children to the afterlife is found among the Kalabari: "Things existing in *teme* (i.e. in the spiritual and immaterial order of existence, H.-J. K.) only can be seen by ordinary people when they are very young, but after the first few years of life the accumulated pollution of the material world spoils their senses and they are no longer clairvoyant. To regain this lost faculty, one must submit to a special herbal treatment known as 'clearing the eyes and ears'." (Horton 1960:15).
24 Cp. Talbot's mention of such stones (1912:96): "All stones rounded by water action into oval form are sacred to Nimm." Cp. Ruel 1969:63.
25 For convenience' sake, in the following witches will be referred to in the feminine form, although men also participate in activities of witchcraft. Talbot (1912:190 ff.) already provided extensive descriptions of witchcraft. Cp. Jones 1956:151 ff.; Ruel 1965; 1969:170, 205, 210 f.; Nicklin 1983:66.
26 Röschenthaler 1993:195.
27 Talbot 1912:192, 230, 232; Ittmann 1957:143, 155; Balz 1984: 322, 364; Koloss 2000:311.
28 References to autopsies are provided by Talbot 1912:193; Staschewski 1917:47; Ruel 1965:11, 15, 18; Ardener 1970:145. Post-mortem examinations were not common in the Cameroon Grasslands (Koloss 2000:324).
29 Thompson 1974:215.
30 This kind of ritual is described by Talbot (1912:193 f.).
31 There is an extensive report about the cremation of a corpse (among the Ejagham of the Ikom Division in Nigeria), after the deceased had been identified as a witch (Onor 1994:109).
32 Koloss 2000:325.
33 Here I also refer to magic figures called *minkisi* or *zinkondi* of the Bakongo, as well as other peoples in the Kongo region (Teke, Yaka, Suku, Songye, Luba and Tabwa). These objects are also made effective through medicines (*bilongo*) and activated against hostile forces (Thompson 1983:101–159; MacGaffey 1986; 1991).
34 Koloss 2000:97; Mansfeld, in: Tunis 1985:502; Talbot 1912: 49 ff.; Talbot 1926:II:79.
35 This pertains to the Cameroon Grasslands as well (Koloss 2000: 57, 98 f., 101, 403, 452 f.).
36 Mansfeld 1908:176 f.; Talbot 1912:174 ff.
37 Likewise in the Grasslands the signs are sent by the ancestors, and in the same way it is the task of the diviner to "read" and interpret these signs correctly. But their divining artefacts are far more diverse than those of their counterparts in the Cross River region (Koloss 2000:311 ff.).
38 Koloss 2000:312.
39 Alligator pepper is essential in many rituals of medicine in the forest area. A first mention of it was made by Hutchinson (1858:170), and a short description is found in Talbot (1932:99): "seeds from the cherry-coloured fruit of the wild ginger (*Aframomum grana paradisi*)".

3 Society and leadership

3.1 Principles and institutions of an egalitarian society

Delegating political power and material concessions to one single person, as practised above all in the kingdoms of neighbouring Cameroon Grasslands with their splendid courtly culture and grand royal palaces, was unthinkable among the Central Ejagham. Although they have always been sceptical of all hierarchical tendencies, social differences as well as positions of leadership do indeed exist in their acephalous and expressly egalitarian social system. Qualities of leadership are attributed in particular to elderly persons (*bakwuianne,* sg. *nnenkwuinne),* who in view of their experiences in life are considered enlightened, rational and wise, despite their diminished physical strength. Like many other African peoples, the Ejagham have numerous aphorisms that express this view, such as: "Age is wisdom.", "What an old man sees when sitting down, a young man can never see, even when climbing up a tree or a mountain.", "The death of an old man is like a library that has been destroyed.", "The words of elders are the words of wisdom.", "Only old people are suitable leaders; it is their task to show their wisdom." Elderly men and women are considered to be especially blessed by God, and it is a known fact that they are close to the ancestors. Thus, they are accorded great authority and esteem. To treat elderly persons disrespectfully or to insult them is seen as very dangerous, for their maledictions and curses are feared. On the other hand, as Agbor emphasises, their words can be very beneficial: "The Keaka people believe that there is a mystical power in words, especially those of parents spoken to their children. The words of parents for example carry 'power' when they are spoken to children, they cause good fortune, success, peace, sorrow or blessing especially when spoken in moments of crisis."[1]

Age is, therefore, the decisive criterion when choosing the successor to a deceased leader, whether in a family, a quarter or a locality. This applies to the sphere of secret societies as well, but with some limitations. There age is a necessary criterion, yet not a mandatory factor for attaining a higher position. Whereas acceptance into a higher rank signifies an influential position, it entails the payment of substantial fees for the person involved. Thus, only wealthy persons are able to meet these costs. At the beginning of the 20th century a person was considered prosperous who owned twelve wives and twelve slaves, as Mansfeld reported in 1908: "Today some chiefs have more, but there are none who own fifty to one hundred slaves and fifty to one hundred wives, like fifty years ago."[2]

Wealth and prosperity were always associated with the renowned *agbokarem,* those women who had undergone long years of initiation rites and who formed an elite society. Today they no longer exist (cp. p. 196 ff.). Only well-to-do families were able to pay the high cost of this initiation. Further, the man who wished to take a *mgbokandem* as wife also had to be wealthy, for the bride price was more than double that for an ordinary woman.

A further important factor for attaining a higher social position is a person's background. Aside from the fact that formerly Central Ejagham women – as almost everywhere in old Africa – were nearly completely excluded from any processes of political decisions, slaves as well had hardly any opportunity for social development. Even members of old established families did not possess the same or equal rights. Thus, today the leading positions among *Mgbe,* by far the most powerful society of the Ejagham, are still reserved for those families who once – as will be discussed in detail below – contributed towards acquiring *Mgbe.*

Even today the funeral ceremony is still seen as a sign of prosperity and reputation. It is a matter of course that the ceremony for a big man must be held in a fitting manner – which means within an elaborate setting. The highest honour for a deceased Ejagham man is the night dance, which is held for elderly and highly esteemed men alone. This dance takes place only rarely, for it entails considerable financial costs. In earlier times a slave was sacrificed on this occasion. Special honours were likewise shown at funeral ceremonies for deceased *agbokarem* in former times. An almost life-sized commemorative figure made of cement (in former times of clay) was erected after their death (cp. p. 200 ff.). This occurred last in 1998.

Men, who have reached a certain age and are provided with wealth, influence and esteem, are usually referred to as big men in English, in the Ejagham language as *arum anne* (sg. *ndum nne*; *ndum* meaning great, noble, important, and *nne* means human, i.e. man). A special title is *Ata*, which always precedes the name of the particular person, a title addressed to honourable men, who are about 70 or older, and to God: *Ata Obasi*.

3.2 The heads of families

The head of a family (*echi ndebenju*, pl. *achi arebeoju*) is the oldest male, which implies that his time in this position is usually not all too long. There is no special ceremony when his successor takes over. The big men do not wear any special insignia. Their social standing is attested principally through the insignia of authority, to which they are entitled as high-ranking members of the secret society *Mgbe*. They may not claim for any special rights or privileges. Like all elderly men, they only have prerogatives in eating and drinking during festive meals, and they may – without question – rely upon respectful manners on the part of boys and younger men, even though this behaviour is not as devout as that in the Grasslands. In this sense Onor once characterised the Ejagham as a whole as follows: "Every family had a head whose choice was informed largely by the principle of seniority. By virtue of his age, he was highly revered by all other members of the family who looked up to him for guidance and protection. He was adjudged a sage who was profoundly knowledgeable in the affairs of society and a potent conduit through which the wishes and directives of the ancestors of the family were communicated to its living members."[3]

The position of the big men of the Ejagham can perhaps best be characterised by comparison with the big men of the Grasslands.[4] The kings and heads of families of that region are distinguished by a number of rights, privileges and insignia. Should one of them die, the most important condition in the selection of his successor is, aside from membership in the "right" family, the ability to lead a large number of people. Upon his installation both a new king as well as a new head of a family must observe a time of seclusion, during which he is familiarised with his future duties and also repeatedly treated with medicines. This time is seen as a period of transformation, that is, the change of an ordinary human being into a king or family head who is furnished with special powers. Only thereafter may a big festival take place, which is intended, on the one hand, to commemorate the predecessor, and, on the other, to introduce the new dignitary to the public. Such festivities last about one week and usually include the entire tribe. The special powers of the dignitary render him "dangerous" for other persons, and therefore they must avoid any physical contact with him. Indeed, the distance that the new dignitary must maintain from his "subjects" is a particular characteristic of his position. This is accompanied by the especially submissive manner maintained towards him by everyone. And this special conduct between heads of families and ordinary men and women corresponds with the explicit will of the ancestors and stands under their guardianship.[5]

Among the Ejagham the head of a family is the eldest man in a family. If this person is not capable of fulfilling this office, he is supported by advisors. His duty is to watch over the family, to cast off dislikes and animosities and to secure or reinstate peace in the family in every imaginable way. The head of the family is responsible for conducting offerings to the ancestors, and it is he as well who resides over meetings of the family members during which all important decisions are made. All major matters are settled in his compound. Moreover, his position is decisively determined by the role which he plays in the *Etek* of the quarter or the village as the representative of his family. His influence is all the greater if he is also a big man in one of the secret societies, in particular of *Mgbe*.

Yet, in spite of all the esteem that a family head receives, his position is not as exalted as that in the Grasslands. When he assumes his office, there is no special installation or ceremony with the aim of creating or transforming him into a "new" person. The qualification for this position usually is founded upon his age alone. The procedure of choosing someone is therefore superfluous, and with that also any incentive for power struggles, which occur often enough in the Grasslands following the death of a king or notable.

In most cases it is a man who assumes the office of head of the family, yet in principle women of corresponding age also have the right to hold it. Throughout time there have always been cases in which no male was present who was suited to be family head, and so a woman had to assume this position. Just as with a male family head, one of her duties was to conduct offerings to the ancestors, a duty which people in the Grasslands would hardly believe possible.[6]

3.3 *Etek*, the assembly of the community

The politically highest forum in a quarter as well as in a village of the Ejagham, in which all important decisions are taken, is the *Etek* (pl. *Ntek*), the council of the people. The term *Etek* designates the assembly or con-

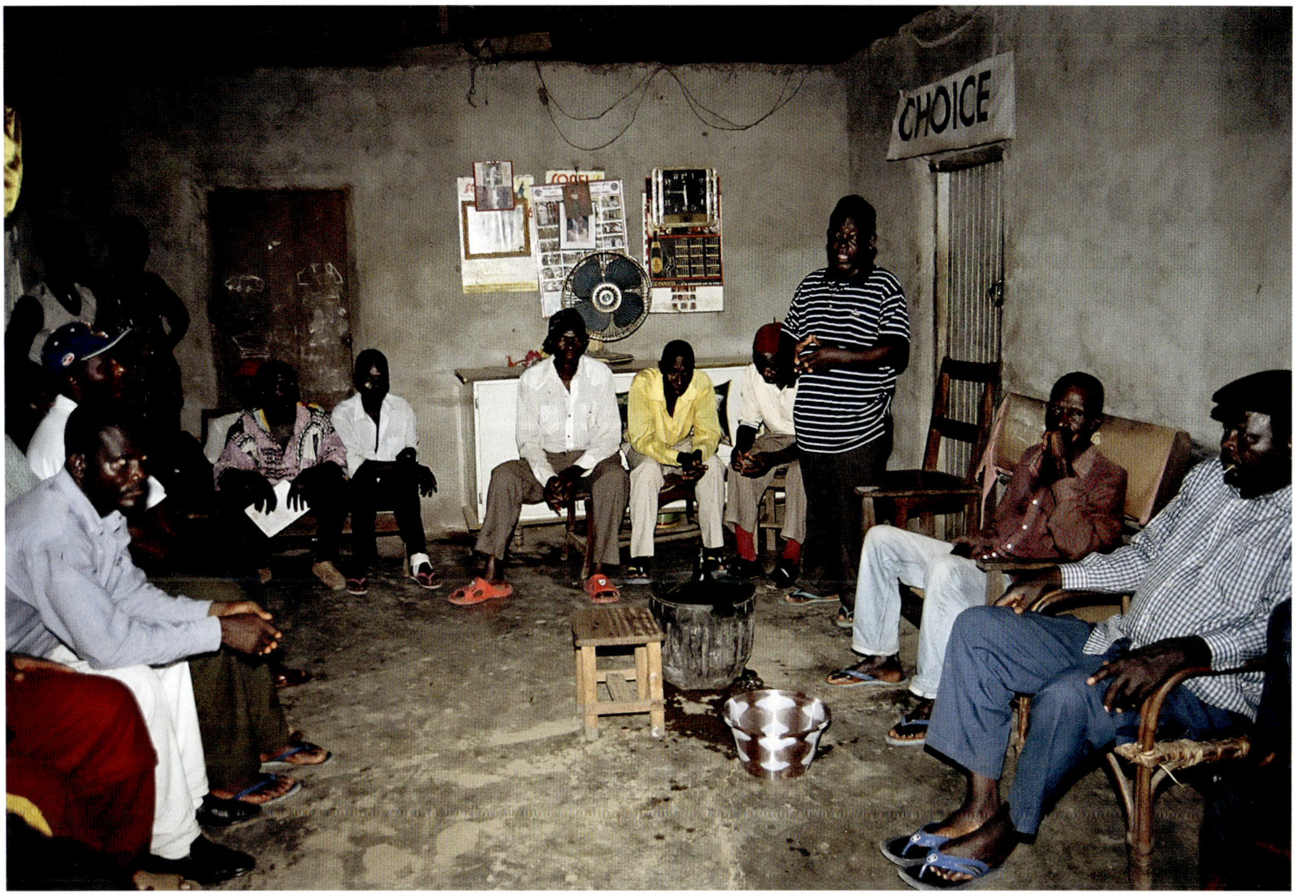

Fig. 38 Meeting of the *Etek* from Nserong quarter. In the centre the jug of palm wine (Kembong, April 2, 2005).

vocation of a community, but also of a settlement, as for instance a quarter, a village, a town or even a province or a country. Cameroon is thus an *Etek*, and *etek akeku* is "the land of the dead people". The concept of *Etek*, of such profound importance for the Cross River region, became generally known through the research of Malcom Ruel among the Banyang at the beginning of the 1960s. His book "Leopard and Leaders" is mainly concerned with the "central concept of Banyang political theory", and consequently – as the author himself noted – could just as well have been entitled "The Notion of *Etek*". As far as I can discern, this concept corresponds to a great extent with the political traditions of the Central Ejagham, especially since both groups have many cultural elements in common.[7]

Among the Central Ejagham – and with them the Banyang – all men have the right to take part in the *Etek*. Only slaves were formerly excluded. Women are also allowed to participate if the problems concerning them are the topic of discourse. However, the *Etek* is not a loosely structured assembly, during which simply recent news or events are exchanged and problems are discussed more or less without any obligatory outcome. *Etek* is far more an official convocation, which is called by the chief of the respective locality, and it follows firm as well as binding regulations. If especially serious decisions are to be taken, it is customary that palm wine is drunk and that the ancestors receive their portion in the form of libations. For it is particularly the inclusion of the ancestors in the assembly that clearly constitutes its official character.

As before a European court of justice, correct behaviour is expected of those participating in an *Etek*. In general, the participants speak only when they are given the word by the head of the assembly, and they must choose their words carefully. Falsehoods and insults are penalised as strictly as any improper actions. Although all persons have the opportunity to present their arguments, it is none too seldom that the elderly, as deciding members of the *Etek*, attempt to guide discussions in the direction of their own particular interests. Yet, often the deliberations end with surprising and unforeseen results. Especially younger people present their arguments in controversial discourse in an aggressive and unyielding manner. Problems are not solved simply through a majority vote; instead efforts are made in all decisions to reach an agreement that is acceptable to all. Therefore, the leader of an *Etek*, usually the head of a quarter or village, must follow the discussion closely and end it with a summarising statement. This conclusion, often in the form of a judgement, is final and binding for everyone. Revisions are difficult –"what has been decided is decided" (fig. 38).

3.4 Chief or head of a village community

Surprisingly there is very little information in ethnological literature about the chiefs or heads of Ejagham communities. As one of the first to research this area, Talbot remarked: "Practically the whole of the country east of the Niger was, until recent times, covered with dense forest, and the population composed of peoples living in independent, unconsolidated and usually small groups, subject to no central government."[8] In the mostly small communities, which were and still are quite characteristic of the Ejagham, there were indeed leading personalities who were viewed as chiefs, yet their powers were rather limited. This position as chief does not imply any "sacred" elements. Just like the heads of families, the chiefs did not have to undergo a "transformation".[9] Their office was not inheritable; it was not the possession of a privileged family.[10]

This acephalous political system was widespread, yet it was not the only form of government among Ejagham groups. Indeed, well into colonial times and foremost in the Nigerian regions of Ikom and Ogoja there was a chief or king with divine attributes, the *ntufam emong*. Onor associates this institution with the Ejagham kingdom, which – according to Onor – came to an end during the 15th century. Completely accordant with the concept of an African sacred king, the *ntufam emong* had to originate from a royal family. His enthronement was exceptionally elaborate and lasted for a long period of time, especially as it was connected with diverse rituals, including in former times human sacrifices. The *ntufam emong* had many insignia of supremacy and the right to special privileges, but he was also bound by a number of taboos: "He was neither to be seen eating nor was his source of drinking water supposed to be known. The top of his head was to be perpetually concealed from the view of other people except perhaps his wives. Finally, he was obliged to render himself somewhat incommunicado in consonance with the awe which accrued to his exalted office. All these taboos, were inter alia, created to mystify the essence of *ntufam emong* and strengthen his authority and power." In the course of the colonial period until the beginning of the 20th century, this system of power was gradually disposed of, "because colonial administrators saw most of its core observances and rituals as antithetical to the ideals and objectives of 'good government'."[11]

In pre-colonial times the chief of a community or hamlet among the Central Ejagham was usually the oldest living male, on condition that he had a good character and was equal to that office.[12] If a chief became guilty of some offends or grew senile he could – in sharp contrast to the Grasslands, where it was hardly possible to depose kings or notables – be replaced by another man. There were several designations for a chief: *ntui mfam Etek, nne echi* (pl. *anne bechi*) (head of people), *nekhi nne* (pl. *bakhi andeh*) (old person) and *etakoko nne* (pl. *betakok andeh*) (old person). It was his obligation to care for the well-being of the community in the fullest sense. In addition to leading the *Etek*, it was his duty to skin leopards with a special knife whenever a leopard was killed; for among many African peoples the leopard is the most important symbol of authority.[13] It was likewise the chief who buried the animal's gall bladder, which was considered extremely poisonous, in a latrine. The same was performed with the gall bladder of a slain python.[14] A large slit-drum was located in the chief's compound, with which deaths and other events were announced. Yet, the chief had no any other rights or duties that surpassed those of the heads of families in the community.

When in former times the leader of a hamlet died and the funeral ceremonies were completed, an assembly – *Etek* – was held in the compound of the successor. This person had to provide food and drink, and afterwards his representative greeted those assembled: "Mr. X. died some days ago and since then we have remained without a *ntui mfam*. Today Mr. Y has invited us to his place. We have come here to make him carry out the functions of late Mr. X. Has anybody to say anything against this proposal? He is the right man." If there was no word of opposition, the drinking continued. The *ntui mfam* received the last glass. Taking it into his left hand, he spoke: "Our fathers, you are dead and have gone. You have left us behind. We are all children, but wherever are children, there must be an older child. Today I have been called to take over the place of late Mr. X. I have not refused. So help me, when I do not know what to do. Also help my people to co-operate with me. Let none of our members suffer from headache and pain." Then he took the glass with his right hand and said: "We have drunk, and now we throw the dregs on the ground for the ancestors." With that the new chief was installed in office. Neither this installation nor that of the new head of a family was followed by a big feast and connected with a "transformation", in contrast to the Grasslands where a celebration is still obligatory on such an occasion. There is, however, another important difference between the kingdoms of the Grasslands and the acephalous societies in the forest area, which will be described in the following.

Today the belief still prevails among the Ejagham that all the deceased persons of a community are ancestors, with the exception of witches and those who led an immoral life, a belief that stands in contrast to traditions in the Cameroon Grasslands. There the ancestors of the village chief alone are considered to be the ancestors of the entire community; likewise, ancestors of the tribe are solely the royal ancestors. Oppositely, among the Ejagham it is not possible for one single family to found a dynasty, and that is one important factor in understanding their acephalous and egalitarian political system. According to the principle of seniority, all families basically have the opportunity that one of their members can act as the village leader.[15]

A political system such as this, in which every member of society can participate directly and with the same rights and obligations in all political decisions, could be designated as "direct democracy", even if it implies the exclusion of women and formerly also slaves. It is quite obvious that this system can only be practiced among small communities; in the larger ones in the Cameroon Grasslands it is absent. There is a representative political system in the Grasslands, in which it is foremost the heads of extended families who make all important decisions (cp. p. 220). The small communities in the forest areas, which had neither chiefs nor kings, were seen by the German colonial masters as being particularly backward and primitive; compare: "The individual villages lie scattered throughout the rain forest like islands in the earth's oceans" and, further, have "completely irregular [social] conditions".[16] Thus, the colonial authorities were convinced that a "remedy" was necessary to improve the situation, and Talbot already reported that the traditional social structure "has been replaced or superseded by new systems introduced since the establishment of British rule."[17] However, it was these changes that were to put the idea and spirit of egalitarian social order totally in question.

The German as well as later the British colonial masters had decided upon an administrative system that designated a mediator for communication with the indigenous population. This person was responsible for all matters in the respective society and had additional duties involving taxation and the selection of workers, who were constantly needed by the colonial administration. This position also gave him the opportunity to exert influence. It was a self-evident and logical step that the traditional chiefs should be chosen for this office, as far as they were accommodating and cooperative; otherwise they were replaced by more "suitable" persons. In the case of tribes, such as the Central Ejagham, which were not accustomed to chiefs or only to those without any special political power, this office was arbitrarily created by colonial officials, which was fundamentally contrary to the political traditions of the people. The intent of the German colonial officials was as follows: "In areas of the rain forest efforts of the government must be to bring order into the thus far completely irregular conditions, so that in larger areas paramount chiefs are appointed, who are supported by the government and who hold a certain local administrative power."[18]

Whereas this measure can be understood as the nullification of a political system, in which the absolute equality of all citizens was the highest of ideals, it was even worse that the Europeans demanded absolute obedience and unlimited commitment in their – the Europeans' – interests from the respective indigenous occupants of this office. Correspondingly, in German times the particular official was furnished with special symbols of authority, such as "official papers, a booklet or a chief's book, a cane, hats, flags and uniforms".[19] Any confirmation of this position of power through the ancestors was, however, impossible. Besides, there is no tradition of a "transformation" among the Central Ejagham.

From its very beginnings, the position of the *ntui mfam okarara*, that is, the "white man's chief", was considered by the colonial masters to be that of a compliant, uncritical straw man and stooge, and he was often seen as such by his own people, as a traitor who had lost his "respect and authority".[20] Many times no one was willing to assume this dubious office, and one of the slaves was forced by *Etek* to present himself as a candidate for the position. With a decision such as this, most serious social problems were implanted, for – as can easily be imagined – the members of the community were not prepared to accept orders from a slave, regardless whether he was officially authorised to give them.[21]

The *ntui mfam okarara* generally had nothing to do with conducting traditional cult rituals. They were normally carried out by the *ntui mfam*, who was the rightfully chosen chief. Additional problems frequently arose when the "new" chief attempted to transfer his office within his own family and so to form a dynasty, an act which formerly was impossible. Once created by colonial powers to bring order to the "irregular conditions among indigenous peoples", the institution of *ntui mfam okarara* ultimately led to a persisting disruption of peace in many communities. Thus, Agbor notes: "Hardly can one find a single village in Central Ejagham where there is no chieftaincy dispute."[22] This corresponds with his opinion of newly appointed chiefs: "The indigenes lost confidence in the chiefs and until today the Keaka Chief is an ally of the government who most of the time acts to have favour from the government rather than protect the people. Most of the Chiefs have become involved in politics today, a legacy left behind by the Germans since they involved the Chiefs in administering the area and collecting taxes as well as recruiting labourers. When the British came, the system continued and it even deteriorated with the independence of the territory."[23]

As stated above, the introduction of the *ntui mfam okarara*, an office from which the chiefs who were installed by the Cameroon government later emerged, has led to considerable problems in the Ngunaya area. Yet nowhere in the Ngunaya area have such dramatic reverberations occurred as in Kembong, which will be subsequently described.

The following list of "Chiefs of Kembong" – the official title – derives from the calendar issued by the Kembong Traditional Council, which was dedicated as follows: "The Installation Coronation of Mr. Alfred Ayuk Ako as Chief of Kembong on the 20th September 1997" (with the addition: "The People's Choice").

1. Ata Nchemti, Nyenya
2. Ata Nfontem, Nserung
3. Ata Ebandip, Nserung
4. Ata Akem, Okem-eh-Benem
5. Ata Tanyi Enow, Ebarensi
6. Ata Awo Minta, Ebarensi
7. Ata Achere Nchung Etta, Okune
8. Ata Oben Anyang, Ayukaba
9. Ata Mbenchang Ayukabang, Okem-eh-Benem
10. Ata Ndip Ebob, Okonyenge
11. Ata Nku Ayo Fang, Okonyenge
12. Ata Tambe Ndip Arrah, Okonyenge
13. Ata Tabe Nyang, Ndengane
14. Ata Acho Okogobe, Ndekwai
15. Ata Arrey Eneke, Okonyenge
16. Ata Tabot Njab, Okonyenge
17. Ata Obenson Bekecheng, Ayukaba
18. Ata Denisenow Tabot, Okonyenge
19. Ata Alfred Ayuk Ako, Ayukaba

The list may impart the impression of an official document, but according to statements from all of my informants neither the names of the former chiefs of Kembong listed nor the sequence of their names are reliable.[24] For example, Kembong did not even exist at the time of Nchemti and Mfontem, who are named here as the first chiefs. Details about the period of office of individual chiefs are not included, just as information is lacking as to who appointed the chiefs, according to what criteria, and whether their selection and installation ran without any problems. By contrast, the conflicts that occurred with the installation of the present Chief of Kembong are still in lively memory. The controversies escalated into an extreme detriment to social accord, whose influence on life in Kembong persisted for 25 years.

Following Denisenow Tabot, the last person in office who died in November or December 1971, two candidates applied as his successor: Alfred Ayuk Ako from Ayukaba and B.T. from Okonyenge. The election of February 25, 1972, resulted in fourteen votes for Alfred Ayuk Ako and only two votes for his opponent. Born in 1920, Alfred Ayuk Ako was installed in the office of "Chief of Kembong" by his community in a traditional ceremony on October 21, 1972. However, he could not exercise this position, officially designated "Second Class Chieftaincy" by the Cameroon government and equipped with the corresponding appanage, until this was formally confirmed by the government in Yaoundé. This meant that for the defeated candidate and his supporters, who were mostly from Okonyenge, the vying for the highest office in Kembong was not yet over. In the meantime the once defeated party presented A.E.B., also from Okonyenge, a new candidate, who even gave up an influential position in the Cameroon Development Cooperation in Limbe, in order to pursue his political goals in Kembong more intensively.

In the course of time A.E.B. succeeded in securing the support of the Senior District Officer (S.D.O.) of the Manyu Division, which today is still regarded as illegal actions or corruption by his opponents in Kembong.[25] It is a fact that in 1978 the S.D.O. sent a letter to the government in Cameroon containing the statement that Alfred Ayuk Ako could not be the rightful Chief of Kembong. Further the S.D.O. was convinced that this was instead A.E.B., who was from the "royal family of Okonyenge", which had always ruled in Kembong, and it was therefore necessary that A.E.B. be installed as the Chief. During my stay in Kembong at the beginning of 1980, the atmosphere among the population was accordingly depressed, even explosive.

Most of the inhabitants with whom I communicated were disappointed in the Cameroon government and felt that they had been treated with great injustice.

The answer from the government came as late as December 1983 and accorded with the suggestion submitted by the S.D.O. in 1978 (I only learned about the events to be described in the following upon my return to Kembong many years later in 2004). When the S.D.O. then installed A.E.B. as Chief of Kembong in April 1984, an uprising broke out, in the course of which many people were wounded and one person was even killed. The turbulence was only brought to an end through the intervention of a large number of gendarmes. In the time thereafter there were tedious hearings and discussions, in which the opponents of A.E.B. – which means the greater part of Kembong's populace – succeeded in proving that neither in Kembong nor in any of the other 27 villages in the Ngunaya area had a royal dynasty or a royal family ever existed. Indeed the position of *ntui mfam* had never been bound to one single family. The eldest male in a community was always chosen as successor to a deceased *ntui mfam*, unless something spoke against him, implying that he did not originate from the family of the deceased. In the course of these discussions A.E.B. was ultimately dismissed from the position as Chief of Kembong in 1985. For many years thereafter the administration of Kembong was under the charge of a caretaker council with the District Officer from Eyumojock as chairman.

After further lengthy negotiations between representatives of Kembong and the new S.D.O. (the final and decisive meeting took place on September 26, 1996), an order from the Prime Minister of Cameroon finally reached Alfred Ayuk Ako on January 21, 1997, announcing: "You have been accepted by your people and the Government, so sit down and start your functions." The official confirmation of the "Enthronement of Mr. A. A. Ako as Chief of Kembong" followed through the order of the Vice Prime Minister on April 21, 1997, and the festive Installation Coronation on September 20, 1997. All of this occurred 25 years after Alfred Ayuk Ako's election by the overwhelming majority of Kembong's population and, thus, in full accordance with the democratic traditions of the Ejagham.

Almost one decade has now passed since Alfred Ayuk Ako entered office, and his actions have been deemed as positive by the majority of the community (figs. 39, 40). It is his duty to represent Kembong at the S.D.O. in Mamfe and at the District Officer in Eyumojock and to carry out the most varied administrative tasks. He may not take the decisions which fall upon him alone on his own authority, but must work hand-in-hand with the Traditional Council, as whose chairman he serves. Members of this committee, which usually meets in his house, are the representatives of the seventeen quarters, that is to say, the respective "quarter-head", a representative each for young people and for women and an elder (fig. 41). The elders are considered to be "notables", and their duty is to act as advisors to the Chief. Furthermore, they alone may choose the successor to a deceased Chief. However, the representative of Obiola had no right to vote in the last election. Established by former slaves, the quarter of Obiola still has no equal rights in this case. Decisions made in the Traditional Council are – and this is quite typical of bygone Old Africa – not passed by the assent of the majority, but through concession. If a problem seems to have been discussed sufficiently, the Chief picks out about five members, who then leave the meeting to work out a detailed solution for proposal. If the proposed solution is accepted by the rest of the members, it is valid.

Hence, the Chief of Kembong is a representative of the government; he is installed by the government and furnished with financial means. At the same time, though, he assumes the functions of the traditional *ntui mfam* and, accordingly, is elected by the people and installed in the traditional manner, he does not have to undergo a "transformation"'. He is likewise the head of all lodges of *Mgbe*, the most powerful of all secret societies, and must take action when a leopard is killed. He must conduct offerings to the ancestors (*ajom Etek*), although there are hardly any corresponding ceremonies for the whole Kembong. The Chief does not have any special insignia or symbols of authority; he simply possesses those which he as a big man in *Mgbe* is accorded.

No special ceremonies are held at the death of the Chief of Kembong, except in honour of him as a big man of *Mgbe*. Only men who originate from "authentic" families of Kembong, in no case descendants of slaves, may be chosen as successor to the Chief. The installation of the new Chief was conducted without any exceptional rituals, in any case in 1972. The oldest of the "kingmakers" raised the new Chief's right hand and set a cap of *Mgbe* upon his head. Then prayers of the Christian dignitaries as well as an offering to the ancestors were carried out by the eldest "kingmaker". During the following night the dance of *Mawu*, the society of women, took place.

Through the new institution "Chief of Kembong" (Kembong itself was established as late as the colonial

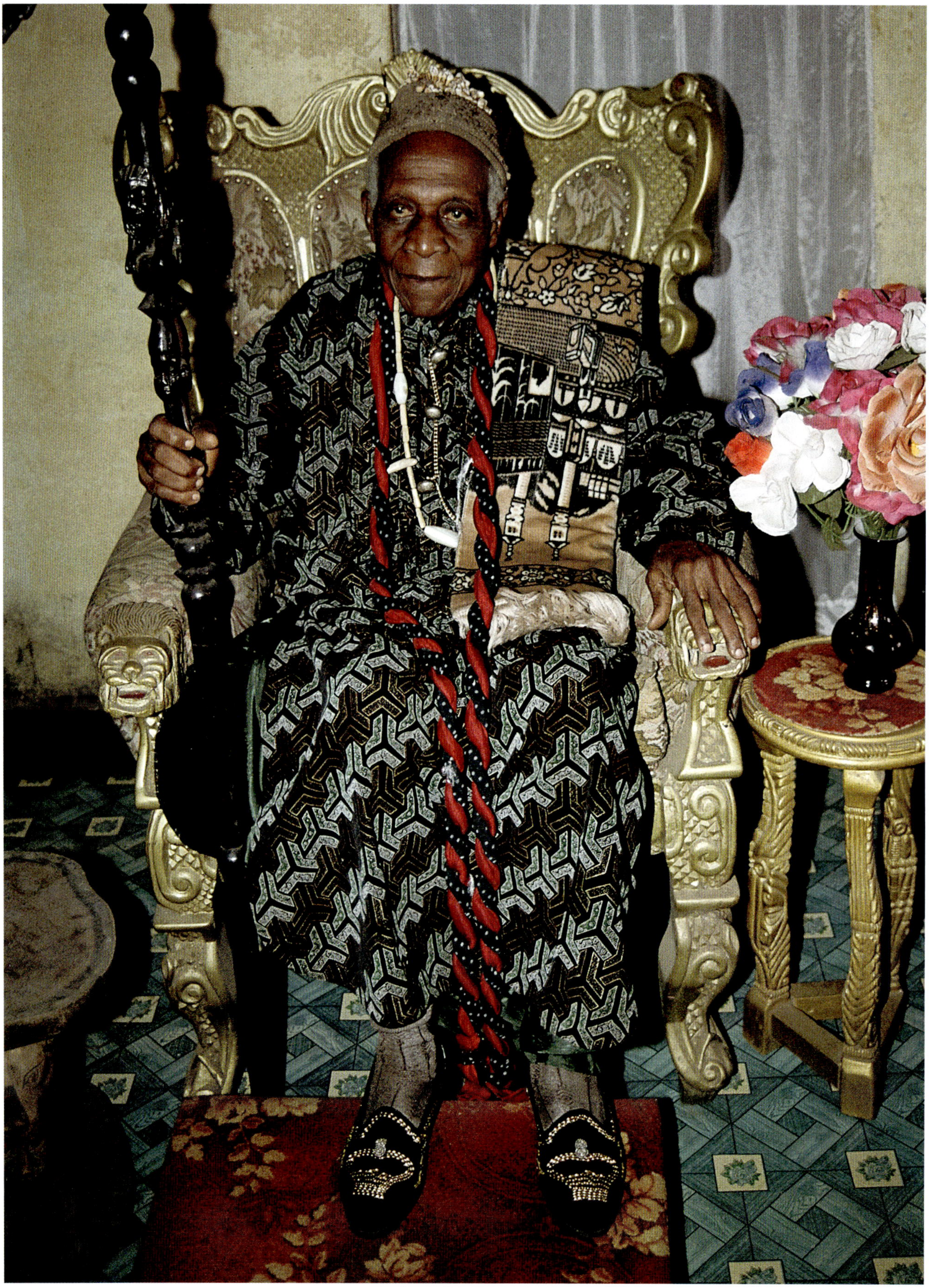

Fig. 39 Alfred Ayuk Ako, Chief of Kembong, seated upon his "throne". In his right hand, the ceremonial staff; over his left shoulder, the towel as sign of a *seseku*, leader of *Mgbe* (Kembong, January 22, 2004).

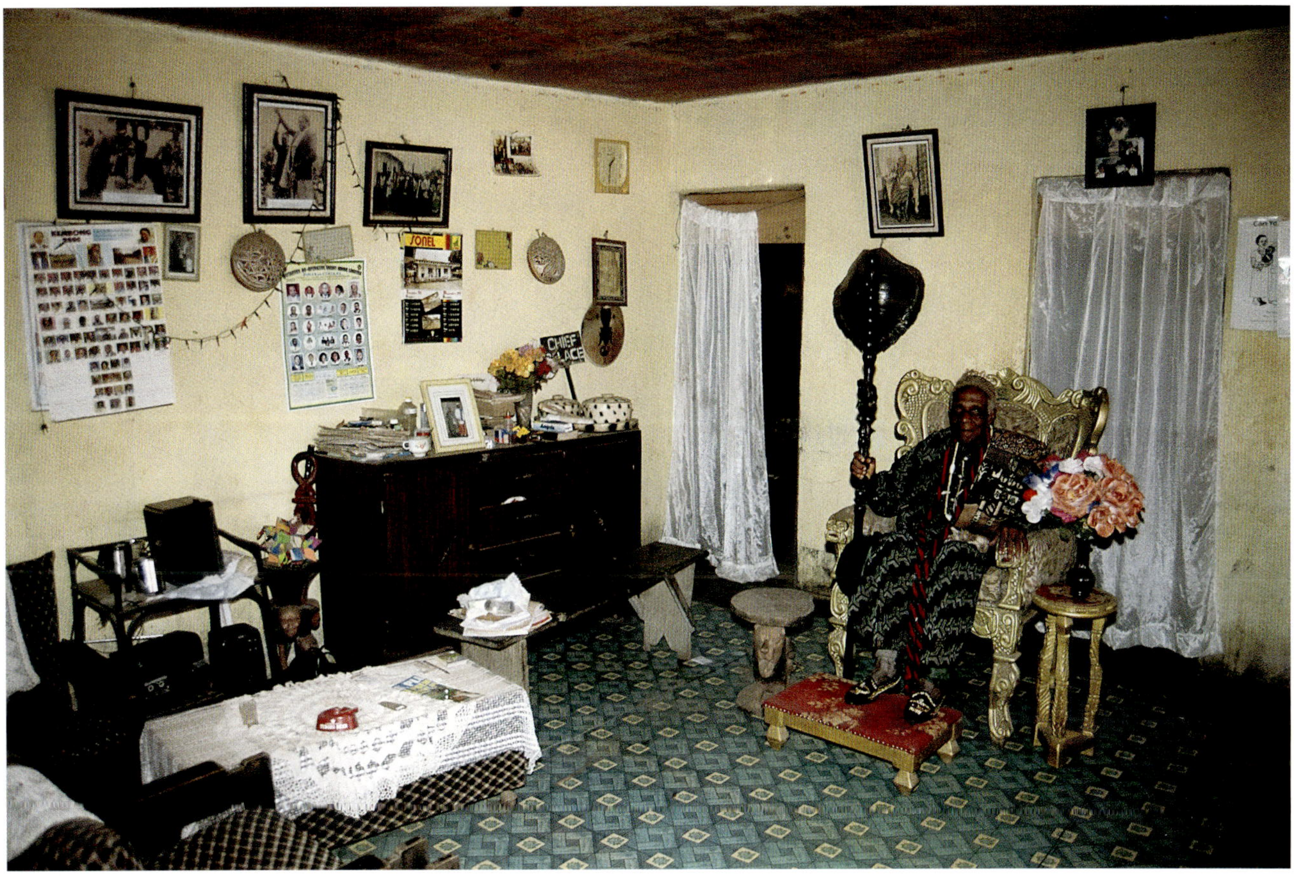

Fig. 40 Alfred Ayuk Ako, Chief of Kembong, in his parlour (Kembong, January 22, 2004).

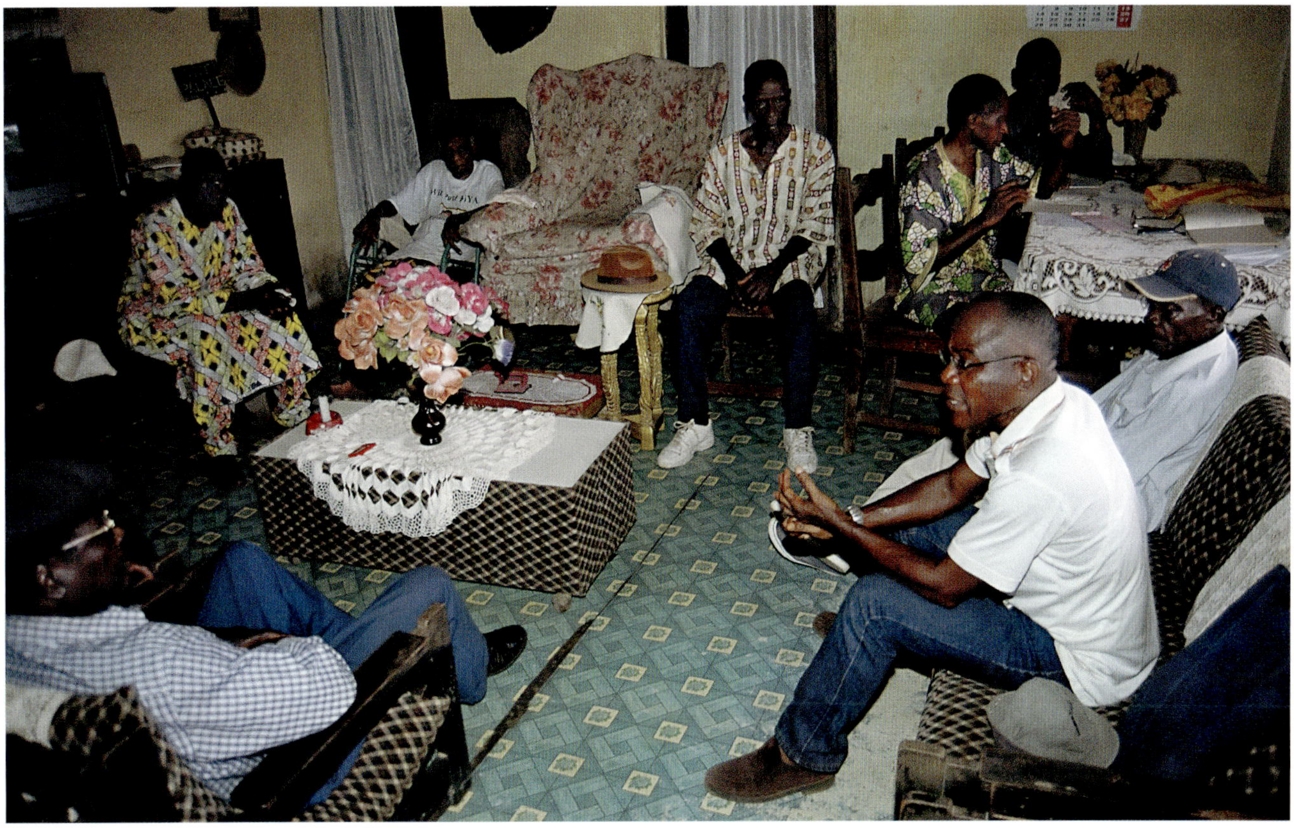

Fig. 41 Meeting of the Traditional Council in the Chief's Palace (the Chief seated top left, to the right of the throne; bottom right, Hon. Rev. Dr. Ayukachale Peter Egbe) (Kembong, April 1, 2005).

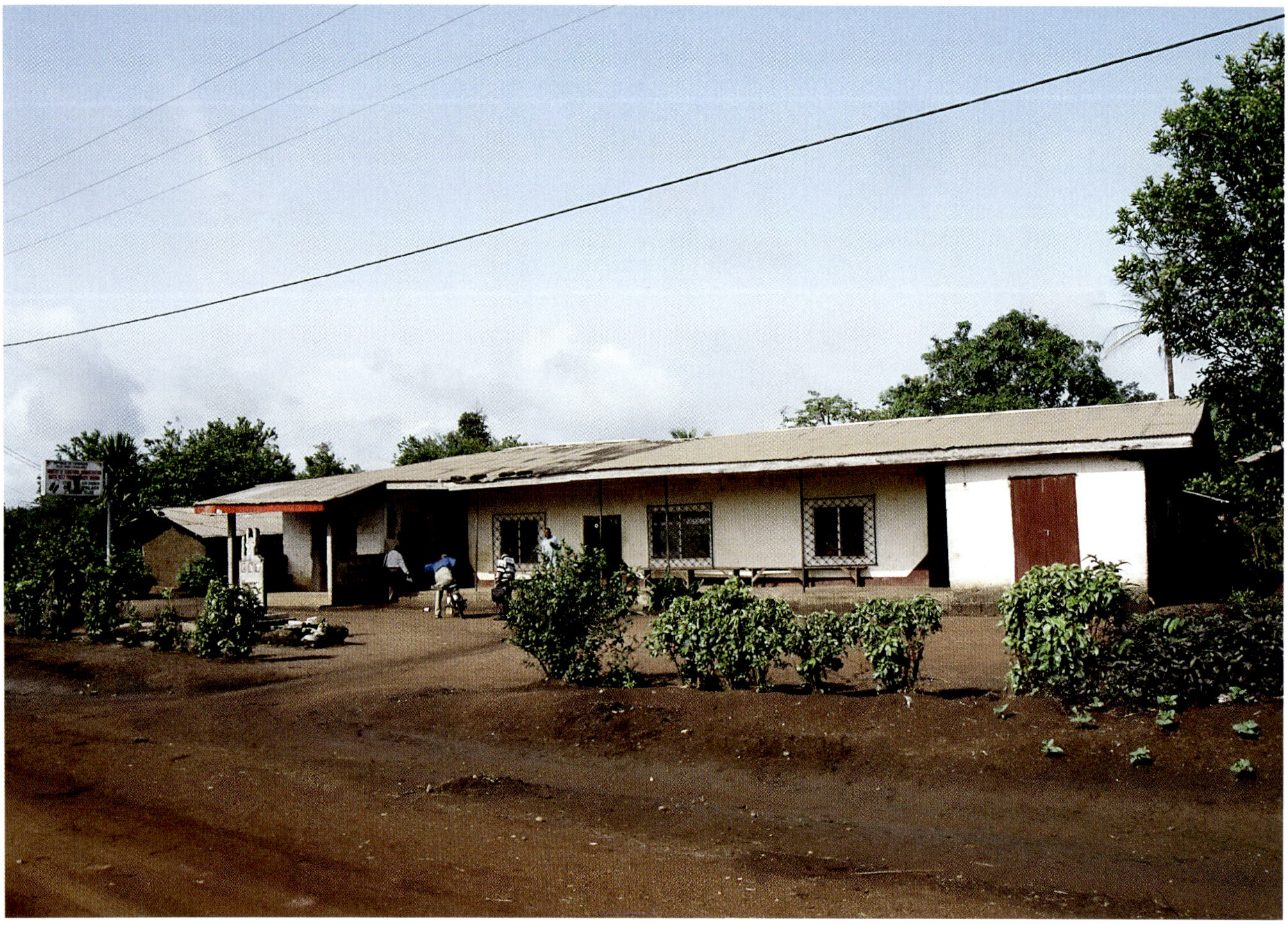

Fig. 42 Chief's Palace, the private residence of the Chief of Kembong (Kembong, January 22, 2004).

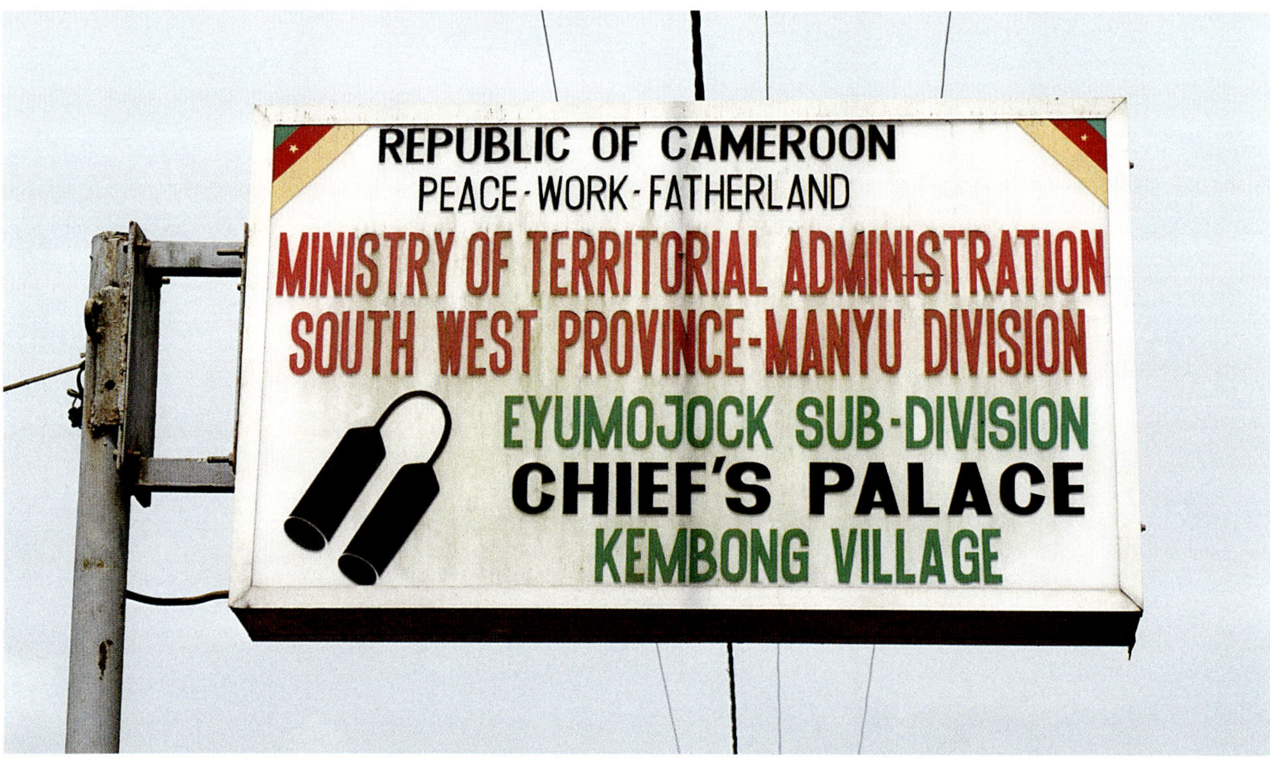
REPUBLIC OF CAMEROON
PEACE-WORK-FATHERLAND
MINISTRY OF TERRITORIAL ADMINISTRATION
SOUTH WEST PROVINCE-MANYU DIVISION
EYUMOJOCK SUB-DIVISION
CHIEF'S PALACE
KEMBONG VILLAGE

Fig. 43 The official sign for the Chief's Palace (Kembong, January 21, 2004).

era – cp. p. 15 f.) the traditional political system underwent a profound change. Even the position of quarterheads (*anne bechi ka quarter*) is not the same as before. It is no longer the oldest male who assumes the position; instead a vote takes place, in which usually a "younger" man is chosen. The confidence no longer exists that older men are capable of meeting the challenges involved in this office nowadays. Nonetheless, quarterheads are still determined by the elders. There is no special ceremony connected with the installation. The eldest male raises the right arm of the new quarterhead and addresses those present with the words: "This is your quarterhead."

Within the sphere of the Chief of Kembong obvious efforts are made in orienting this office towards the kingdoms of the Cameroon Grasslands. Thus, not only is the term "kingmakers" employed, but also "palace" and "throne". However, in the case of "palace", this is the private home of the Chief (*ochantui*) (figs. 42, 43) and not a complex encompassing some one dozen buildings, as in most Grassland kingdoms, which in addition is not the private property of the king but of the people. There are efforts in Kembong towards erecting a large representative palace as residence for the Chief, which are supported by the whole population. But in contrast to the Grasslands, there will never be a royal dynasty among the Central Ejagham – that is above all doubt – which in Africa always includes royal ancestors. In addition to these differences, the Chief does not possess any "sacred" traits nor is he greeted in a subservient manner. It is hardly possible that monarchical traditions like those that have developed throughout centuries in the Grasslands could be transferred to a society, in which positions of exceptional power have scarcely emerged in the long course of time.

3.5 Secret societies – organisation and functions. An initial overview

In many African communities secret societies and associations are of extraordinary significance, and this applies to the Ejagham, too. As Talbot already noted: "The whole country is honeycombed with secret societies."[26] There are secret societies for men as well as for women; however, societies for men hold more power and importance, and they appear in public far more often than those for women. The general term for secret societies or associations – even for Christian congregations – is *akum* (sg. *okum*).[27] From a European point of view, medicine societies – *ajom* (sg. *njom*) – are also secret societies. Both terms, *okum* and *njom*, do not imply any kind of secrets as do the European designations "secret society", "société secrète" or "Geheimgesellschaft". Membership in the associations is not at all secret; anyone is able to find out the society to which a person belongs. Still, as in many social groups in the world, there are spheres within a society, about which outsiders should or even must not be informed. The degree of secrecy varies. The secrecy kept among the societies of the Ejagham as a whole differs considerably from that of societies in the Cameroon Grasslands, which by comparison are far more stringent. But I shall return to this point later (cp. p. 59, 189, 221). Secret societies are in principle open to all male members of a community, with the exception of slaves in former times. They can be understood as a tie between different extended families, but – in view of their broad regional occurrence – they also serve as a support to relationships and contacts with neighbouring communities and tribes.

In the following overview, which starts with the societies for men, it can be stated at once that the most important of all secret societies is *Mgbe*, and this applies everywhere among the Central Ejagham, including Kembong. At least in former times it was the role of *Mgbe* to punish lawbreakers and wrongdoers, and today the society still preserves order and peace and is responsible for enforcing laws and regulations that are decided by *Etek*, the community assembly. In addition, *Mgbe* appears at funeral ceremonies for deceased members, where its masks carry great significance. These performances occur relatively frequently, for now as before many men in Kembong are members of the society.

The duty of the society *Angbu* is to take care of unpleasant and in the broadest sense bad things, that is to restore order. With its mask this society is in the position of warding off dangerous powers. Its special task is that of conducting autopsies, which particularly in earlier times was commonly practised in cases of death; today this allegedly occurs only occasionally.

Of all the *akum* in Kembong, *Mgbe* and *Angbu* are the only societies that have an "evil forest", the English designation for their special grove. The "evil forest" is an area in the bush outside of the village, which is forbidden and dangerous to outsiders and where important and secret ceremonies are conducted and magical plants are grown. These activities are always held in strict secrecy, for which reason at their initiation new members must take an oath to preserve the secrets of the society.

The other *akum* do not have medicine rituals like *Mgbe* and *Angbu*, and they have nothing that must be kept secret. Among these rather "harmless" associations is *Obon*, whose members usually meet when new members are admitted and at death ceremonies for deceased members. Further, some groups are known as "dancing societies". One of these is *Nkanda*, an autonomous society in Kembong, whereas in other communities it is a section of *Mgbe*. Other societies include those which own a mask covered with skin, such as *Nchebe* and *Mkpe*. They are masks, which European and American art-circles consider to be among the most remarkable works of art ever created by Old Africa. Owned by private families, the domain of *Nchebe* and *Mkpe* are the night dances, which are exceptionally expensive and therefore hardly performed anymore. After a long pause in time these masks performed once again in Kembong in 2005 (cp. p. 119 ff.). The masks of these dancing societies, including *Njom Ekpa*, the mask of the women (not represented in Kembong), have nothing to do with medicine and are therefore "harmless". They mostly appear at commemorative ceremonies, but not only for deceased members of their own society. The masks can also be engaged by non-members "to make their ceremonies heavy and important".

The few medicine societies – *Mfam*, *Amok* and *Okeboho* – must be counted among to the secret societies as well. Their function is to pursue and destroy the greatly feared witches with the use of their strong and dangerous medicines, and in this way they serve to protect the people and to maintain the social peace. Like *Mgbe* and *Angbu* some of them also have special groves for conducting their medicine rituals, and here it is understood that the groves are strictly taboo for outsiders. The associations are designated as *ajom* (sg. *njom*), yet in a very general sense they can be counted as *akum* as well. The most prominent *njom* is a mask: *Obasinjom*, the "God of medicine".

The single society of women in Kembong of today is *Mawu*. It is concerned with the interests of women, but seldom appears in public. The society is feared for its nocturnal dances, when its members "swear medicine" against men found guilty of attacking a woman. The former highly esteemed women's society *Ndem* no longer exists in Kembong nor in the surrounding communities. Its members were the *agbokarem*, who came from wealthy families. They had to complete an initiation that lasted several years, and as a whole they formed an elite group.

These associations, in particular *Mgbe*, *Angbu* and *Obasinjom*, do not represent units of a homogenous character. On the contrary, they are constituted by several ranks or levels, the ascent in which is characterised by the gain in knowledge and rights, and also the influence upon decisions as well as responsibility and prestige. Upon their acceptance into the society the new, usually young members are called "small children", who know nothing and must first learn how to behave. In contrast to many other African peoples, there are no "bush schools" among the Ejagham, in which young people are acquainted with the traditions of their tribes. Thus, it is mainly the part of secret societies to assume this function. The initiates acquire the status as full members only after many years, and only then do they receive the right to partake in important and secret rituals. Very few have the chance to attain the status of a chief or big man, who is informed about everything that concerns the society and who participates with authority in all decisions. On the one hand, achieving a higher position depends upon age – the principle of seniority also prevails in secret societies. On the other hand, it depends upon the diligence of the respective person, that is, his mental and physical traits, as well as his financial situation. Membership in an association, especially a high position in *Mgbe*, is thus the fundamental sign of an esteemed and successful man. A rise in status, which is based upon achievements and diligence, is only possible within secret societies. In families, however, normally age alone counts; there it is predominately older men and women who exert the greatest influence upon important decisions.

Admission into the society as well as into the circle of full members of *Mgbe*, *Angbu*, *Obasinjom* and the other medicine societies (*ajom*) is connected with a special ritual, which usually involves an oath to preserve the secrets. Initiation rituals of this kind are not obligatory among the "harmless" secret societies (*akum*), but high fees are demanded by most societies upon entering and for acceptance into higher ranks. The fees are seen as the price for the new knowledge acquired, above all for the right to participate in feasts that are held within the new rank. In this respect, membership in an association can be viewed as a kind of old-age security: whereas a younger person endeavours to pay the sometimes high fees, the person of advanced age can profit from these investments. Simultaneously, membership in associations is always connected with the certainty of support and protection in times of need. In particular, high ranking members are seldom in jeopardy of being accused of illegal activities connected with witchcraft.

Just as family units, these secret societies feel an indebtedness to the ancestors. Indeed, they are completely aware of the truth that without the ancestors the societies would never have come into existence nor could they exist at all. The ancestors are not only to thank for the organisational form and rules of conduct, but also the medicines and the masks. All prayers of the secret societies are directed to the ancestors alone – here demons or spirits play no role whatsoever.[28] It is a matter of fact that the ancestors are commemorated at all important meetings. When palm wine is drunk on official occasions, first the ancestors receive their portion in the form of a libation, and this offering is repeated at the conclusion of the occasion. It is likewise the task of secret societies to participate in death ceremonies for their deceased members; indeed, it is precisely their appearance that renders a decisive mark to these important festivities.

As mentioned above, medicines for surmounting problems in life play a role in secret societies, and they as well, together with the masks, are indebted to the ancestors. This also applies to many parts of traditional Africa, yet their use and meaning are not the same everywhere. This is clearly illustrated by a comparison of the *jujus* from the Cross River region with those in the Cameroon Grasslands.

Typical of secret societies in the Cameroon Grasslands is a bad medicine that is found in so-called medicine corners in the mask or medicine houses. This medicine pursues all those who transgress against the laws of the *jujus*. For example, it punishes members who have revealed secrets of the societies, as well as non-members and above all women who have seen things forbidden to them by the *jujus*. Through this bad medicine the masks and the so-called sacred musical instruments, which are played at nightly rituals, are imbued with powers. Non-initiates may view the masks only during their public performances, but it would be dangerous for them to see the secrets of the masks and medicines and – for instance – attempt to approach their prohibited houses. If this were to happen, the person(s) would have to reckon with being pursued by the medicine and becoming ill, even dying. Allegedly, in earlier times women did not know that the masks, in fact, were danced by men. They believed that the masks were of divine origin, from heaven or water.[29]

A bad medicine of this sort is unknown among secret societies in the Cross River region, which signifies that the societies cannot isolate themselves from non-members in a similar extreme fashion as in the Grasslands. In the Cross River region everyone knows what a mask is; there are no special secrets connected with its significance. As will be discussed in detail below, the mask bearers in some societies don the mask garment in public view (figs. 153, 154, 185–187, 201, 202). Sometimes one can see a mask garment laid out to dry in the sun (figs. 72, 161; cp. figs. 124, 159, 160, 164, 166, 181–184, 196, 197–200), and it is not unusual for women to make mask garments. Among the Ejagham the number of objects that are taboo and dangerous for outsiders is few, especially compared with the Grasslands, and correspondingly there is no need for special mask and medicine houses, whose vicinity no unauthorised person would dare approach, as in the Grasslands.

The so-called dangerous societies of the Ejagham, *Mgbe*, *Angbu*, *Obasinjom* and other *ajom*, also conduct ceremonies from which the general public is excluded.[30] They usually take place in the respective society's "evil forest", which is strictly taboo for non-initiates. To this day very little is known about the course of these significant events, which involve offerings and other rituals. In view of my own experiences in the Grasslands, I would presume that the so-called sacred musical instruments are played, which constitute both the most important and utmost secret ritual objects of every secret society, such as bull-roarers, mirlitone flutes and pipes made of crab claws.[31] The greatest secret among the Ejagham is the instrument with which *Mgbe* imitates the sound of the leopard. Large drums and slit-drums are of special importance in many societies in southern Cameroon and southern Nigeria. Offerings are made to them, and it is said that "great drums have souls".[32]

If an outsider to the secret societies of the Central Ejagham should by chance observe an event which is forbidden to him, he must "only"reckon with a purely mundane punishment. He must pay fees to the respective association, the same as those required from new members. In fact, the guilty person recognises the punishment as such if he decides to enter the association, which is often demanded in such cases. However, it has always been dangerous for non-members and outsiders in general to approach the "evil forest" and all the more so to set foot in it. Thus, Talbot reported that once two young girls of the Ekoi mistakenly entered the "evil forest"; for this "crime" they were hanged immediately by the *Mgbe*: "Their brother, who was a member of the highest grade of the society, was allowed, as a great favour, to be present at their death and afterwards to carry home the bodies to his family. Of redress, in such a case, there could be neither hope nor thought."[33] Penalty through medicine as practised in the Grasslands, which can lead to illness and death, is – by contrast – not found among the Ejagham. Yet, in this respect *Mawu*, the society for women, presents an exception. Should a man attempt to spy upon their night dances, he runs the risk of becoming impotent or seriously ill through their medicine.

3.6 Age-groups

So-called age-groups (*okan*, sg. *nkan*), which have "always" existed among the Ejagham, belong to the *akum*, that is to say, the societies.[34] The age-groups are principally concerned with upkeep and provisions, also with assistance and support among themselves, with the result that these groups are founded upon friendship, trust and solidarity. Hence, one could rightfully say that they form the basis of society.

Members of an age-group include men and women from the entire area of Kembong, who were born within the same year. That is to say, members of the respective groups are usually of the same age. The eldest member – no matter whether male or female – is the head of the group, and their meetings take place in his or her compound, normally once a month. An individual group is referred to by its own members as *nkan*. Its activities centre around singing, dancing and games, but also aiding in farm work, house construction and other difficult tasks. Another frequent responsibility of an age-group is to provide support in financial matters by organizing a conjoint savings program in the sense of a "rotating credit association". Every participant pays a specific amount into the joint savings at meetings, which are at one member's disposal for larger acquisitions or undertakings. If a group has a total of x members the savings are replenished after x meetings. Diverse secrets or religious activities, as in some secret societies, are unknown among the age-groups. Upon the death of a member it is customary to provide support for the family of the deceased. Today age-groups have very little significance; at present there are only about three age-groups in Kembong, who meet regularly.

Footnotes

1 Agbor 2001:14 (cp. Koloss 2000:450 f.).
2 Mansfeld 1908:162.
3 Onor 1994:87. This also applies to the Efik (Nair 1972:13).
4 Koloss 2000:67 ff., 150 ff.
5 Koloss 2000:70 ff., 159 ff., 165 f.
6 Talbot also noted: "The Ekoi are a polygamous people, but till several years after my arrival, the chief wife, not the husband, was regarded as head of the house" (1912:97). Whether or not women also have the right to carry out ancestral offerings could not be found out with certainty, according to Röschenthaler (1993:234).
7 Ruel 1969:XII. Accordingly, *Etek* among the Banyang signifies three aspects: "'settlement', 'community', and 'a body of persons representing a community' – (they) are closely interrelated" (1969:20).
8 Talbot 1926:III:562.
9 Already in the reports of the very first explorers, who penetrated into Cameroon's interior about 1890 (Eugen Zintgraff and Franz Hutter), the chiefs of the forest area were characterized as men of little influence, who made a poor impression ("ärmliche" bzw. "jämmerliche Dorfschulzen") (Zintgraff 1895:46, 184 f., 204; Hutter 1902:264). There is a striking contrast between these reports and those on the kings of the Grasslands, who were presented by them in a by far more positive and respectful light (Zintgraff 1895:183 ff.; Hutter 1902:335 ff.). Jones points out the "weakness" of the chiefs of the forest area as well (1956:126). The same applies to the chiefs of the Bakossi, who likewise belonged to egalitarian societies. For them "chieftaincy is not known in the early period of Bakossi history" (Balz 1984:53). It was only in colonial times that a chieftaincy developed, but "a 'chief' … could traditionally be nothing else than a speaker of the Ngwe-elders" (Balz 1984:202). They were "by no means sacred persons" (Balz 1984:129). Correspondingly, it is said in "Bakossi Area: Assessment Report 1931": The village chief or "king" "was probably a quite unimportant personage in pre-European times: for instance he could not even order the clearing of the village without first calling the meeting of the old men called Ngwe … and receiving their sanction …" (Balz 1984:203 f.).
10 Mansfeld 1908:161; Staschewski 1917:16; Ruel 1969:66; Nicklin 1983:67; Röschenthaler 1993:162.
11 Onor 1994:93 ff.
12 Cp. also Talbot 1912:322.
13 For a detailed description of this ceremony, see Ruel 1969:49 ff.
14 Talbot 1912:27, 333f., 408; Ruel 1969:53.
15 After this exposition it does not make sense to refer to the small tribes in the western part of the Grasslands, such as the Meta' or the Moghamo, as "acephalous" (Fowler and Zeitlyn 1996:3). For in contrast to the really acephalous societies of the Cross River region their political system shows the monarchic, and that means "cephalous" features typical of the Grassland tribes, namely "transformation" and "heritability". As Dillon (1990: 125 ff.) points out in detail, among the Meta' the king (*Fon*) has supernatural powers, which he is endowed with during his installation; moreover, that office is regularly bound up with one of those families, which once founded the locality. The title *Fon* has a ring of the Grasslands anyway. Even though Dillon calls the Meta' society "acephalous" (1990:1, 199, 265), apparently because the *Fon* is neither sacred nor omnipotent, the fact remains that the kings of the "classical" Grassland monarchies can by no means be regarded as sacred and omnipotent either – and yet they are recognized as "kings" (cf. Koloss 1992; 2000: 171 ff.).

16 Langheld 1909. Lord Lugard, who had successfully introduced "indirect rule" in northern Nigeria referred to southern Nigeria as "chaotically administered" (Crowder 1962:199); Sigrist (1978: 29) also notes: "The 'primitiveness' of tribal societies was seen precisely in its lack of political institutions."

17 Talbot 1926:III:562.

18 Langheld 1909:545.

19 Ngoh 1996:76.

20 Agbor 2001:28.

21 Mansfeld (1908:19 f.) gives an account of such a case. Similar difficulties caused by the decision of German colonial officials to establish the office of a chief in a traditionally egalitarian, acephalous society arose not only in the Cross River region, but also in other regions in Cameroon. Matiba (1966:47), he himself a Bassa from southern Cameroon, provides a moving description of such a fatal situation among his own people: "The Germans made 'chiefs' (out of members of the former class of slaves); they served as mediators between the military administration and the people. They were given a uniform with striking red shoulder-pieces, a helmet and a cane as a sign of their power and privilege. In that way they were conspicuous and differed from the people. It is said that most of them belonged to the lower levels of society, and their appointment to this position was all the more unbearable for us. They made innumerable follies, mistakes and outrageous things; for as a person of respect, which a chief indeed is, they disposed over a certain freedom of actions. Of course, thereby they could not damage the interests of the colonial powers. Thus, the chief demanded submission to the law and could harass us thoroughly with any kind of chicanery." The same situation existed by the Bakossi. There as well with the arrival of Europeans slaves were "used" to "play" the role of the chief (Balz 1984:115, 192).

22 Agbor 2001:27. The same problems arose in particular in southern Nigeria with the introduction of "indirect rule" by the British. The installation of an "artificial" chief in tribes with an egalitarian political system led to conflict, for example, a threatening uprising among the Igbo in 1929. "Indirect rule" in that region proved to be unachievable and was given up during the 1930s (Meek 1937:328 ff.; Crowder 1962:211 f.; 1977: 158). We owe Geschiere (1993) thanks for his extensive analysis of the problems that resulted among the Maka and Bakweri, both originally likewise acephalous, from the colonial administration's introduction of the office of chief.

23 Agbor 2001:28.

24 *Ata* Ebandip and *Ata* Akem (no. 3 and 4 in the list) are also mentioned by Mansfeld (1908:15).

25 Thus, Agbor (2001:27) remarks: "Until today, the 'kingmakers' are still influenced either by money or goods and it is very difficult for them to arrive at an unanimous decision as to who should be appointed chief."

26 Talbot 1912:37.

27 Cp. Talbot 1912:198, 410 ff.

28 I studied the same dominant position of the ancestors for secret societies in the Cameroon Grasslands (Koloss 2000:97 ff.). It was therefore of interest to me that the same is reported about the Bakossi: "The departed founders' souls ... are the only 'spiritual' non-material element in the secret Ahon ritual. There is no spirit of Ahon above or behind them... Ahon is not a spirit" (Balz 1984:231). *Ahon* is the secret society among the Bakossi that represents wealth and prestige.

29 Koloss 2000:99 f. As Ottenberg notes, it is also dangerous for women of the Ifikpo to view forbidden activities of a secret society: " ... she is defiled and will no longer become pregnant; to atone for her error, she must make a purifying sacrifice at the spirit shrine" (Ottenberg 1975:9).

30 This applies especially to women. Correspondingly, in his study of masquerades in southeastern Nigeria O. Nzekwu states: "Women have been excluded from sharing in the secrets for they are weak and fickle and are therefore not fit to take part in them. They are also mysterious and sometimes unclean. They cannot therefore approach these ancestral manifestations, whose character is diametrically opposed to their own. Any meeting between them would have adverse effects on both parties. Much harm would come to the women and masquerades would lose something of their virtue" (1960:135).

31 Bull-roarers have a wide distribution in southern Nigeria and the Ejagham use them as well (Talbot 1912:221 f., 284; 1926: III:758 f., 769, 780; Jeffreys 1949). In the Cameroon Grasslands they are mostly in the possession of military societies (Koloss 2000:99, 206). Mirlitone pipes (wooden pipes, one end covered with a membrane) are employed in the secret rituals performed in many African societies (Jeffreys 1949; Boston 1960:60 f., 64; Nzekwu 1960:138; Lifschitz 1988). In the Grasslands they usually belong to the mask societies of extended families (Koloss 2000:99, 338). Musical instruments of special importance among the Ejagham are pipes made from crab claws (Talbot 1912:55, 408).

32 Corresponding information is provided by Talbot (1912:297; 1932: 271); Weston (1984:147) and Röschenthaler (1993: 163).

33 Talbot 1912:43 f.

34 Detailed information about the age-groups among the Banyang is supplied by Ruel (1969:206 ff.). For more information, see Talbot 1912:108, 283; 1923: 215; 1926:III:543; Ittmann 1954/1955; Anonymous 1957:169; Horton 1971:42; Röschenthaler 1993:158 ff.; Onor 1994:91 f.

4 *Akum* – the secret societies

4.1 *Mgbe*

4.1.1 History, dissemination and general characteristics

For the Central Ejagham *Mgbe* is the most important, influential and feared secret society of all.[1] Widespread in large areas of southeastern Nigeria and southwestern Cameroon, this society emerged in the coastal region as early as the 17th century and at that time already was considered to be "most powerful and influential".[2] The society's name differs among the various peoples. The name *Nyampkwe* is also widespread.[3] Further, the majority of the other Ejagham groups and the Banyang call the society *Ngbe*; the Efik name is *Ekpe*; in Pidgin-English it is *Egbo*.

Mgbe, *Ngbe* and *Ekpe* are designations for the leopard, the most dangerous animal in the region, and – as its members always insist towards outsiders – it is precisely the strength of this animal from which the society of the same name draws its powers.

Yet research and documentation of this secret society are confronted with considerable difficulties, so that any statements pertaining to it must be regarded with a certain caution. This is due to the fact that even today all actions that occur within *Ngbe/Ekpe* are strictly taboo for non-members. The hope uttered by C. Partridge as early as 1905 that one day "one of the initiated members of this interesting Egbo society will come forward and tell us in a book all about it" has not been fulfilled to this day.[4]

It is said that *Ngbe/Ekpe* was founded in southwestern Cameroon,[5] either among the Ejagham, as thus far assumed, or in Isangele in the area of the Balondo, as later research by K. Nicklin revealed.[6] There are many mythical-historical traditions, according to which a woman discovered the secrets of *Ngbe*.[7] All diversities in details aside, the basic precept is the same. According to Nicklin's account: "A magical fish with a leopard's voice is caught by a woman before being brought under the control of men for the purposes of firm government."[8]

Ngbe was acquired by the Efik, when they abandoned their old settlement area west of the Cross River and resettled in Calabar. When trade in slaves and palm oil came to dominate the economy, *Ekpe* – as the society was called by the Efik – attained exceptional significance. Until then there had been no central political organisation among the Efik, and so *Ekpe* developed into an institution, in which all important political decisions were taken. Above all *Ekpe* became known for its correct management of business matters. *Ekpe* levied high penalties when contracts were not kept, and it had the responsibility and power for collecting debts. In addition, *Ekpe* was viewed as an institution that held slaves and women as well under control.[9] *Ekpe* spread from Calabar to neighbouring areas. Before the colonial era began, the society had reached the Central Ejagham and Banyang[10] and later Bangwa.[11] The fundamental elements of the association with the leopard as a symbol of unlimited power and the responsibility for the well-being of the community were the same everywhere. Yet, there were considerable regional differences, primarily in the forms of organisation, which will be discussed below.[12]

4.1.2 The 32 *Mgbe* lodges in Kembong

When the inhabitants of the surrounding hamlets were resettled in Kembong, they already owned *Mgbe*. The 32 *Mgbe* lodges (*ocha Mgbe*, pl. *acha Mgbe*, "lodge of *Mgbe*" or "parlour of Mgbe") that exist in Kembong at present can be divided into two groups, according to their origin.

The first group originated in Ayiko in Ndian and is constituted by eleven lodges. Achere Benem, the brother of the great-grandfather of Dr. Ayukachale, my companion and translator, acquired *Mgbe* in Ayiko presumably between 1850 and 1870. Later the society was sold to other communities.

The following is a list of the lodges and their leaders (*boseseku*) in Kembong in 2005:

Seseku (Chief of *Mgbe*)	Quarter
1. Ayuk Sampson Eno	Okemebenem
2. Ayuknsok Isaac	Okemebenem
3. Akemodu (died in February 2005)	Okemebenem

4. Arrey Baracle	Nserong
5. James Awoh	Okangku
6. Deba Thompson	Okangku
7. Ojongndang Peter	Okangku
8. Mbeng Mathias	Okangku
9. Ndip Jacob Ebotmbu	Okangku
10. Takang Samuel	Abotabe
11. Moses Ashu	Nyenya

The second group came from Echoko in Upper Ekwe and was acquired together by Tanyi Enow and Oru Ogum from Ebarensi. This group is composed of 21 lodges:

Seseku (Chief of *Mgbe*)	Quarter
1. Kofi Tabe	Ndengane
2. James Ayuknchiobo	Ndengane
3. Oben Isaac	Ndengane
4. Ateke Johnson	Takpang
5. Akoachere E. B.	Takpang
6. Ojongndip John B.	Takpang
7. Akobenem Sampson	Mbiofong
8. Ernest Array Ayuk Tarkang	Nkonghobe
9. Nso John Agbor	Ebarensi
10. Arrey Joseph	Okune
11. Ojong Samuel Ebot	Okune
12. Ojong Samuel Tabe	Okemnjemeba
13. Otto Agbor Ntui	Ayukaba
14. Ako Besem	Ayukaba
15. Eta Sampson	Ayukaba
16. Dan Nkongho	Ayukaba
17. Tabe Etengeneng	Ayukaba
18. Tabe Ndepaya	Okonyenge
19. Elias Tanyi	Okonyenge
20. Dr. Moses Besong	Okonyenge
21. Dr. Agbor Besong Ben	Okonyenge

The costs for *Mgbe* were once, when the people still lived in the hamlets, raised collectively, but not all families participated in the purchase. The decision of families for or against the acquisition of *Mgbe* had far-reaching consequences, and these will continue as long as *Mgbe* exists. The reason is that only a member of a family who took part in the purchase of *Mgbe* may become chief of *Mgbe*, that is, a *seseku*. Hence, those members of *Mgbe* who do not belong to these privileged families are excluded from the position of the chief of *Mgbe* forever.

Although the individual lodges claim to be broadly autonomous, *Mgbe* is generally regarded as the sum and fellowship of not only the 32 lodges in Kembong, but also the *Mgbe* lodges in other regions. Close contact is generally cultivated between neighbouring lodges and especially those with a common origin. Thus, not only are reciprocal invitations to important ceremonies a matter of course, but specific ceremonies, such as the initiation into the level *eteme Mgbe* ("grove of *Mgbe*"), are even conducted jointly. Moreover, serious transgressions are never dealt with by a single lodge, but are requited in principle by the big men of several lodges together. A member of *Mgbe* has access to all *Mgbe* lodges, wherever he may be. However, the guest must prove his membership through his correct knowledge of the sign language used in all *Mgbe* societies.[13]

4.1.3 Ranks in *Mgbe*

As is typical of African secret societies, *Mgbe* is organised in several ranks connected with special duties, which are basically characterised by an ever increasing amount of knowledge and rights as well as responsibility.[14] Yet it is strictly forbidden to write down anything taught in the different levels; all teaching in *Mgbe* is oral. Although the most important ranks are clearly defined, there is also a plenitude of special rights in conduct and in the use of status symbols, for which additional fees must be paid. This accords well with the saying: "You can never finish *Mgbe*."[15] Altogether the ranks and special rights determine not only the actual position of the individual member, but also the form in which *Mgbe* will conduct the funeral ceremony for him.

Mgbe is an important and esteemed society, yet not all of the men in Kembong belong to the society, nor did all in former times. Moreover, many members work in one of the cities in the south and, consequently, can return to their hometown only seldom. This has also led to the consequence that the society of *Mgbe* has become less important. Nowadays there are some lodges whose members number no more than six. Principally, all men have access to *Mgbe*, even boys who are old enough to preserve the secrets of the society. This applies also to men who allegedly have a bad character. The latter are even welcomed when they go to *Mgbe*, for – it is said – there they can be disciplined.[16] Slaves were formerly accepted as members, but only into the lower ranks.[17] It was often the task of slaves to guard the house of *Mgbe*. They were entrusted with as few secrets as the woman, who today still represents the interests of women in corresponding negotiations in *Mgbe*.[18] But now as before all women are excluded from *Mgbe*.[19]

4.1.3.1 *Abo Mgbe*, the "young people of *Mgbe*"

Members of the lower levels are designated *abo Mgbe*, the "young people of *Mgbe*". Although most of them have already seen the greatest secret of the society, in the sphere of *Mgbe* they may behave only "like a thief", meaning they know nothing; their knowledge is like that of women. On the other hand, they are not made fully responsible for their actions. The punishment for any offences committed by them against the laws and regulations, about which they have not been sufficiently informed yet, is usually mild.

4.1.3.1.1 *Bekundi*

Fees are required to enter the various ranks of the society of *Mgbe*. For the level *bekundi* the fees include: one goat, four "animals" (*oya*, sg. *nya*) (one "animal" means the leg or joint of a deer), 30 litres of palm wine, two bunches of plantains, two bottles of palm oil, two cups of salt and two cups of pepper. *Bekundi* is the first level of *Mgbe*. A person who wishes to enter *Mgbe* first contacts the *seseku*, the chief of *Mgbe*. In case the candidate is still too young – sometimes boys as young as 15 years of age are accepted into *Mgbe*, if they display the corresponding maturity – contact is made by his father. The *seseku* discusses the case with the elders of the society, and thereafter he informs the candidate about the fees to be paid and sets a date with him for admission into the society. Usually several other – three or four – young men are initiated at the same time. This takes place either in the house of the *seseku* or during a funeral ceremony in the compound of the deceased person. First a white stripe is made on the nose and a red stripe on the temples of each new member. A red and a white circle are drawn around the breast nipples of each person. The application of these signs is called *aseng wa Mgbe*: "They have written *Mgbe* on you." The initiates are not treated with medicine, as by contrast is still practised in the secret societies of the Cameroon Grasslands; for *Mgbe* does not own any medicines, as was repeatedly emphasised to me, and, moreover, it does not wish to have anything to do with medicines.

4.1.3.1.2 *Okat Mgbe*, "curtain of *Mgbe*"

Fees: one goat or two "animals" and 30 litres of palm wine.

Acceptance into this rank may take place one day after admission into the first rank, *bekundi,* at the earliest. As the designation of the level intimates, the new members are entrusted with *Mgbe's* greatest secret – they are shown the instrument with which the voice of the leopard is imitated.[20] Only thereafter are they deemed real members of *Mgbe* and also from that moment on they may visit any other *Mgbe* lodge. Beforehand though they must swear an oath upon a medicine (*njom*), such as *Okeboho* or *Mfam,* that they will preserve all secrets of *Mgbe*. Christian members are allowed to swear upon the Bible: "As I have become a member of this society today and as I have entered this stage today, should I release a secret to someone who is outside the society, let me suffer the penalty of this oath." At the same time the new members are admonished adamantly to observe the following commands under all circumstances: no fighting, never to raise a cutlass against someone, and never to commit adultery. It is made clear to each new member that whoever transgresses these laws must reckon with severe punishment.

4.1.3.1.3 *Okongo*

This section of *Mgbe*, which appears at nocturnal funeral ceremonies with secret musical instruments, requires special fees: two "animals" and 30 litres of palm wine. This ensures that upon his death the respective member will be buried by *okongo*.

4.1.3.1.4 *Ebongu* and *Ema*

The level of *abo Mgbe* is connected with *Ebongu* and *Ema*. They constitute the only sections in the society of *Mgbe* among the Central Ejagham that have masks, unlike in other regions where *Mgbe* has more masks.[21] Once a person is initiated into the *bekundi* level, he automatically becomes a member of *Ebongu* and *Ema*. At his death celebration *Ebongu* and *Ema* perform in his honour. These masks are the forerunners of *Mgbe* and the only masks connected with the main structure of *Mgbe* society. They are not treated with medicine (*njom*) nor are they charged with the pursuit and punishment of offenders and witches. They appear only during death celebrations for members of *Mgbe* and during the day; they cannot be seen on any other occasion (figs. 61–63, 73, 76, 81, 85–91).

Among the special features of *Ebongu* and *Ema* in the Ngunaya area is the fact that they use the same mask garment. At funeral ceremonies *Ebongu* appears first, holding a lightweight raphia pole in the right hand. After the offering is made to the ancestors, the same mask appears again, but now it acts as *Ema*. It differs from *Ebongu* in that in place of the raphia pole, it holds a whip in its right hand. Nowadays this alternation does not always occur. *Ema* is the more dangerous of the two masks. *Ebongu* and *Ema* hold medicine leaves in the left hand (figs. 62, 87, 91), which are called *efune Mgbe*. There is no translation for the word *efune*, but it also appears in association with the mask *Obasinjom*: this mask also holds medicine in the left hand, a small piece of wood called *efune Njom* (cp. p 160 f.).[22]

Ebongu and *Ema* wear a knitted dress covering the head and arms, extending down to the ankles; it has no carved headpiece like other masks of the region.[23] The dress is knitted out of a type of local thread with small sturdy sticks. The garment is basically in hues of reddish brown and yellow. Stripes and larger sections in the same colour are in horizontal arrangement. A circle of fibres hangs round the neck, falling to the shoulders. Similar circles of fibres are attached to the feet. Especially typical for *Ebongu* und *Ema* is a large bell that hangs around the waist on the back, falling loosely over the buttocks to allow a clear jingling sound (figs. 61, 89, 91). Also worn on the upper back is a disc consisting of two halves and covered with cloth, to which a mirror called "*efe Ebongu/Ema*" (mirror of *Ebongu/ Ema*) is attached (fig. 89). Today merely a decoration for most people, the disc was originally of significance. This is indicated at least by the symbol of a chameleon near the mirror, an animal that can see in "all" directions. Possibly this is associated with "extra eyes", as R.F. Thompson noted among the Banyang: "The mirrors guard his back, imparting magic vision."[24] A "mirror" also belongs to the medicines of the widely renowned mask of *Obasinjom*. *Efe Njom* is at the back of its head and is regarded as the mask's "brain-box". All the decisions taken by *Obasinjom* originate from there (cp. p. 160). A stick of beautiful feathers hangs loosely from the head of *Ebongu/Ema*, and these feathers are taken from the walking staff of the *seseku* (figs. 52, 71). *Ebongu* and *Ema* are masks with agile movements, and so they are also known as "jumping cat" (*angwa ribo)*. Mask outfits, which are very expensive, are usually not the possession of a single lodge, but are acquired by several lodges together.

Even today the performance of *Ebongu* as well as *Ema* includes chasing children and attacking men, as a measure to encourage them to join *Mgbe*. However, the masks are not nearly as aggressive as they were in former times. Then they were shown far more respect by non-members and were feared to an even greater extent.[25] Although no secret medicine rituals are required for *Ebongu* and *Ema*, as is the case with *Obasinjom* (cp. p. 160 ff.) and *Angbu* (cp. p. 131), outsiders are not permitted to watch the dancer assume the mask outfit. However, the chance possibility of looking at the mask, when it has been laid out to dry in full view of the public, is of little matter (fig. 72). Furthermore, women are usually the ones who make the mask garments.

Opposite the members of higher ranks, the *abo Mgbe* have a very limited number of rights. They are not allowed to wear caps and shoes in the area of *Mgbe*,[26] and the use of a walking staff is principally forbidden to the young people. Likewise forbidden are all objects of European production, such as trousers, watches, flashlights and mobile telephones. As the *abo Mgbe* do not yet have their own names in *Mgbe*, they may only take part in official discussions, when they have asked a higher ranking member to greet *Mgbe* for them. Everyone who wishes to speak at the official assembly must first clap his hands two times and greet *Mgbe*.

The youngest members of *Mgbe* already receive various small tasks to carry out, for example, to deliver messages or to play the drums. Yet, they do not have access to the ceremonies in the grove of *Mgbe*. *Okina*, messenger of *Mgbe*, comes from the *abo Mgbe* as well (figs. 44, 63, 76, 81). With his "rifle", a zigzag-shaped staff, he "shoots" at the person whom *Mgbe* wishes to see: "Bum, bum, *Mgbe* needs you." Only clever and intelligent men are chosen for this position. And because *okina* is used as jester and fun-maker during performances of *Ebongu/Ema,* needless to say he should be a person of good humour and not solemn or ill-humoured. *Okina* is not required to pay any fees, for he is employed by *Mgbe*.[27]

4.1.3.2 The full members of *Mgbe*

4.1.3.2.1 *Eteme Mgbe*, "grove of *Mgbe*"

Fees: one goat, two "animals", 70 litres of palm wine, two bunches of plantains, two bottles of palm oil, two cups of salt, two cups of pepper, 5,000 Francs CFA.

Initiation into this rank is a very significant event, for it is the level of full membership. Whoever has seen the grove of *Mgbe (eteme Mgbe* or *ekot Mgbe)* – and initiation is precisely that which enables entrance into the grove – knows the most important secrets of the socie-

Fig. 44 *Okina*, messenger of *Mgbe* (Samuel Tanyi Tambe, Okonyenge) with his zigzag-shaped staff, special cap and raphia bag on an official mission (Kembong, February 24, 1980). ▶

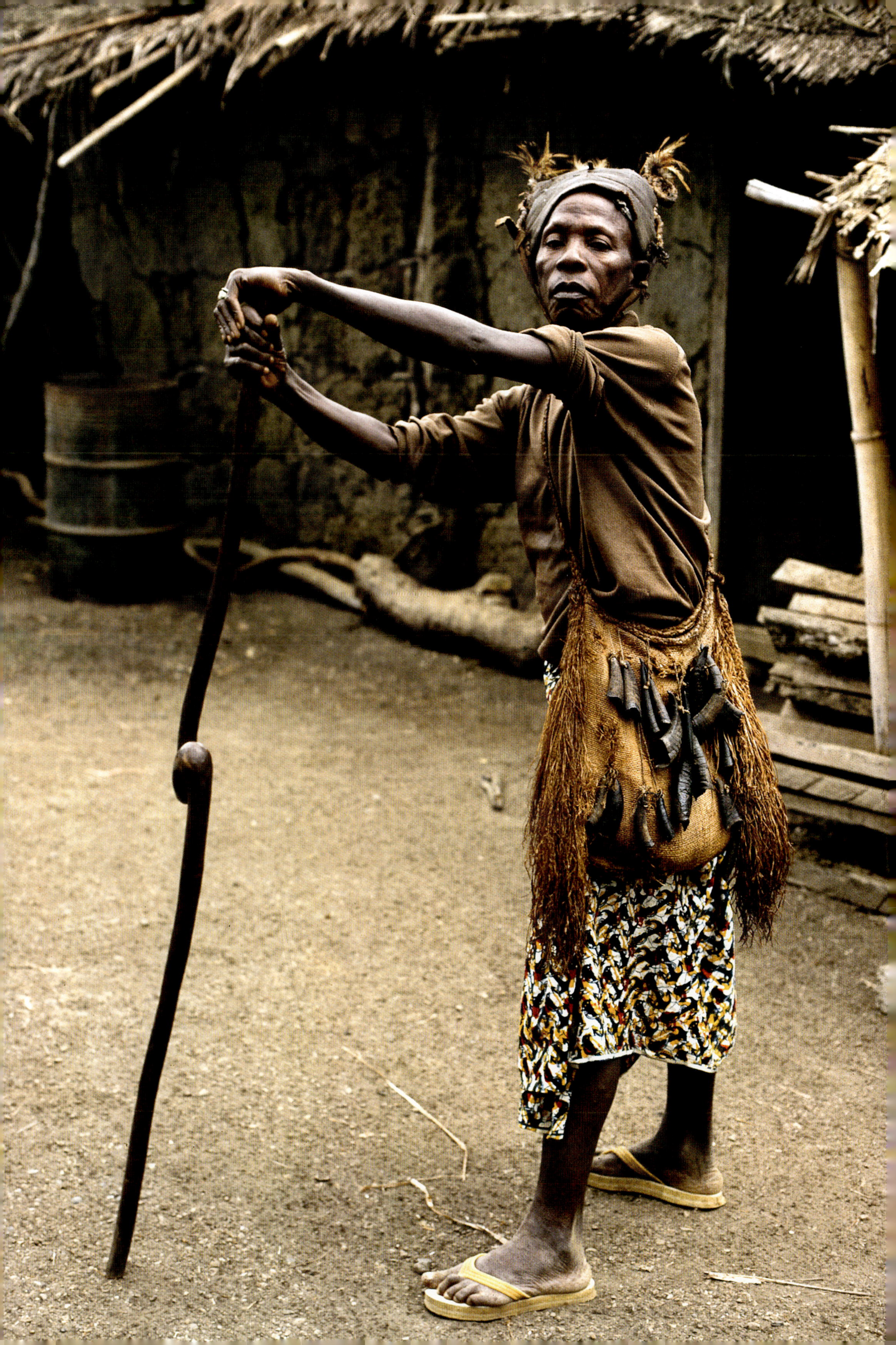

ty. For this reason before entering this level the person must swear a further oath: to preserve the secrets in all circumstances, just as at his acceptance into the society. Initiation into *eteme Mgbe* is usually conducted by several *Mgbe* lodges together, specifically lodges of the same origin. Thus, *eteme Mgbe* is the union of *Mgbe* at an inner-village level and even an inter-tribal level. In earlier times the initiation took place very rarely, in fact sometimes only once in a generation. Nowadays it is held regularly every few years.

Initiation into *eteme Mgbe* lasts about five days. It takes place in the grove of *Mgbe*, but the participants sleep in their own compounds at night. On the evening prior to initiation there is a big meal with lots of food and drink in the compound of the *seseku*. On the next morning the initiates march in a long line, led by the *seseku*, to the *eteme Mgbe*. There the *seseku* turns to the first ancestor in prayer: "*Ata* X., we have assembled here to initiate these men into the stage of *eteme*. We give you this water, take it and meet also the other big men. If we have had bad intentions, let ill luck follow us. But if we have done, as you have taught us, let everything go well. Here is your food – plantains and meat. When we ourselves will eat later, may our head and neck not pain." After drinking palm wine he offers the last sip to the ancestors: "Here are the dregs, *Ata* X., take them and meet those whom I know and also those whom I do not know. And let our celebration be peaceful." The ceremonies that then follow belong to the most profound secrets. "Whoever wishes to go into the evil forest", according to one of my informants, "must be strong. For there he will see terrible things – amongst others, his ancestors."[28]

During initiation the initiates are regarded as "widows" (*akekwet*, sg. *nkekwet*), and they must perform all tasks that are requested of them. At this time they should become well-acquainted with the "real *Mgbe*", and that involves not only the most important secrets of *Mgbe*, but also the principles and rules for correct behaviour by which all must abide. Accordingly, the initiates are entrusted with the secrets that concern the "table" (*efem Mgbe*), which is erected for every deceased member of *Mgbe* (fig. 69). One of the highlights of initiation is the entrustment with the secret sign language, which is called *nsibiri* or *nsibidi*. It is employed for transmitting confidential messages and for proving his own membership in *Mgbe* when entering other, foreign *Mgbe* lodges.[29] Instruction in sign language usually continues after the period of initiation has ended, and private teachers are also engaged in this. As the saying goes, one should make use of every opportunity to learn new signs.

Further, the initiates learn new songs and dances, and special importance is placed upon social conduct: "how to behave in a community". They should understand that all laws are ultimately meant to maintain peace in the community and especially to protect women and all those who are dependent upon help. If a full member of *Mgbe* should commit an offence in the future, he must reckon with harsh punishment, because now he is knowledgeable of the laws and rules. As the saying goes: "You have been warned".

4.1.3.2.2 *Eyume Mgbe*, "voice of *Mgbe*", or *okahah Mgbe*, "to answer *Mgbe*"

During the last night in the grove, dances take place that last until dawn. After that the members return to the compound of the *seseku*, where a further ritual is conducted, the admission of new members to the rank of *eyume Mgbe* ("voice of *Mgbe*") or *okahah Mgbe* ("to answer *Mgbe*").[30] Acceptance into this level is connected with more fees: two "animals", 30 litres of palm wine, two bunches of plantains, two bottles of palm oil, two cups of salt and two cups of pepper. There are dances on this day as well. During the festivity the new members dance upon mats and look forward to receiving gifts from relatives, friends and acquaintances.

The ritual gains even more significance, for at this time each of the initiates receives a new name. It is frequently used in the lodge by other members as a way of praise and congratulation to the newly initiated. Yet, they still maintain their old names in normal life. In fact, non-members must not even know those new names. With his new name each initiate has the right to greet *Mgbe* and with that to partake in official discussions in *Mgbe* without special permission, as is the case with *abo Mgbe*.

Acceptance into *eteme Mgbe* and *okahah Mgbe* signifies a person's full membership in *Mgbe*. The members have access to all important activities of the society; they have the right to speech in discussions; and they are no longer bound to the numerous restrictions, which they had to observe as *abo Mgbe*. They have the right to a walking stick and a head covering; their special symbol is a white cap, which is decorated with various things, such as cowrie shells, elephant hair, porcupine quills and eagle feathers (figs. 45–47, 49).[31] Members may also choose to wear a red cap (*ebiolak*, pl. *abiolak*), which is worn by higher ranking members of *Mgbe* as well (figs. 48, 50–53).[32] Finally, the new members are permitted to wear shoes and to utilise objects of European provenience in the vicinity of *Mgbe*, rights which, as mentioned above, are prohibited to *abo Mgbe*.

High-ranking members of *Mgbe* in Kembong (figs. 45–47).

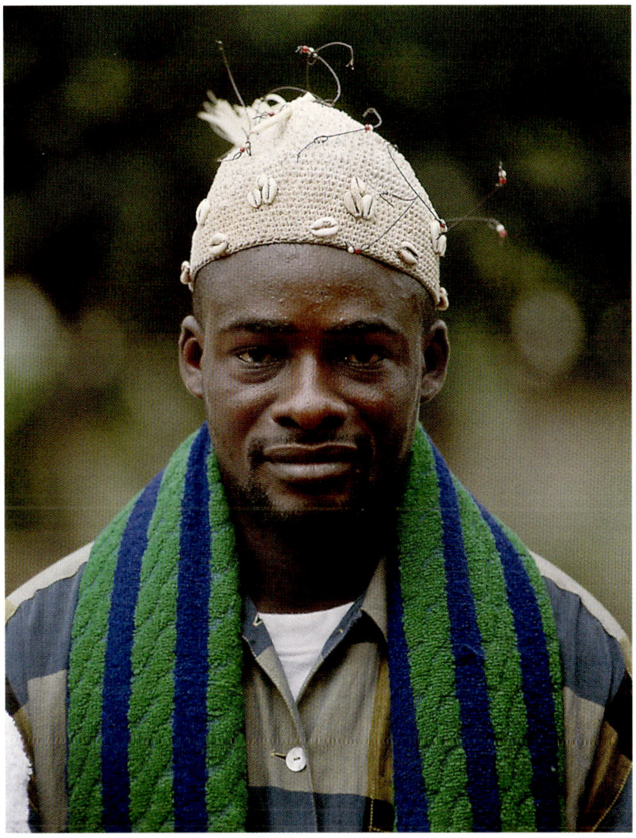

Fig. 45 Ateke Maurice Manyi (Kembong, January 21, 2004).

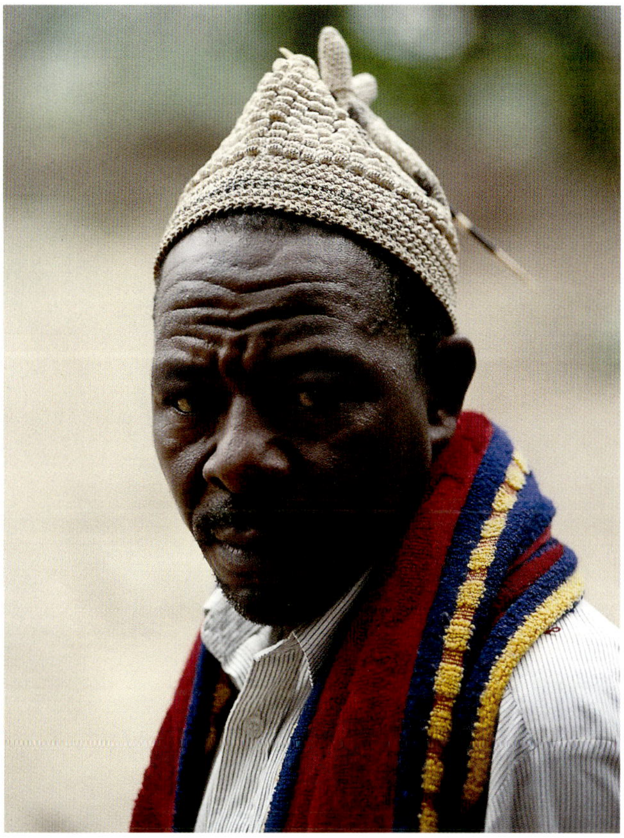

Fig. 46 Atmeyo Petro (Kembong, January 21, 2004).

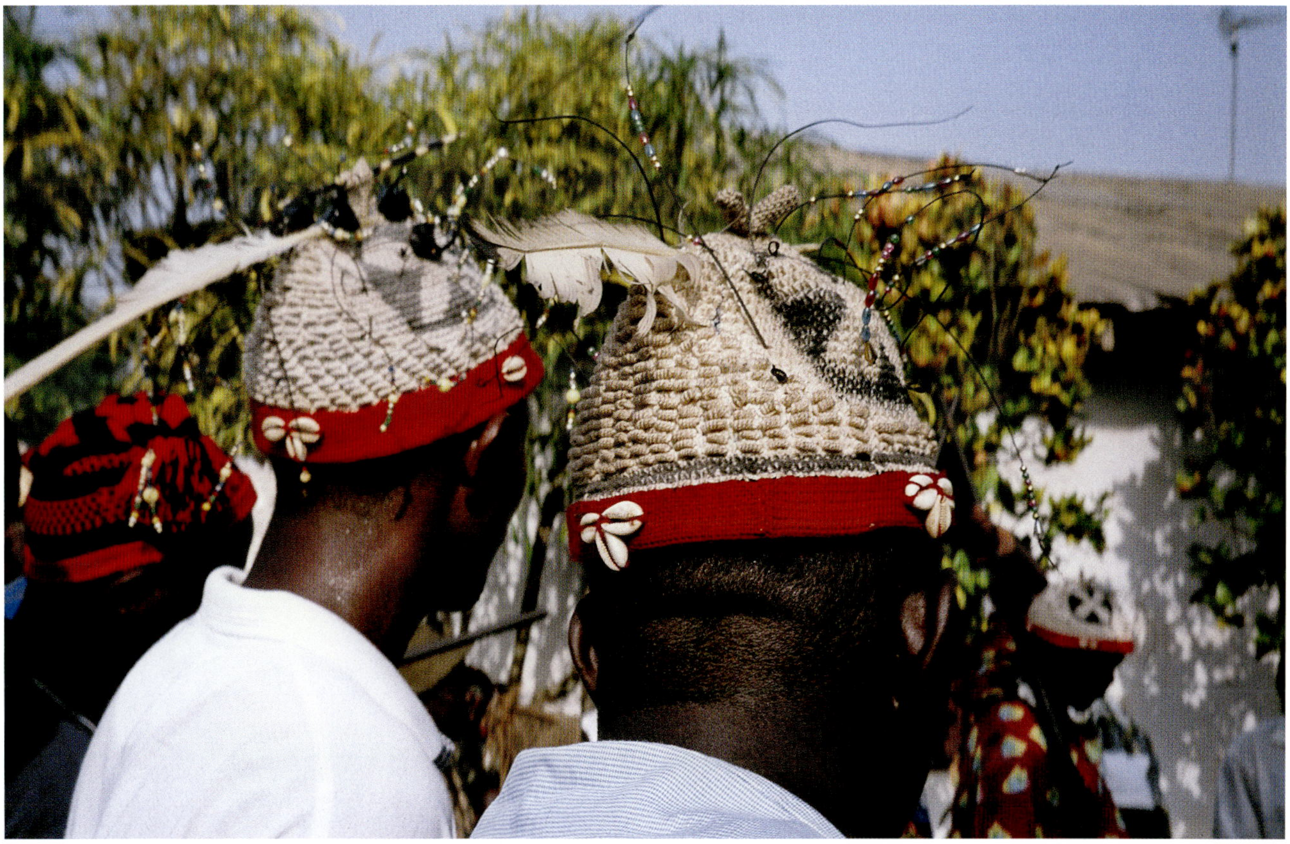

Fig. 47 Unknown (Kembong, March 27, 2005).

Four *boseseku*, leaders of *Mgbe*, in Kembong (figs. 48–51).

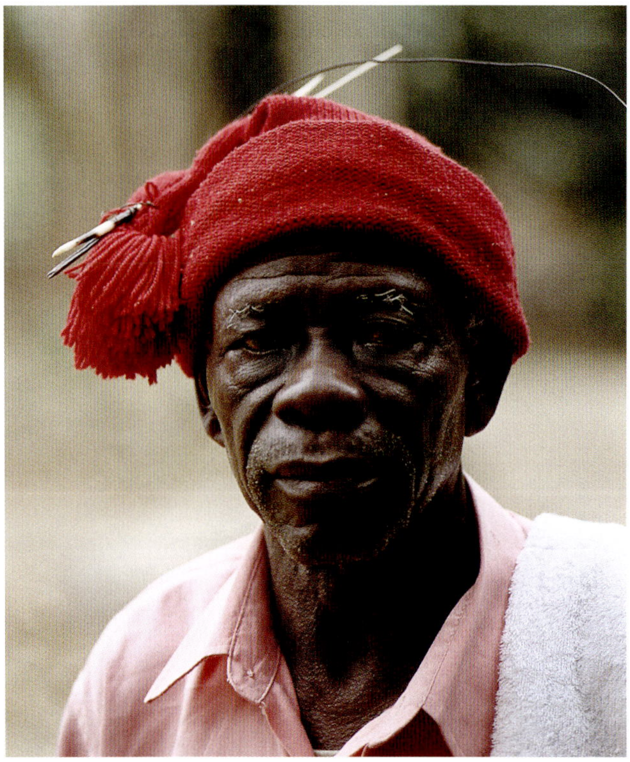

Fig. 48 Johnson Ateke, Takpang (Kembong, January 21, 2004).

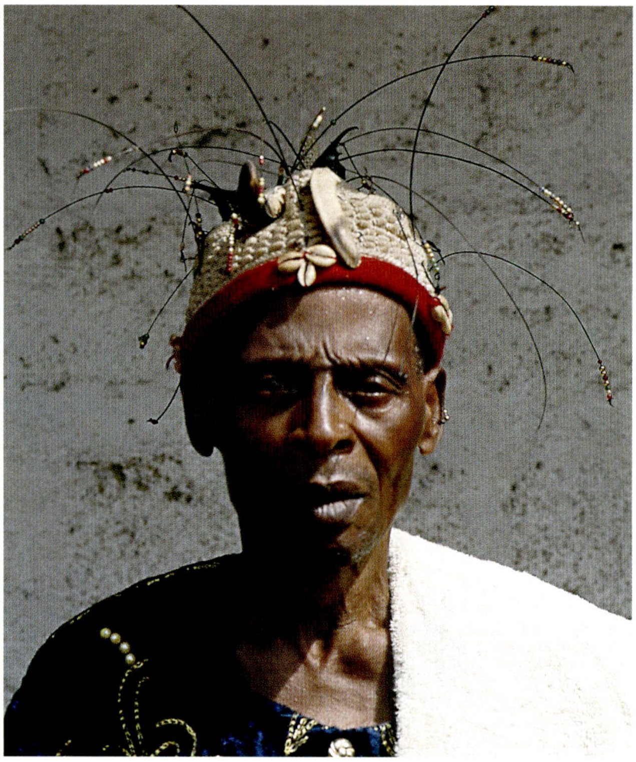

Fig. 49 Ayuk Sampson Enow, Okemebenem (Kembong, April 3, 2005).

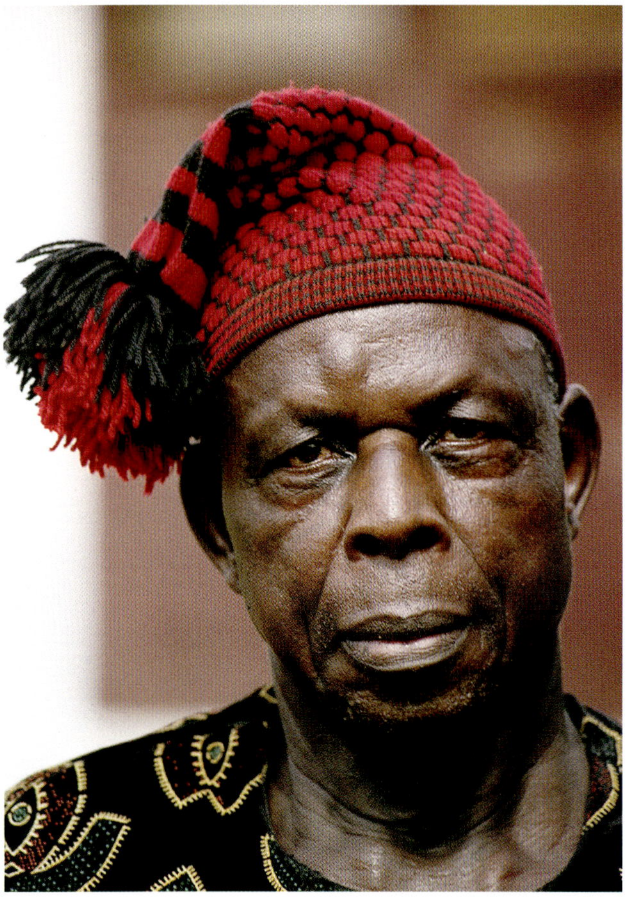

Fig. 50 Elias Tanyi, Okonyenge (Kembong, January 26, 2004).

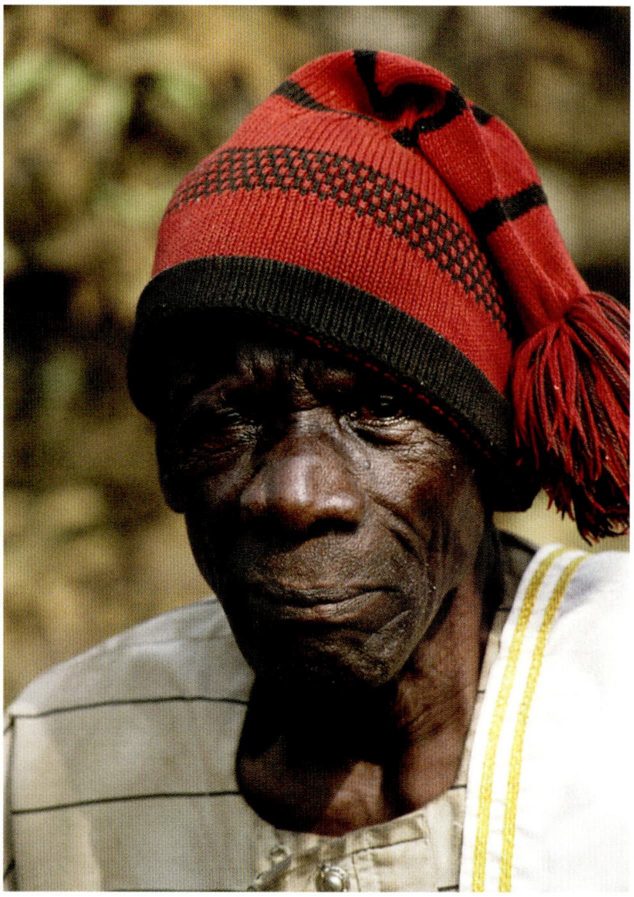

Fig. 51 James Awoh, Okangku (Kembong, January 28, 2004).

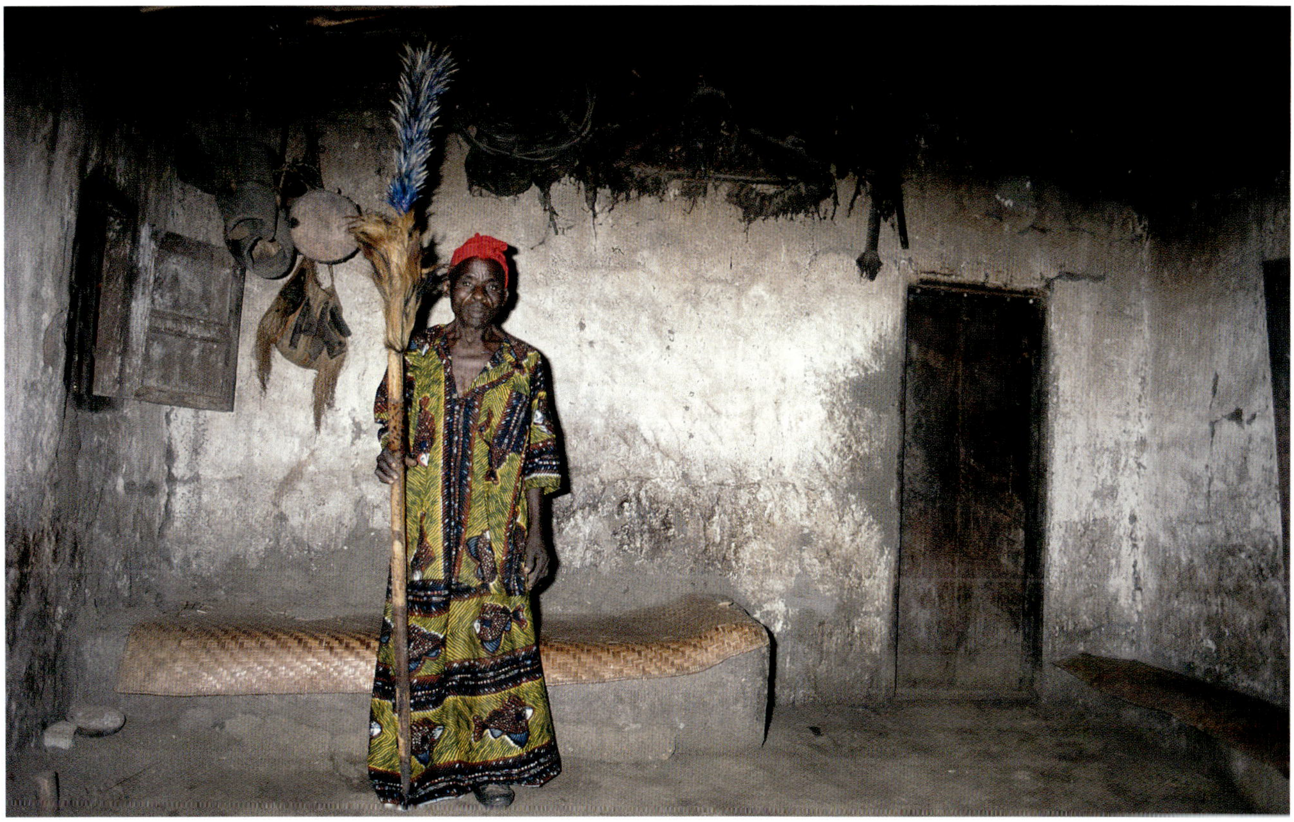

Fig. 52 A *seseku* (Njock Besem Takor, deceased) in his house. He holds the ceremonial staff, *monyo*, in his right hand. Rather indistinct on the wall, left above the door, hangs the "board of *Mgbe*", *orongho Mgbe*. Below covered by the traditional mat is a mud-bed, scarcely extant today (Kembong, February 1, 1980).

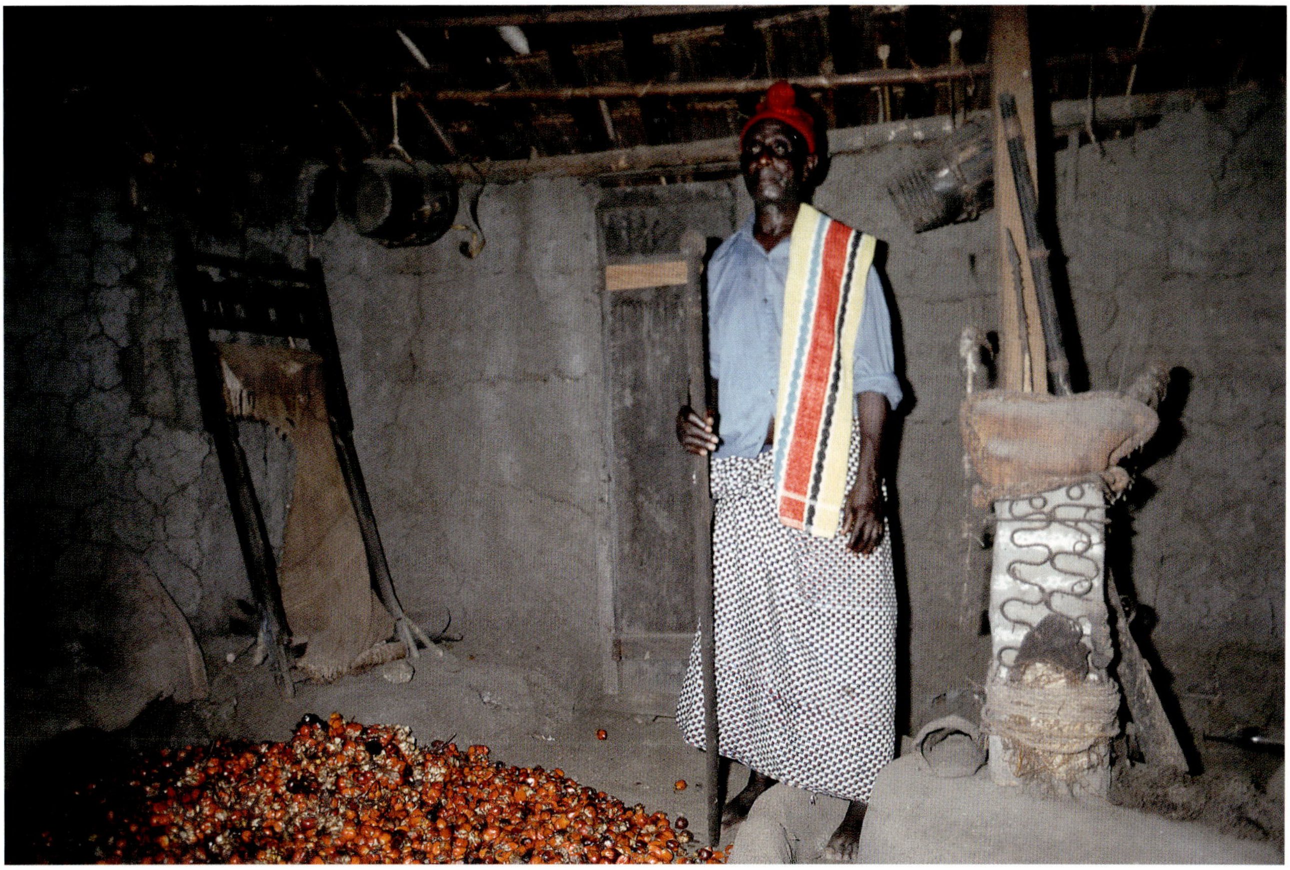

Fig. 53 John Etchu, a *seseku* from Okune and one of the leaders of *Obasinjom* (d. 1996) in his house. Next to him the all important "stone of *Mgbe*", *eteh Mgbe*. This was presumably the last "stone of *Mgbe*" in the possession of a *seseku* in Kembong (Kembong, February 26, 1980).

4.1.3.2.3 The *dikaba*

An important position in *Mgbe* is that of the *dikaba*. This person is the speaker of the society, and he is also the person who counsels the young members and instructs them about the most important rules. Moreover, the *dikaba* is responsible for the distribution of palm wine, food and money. He decides which palm wine is good for *Mgbe* and which should be rejected. When there is a major ceremony, he sits in the room behind the curtain, where the voice of the leopard can be heard. There can be two or three *bodikaba*, according to the size of the lodge. One of them is responsible for the internal sphere, the other for ceremonies that take place outside. If the office is vacant, one of the full members is appointed by *Mgbe*. He does not have to pay any fees, but he is expected to contribute a case of beer.

4.1.3.3 The big men of *Mgbe*

Okume eboho Mgbe ("sitting on the mud-bed of *Mgbe*") is the highest level in *Mgbe*. It is the level of the *achi Mgbe*, "the heads of *Mgbe*" and refers to the core members of a lodge. There are about three to six members depending upon the size of the lodge. One of them is the *seseku*, the president, while another title bearer is *osongaribo*, his representative. The *achi Mgbe* are informed about all matters concerning the society and make all of the important decisions. In contrast to the other members, they alone have the right to drink palm wine while seated. At gatherings all of these big men sit on a special bench, formerly on the mud-bed (fig. 52), which is at the front of the room and faces the ordinary members.

The fees to be paid for this level comprise one goat, 30 litres of palm wine, two bottles of palm oil, two cups of salt and two cups of pepper.

4.1.3.3.1 *Osongaribo*

Fees: two "animals", 30 litres of palm wine, two bunches of plantains, two bottles of palm oil, two cups of salt and two cups of pepper.

The *osongaribo* is the representative of the *seseku*. When the latter makes an offering, it is the *osongaribo* who assists him. And at the performance of *Ebongu*, the *seseku* who leads the group is constantly "threatened" by his *osongaribo* with a cutlass, symbolising that the *seseku* should be "killed", so that the *osongaribo* can take over his position (figs. 59, 75).[33] Yet, in fact, an *osongaribo* automatically succeeds upon the death of "his" *seseku*.

4.1.3.3.2 The *seseku*

The chief or "president" in every lodge of *Mgbe* is the *seseku* (pl. *boseseku*) (figs. 38, 48–53, 57, 59, 60, 64–66, 68–71, 75, 77–80, 85, 91, 93, 94). He is also designated *eyamba*, but only few persons know this name and it is seldom used.[34] The *seseku* is generally respected and honoured as a figure of authority, regardless of his age. He is of course well informed about all matters pertaining to *Mgbe*, he conducts offerings to the ancestors, and without him sitting upon his seat no important decision of the society can be made – the *seseku* has the last say in *Mgbe*. The *seseku* sits in a central position among the big men, and he receives the first and always the largest share in wine, food and money, when such is shared amongst the members. If the leopard is present at a meeting of *Mgbe*, it turns to the *seseku* alone when greeting the members.

A sign of a *seseku* is a towel or a similar cloth (*mbom*, pl. *abom*), which he wears over his left shoulder (figs. 38, 53, 57, 69–71, 85, 91, 93). All those who have attained full membership may wear the towel around their neck. The use of the towel is as old as *Mgbe* itself, but as there were no towels in early days, pieces of cloth or woven materials were used instead. A special sign of a *seseku* is the ceremonial staff called *monyo*, which is wrapped with pieces of hide of various animals – leopard, antelope, cow, sheep – and crowned with colourful feathers. The staff is used only at ceremonial events and not in daily life (cp. p. 93) (figs. 52, 71).[35]

One of the most important possessions of a *seseku* is the *orongho Mgbe* (pl. *arongho Mgbe*), the "board of *Mgbe*", and *eteh Mgbe*, the "stone of *Mgbe*". All *boseseku* have the right to these holdings. The *orongho Mgbe* consists of a mat, square or rectangular with a side length of 100–130 cm, to which animal skulls and other objects are attached (figs. 52, 54, 55).[36] The board is the property of the lodge and in the possession of the respective *seseku* at the time; it is both of profound meaning and an indispensable sign of authority. The *orongho Mgbe* usually hangs on the wall in the *seseku's* living room, where the curtain of *Mgbe* is hung during death celebrations. And it is precisely this curtain behind which the leopard abides during these celebrations. Various objects are fastened to the mat. The aforementioned animal skulls are from bovines, goats and antelopes, among others, which were slaughtered and eaten at the

Two examples of the "board of *Mgbe*", *orongho Mgbe*, the most precious object of *Mgbe* (figs. 54, 55).

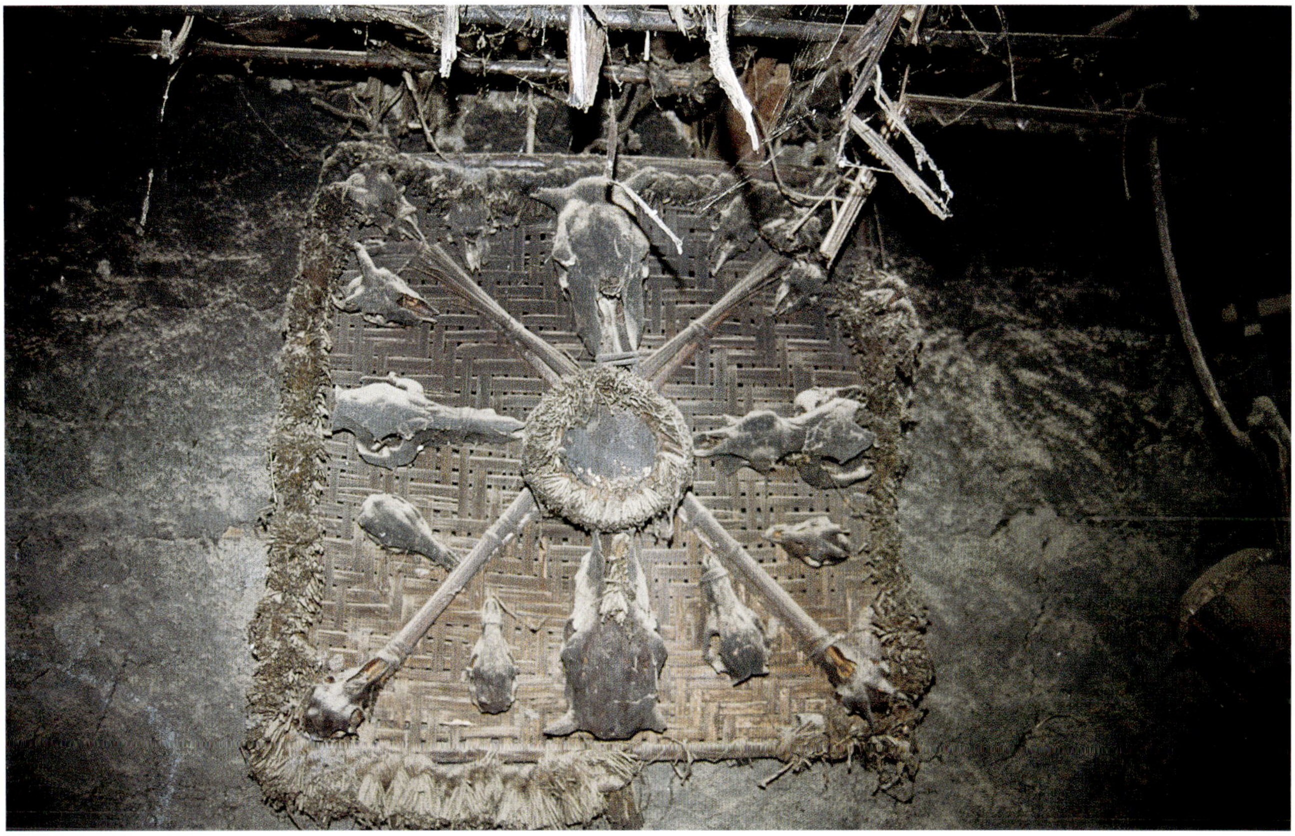

Fig. 54 The *orongho Mgbe* of Elias Tanyi, Okonyenge (Kembong, January 19, 2004).

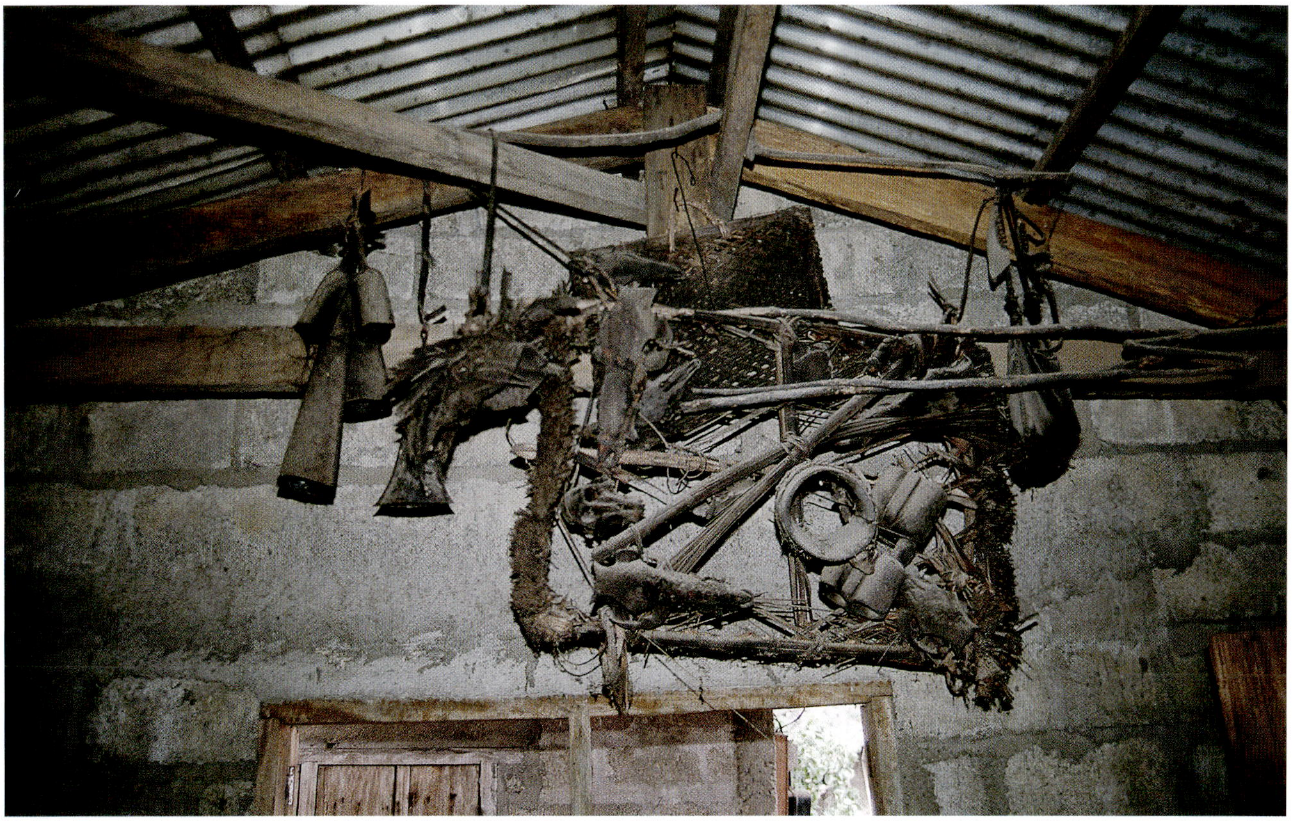

Fig. 55 The *orongho Mgbe* of Ayuk Sampson Enow, Okemebenem (Kembong, April 3, 2005).

feast on the occasion of the installation of the respective mat. Attached to the mat as well are musical instruments, in particular drums and rattles used by *Mgbe*. The drum is especially meaningful, as it contains magic medicines to fend off hostile forces. Typical of the *orongho Mgbe* are two brooms, fastened diagonally, small calabasses, bags and the like. Details about these are unknown to the public, for the secrets surrounding the *orongho Mgbe* are strictly preserved. The *orongho Mgbe* are never utilised in ceremonies or rituals; they are exclusively the insignia of the *boseseku* and in their safekeeping. Upon the death of a *seseku*, his successor takes over the *orongho Mgbe*. Additional fees are not required, for the assumption of *orongho Mgbe* is part of the installation of the *boseseku*. Since the 1970s great numbers of *orongho Mgbe* have been purchased by dealers, for they were in great demand on the international art market.[37]

The "stone of *Mgbe*" (*eteh Mgbe*, pl. *ateh Mgbe*) is the most important ritual object in the sphere of *Mgbe* (fig. 53).[38] Only the *boseseku* are entitled to its possession, but at present no *seseku* in Kembong has acquired the stone as yet. One reason for this are the high fees required (one goat, 50 litres of palm wine, two bundles of plantains, two bottles of palm oil, two cups of salt, two cups of pepper), and the other reason is the prevailing fear that the *seseku* who acquires the "stone of *Mgbe*" will not live very long. The setting of the stone represents the highest level in *Mgbe*, and this is only achieved after attaining all other levels, usually two to four years following initiation as *seseku*. In addition, the person must have reached a certain age, he must possess a strong heart, and he must be honest, reputable, trustworthy and courageous. Moreover, acquisition of the stone is connected with a further condition, to which the respective *seseku* is strictly bound: He may plant the stone only after he has gained five to ten new members for his lodge.

Setting the "stone of *Mgbe*" involves an elaborate ceremony, in which the members of all befriended *Mgbe* lodges partake. First the necessary medicine plants must be sought in the bush. Of special importance is the bark of a certain tree. Upon finding this tree, the leader of the *Mgbe* members spits on it with alligator pepper and says: "We have come to take you, because you are the stick for *eteh Mgbe*." He then takes a chicken with his left hand, saying: "This is your fowl" and lays it at the trunk of the tree. He takes the chicken again and swings it in the air three times, saying: "This is your fowl. We have come to take you, because you are the stick for *eteh Mgbe*." Now the leader holds the chicken with his right hand, swings it in the air four times and repeats the words. With a cutlass, held first in the left hand and then in the right hand, he removes some bark and lets it fall onto the ground. The pattern made by the falling pieces of bark serves as an oracle, announcing the ancestors' acceptance or refusal of the whole ritual. If the oracle is negative at first, the aspirant must be treated with a special medicine: "In the bush this stick saw some trouble with you and you have now accepted your trouble. Now I bless you, so that you may plant this stone. If all is well, let the oracle accept it."

Setting the stone (*eteh Mgbe*) takes place in the evening. After digging a hole the new owner secretly places a small stone, the so-called heart of *Mgbe* in it. This is a secret known to only few of the men.[39] Then a goat and a dog are slain, and their blood is directed towards the hole. When *eteh Mgbe* has been set into the hole, the new owner rubs it with medicine: "Mr. X, you have died, and this stone, although lying on the ground, still has your marks on it. Today we want to install it in the name of Mr. Y (his own name). I therefore wash your marks on the stone (rubbing it with his left hand). Here is your food, here is your meat, and here is your wine." The medicine that he takes into his right hand is meant for the living: "I wash the stone now as I have been accepted by the society to be the new chief and now I install it." At this point the *eteh Mgbe* can be set upright: "As this stone has been installed, we are praying for the birth of children, for good catches during hunting-expeditions and for peace in the entire community." He rubs white and yellow pigment upon the stone, for it should be pleasing in appearance. In addition, the stone is decorated with various objects: a cutlass, a rifle, a cord with medicine plants wound about it, a spear, a tortoise shell and a feather. A cap is set upon its "head", and the chest is formed by iron rods. The stone is placed so that persons entering the room see it immediately.

The stone has no direct use in ceremonies and rituals; it is primarily the sign of a big man. But once a year it is the centre of attention, namely when a ceremony of offerings is made for the ancestors. In the case of serious problems and grave failures a person can direct a prayer to God by standing next to the stone and speaking: "*Obasi*, you sent us on earth and taught us how to do these things for our well-being. Help us, therefore, as we carry out this act and plea with you on behalf of the hunters. We received these things from you, now we want to assure you that they will not be lost. Take this food and wine and eat and open the eyes for our hunters to see animals. And let the guns shoot without missing."[40]

When a *seseku* dies, the respective *osongaribo* assumes his office immediately. It is this new *seseku,* who leads the group of *Mgbe* to the grove of *Mgbe* to get the leopard. The ensuing offering to the ancestors – the rituals of death held by *Mgbe* will be discussed in detail later – is already the duty of the new *seseku* (cp. p. 79, 85, 89). Nonetheless, before this activity can be carried out at all, the vacant position of the *osongaribo* must be filled. Only those members who have reached the level of *okume eboho Mgbe* or *eteme Mgbe,* can be considered for this. Above all, the candidate must stem from one of the families, who once contributed towards the acquisition of *Mgbe*. In order to preserve the claim of the founding families to leadership of *Mgbe*, the investiture of a new *osongaribo* – and with it that of a new *seseku* – follows the principle of rotation.[41] This signifies that the *seseku* and the *osongaribo* may not stem from the same family. However, all members of *Mgbe,* whose families are not among the founders, are excluded from the position of *seseku* and *osongaribo* forever.

The fees which a *seseku* must pay to *Mgbe* consist of one goat, 100 litres of palm wine and one bottle of European whisky.

4.1.4 The activities of *Mgbe*

There are no specific days upon which the members of *Mgbe* gather. They meet in the house of the *seseku* only on important occasions: initiations and discussions about matters of law and other problems, and in the house of the deceased for death ceremonies. After Kembong was founded by the Germans – through the fusion of the surrounding hamlets –, the *Mgbe* lodges never had their own house, as is still the normal case in the other regions.[42] Only the quarter of Okonyenge has its own "*Ekpe* Hall" (the hall of *Mgbe*) (figs. 102, 123).

All meetings commence with the official drinking of palm wine.[43] The *dikaba* receives the first glass. He greets *Mgbe* and tests the wine. If he announces that the wine is good and can be drunk, the next glass is given to *okina*, the third glass to *nkakamem* who pours the wine, and the fourth to the *seseku*, who pours some of the wine onto the ground in offering to the ancestors: "I am opening this meeting, because you taught us *Mgbe*. This is your own share." He drinks half of the glass's contents and passes it on to his deputy. He in turn is followed by the members of the other levels. The *seseku* receives the last glass, which he drinks empty and gives to the *nkakamem*. Afterwards the discussions and negotiations begin.

The assembly also concludes with drinking. Everyone may drink as much as he wishes. The last glass is again for the ancestors. The *seseku* first holds a glass in his left hand and addresses them: "*Ata* X, this is your *Mgbe*, which you once started. We have finished our discussions and the wine we have taken. These are the dregs, we give them to you." Then he takes the glass with his right hand, saying: "For those of us who are still alive. Let no one have pains in the head or the neck." At the end of the ritual he holds the glass in both hands and allows the wine to flow onto the ground: "We have drunk. We now throw the wine for you." Then the *seseku* gives the empty glass to the *dikaba*, greets *Mgbe* three times and says "*eoso*" in departing. With that the meeting is brought to an end. If food is to be shared, the *seseku* is given his share first, then the *osongaribo*. The rest of the food is shared amongst the persons present, irrespective of their rank.

The actual function of *Ngbe/Ekpe* is always and everywhere to safeguard social order,[44] and this applies to *Mgbe* in Kembong as well. As mentioned above, in Old Calabar *Ekpe* was "a centralizing legislative, political and executive body".[45] In particular, *Ekpe* was indispensable for the credit system introduced by the Europeans, for it held the authority to collect debts.[46] At the same time *Ekpe* had the power to make laws and thus to function as a governing body.[47] Further, *Ekpe* was the only institution in Old Calabar, which was "capable of maintaining peace between different groups or of stopping fights."[48]

In Kembong *Mgbe* watches over social order, but it is not in charge of making political decisions in a broader sense, as is the case especially with larger ethnic groups.[49] In Kembong this is the matter of *Etek* alone, the assembly of the people; however, only *Mgbe* is capable of enforcing the orders decided upon in *Etek*.[50] Therefore, a trusting cooperation between the two institutions is indispensable. There is further reason for the close association between them, because in Kembong basically the same persons make the decisions: on the one hand, as big men in *Etek* and on the other, as big men in *Mgbe*. Yet, the institution that is of greater significance is *Etek*, for it embraces all men as well as women – it represents the people, indeed *Etek* is the people itself. And aside from that, it was *Etek* that at one time made the decision to acquire *Mgbe*.

It is the responsibility and duty of *Mgbe* to enforce resolutions and orders made by *Etek*, which means that its own members are not only subordinate to *Mgbe*, but at the same time all men and women are under its protection. Whoever suffers injustice can turn to *Mgbe* for

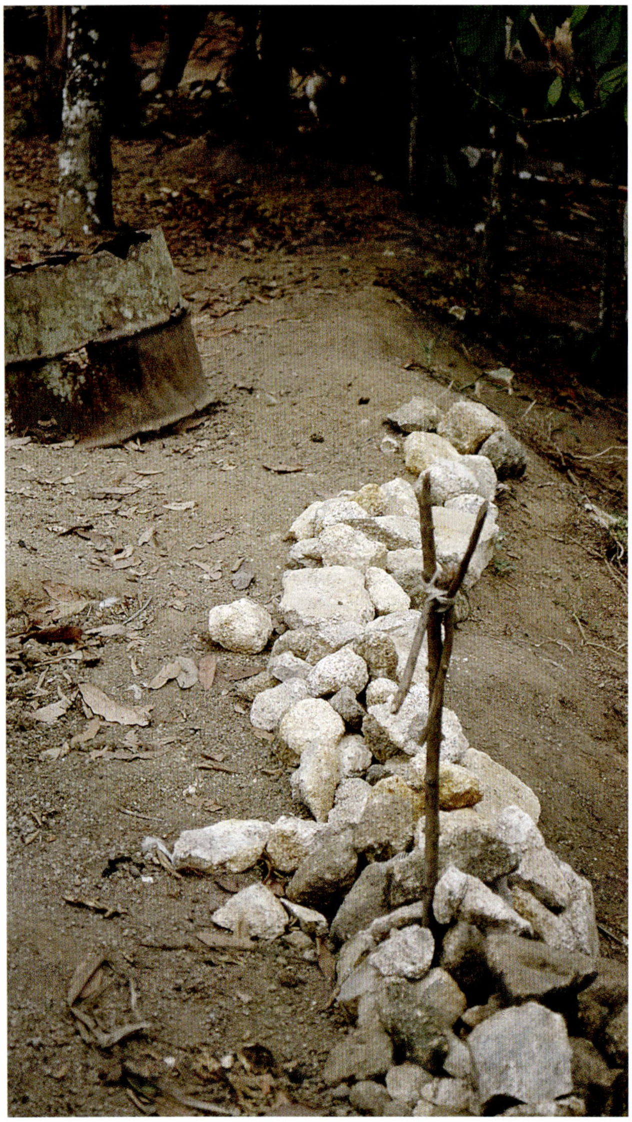

Fig. 56 *Bekundi*, the taboo-sign of *Mgbe*, made of sticks. It was set in place following a conflict about the stones, signalling that they must not be touched until the problem is solved (Kembong, January 21, 2004).

aid.[51] With the assistance of *okina*, the messenger of *Mgbe*, the *seseku* has the right to order a person to appear before *Mgbe* at any time. In cases of serious conflicts the *seseku* can order the drum of *Mgbe* to be sounded, and thereafter the conflict must halt immediately. If the conflict involves an object, *Mgbe* marks the item with its special sign – *bekundi* (fig. 56). No one dares to touch the object, until *Mgbe* has passed judgement in the case and *bekundi* is removed. It is worthy of note that this object is not treated with medicine, as would be the case in the Cameroon Grasslands;[52] with the Ejagham it is purely secular.[53]

When *Mgbe* deliberates on a case, this usually occurs "behind closed doors", that is, with the exclusion of the public. Occasionally non-members are called to the hearings: plaintiffs, the accused or witnesses. Minor offences are tried before the general assembly of *Mgbe*, and all members may participate in the discussions. Serious conflicts and major offences are not a matter for a single lodge, but several, and only the big men pass judgement. In especially difficult cases the discussions take place in the grove of *Mgbe*.

In earlier times, major offenders were either sold as slaves or sentenced to death – they were executed with a cutlass or hanged. Aside from the fact that serious violations have long been the matter of the public courts, today penalties imposed by *Mgbe* mainly involve payments of animals, palm wine and money.[54] In such cases the penalisation for various transgressions and malevolent acts is not clearly defined; instead it is oriented towards the social status and financial potential of the perpetrator. Those who are wealthy must reckon with higher penalties than persons who are less affluent or poor. This accords with a prayer of *Mgbe*, which will be presented in its entire length below (cp. p. 89): "Let there be plenty of food and drinks. We want defaulters to be rich people and not poor people."

Sentences ordering social isolation are the consequence of serious offences.[55] In such cases *Mgbe* announces that every form of contact and cooperation with the censured person is prohibited; further, the person is not permitted to go to the market. No one may speak to the person or – much less – visit him or her. Thus, the sentenced person is cast out of society: "If he proves to be more than the people, let him go." Social isolation as punishment is not restricted to *Mgbe* alone, but can be decreed by *Etek*, the assembly of the community, as well as by *Mawu*, the women's society.

In Kembong *Mgbe* still maintains social peace and harmony today. For example, when conflicts involving physical attack between two women broke out on November 19–20, 2005, in the quarter Okemebenem, *Mgbe* took action. In the night of November 21, 2005, the beating of the tortoise shell (*nkwui*, pl. *okwui*) could be heard, calling the members of *Mgbe* to meet in the house of the *seseku*; *Mgbe* had to confer on this incident. The complaints of the women involved in the conflict and of some witnesses were heard, and the judgement was announced on the following morning. Both women were convicted, and each had to pay a fine of 10,000 Francs CFA (c. 15 Euro). The fines ordered by *Mgbe* had to be paid immediately, which one of the women obeyed. Meanwhile, the other woman, as was later discovered, had left Kembong in a taxi. It was presumed that she fled to one of the towns in the south. Yet, *Mgbe* did not retract the punishment.

Quite the opposite, as is common in such cases, her family was made responsible for payment of the fine; it was her father who had to pay the 10,000 Francs CFA. The general conviction among the populace was that the woman who had fled from *Mgbe* would never dare to return to Kembong. If she were to do so, she would have to reckon with being socially isolated or outcast. The 20,000 Francs CFA-fine was not utilised for purposes in the interest of the community; quite the opposite, it was *Mgbe's* alone and was used to buy beer.

If non-members should happen to see things or actions that are otherwise prohibited to them, they are obliged to enter *Mgbe*. Their penalty is then reckoned as part of the fees for their initiation. As I was repeatedly assured, women are never in danger of getting near the secret activities of *Mgbe*. For example, when *okongo* appears, it is the duty of some of the members to ensure that no unauthorised persons disturb the dances. Over and above, the evil forest is absolutely taboo for all non-members and outsiders.

Offences against the internal rules and laws of *Mgbe* by members of the society itself are harshly punished. Nonetheless, a measure of clemency and leniency is shown to younger members, who are not yet well-informed about all of the regulations and customs. Members of *Mgbe* societies in other areas, who are convicted of an offence in Kembong, are not punished in Kembong, but by their own society after it has been informed of the proceedings by *Mgbe* in Kembong. Information is sent by messengers, telephone, telefax or, as expressly stated, by e-mail.[56]

4.1.5 *Mgbe* and its association with the leopard

Especially in former times *Mgbe* held practically unlimited authority over the population, that is, over non-members as well as its own members. For non-members *Mgbe* is still an incalculable and – for those in guilt – a merciless power; non-members are ignorant of who *Mgbe* is and in which manner it acts. The basic concept of many secret societies in Africa is that they consult and make decisions in seclusion and secrecy and are not prepared to hold any public discussion. Hence, outsiders are principally forced to follow *Mgbe's* orders without comment and to avoid its proximity.

The immense authority of *Mgbe* is foremost a consequence of its association with the leopard, to which its name refers. The leopard forms the absolute centre of the society. Most secrets of *Mgbe* pertain to this animal. Even today, when the voice of the leopard sounds, all people should be aware of the presence and power of *Mgbe*. While the real animal itself is considered to be extremely aggressive and dangerous, this applies all the more to the leopard of *Mgbe*. It is associated with all the attributes of the animal, and at the same time is believed to be a supernatural creature, which no outsider has ever seen. For the abode of this leopard is the "evil forest", which only high-ranking members of *Mgbe* may enter upon special occasions. When the leopard is brought into the community – death celebrations for deceased members may not be held without the presence of the leopard –, its voice alone is heard. The leopard is invisible to non-members, thus appearing all the more uncanny and threatening. Even the masks of *Mgbe* are not associated with leopards in any way, as will be discussed below.

This characterisation of the most important and at the same time most feared secret society of the Ejagham – with special emphasis upon the supernatural powers of the leopard – can be understood as the official version of *Mgbe* about itself, which is continually circulated among non-members in order to demonstrate its power and authority. But not everyone in the community supports or abides by this completely. Nevertheless, it is *Mgbe's* self-depiction that has found its way into ethnographic literature. Talbot was one of the first who attributed the might of *Ngbe/Ekpe* to the strength of leopards: "On account of the superior craft and power of the animal it would naturally draw to itself the largest following."[57] However, the information that *Mgbe* imparts to non-members does not suffice at all for a somewhat reliable description and explanation of *Mgbe's* actual practices and concepts – outsiders are intentionally misled.[58]

Promptly during the first phase of their initiation young members of *Mgbe* already learn about an essential sphere of knowledge of the esoteric, which is indispensable for correct conduct among the members themselves, but equally necessary for the scholarly comprehension of the meaning and purpose of *Mgbe*. They are confronted with the greatest secret of *Mgbe*, namely the secret instrument with which the voice of the leopard is imitated. They learn that it is not a "real" leopard, whose voice is heard at death celebrations and which means that its presence is only simulated for non-members. All of my informants on *Mgbe* declared unanimously that no one in *Mgbe* has ever believed in the existence of the leopard in the grove of *Mgbe*. Further, every rational person in the community, who is not a member of *Mgbe*, knows that no leopard exists in the grove of *Mgbe*, and that it is only a "game", when it is announced that the leopard will be brought into the community (figs. 57, 58). However, it is a game with firm rules, and everyone is well-advised to observe them exactly. Whatever the individual may personally think about this game, that is, how he may imagine the figure of the leopard, is of less significance; he must follow the orders and rules of *Mgbe*.

Nevertheless, the society does not identify itself with the leopard without reason. Indeed, it is no doubt a very dangerous animal, which in addition acts in concealment and only seldom comes into human view. The message, therefore, is obvious for all: whoever opposes *Mgbe* is making a big mistake. The same relates to many other African peoples. For them the leopard is also the most important and meaningful symbol of authority and power, and this applies especially to the Cameroon Grasslands.[59] By contrast, in *Mgbe* there is absolutely no ritual connection to a leopard spirit, to whom offerings are made and prayers addressed. All of the prayers that I heard in *Mgbe* were directed solely to God and the ancestors and deceased, just as in associations with magic medicines (*ajom*). Talbot, who as mentioned, traced the power of *Ngbe/Ekpe* to its association with the leopard, nonetheless concluded: "The name of Obassi is invoked before every sacrifice, and an oblation of food and drink is laid in front of the Etai Ngbe (leopard stone)."[60]

In complete conformity with the conviction that *Ngbe/Ekpe* owes its power and strength to the leopard spirit, throughout ethnographic literature its masks are also understood as representations of spirits,[61] probably in conjunction mainly with Talbot, for whom a mask was "a spirit summoned from the woods, and bearing assumption of a sylvan character by carrying a branch of a tree in the hand not engaged with the whip."[62] However, the question still arises as to whether the many studies that approach the existence of a "leopard spirit" in a matter-of-fact attitude are actually based upon intensive and lengthy research, which is essential for such a difficult and important object of research as comprehending *Mgbe*.

As will become clear in association with masks of other secret societies, masks in the Cross River region are not at all representations or incarnations of various spirits; they are, as I could also ascertain in the Cameroon Grasslands, beings in their own right. Although most masks display attributes of the human body or of animals, they do not depict any natural or supernatural beings. *Ebongu* and *Ema* are not seen as an embodiment or a representation of leopards. Instead they are independent beings, new creations that are taken over from the ancestors and towards whom special behaviour is shown on the part of all, that is, by members of *Mgbe* as well as non-members. Explanations as to the form of their existence are superfluous – *Ebongu* is simply *Ebongu*, and *Ema* is *Ema*.

As mentioned above, the sphere of masks in the Cross River region is not connected with extreme secrecy, as is the case in other regions of Africa, for example in the neighbouring Cameroon Grasslands. In the Cross River region there are no secrets of that nature. The masks of *Mgbe*, *Ebongu/Ema* and *Nkanda* (cp. p. 65 f., 106) are not even treated with medicine and, furthermore, they are not used in the pursuit of witches nor in the chastisement of wrongdoers. These masks perform solely at funeral and commemorative ceremonies for deceased members of *Mgbe*. It is expected that they dance beautifully, but at the same time the masks are to demonstrate the strength and unlimited power of *Mgbe* in the community. However, the masks are neither dependent upon a leopard spirit nor do they represent a leopard.

In his study on the political and social foundations of the Banyang, Ruel clearly refuted other authors' attempts to correlate the power of *Ekpe* with "the cultic control of a forest 'spirit' or similar supernatural agency." He, on the contrary, referred to the significance of the ancestors and medicines in the sphere of *Ngbe*: "Whenever I have suggested to Banyang that the power of Ngbe was supernatural this has been strongly denied. Association activities include a ritual or supernatural element, as do most aspects of Banyang life: the blessing of the dead may be asked for in an association context; 'medicines' are used to protect the rights of association members or as a test of truth. But the central purpose or power of Ngbe is in no way supernatural. 'Ngbe', the leopard-like creature that gives its name to the association, is a secular and not a religious symbol."[63] The decree of the Presbyterian Church in c. 1979 – and later other churches – can be viewed as a certain confirmation of this theory: Members of *Mgbe* were accepted into the Christian Church. By contrast, this tolerance has not been bestowed upon the medicine societies (*ajom*) to this day. They are considered to be heathens and their practices as incompatible with Christian beliefs.

4.1.6 Funeral rituals in *Mgbe*

Mgbe is not only an institution, whose principal responsibility is to safeguard social peace and harmony; it also has the obligation – just as many other secret societies in Africa of comparable significance – to conduct funeral ceremonies for its deceased members.[64]

Death celebrations are among the most important religious ceremonies in general. The specific purpose of a death celebration is to ensure that the deceased is buried correctly, that is, that the deceased person is clothed, furnished and "treated" in such a manner that his soul is able to enter the afterlife. There the soul can find its peace and provide the survivors with protection and assistance. The "correct" funeral ceremony must be conducted in an elaborate and painstaking manner that corresponds to the prestige and political influence of the deceased.[65] With the funeral ceremony a family demonstrates its own esteem and wealth, which can often mean that the expenditures involved in such ceremony leave a family almost impoverished.

4.1.6.1 *Ofu akeken nkeku*, "day of burying the corpse"

Rituals of death are by no means the same for all members of *Mgbe*, but are oriented towards the rank that the deceased once held in the society. In principle, during the course of the burial ceremony, *ofu akeken nkeku*, the surviving family must pay *Mgbe* once again the fees for all of the ranks that the deceased achieved and paid for during his membership in the society.[66]

When a member of the *Mgbe* society dies, the chief of the quarter is informed. He in turn orders the women of the family to prepare the body for burial. The corpse is washed with warm water and carried to the main hall in the deceased's compound and – in former times – laid upon the mud-bed (*eboho Mgbe*) (fig. 52). The dead man is dressed by close relatives, who are members of *Mgbe*. Meanwhile the *Mgbe* members are called together, and *okina*, the messenger of *Mgbe*, is sent to the other *Mgbe* lodges in the village. When the corpse has been clothed, the curtain (*okat Mgbe*) is hung on the wall where the corpse lies. Then the table of *Mgbe* (*efem Mgbe*) is decorated for the deceased (fig. 69). However, there is a difference in the setting of the table as well as the hall: *Mgbe's* ornamentation is in full display only at the death of a senior member. And in case he had a stone (*eteh Mgbe*), it is removed. In the meantime other members of *Mgbe* have arrived. All of these differences are only noticeable to members of *Mgbe*. Other people may not enter the room where the corpse lies. The *seseku* is given a cock, and then *Mgbe* prepares to go to the grove of *Mgbe*. The big man leads the procession, holding the cock in his hands. Their intent is to capture the leopard, which will stay in the dead man's compound for one or two weeks.

In the vicinity of the grove the *seseku* swings the cock with his right hand, and when it makes a noise he addresses the leopard: "I am the one approaching your forest to invite you to the village for the celebration of Mr. X's death who has left us today. We have come to take you to the village. Do us no harm as we approach you". The chief and other members, who have attained the level of the bush (*eteme Mgbe*), then enter the forest to collect herbs for the medicine. The other members wait at the entrance.

When returning to the entrance of the grove – the herbs gathered in a bag –, the *seseku* performs a ritual called "taming or placating the leopard". A thick leaf of underbrush called *ngilako* (broad-leafed, colourful and fragrant) is cut and placed upon the ground at the entrance. An egg is then crushed upon it and the *seseku* invokes the dead man: "Mr. X, you have died and we have come to catch the leopard from the grove for your celebration. May your celebration be peaceful." After this the members of *Mgbe* are led back to the deceased's compound by the chief, who holds the cock in his hand (fig. 57). At the end of the group are members with musical instruments: a drum, an iron bell and a tortoise shell (*nkwui*, pl. *okwui*), which is also played as a percussion instrument. The last man in the group carries a branch from a succulent plant (*ekong*, pl. *bekong*), which is used later by the *seseku* in a special ritual. This particular ritual is practised only in *Mgbe* lodges that originate from Echoko; lodges that stem from Ayiko, for instance, are not familiar with it. The last man also carries a bag over his shoulder, in which – as *Mgbe* officially declares – the leopard is concealed. In reality the bag contains herbs (fig. 58).

After *Mgbe* has brought the leopard into the house of the deceased, two *ngilako* leaves from the medicine herbs, which were collected in the grove of *Mgbe,* are placed upon the corpse; they will be used later in an important ritual called "washing of the dead" (*asu Mgbe*). Preparations are made for the appearance of *Ebongu*, which is obligatory at the death of every member of *Mgbe*. This takes place after a drum has been beaten seven times and the leopard has answered seven times.[67]

Then the members of *Ebongu* start dancing together with their mask (figs. 59–63, 75, 76). The mask *Ebongu* appears with its heavy bell, worn at the waist, and makes graceful movements inside and outside the dancing group. The group of *Ebongu* members is led by the *seseku*. He holds a leaf in his mouth, which is to hinder his speaking: "He should not carelessly speak." (figs. 60, 75)[68] In his right hand he holds *ekong* (that is, if his lodge stems from Echoko), the medicine plant that grows in the grove (figs. 59, 60, 75). The *seseku* is

Death celebration for Gregory Ayuknchiobo from Ndengane (Kembong, April 10–16, 2004) (figs. 57–74).

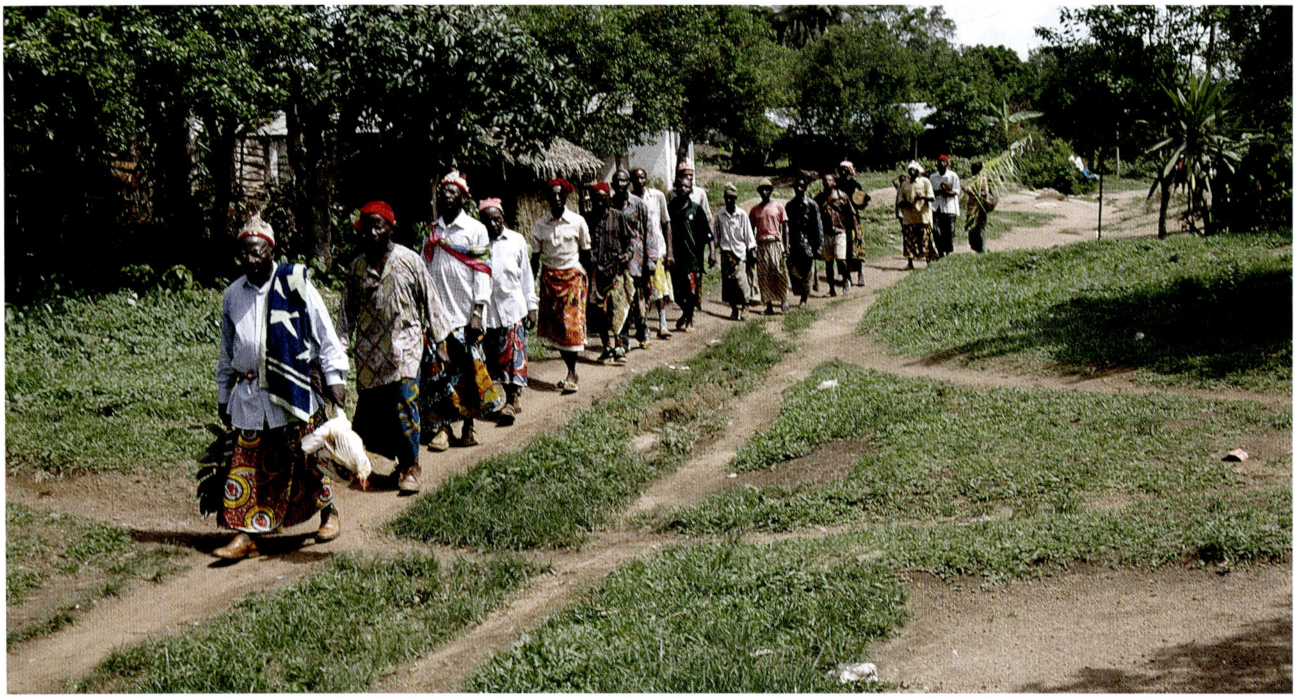

Fig. 57 *Mgbe*, led by the *seseku* Ojong Samuel Ebot from Okune, returning from the grove of *Mgbe*. There the leopard was caught and is now being taken to the house of the deceased (Kembong, April 10, 2004).

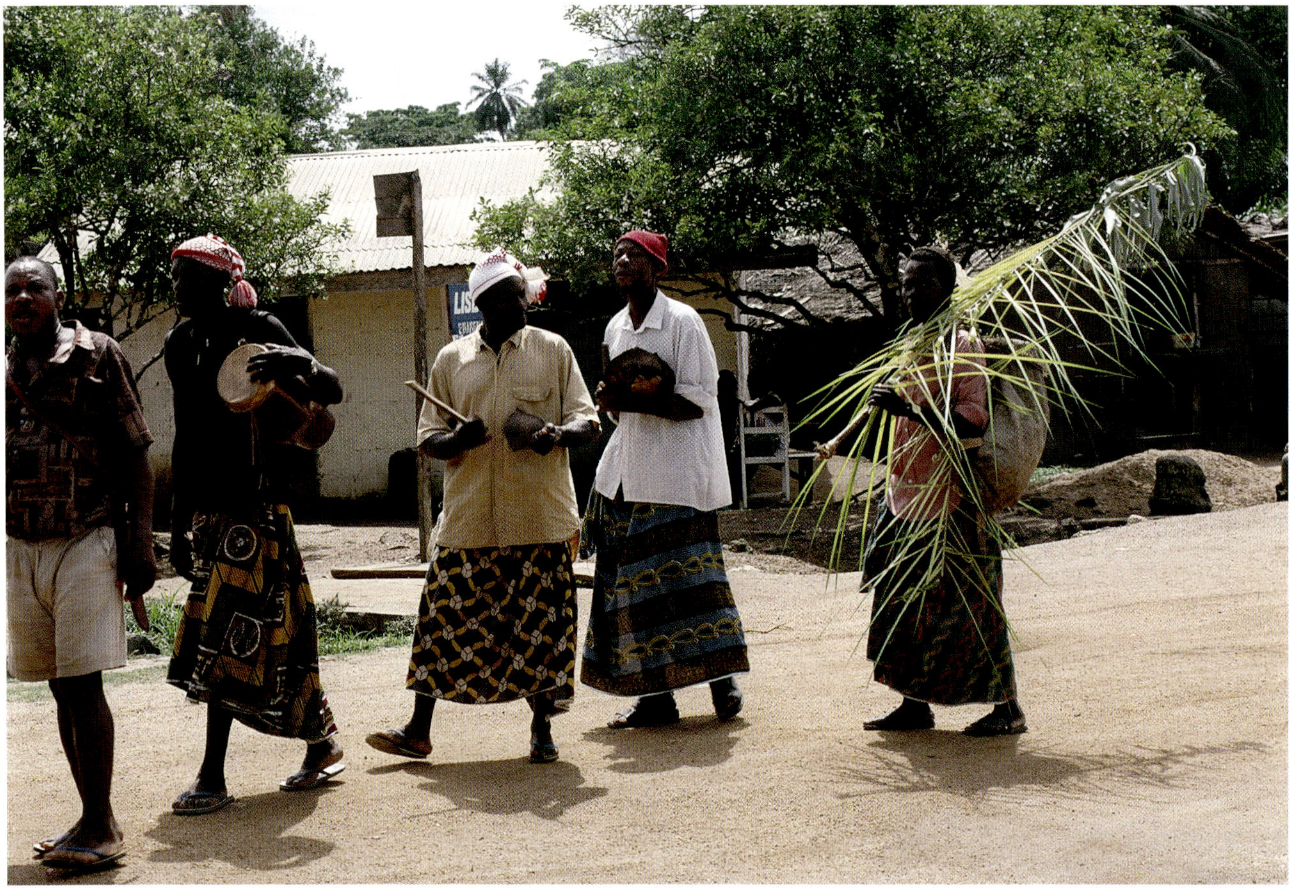

Fig. 58 The last person in the line carries the bag with the captured leopard and the medicine plant *ekong*, also indispensable for this ceremony (Kembong, April 10, 2004).

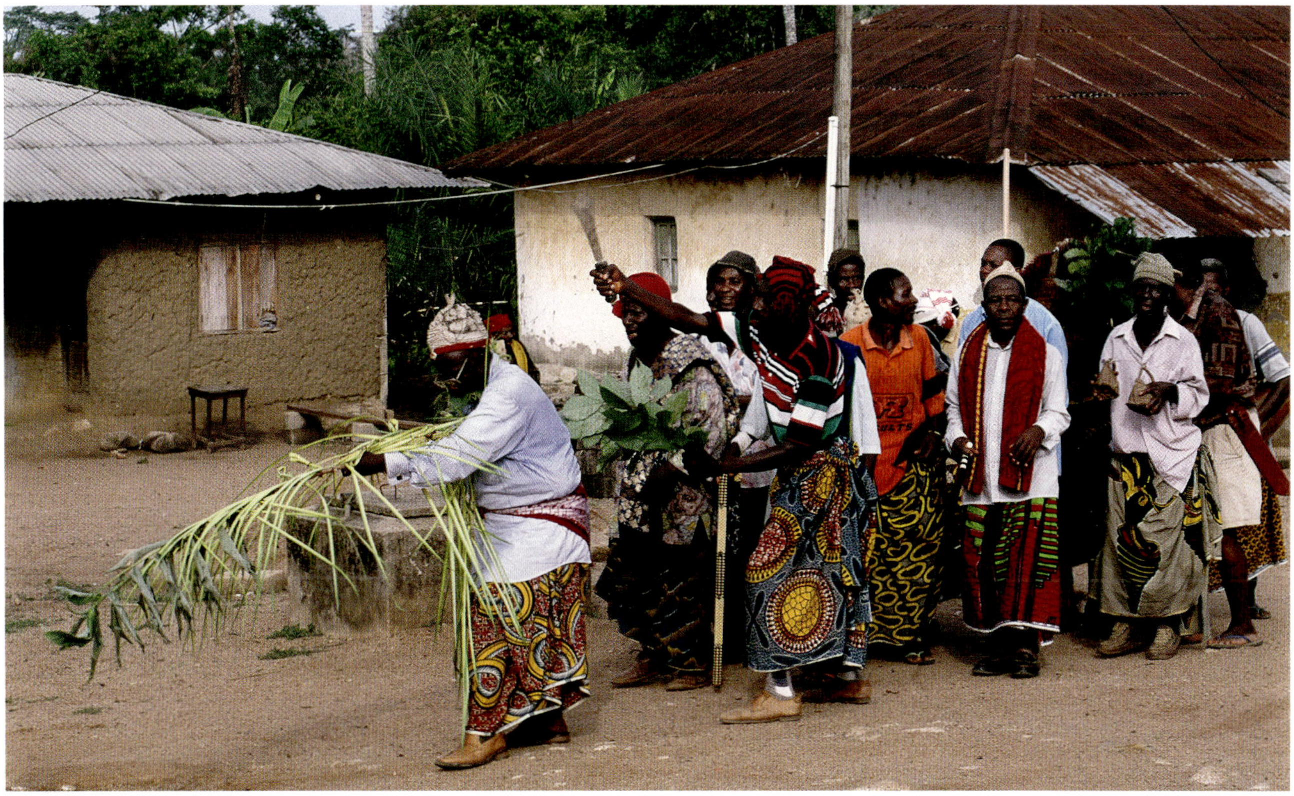

Fig. 59 Performance of *Ebongu* with the *seseku* in the front holding *ekong* in both hands. According to tradition the *seseku* is "threatened" by "his" *osongaribo* with a cutlass (Kembong, April 10, 2004).

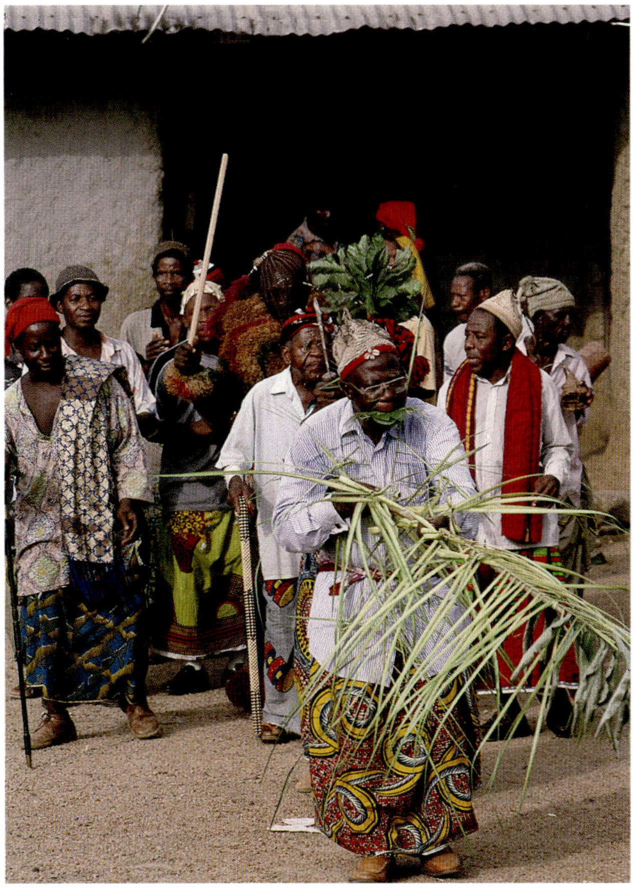

Fig. 60 The *seseku* holds a leaf in his mouth: "He should not carelessly speak" (Kembong, April 10, 2004).

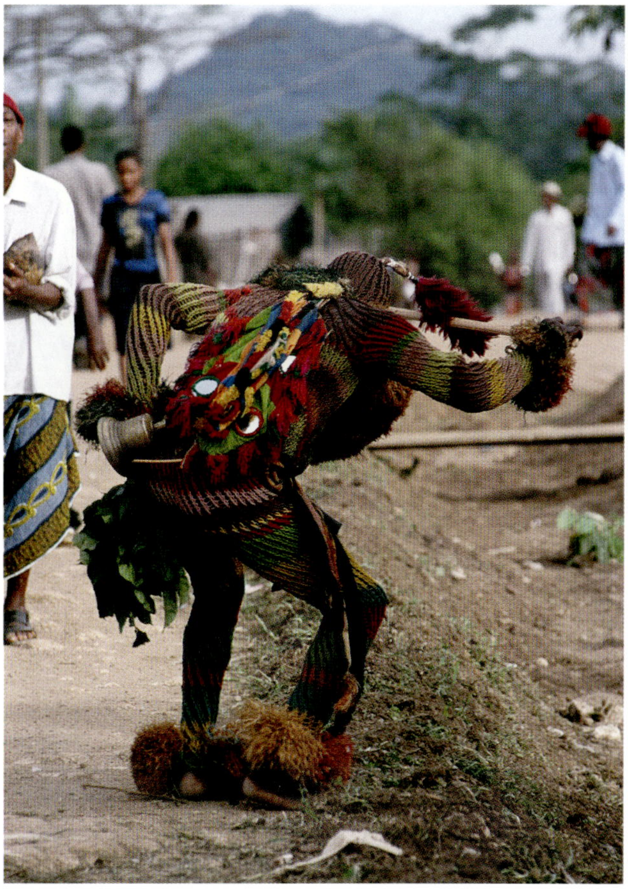

Fig. 61 The highlight of *Ebongu*'s performance is the dance of the mask, clothed in a knitted garment (Kembong, April 10, 2004).

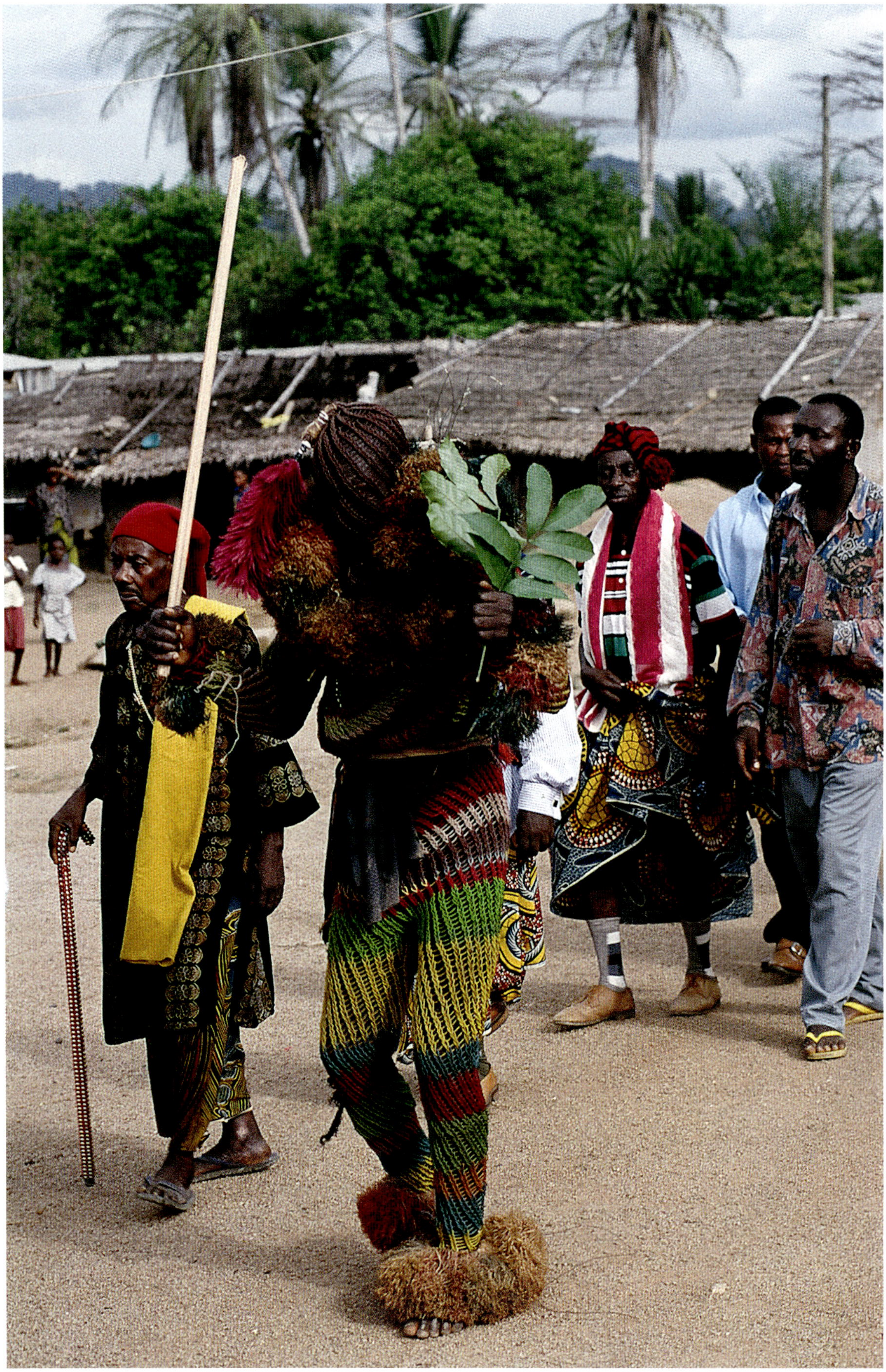

Fig. 62 *Ebongu* at the head of the procession. It holds a stick in the right hand and medicine leaves (*efune Mgbe*) in the left (Kembong, April 10, 2004).

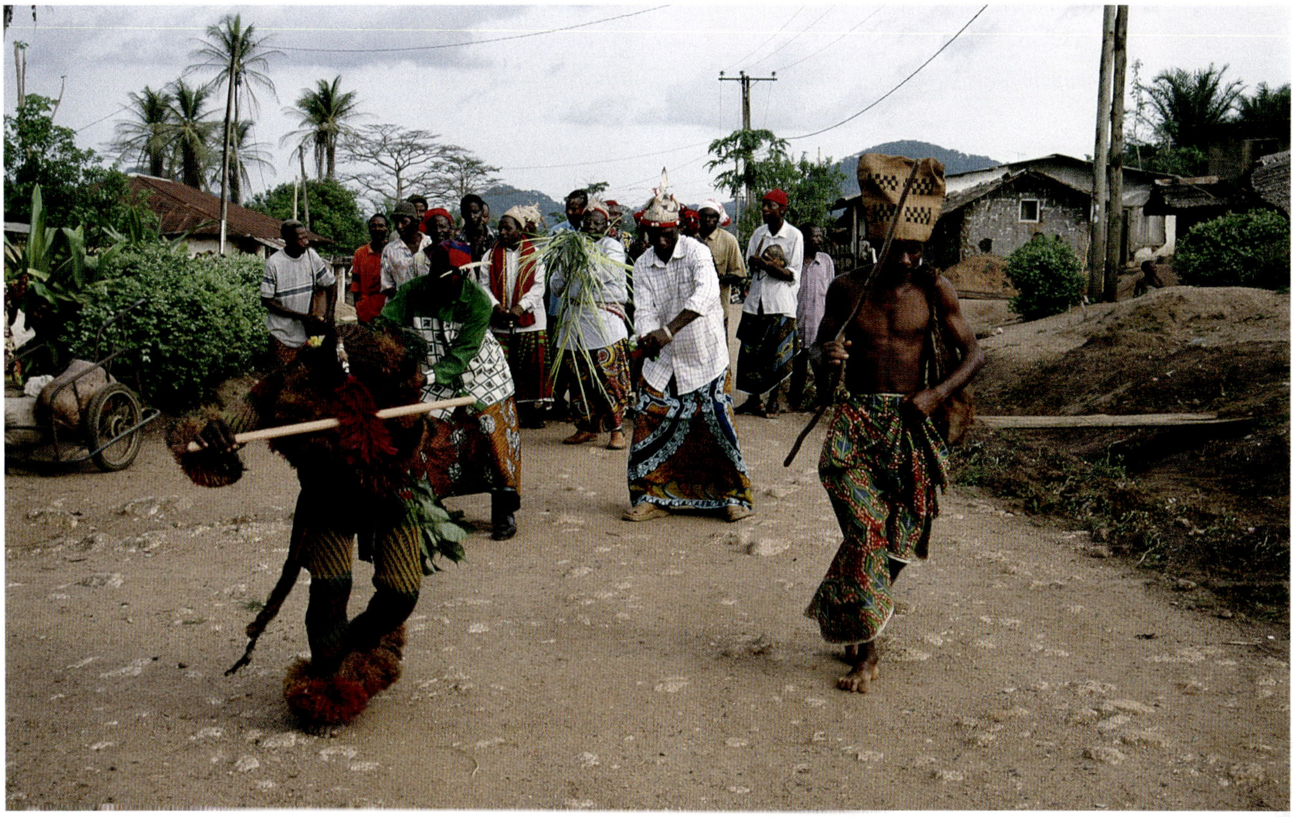

Fig. 63 *Ebongu* in procession with the mask and *okina*, here as a jester, in the foreground (Kembong, April 10, 2004).

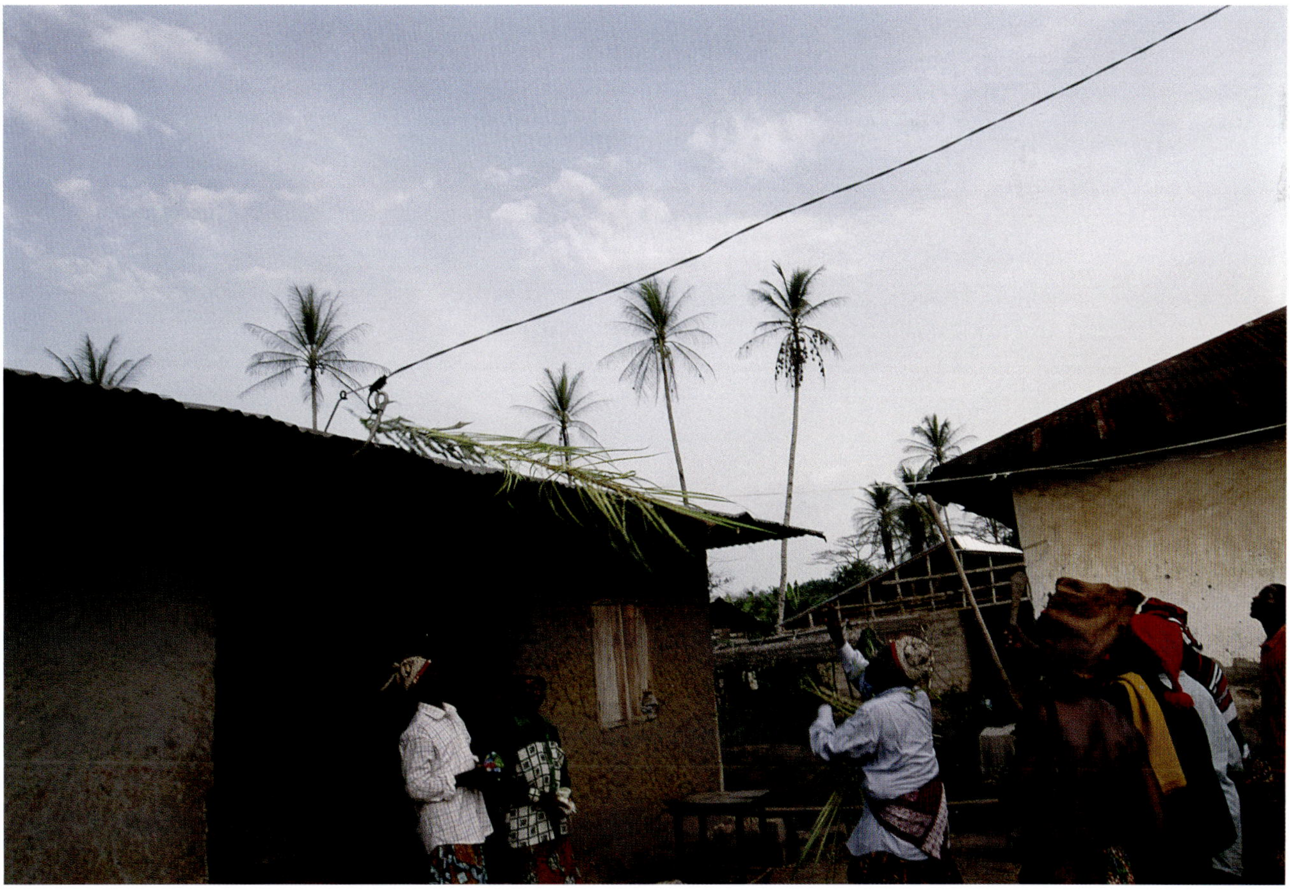

Fig. 64 An important role of the *seseku* (Ojong Samuel Ebot) in the death celebration is to throw *ekong* onto the roof of the deceased's house. When it remains upon the roof, as in this case, all those present are relieved (Kembong, April 10, 2004).

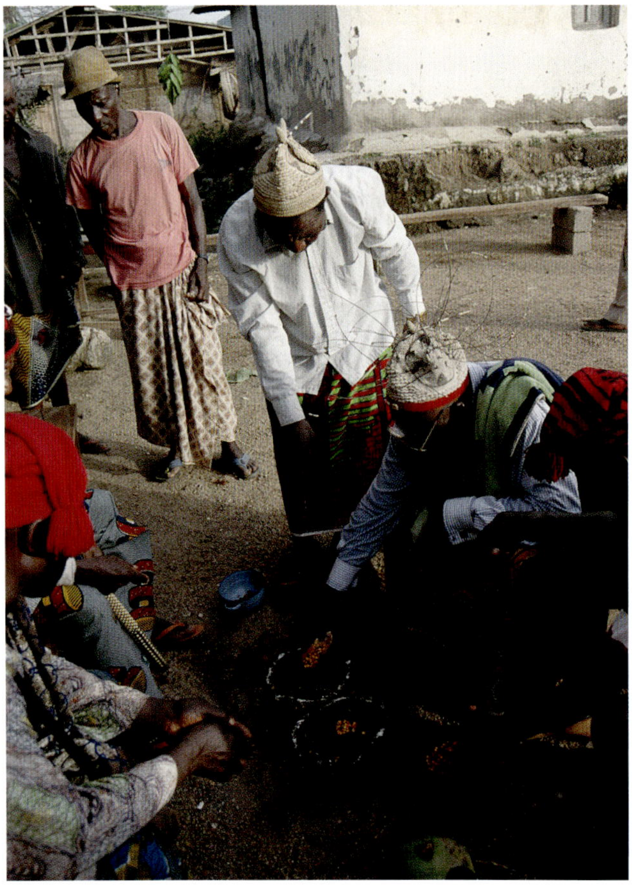

Fig. 65 The *seseku* offers maize in his right hand (Kembong, April 10, 2004).

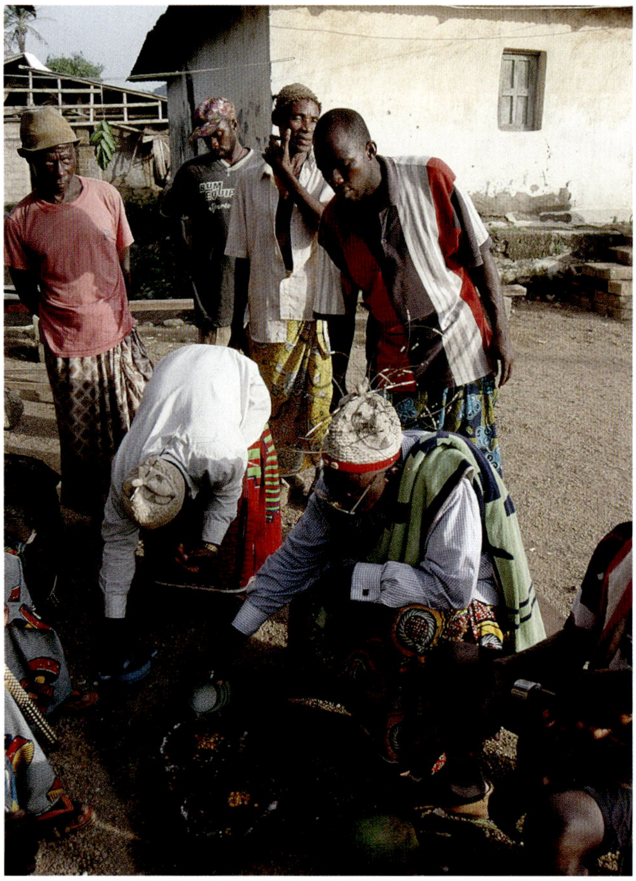

Fig. 66 The offering of palm wine (Kembong, April 10, 2004).

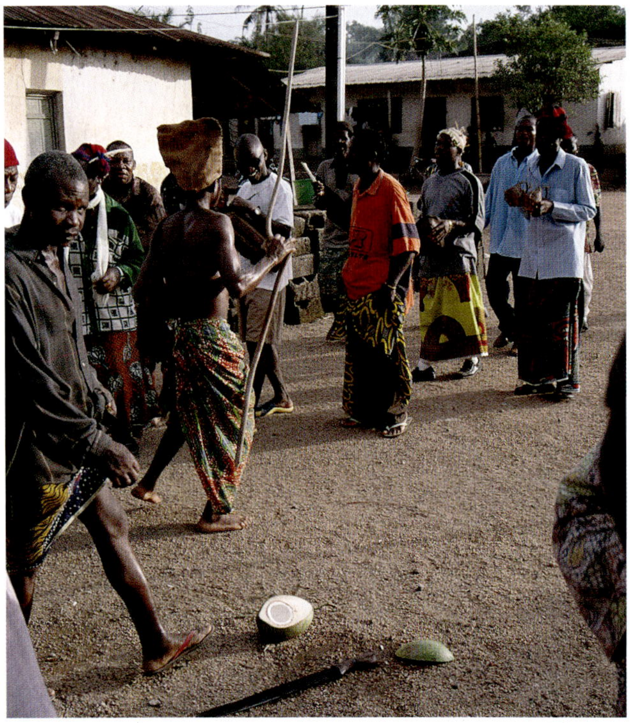

Fig. 67 Oracle with a coconut. For this oracle, a young coconut is cut in two halves with a single stroke of a cutlass. One half lies with the exterior surface upwards, the other half with the inner side upwards: the ideal result, meaning that the ancestors have accepted the offering (Kembong, April 10, 2004).

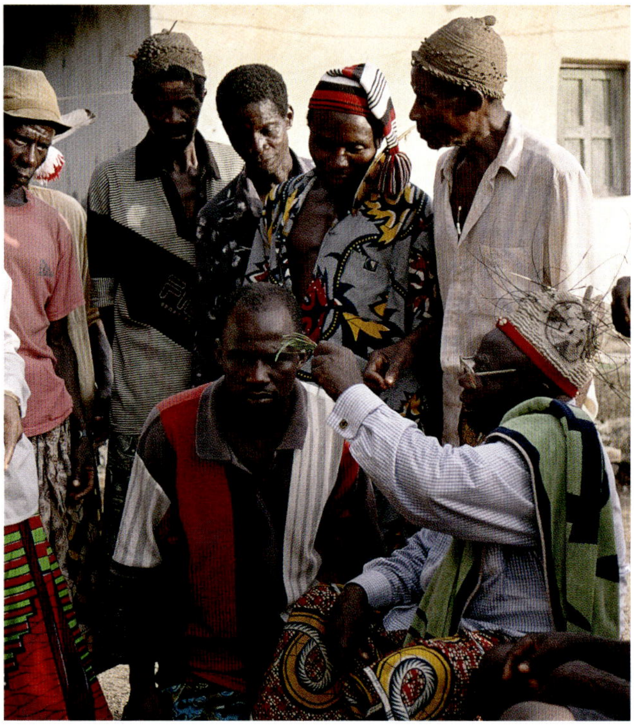

Fig. 68 The "washing of the living" follows the offering to the ancestors. Whoever wishes is treated with medicine for his well-being (Kembong, April 10, 2004).

followed by his *osongaribo*, who constantly "threatens" him with feigned attacks (figs. 59, 75). The *osongaribo* raises his cutlass against the *seseku* again and again with the message that he should leave so that the *osongaribo* can assume his position. A further outstanding figure is that of *okina*, who appears as a jester (figs. 63, 76, 81). The group of *Ebongu* proceeds some 100 to 200 meters to both ends of the village road and then returns to the deceased's house. One of the highlights of the ceremony is when the *seseku* throws *ekong* onto the roof of the house (figs. 64, 77). If *ekong* remains upon the roof, this is a very positive sign, and the people present clap their hands, but if it falls down to the ground, this is interpreted as an extremely bad omen.

The members of *Mgbe* continue dancing together with the mask, which is now *Ema* (fig. 73), while the *seseku* and other big men of *Mgbe* prepare the sacrifice of *Mgbe* (*ajom Mgbe*) for the dead member and for the ancestors. The sacrifice is made in front of the deceased's house. First the ground is cleaned, so that two circles, each about 30 cm in diameter, can be marked with a substance consisting of chalky earth and yellow camwood. They are intended for offerings: the left circle meant as male, the right as female. The sacrifice is conducted in the same manner as is customary for ancestral offerings, and this is the charge of the *seseku* (figs. 65, 66, 78). Now is the moment of "washing the living and the dead" (*asu Mgbe*) (figs. 68, 79, 80), likewise the charge of the *seseku*.

Through the ritual washing of the face, misfortune and guilt are believed to be removed from both the living and deceased persons, and they can begin a "clean" new phase in life. This ritual is of especial importance for those members of *Mgbe* who wish to attain a new rank in this society. Other persons also partake in this act – in most cases in order to gain economic advantages. It is hoped that through the ritual deceased persons will be able to encounter the ancestors freely without any burden. The herbs which were collected in the grove of *Mgbe* are used for this medicine. One part of the medicine is intended for the living members (figs. 68, 79), the other for the dead person (fig. 80). The *seseku* squeezes the herbs and puts them in a bowl; yellow and red camwood is added as well as palm wine. First the living are blessed outside in front of the house of the deceased, whereas the "washing of the dead" follows inside the house. Here the *seseku* addresses the deceased: he wishes him lasting peace and that his face be so clean that the ancestors accept him into their sphere. At the same time the *seseku* entreats him to bestow good fortune and well-being on the living. The *seseku* then rubs the face of the deceased with two *ngilako* leaves and sprinkles yellow camwood and white chalky earth upon it.[69] The *ngilako* leaves remain upon the face of the dead person; should they be removed, the bereaved family must pay 30 litres of palm wine. My informants stressed that the leaves are not intended to cover the face in a manner similar to covering the head of a slain leopard. The leopard's "face" may not be seen, above all by women and children, for the leopard is too wild a beast.[70] On the other hand, the leaves that are used in *asu Mgbe* are considered in public as "tiger's leaves" and the face of the deceased as "tiger's face". Reference has already been made that the word "tiger" when used in English conversation stands for "leopard" (cp. p. 134, fn. 1).[71]

On April 10, 2004, a sacrifice took place as part of the funerary ceremony for Gregory Ayuknchiobo, who held the position of *osongaribo* in *Mgbe* in the quarter of Ndengane in Kembong. Gregory Ayuknchiobo, unmarried, had died earlier in February at the age of c. 60, but *Mgbe* was able to "celebrate" his death only at this later time (figs. 57–74). In this regard, it was not a customary burial. After the leopard had been "captured" and brought from the "evil forest" (figs. 57, 58) and *Ebongu* had performed (figs. 59–63), the *seseku* threw *ekong* onto the roof. It remained on the roof and this was a very positive sign (fig. 64). Thereupon another highlight of the day took place: The *seseku* conducted the offering to the ancestors (*ajom Mbge*). He commenced by addressing God and the deceased person: "*Ata Obasi*, *Mma Obasi* and Gregory Ayuknchiobo, I am calling you. You know your celebration is going on. Let your celebration be quite normal and without any problem. We do not want problems, but everybody who wants problems shall follow you." This was followed by an offering of maize. Taking some grains in his left hand the *seseku* spoke: "*Ata Obasi*, *Mma Obasi* and Gregory Ayuknchiobo, you and all those who are dead in our family. Carry this corn to those ancestors whom I know and to those whom I do not know." Then the *seseku* took some grains into his right hand (fig. 65): "This is food from us, the living. We have eaten our own, and this is your part. Share it with those whom I know and with those whom I do not know." Proceeding in the same manner and with prayers like those for the grains of maize, the *seseku* offered the deceased and the ancestors pieces of meat, palm wine (fig. 66) and water. Then he offered whisky: „Gregory Ayuknchiobo, this is the white man's *mimbo* ("alcoholic drink"). Give it to those, who drink palm wine and to all the others. All of us should be in fellowship." The offering of two pieces of a colanut was at the same time an oracle: "Gregory Ayuknchiobo, following our culture, if a stranger enters our house, you

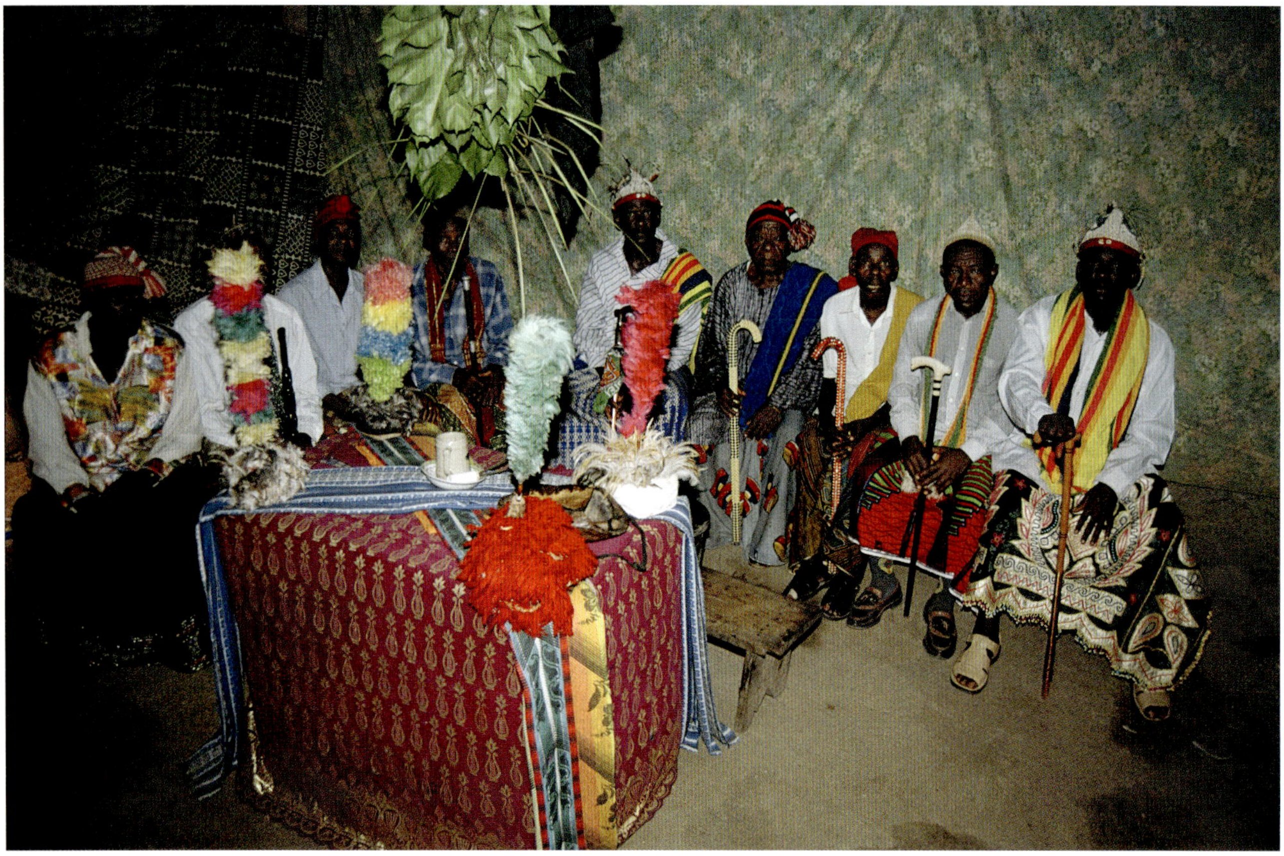

Fig. 69 A table, *efem Mgbe*, is decorated in the house of the deceased in his honour. The details are among the strictly guarded secrets of the society. The men in view are the *boseseku*; in accordance with their position they wear a towel over their left shoulder (Kembong, April 10, 2004).

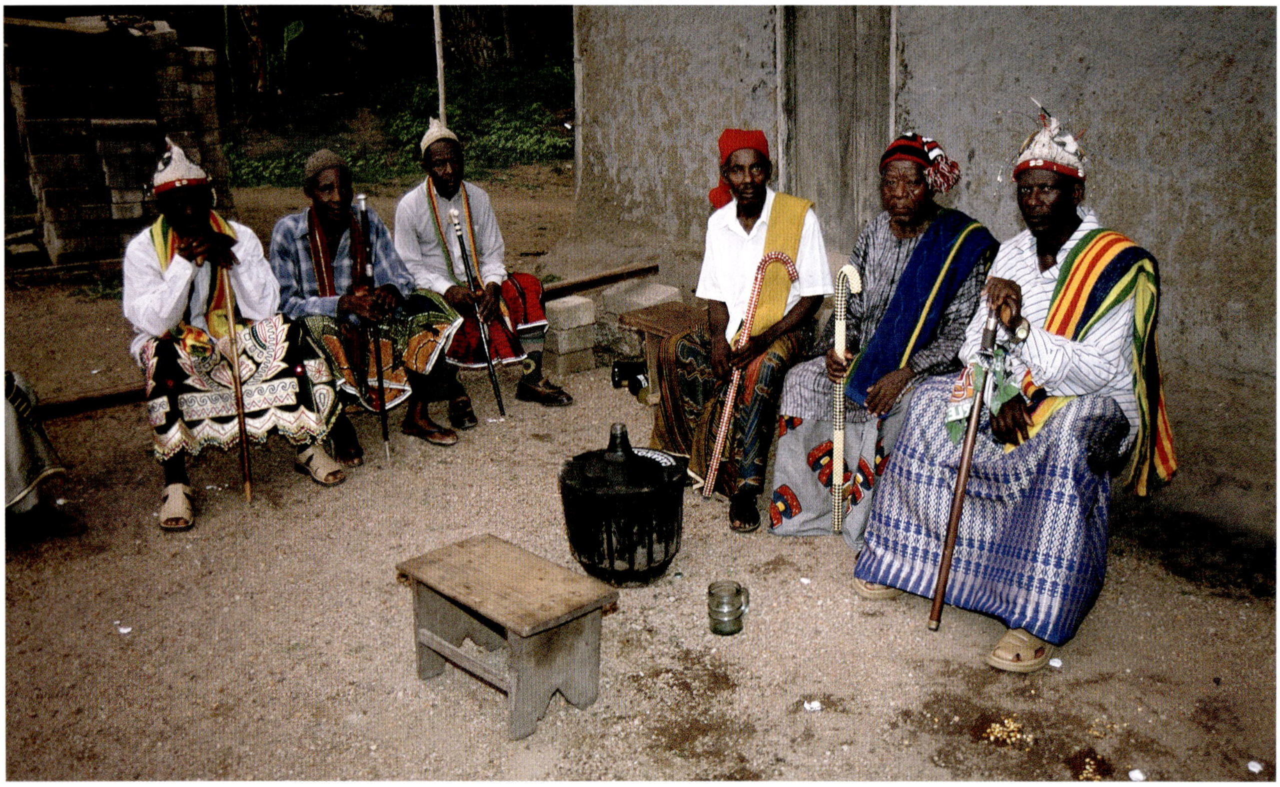

Fig. 70 *Mgbe* remains in the compound of the deceased until the end of the death celebration. Here three *boseseku* (left to right: James Ayuknchiobo, Kofi Tabe, Ernest Array Ajuk Tarkang) and three other high-ranking members (left) have gathered to drink palm wine (Kembong, April 11, 2004).

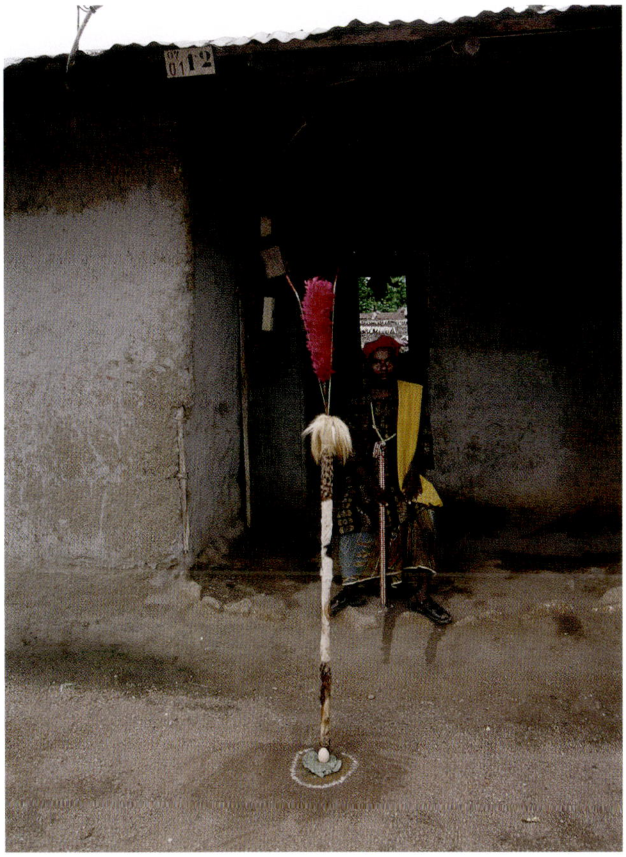

Fig. 71 The ceremonial staff, *monyo*, implanted in front of the deceased's house, indicates the presence of *Mgbe*. At its base is a chicken egg, which is carefully guarded by all – in this case by the *seseku* James Ayuknchiobo (Kembong, April 14, 2004).

must first of all break him a colanut. We have eaten our own, this is yours." He threw the two colanut pieces onto the ground, and their position proved that the ancestors were happy. Though they had shown their satisfaction in this way, another oracle was carried out with a young coconut. One of the men proceeded to cut it into two parts with the single stroke of a cutlass: one side lay upwards, the other towards the ground. The position was ideal and meant that the ancestors had accepted the offerings (fig. 67). Similar to the oracle with two leaves *ebanghaah* (cp. p. 34 f.), if both segments had landed with the sides upwards, it would have been a sign that the ancestors were laughing. Had both sides been downwards, it would have been a very unfavourable sign, for with that the ancestors would have shown their dissatisfaction and anger. In the case of the latter position, the *seseku* usually hits the segments of coconut with a stone and appeals to the ancestors: "Oh, ancestors, if you are not happy, we apologise to you, whether we know you or not. We are your children. We plead for forgiveness. Accept our fervent prayer." Following this the "washing of the living" took place (fig. 68). The "washing of the dead", however, was not possible, for the deceased person had long been buried.

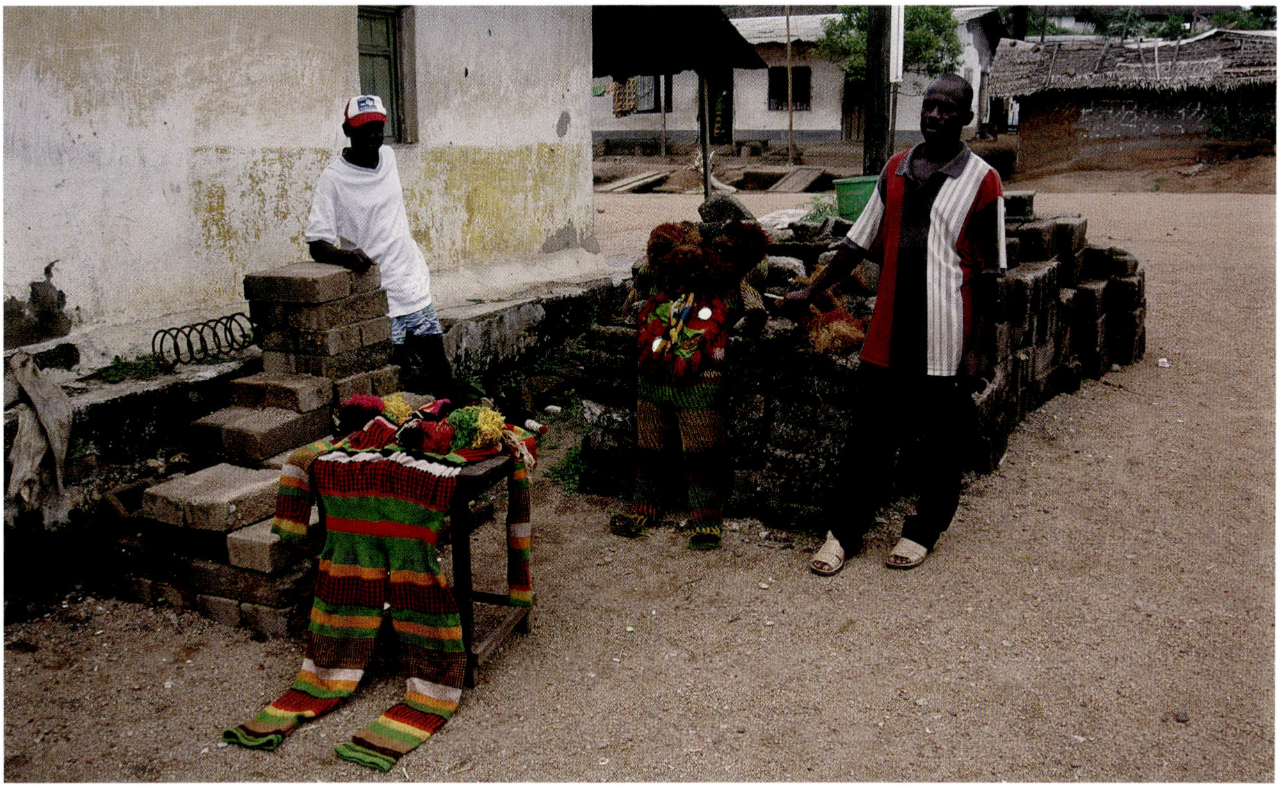

Fig. 72 Mask garments of *Ebongu/Ema* are spread out to dry in the compound of the deceased in full view of the public (Kembong, April 15, 2004).

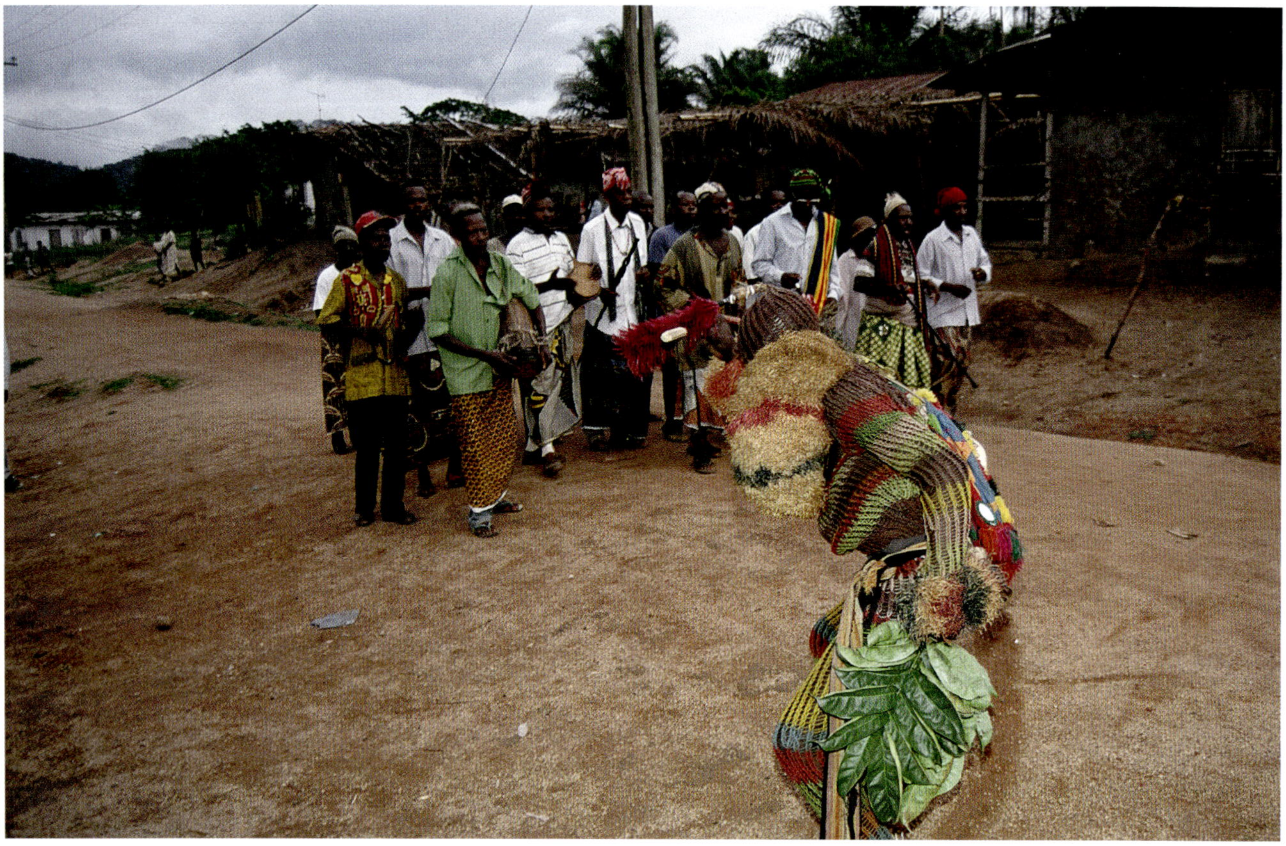

Fig. 73 The participation of *Mgbe* in the death celebration ends with the performance of *Ema* (Kembong, April 15, 2004).

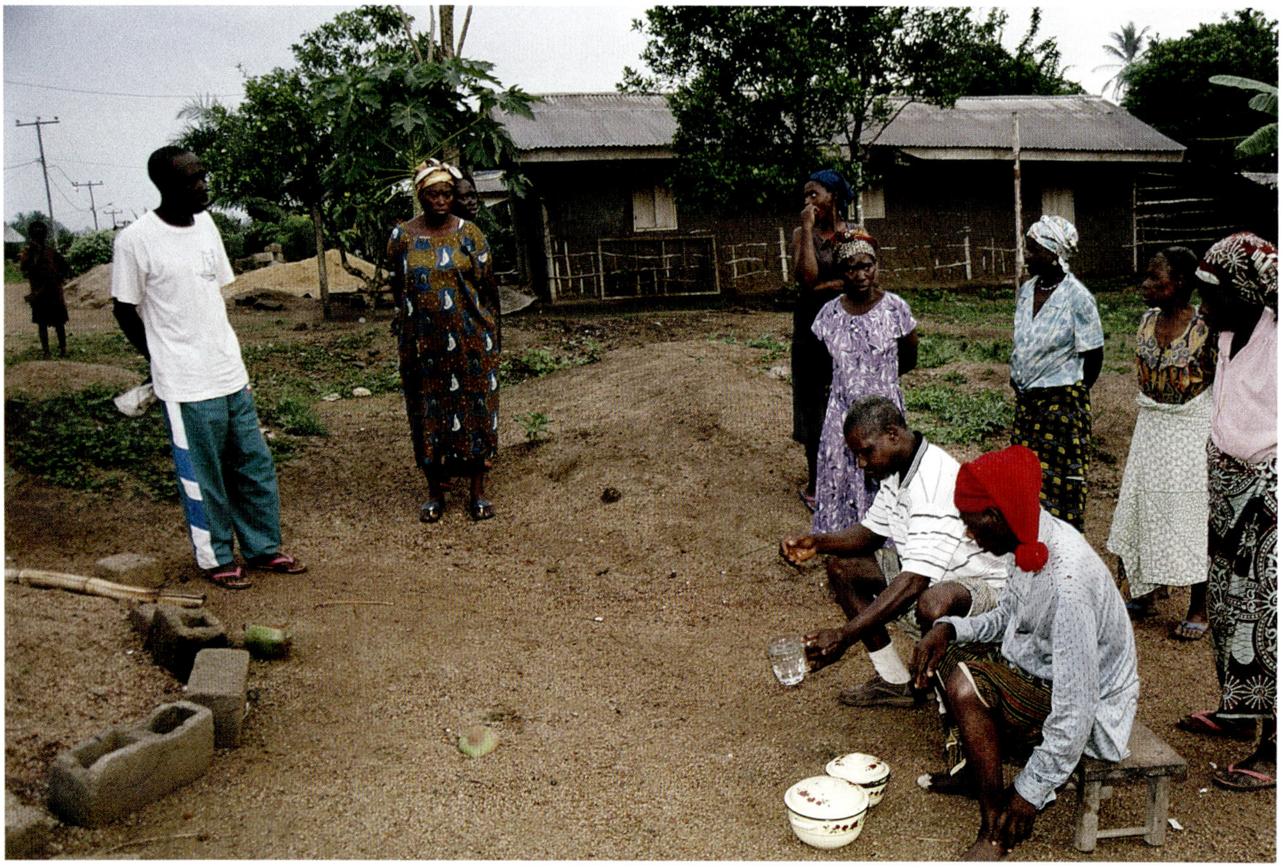

Fig. 74 The death celebration concludes with the sacrifice to the ancestors, the *etaah nji eyatek*, which is conducted by the head of the family (Kembong, April 16, 2004).

I was able to experience another death celebration in Kembong on April 17, 2004. It was held for Martin Mbo Agborya from the quarter of Ebarensi, who had died one day before (figs. 75–81). Martin Mbo Agborya was about 80 years old and had held the rank of *osongaribo* in *Mgbe*. Following tradition *Mgbe* fetched the leopard from the grove and took it to the Unity Hall, where *Mgbe* resided during the ceremony. When the mask *Ebongu* appeared in the compound of the deceased, the corpse had already been laid in a coffin. The family had decided to carry out the burial earlier than usual for hygienic reasons. *Ebongu* placed the two medicine leaves that were meant to cover the face of the deceased *osongaribo*, upon the coffin. After the public performance of *Ebongu* (figs. 75, 76) the *seseku* threw the *ekong* plant upon the roof of the Unity Hall (fig. 77), and this was followed by *ajom Mgbe*, the sacrifice of *Mgbe* (fig. 78).

Thereupon the *seseku* commenced with the offering of maize: "Martin Mbo, you are dead and I am giving you this *ebone*. This is the food of *Mgbe* (*ebone*), which we have come to give to you. We also call the ancestors of the whole quarter to take the food. Let the ceremony be very fruitful. Some of us escaped (left) from *Mgbe* in those days and now we have come back. Let the ceremony *Nyampkwe* bear more fruit. Take this food and meet people like Peter Ako and Ayuknchiobo and those I know and those I do not know." He took grains of maize in his right hand, saying: "This right hand is for us, the living. Give us prosperity." When offering a colanut, he addressed the ancestors anew: "When ancestors eat, they also need colanuts. This colanut is broken for you, the ancestors, and for us, the living. Right from the hamlets (that is, inhabitants of hamlets at the time prior to the arrival of Europeans) there is a saying: An old man falls only from a colanut-tree and never from another tree." When offering palm wine he continued: "The ancestors have eaten, they also drink wine. The wine should make us peaceful. As all of us have taken this wine, let there be blessings on all of us from *Mgbe*." When offering whisky he spoke the same words. As is customary at death celebrations, the offering of an unripe coconut was associated with an oracle: "This coconut is to be given to you and to us to eat. If this blessing is acceptable to you, who have eaten the food, let the coconut agree or accept our offer. If not, let there be a negative answer." With a single blow with a cutlass the coconut was divided in two, but both halves lay with the inside upwards. This was a negative result, so he addressed the ancestors once more: "The ancestors should not be angry. We the living are happy. Let them also be happy for the purpose of cooperation and mutual understanding." Now he threw both halves into the air, and they landed positively. The ancestors showed their satisfaction, and so the group could begin with another ritual: washing the living and the dead (*asu Mgbe*).

He began by blessing the living members. First he took the liquid medicine with his left hand and rubbed it on his own forehead with the words: "I wash my face with my left hand. May all ill-luck go away." He did the same with his right hand: "I wash my face with my right hand. May I remember all the *Mgbe* (laws) which I have learnt and may I never forget anything." The *seseku* then proceeded by washing the members' faces, one after the other, each time with the words: "I wash your face. May you remember all the *Mgbe* (laws) you have learnt and never forget anything." He said this to all members that they might prosper in their respective occupations. To a civil servant he said: "I am washing your face for you to be strong at your job. Let your officials receive you at your job with clean hands. Let them give you promotions in order that you should have your regular salary" (fig. 79).

Finally *Mgbe* entered the house of the deceased, where the "washing of the dead" should have taken place. Since the corpse was already in the coffin, the deceased was represented by his cap, which lay upon his bed (fig. 80). The *seseku* addressed the dead man: "You are dead. If your death was caused by somebody, let the person follow you in less than no time. But if your death came from your own hands or from Almighty God, we wish you a save journey. We are coming behind you, because death is for all of us. Give us luck to carry away all our sicknesses, from which we are suffering. I am washing your face. If in your life-time you had any bad luck, let your face be clean, so that you can join your ancestors." The *seseku* took medicine into his right hand: "May our faces also be bright, so that we can continue to teach young people what has been handed down to us." He took the feather from the deceased's cap, which he normally would have placed upon the head of the dead man. In this case the *seseku* placed the cap where the head would have rested: "This is your *Nyampkwe*, which I am washing. Let the *Nyampkwe* be a peaceful one. Let there be plenty of food and drinks. We want defaulters to be rich people and not poor people." Then he took the *ngilako* leaves and covered the "deceased's face". After this the *seseku* sprinkled white chalk over the "face" of the deceased and after that yellow camwood. During all of these actions he named the ranks of *Mgbe*, like *bekundi*, *Ebongu* and *okongo*, in which the dead person had been a member. Whenever he named a level, he made a *Mgbe* call and the members of *Mgbe* answered. This was, however, not the only

Death celebration for Martin Mbo Agborya from Ebarensi (Kembong, April 17 and 21, 2004) (figs. 75–81).

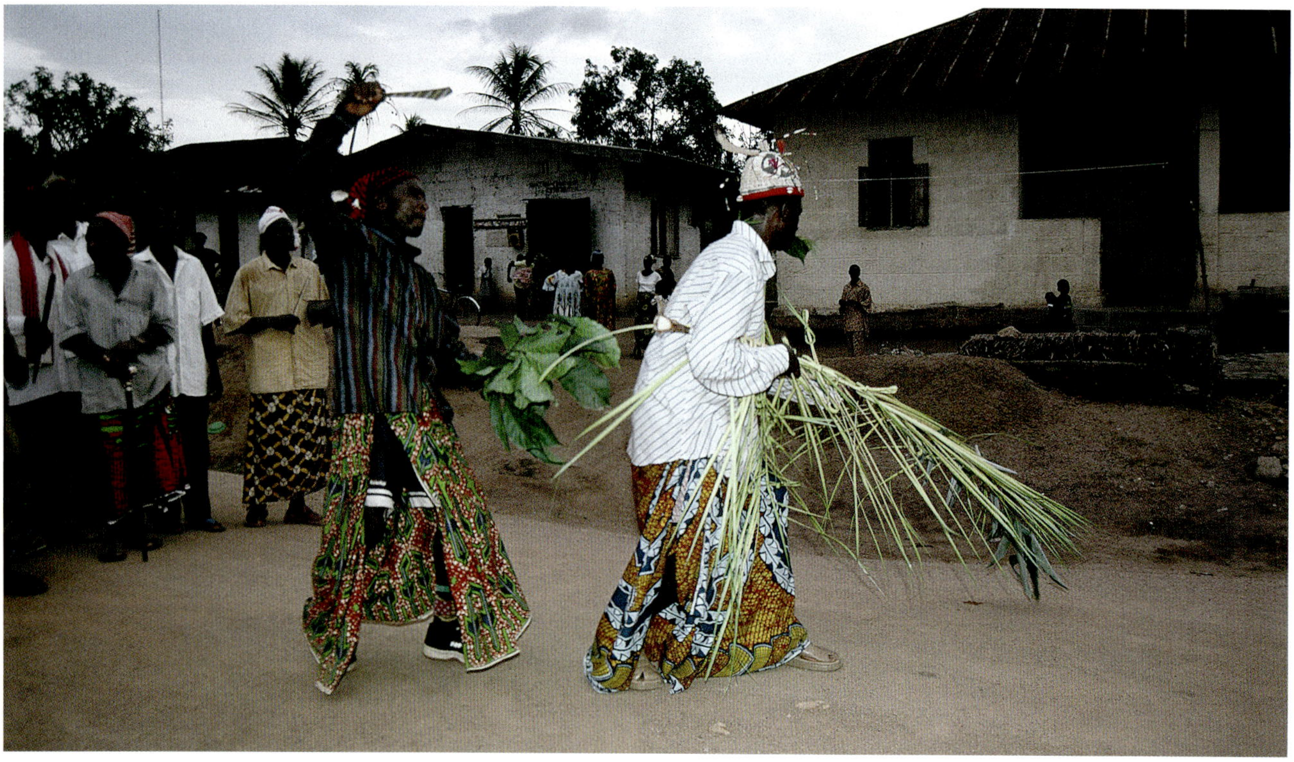

Fig. 75 Performance of *Ebongu*, in the foreground a *seseku*, Ernest Array Ayuk Tarkang from Nkonghobe, carrying the medicine plant *ekong* and followed by "his" *osongaribo* "threatening" him with a cutlass (Kembong, April 17, 2004).

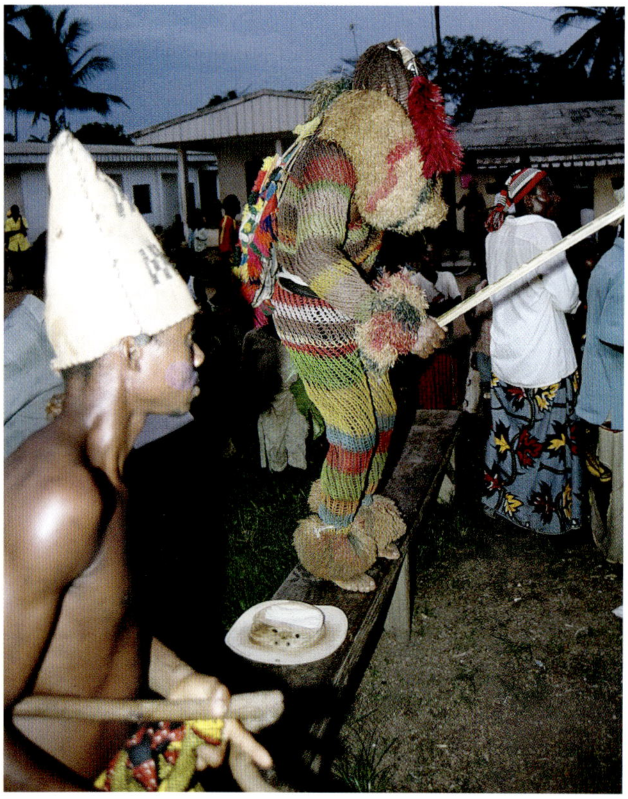

Fig. 76 The mask *Ebongu* and *okina*, the messenger of *Mgbe* (left foreground) (Kembong, April 17, 2004).

reaction from *Mgbe*; simultaneously the voice of the leopard sounded – it was also responding. It was happy that the corpse had been washed and dressed and that all preparations were made for the burial.

Only when the ritual of washing has taken place is the family of the deceased allowed to begin with its own grieving.[72] It is *okina* who informs the women that the ritual has been finished and that they should begin to lament. At the same time dances for the general public begin, continuing until around midnight. At that time the "call of *Mgbe*" sounds, meaning all who are not members of *Mgbe* "should go to their homes and sleep". When all have left, *okongo*, a section of *Mgbe* which is responsible for death celebrations, appears. Its nocturnal rituals are strictly forbidden for outsiders. Around four o'clock in the morning preparations for the inhumation commence. After the deceased is buried, his successor takes leave at the open grave: "Mr. X, you have died, and now we are burying you. If your death was caused by someone, turn your eyes and look at the person." Taking small lumps of clay first into his left hand, and then in the right, he continues in prayer: "But if your death comes from God, go in peace." Thereupon he throws small

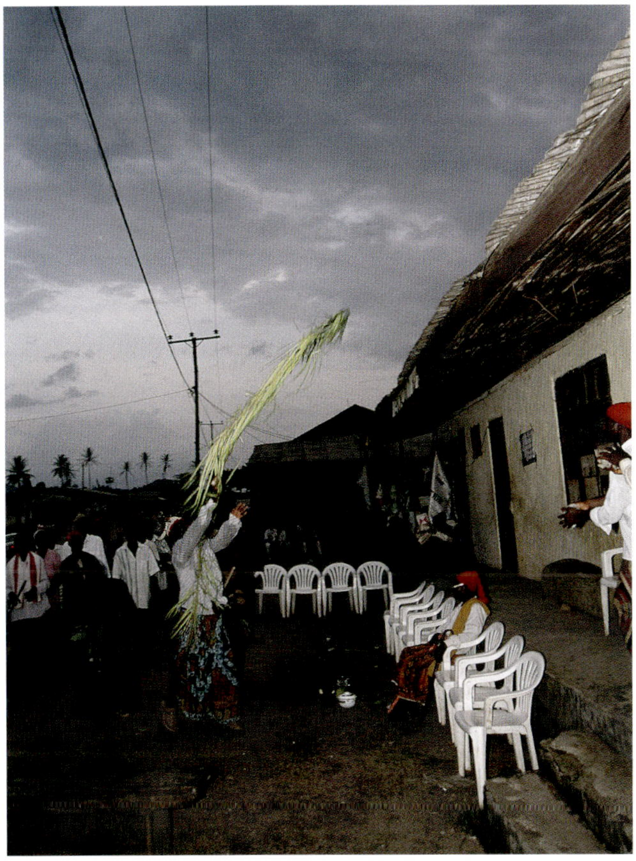

Fig. 77 The *seseku* throws *ekong*, the medicine plant, onto the roof of the Unity Hall, where the death celebration takes place (Kembong, April 17, 2004).

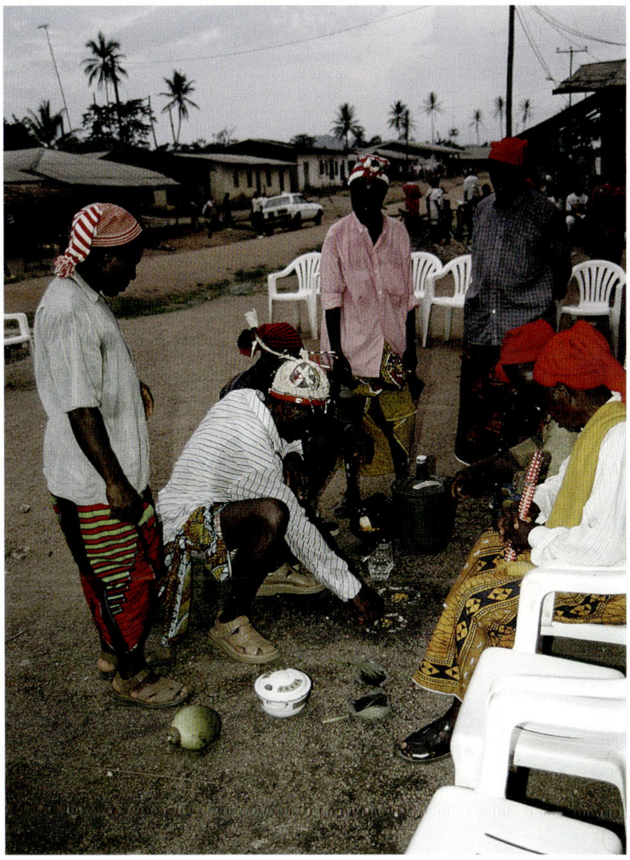

Fig. 78 The *seseku* carries out the offering to the ancestors, *ajom Mgbe* (Kembong, April 17, 2004).

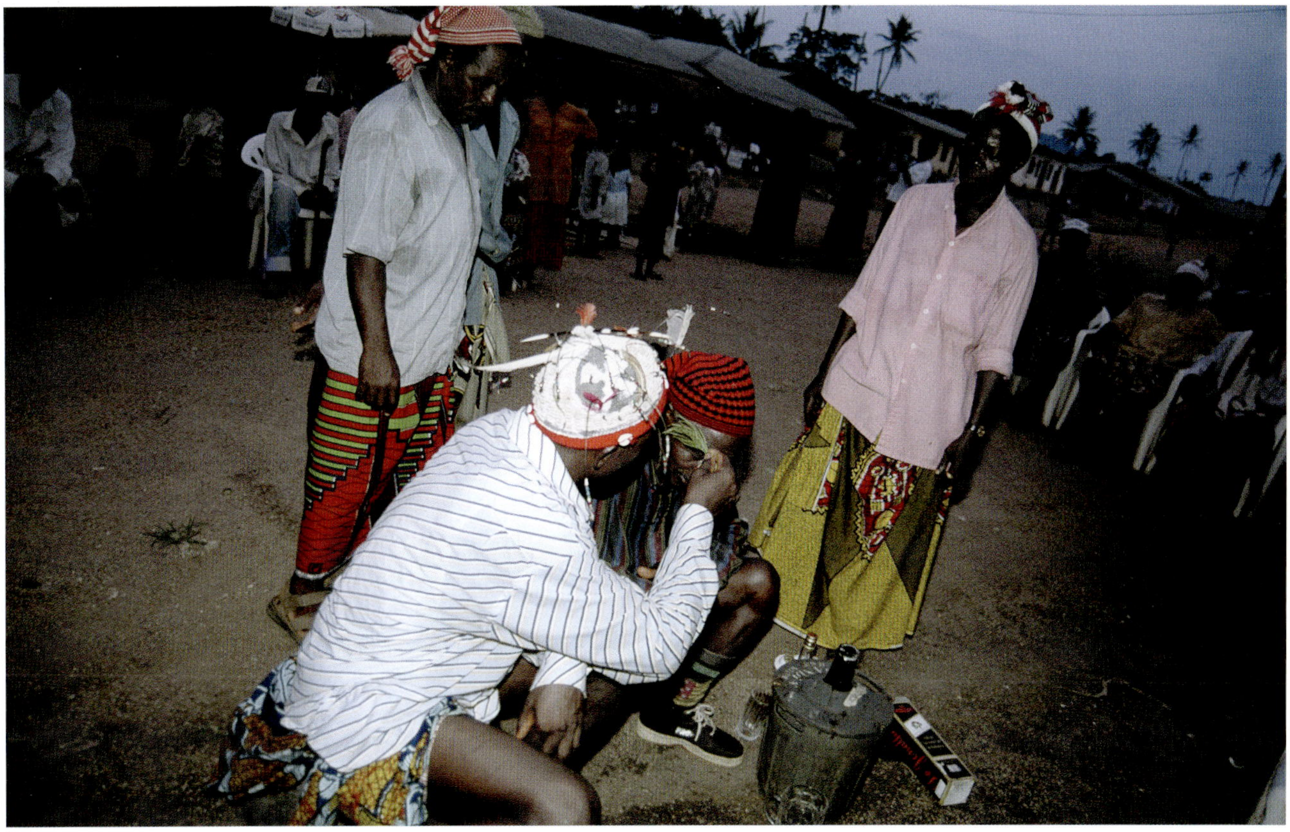

Fig. 79 The ritual "washing of the living" (Kembong, April 17, 2004).

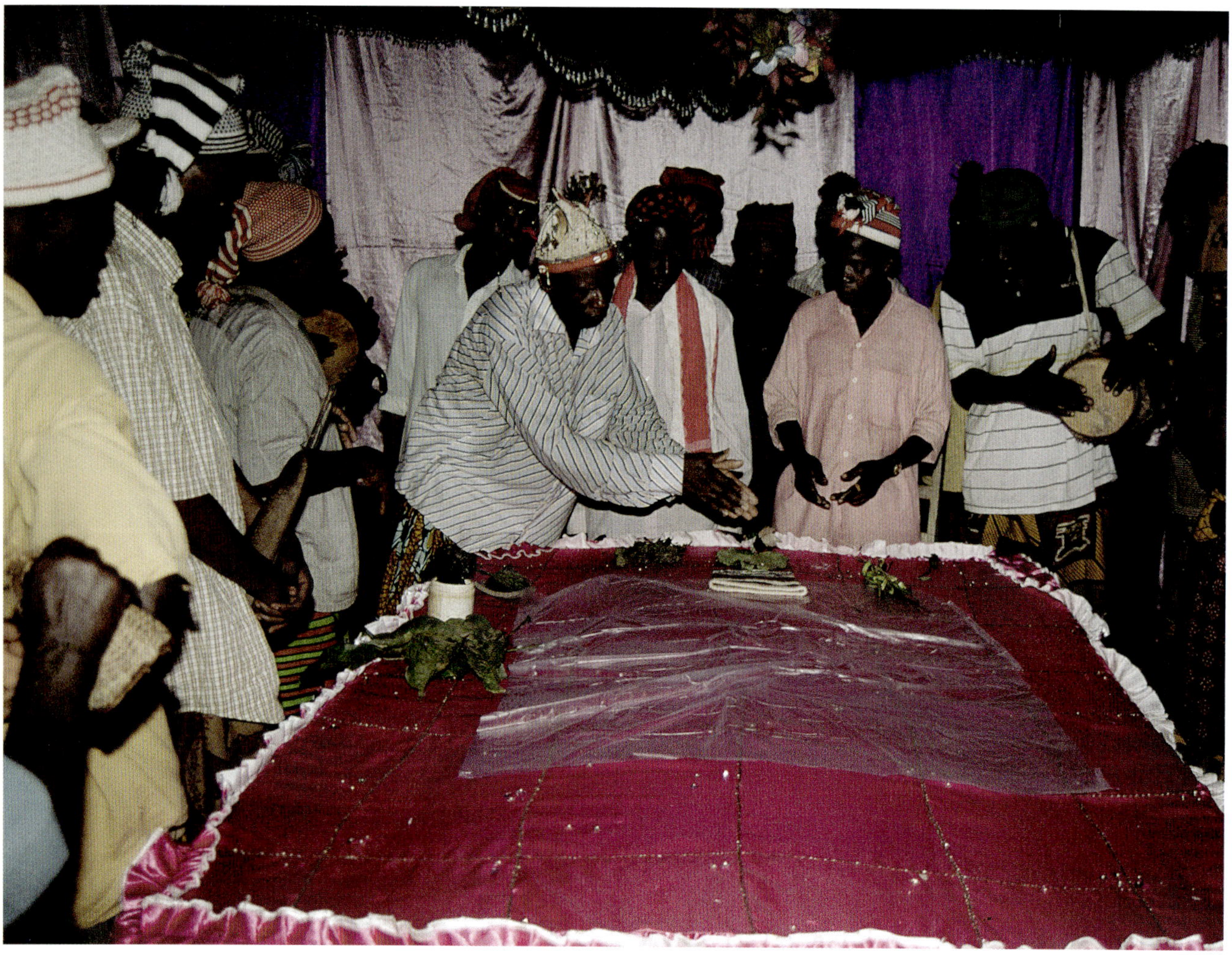

Fig. 80 The ritual "washing of the dead". Since the deceased has already been buried, his cap is treated with medicine in his place (Kembong, April 17, 2004).

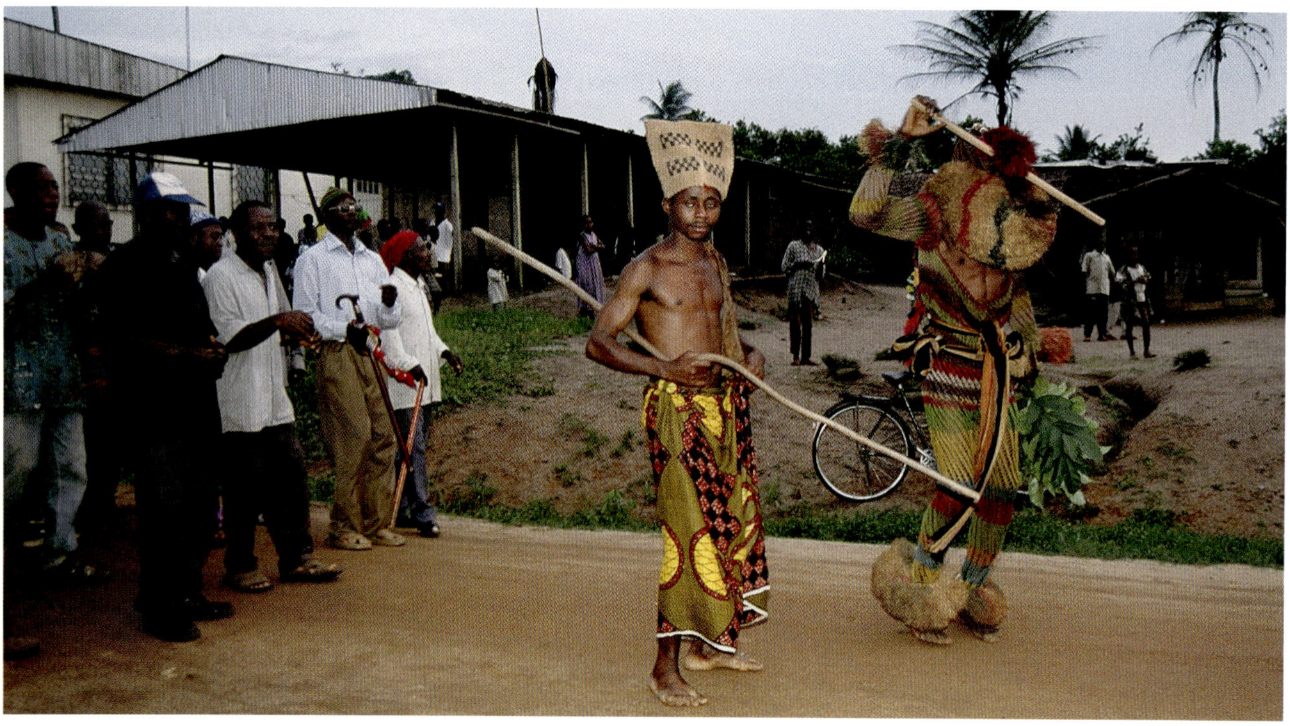

Fig. 81 Performance of *Ema* with the mask and *okina* (Kembong, April 21, 2004).

lumps of clay into the grave. Meanwhile complete silence dominates the scene.

While the grave pit is being filled with earth, *okongo* and *Ema* appear once more. In dance they move along the main street from one end of the village to the other. By the time they return to the compound, the grave must be completely filled. *Ema* performs again in conclusion of the burial ceremony. The mask dances upon the grave and in the name of *Mgbe* makes a final farewell to the deceased.

The burial ceremony is only the first part of the death celebration, with which every deceased person is honoured and to which everyone has a right. If the celebration is not correct in any way or not even conducted at all, the surviving family must reckon with the wrath of the deceased. The second part of the death celebration is *aboku*, the actual day of celebration or the "feasting day". It can follow directly upon the burial, or it can also be held a few months or even years later, if the respective family does not have the financial means to celebrate in the appropriate form, that is, with a generous reception for guests.

During the morning after the burial, the family of the deceased meets to decide upon the date for *aboku*. If it can be held in the coming one or two weeks, which is normally the case, *Mgbe* remains in the compound of the deceased and with it the leopard. During this time there is absolute peace and quiet in the respective quarter. Should conflicts or serious problems arise, the leopard would flee into the grove of *Mgbe*. Those who have disturbed the peace and thus caused the leopard's flight must reckon with a large fine in order to bring the leopard back to the compound of the deceased.[73]

The reception hall in the deceased's compound is continuously occupied by members of *Mgbe*, and they dance in the mornings and evenings. The occupancy of *Mgbe* in the compound is visibly demonstrated by the presence of *monyo*, the ceremonial staff of the *seseku*, which is implanted in the ground in the courtyard. Prior to this the feather crown has been removed from the staff and fastened to the headdress of the mask *Ebongu/Ema* in such a manner that it dangles from the mask's face. An egg is placed upon two medicine leaves next to *monyo* and closely guarded. For should the egg disappear, for instance, be taken by a dog, *Mgbe* can demand a goat as a fine. At the death of a *seseku* the ceremonial staff is left standing in the courtyard during the entire period of celebration, that is, for several days. In the case of an ordinary member, *Mgbe* appears only one single day (fig. 71).

The members of *Mgbe* eat their meals together. The *seseku* receives his share first and then the other members are given their portion. Yet, a "good" and "friendly" *seseku* waits until all have been served before he begins to eat. If there is not enough food for all of the members, he offers his share to them. At initiation celebrations the portions of food differ in amount: the largest portion goes to the *seseku*. Upon the second day after the burial, the table of *Mgbe*, which was set up in honour of the deceased in his reception hall, is removed (fig. 69).

4.1.6.2 An excursus: *aboku*, the feasting day

In contrast to the day of burial, during which of all the secret societies only *Mgbe* performs (that is, for its own members), on *aboku* all members and institutions of the community have the opportunity to commemorate the deceased and to honour him in dance and other presentations. The entire quarter is entertained on the day of *aboku*, the feasting day of the death celebrations. And it is customary that the hosts provide generously for the guests.

Aboku always begins with the performance of the mask *Nchockandah* (figs. 82–83, 95–99), which belongs to the *abonche*, boys between four and twelve years of age.[74] There is no further information about the name of the mask, *Nchockandah*, which literally means "puller of testicles". Although it "only" consists of branches and leaves, no *aboku* may take place without the performance of this seemingly "harmless" mask. Women may not be present when the mask bearer puts on the mask costume, which is usually on one of the farms at a distance from other houses. *Nchockandah* dances in the compound of the deceased for about ten minutes. The rest of the boys accompany it by singing songs and beating sticks together in rhythm (figs. 95, 96). One of the boys, who like the mask wears parts of plants on his body, acts as *okina*. And just like his "colleague" in the performance of *Mgbe*, he plays the role of a jester (fig. 95). After the dance the mask goes to the grave of the deceased, where the mask bearer takes off the mask garment (figs. 83, 98). In contrast to donning the mask costume, this occurs more or less in full view and may also be seen by women. The mask garment is left lying upon the grave until it has rotted away (fig. 99). Following the performance the youths of *Nchockandah* are the first to receive their share of the feast. As mentioned above (cp. p. 38) they must decide whether or not the food is good and sufficient. Should their judgement be negative, which, however, is seldom the case, *aboku* may not take place (figs. 100, 101).[75]

Aboku, the feasting day, for James Besem Ashu Tambe from Nyane (Kembong, January 18, 2004) (figs. 82–94).

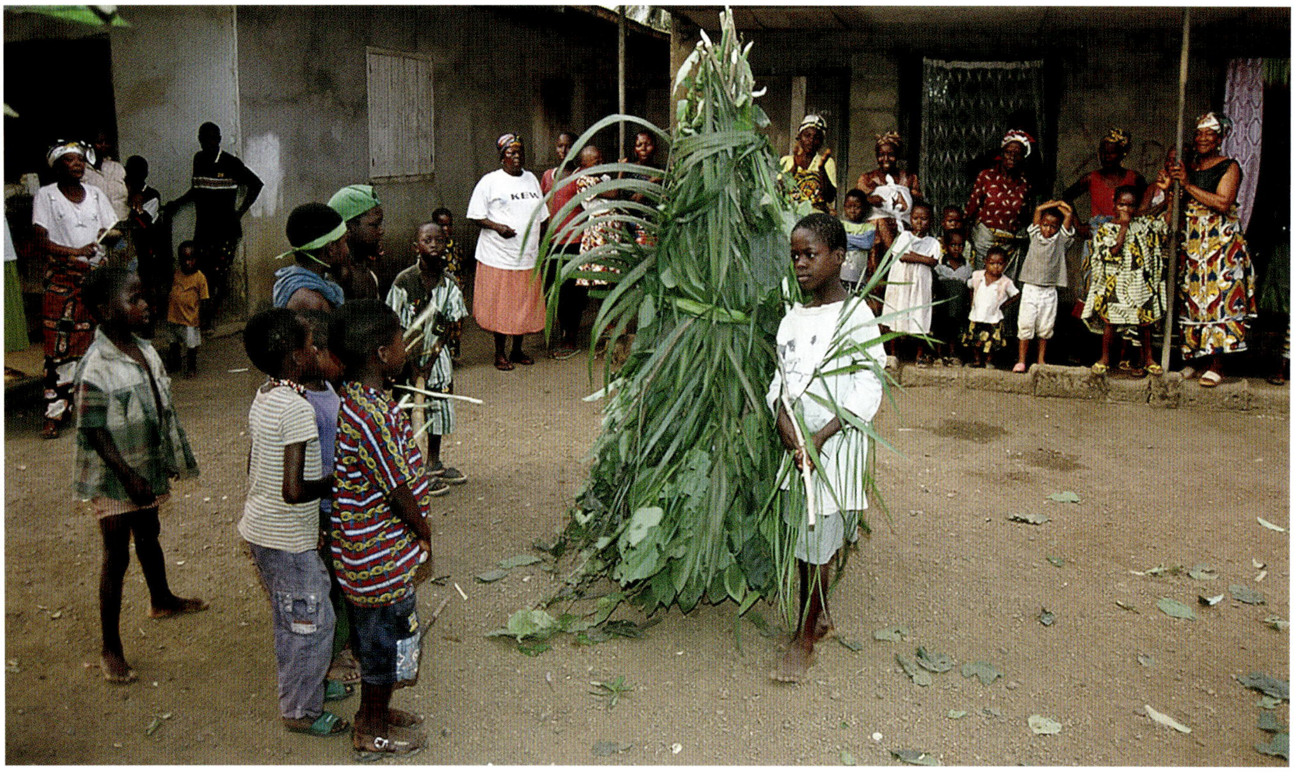

Fig. 82 *Aboku* always begins with the appearance of the mask *Nchockandah* which belongs to young boys and is made of grass and leaves. (Kembong, January 18, 2004).

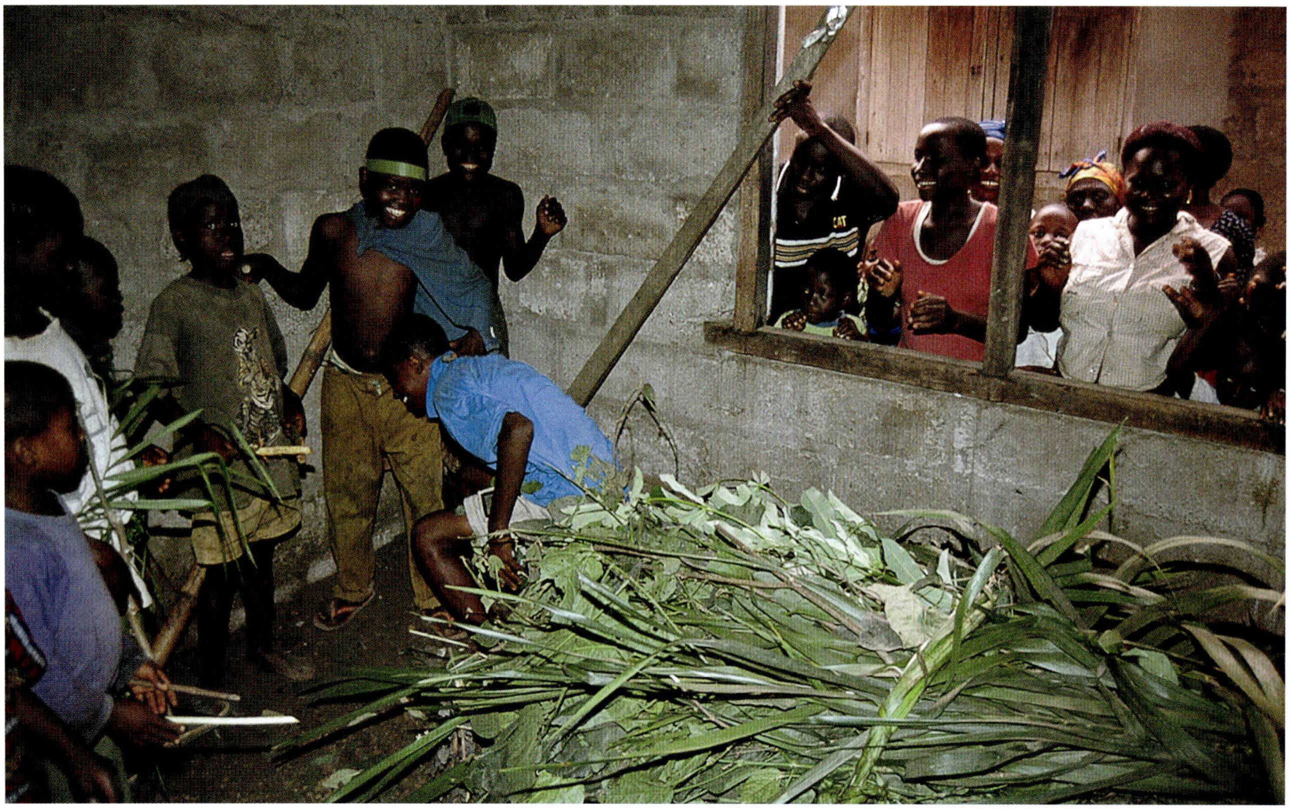

Fig. 83 In public view the young mask bearer leaves the mask "costume" upon the grave of the deceased, which is located inside the person's house (Kembong, January 18, 2004).

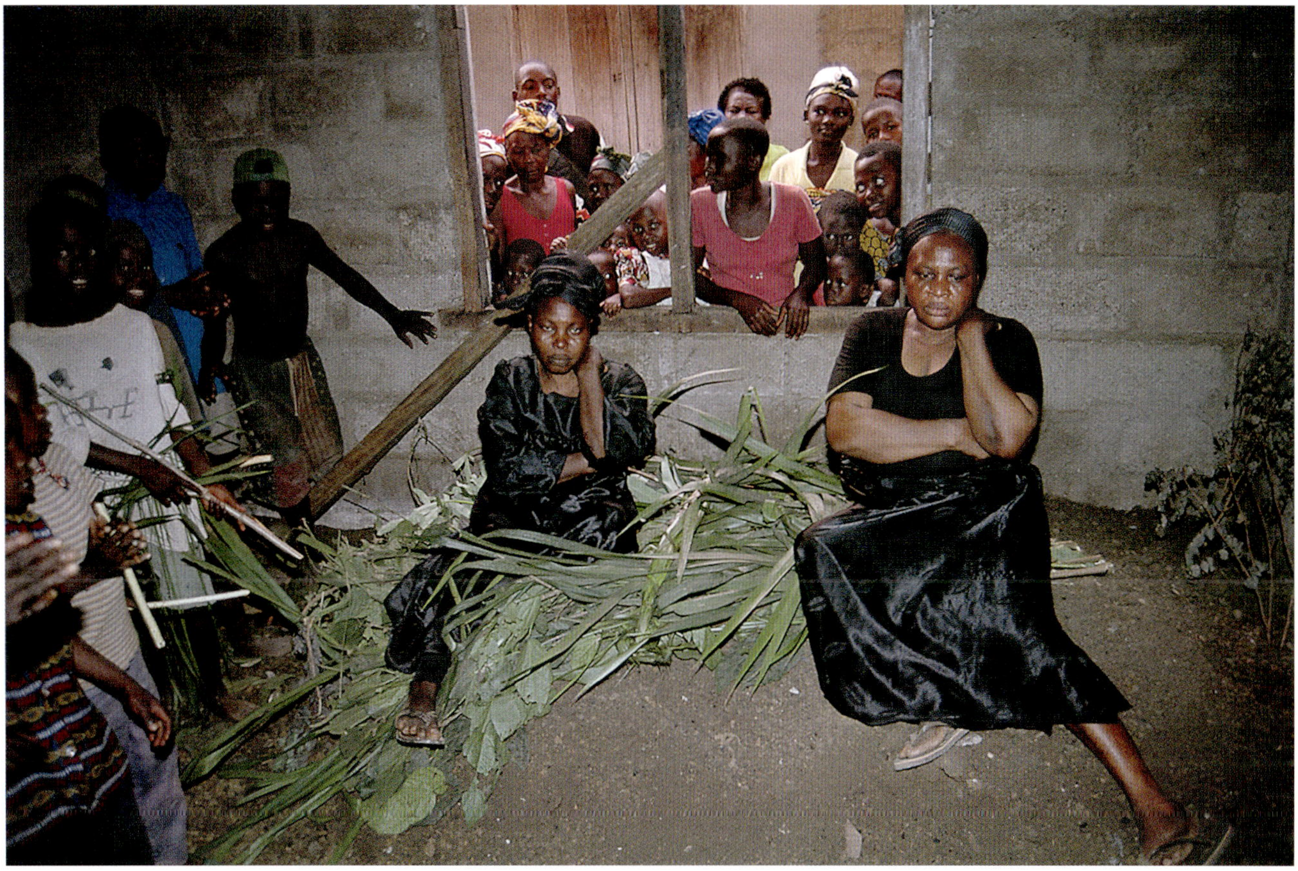

Fig. 84 Seated upon the mask and the grave the widows of the deceased demonstrate their grief for the deceased husband (Kembong, January 18, 2004).

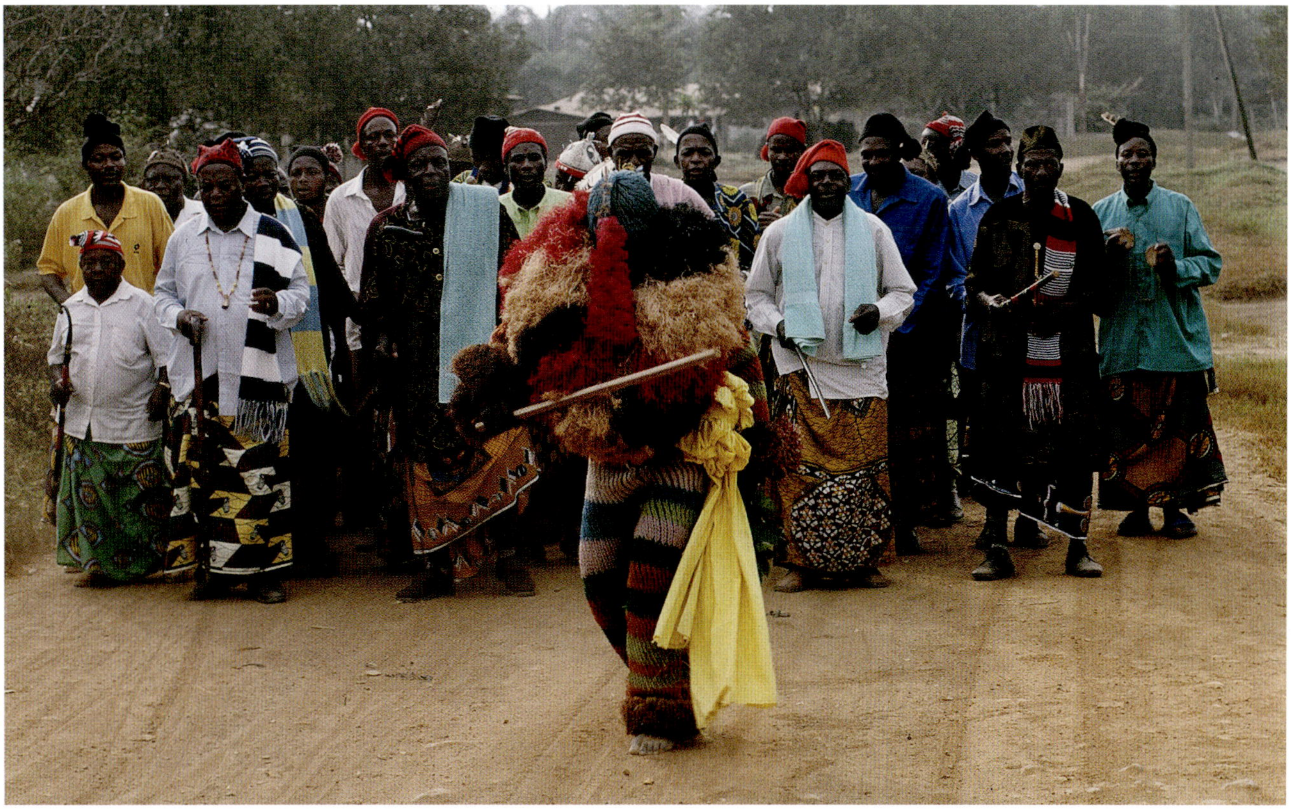

Fig. 85 Performance of *Ema* and its mask (Kembong, January 18, 2004).

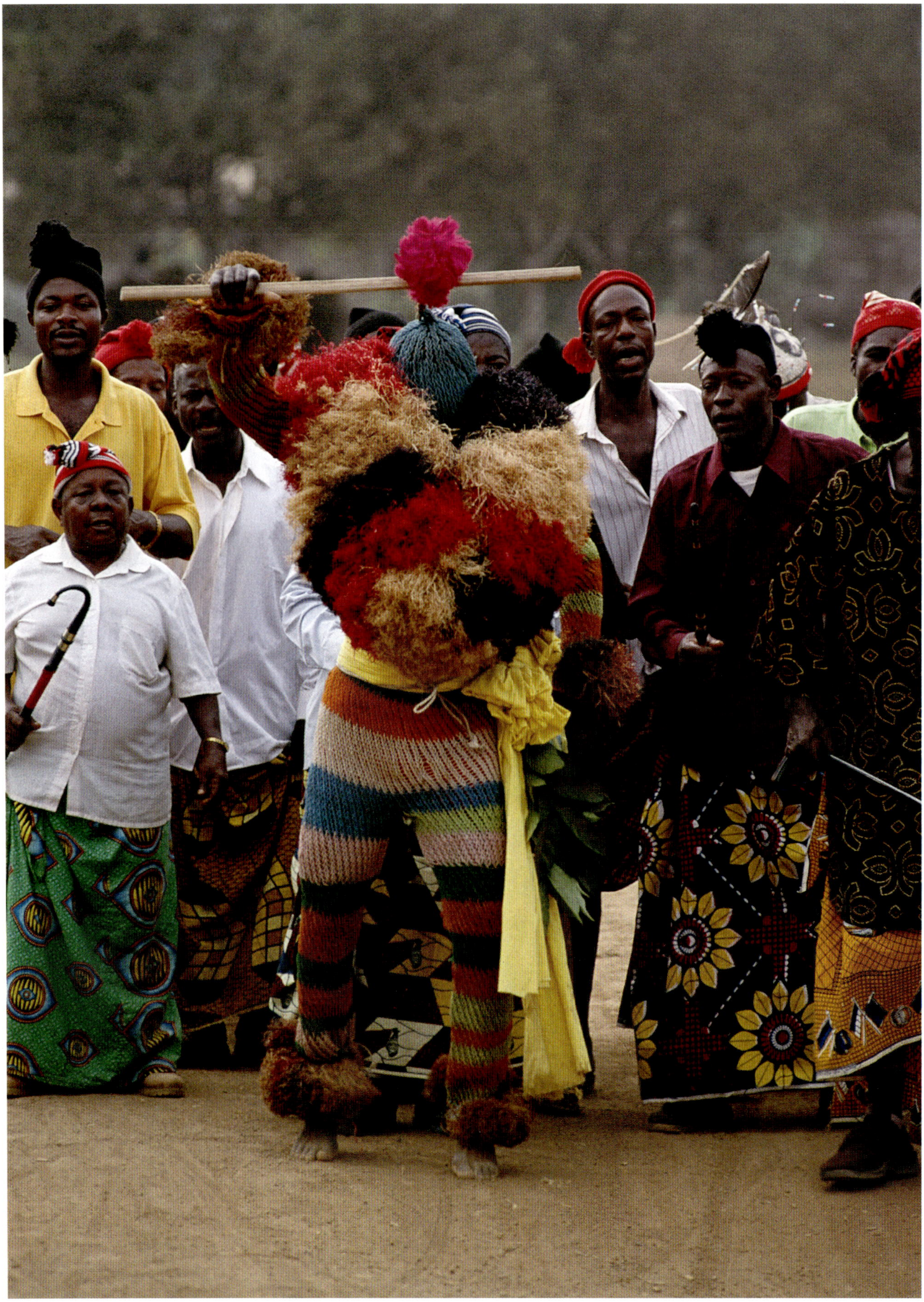

Fig. 86 *Ema* at the head of the procession (Kembong, January 18, 2004).

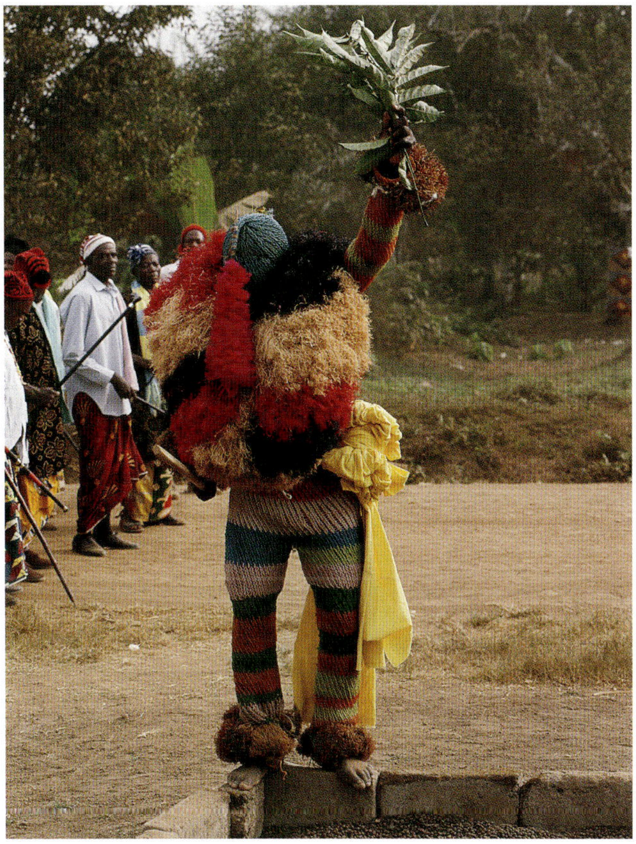

Fig. 87 *Ema* in performance, self-confident and demonstrative (Kembong, January 18, 2004).

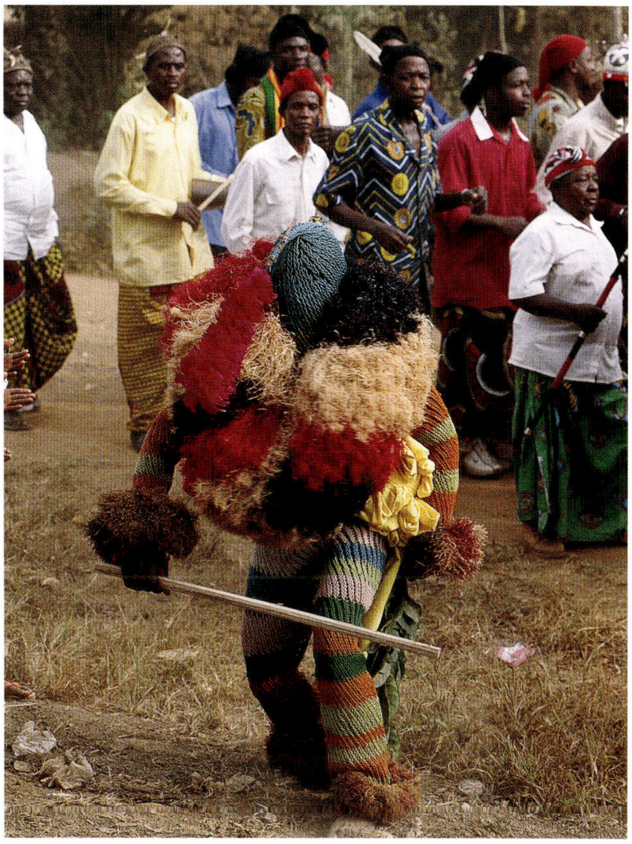

Fig. 88 *Ema* with a stick in its right hand (Kembong, January 18, 2004).

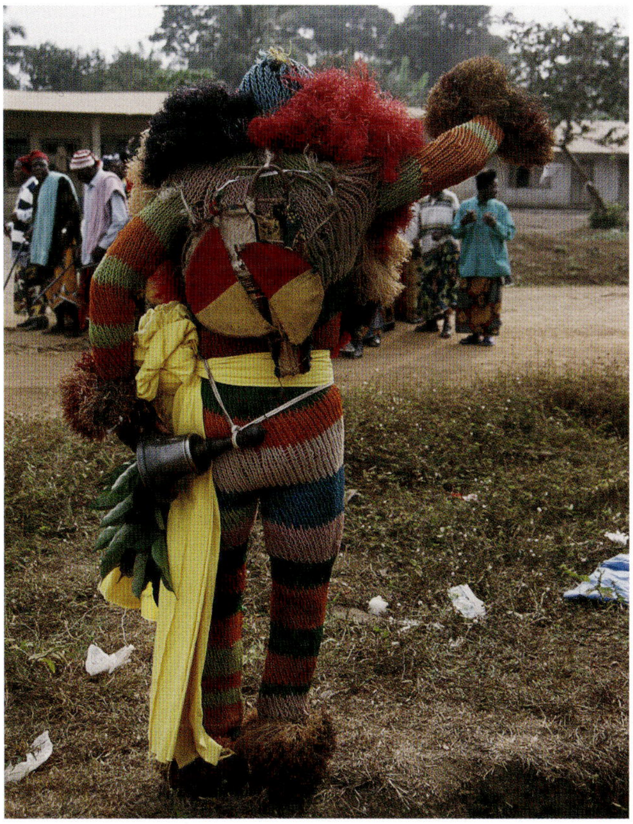

Fig. 89 On its back *Ema* carries a large brass bell of European production, which it occasionally rings to the accompaniment of the drums (Kembong, January 18, 2004).

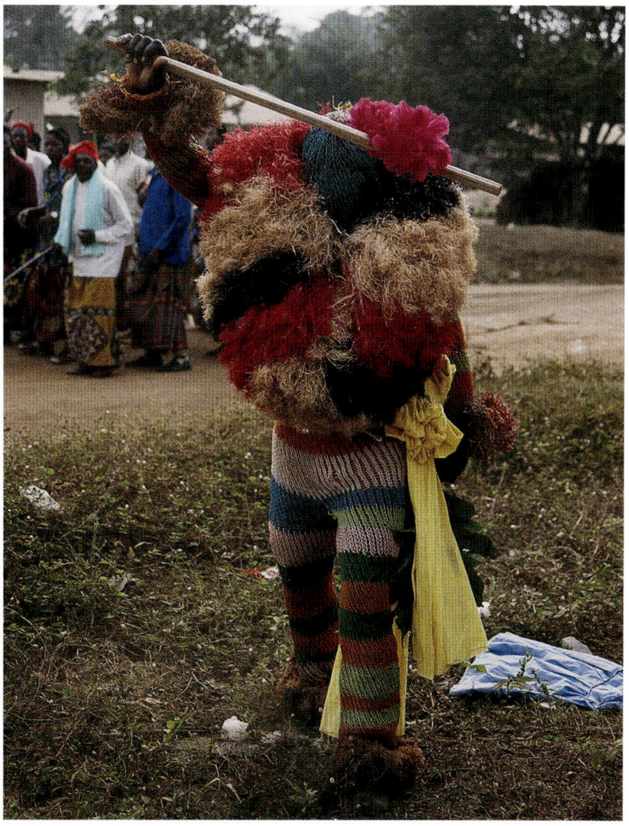

Fig. 90 A circle of fibres hangs round the neck of *Ema* (Kembong, January 18, 2004).

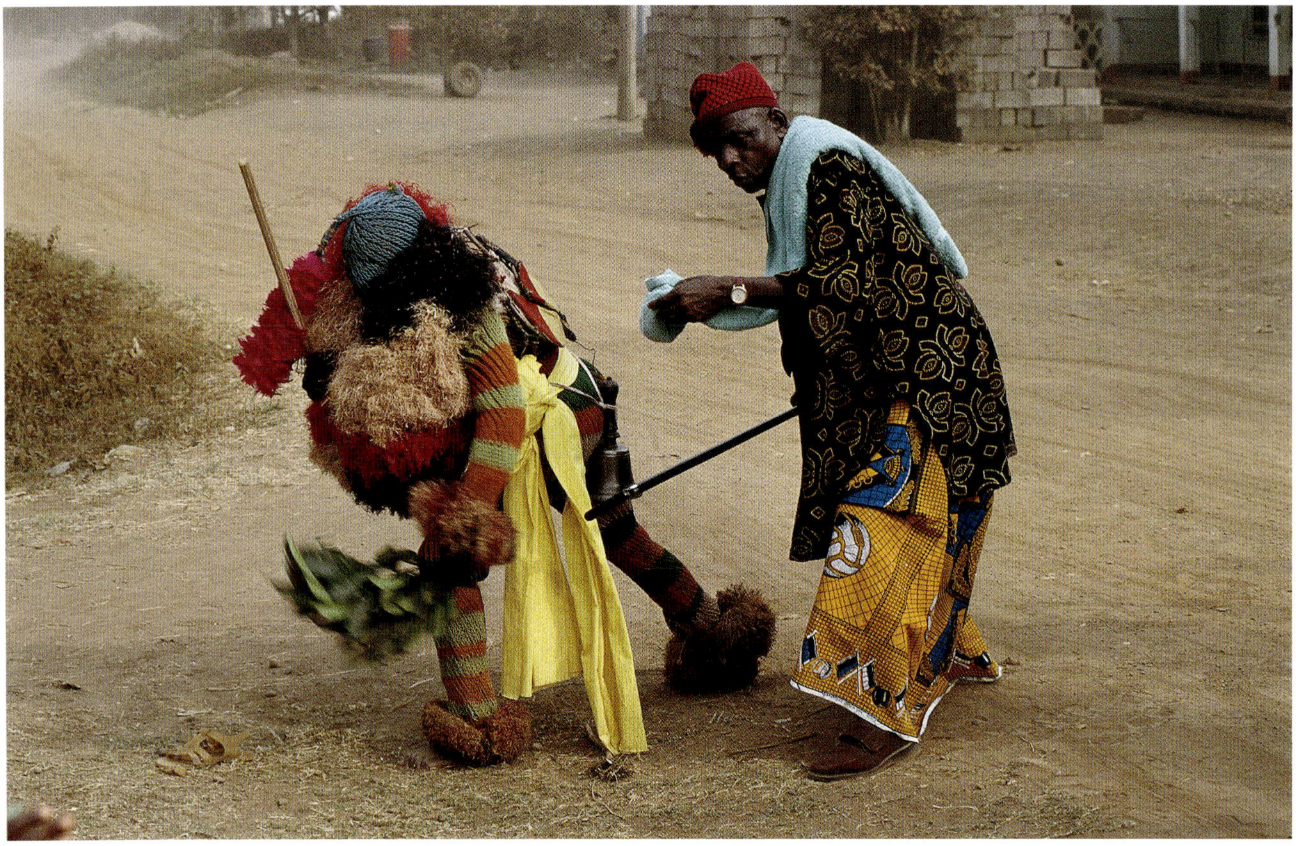

Fig. 91 Dance of the *seseku*, Elias Tanyi, with *Ema* (Kembong, January 18, 2004).

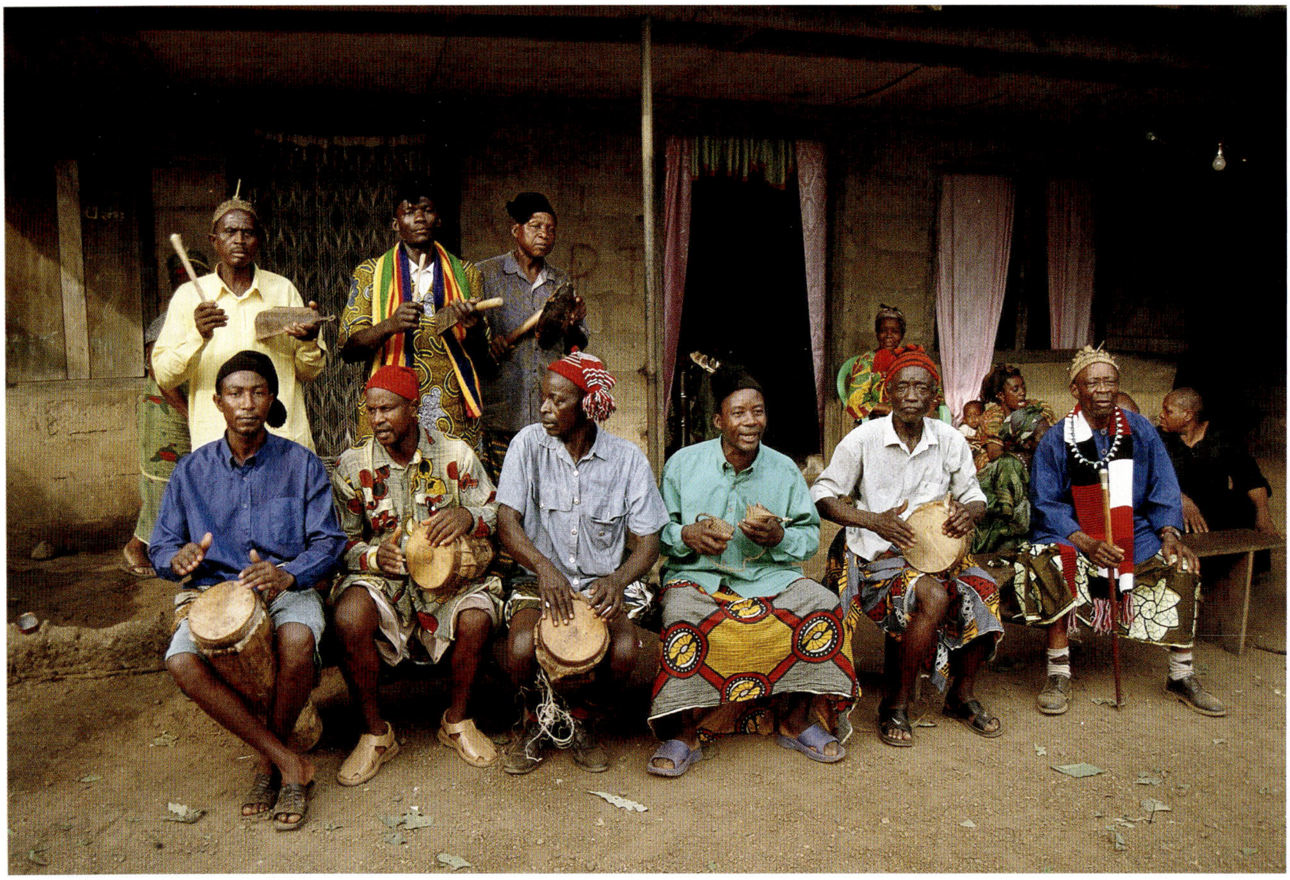

Fig. 92 The musicians of *Ema* with their instruments: small drums, hand rattles, iron gong and a tortoise shell (Kembong, January 18, 2004).

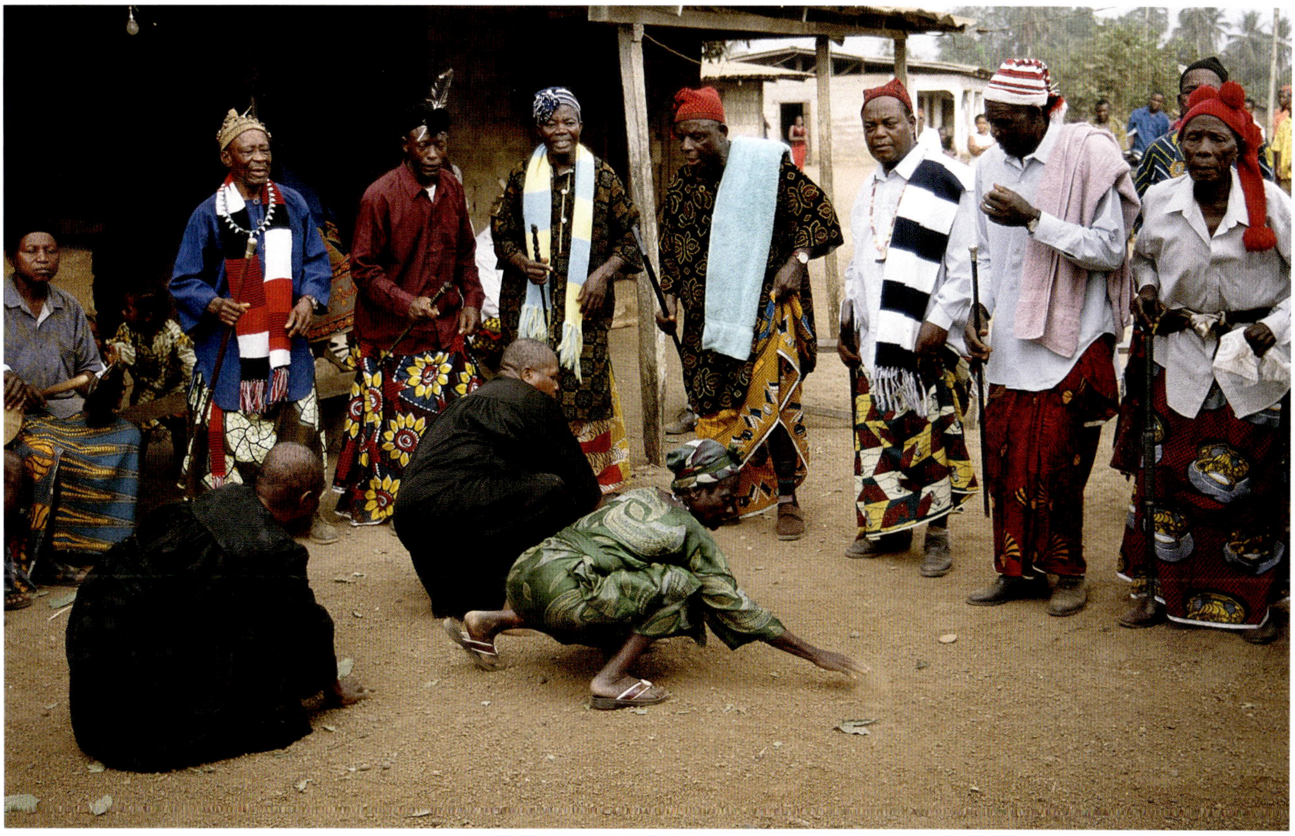

Fig. 93 The widows and a sister of the deceased clean the ground in the courtyard, according to tradition (Kembong, January 18, 2004).

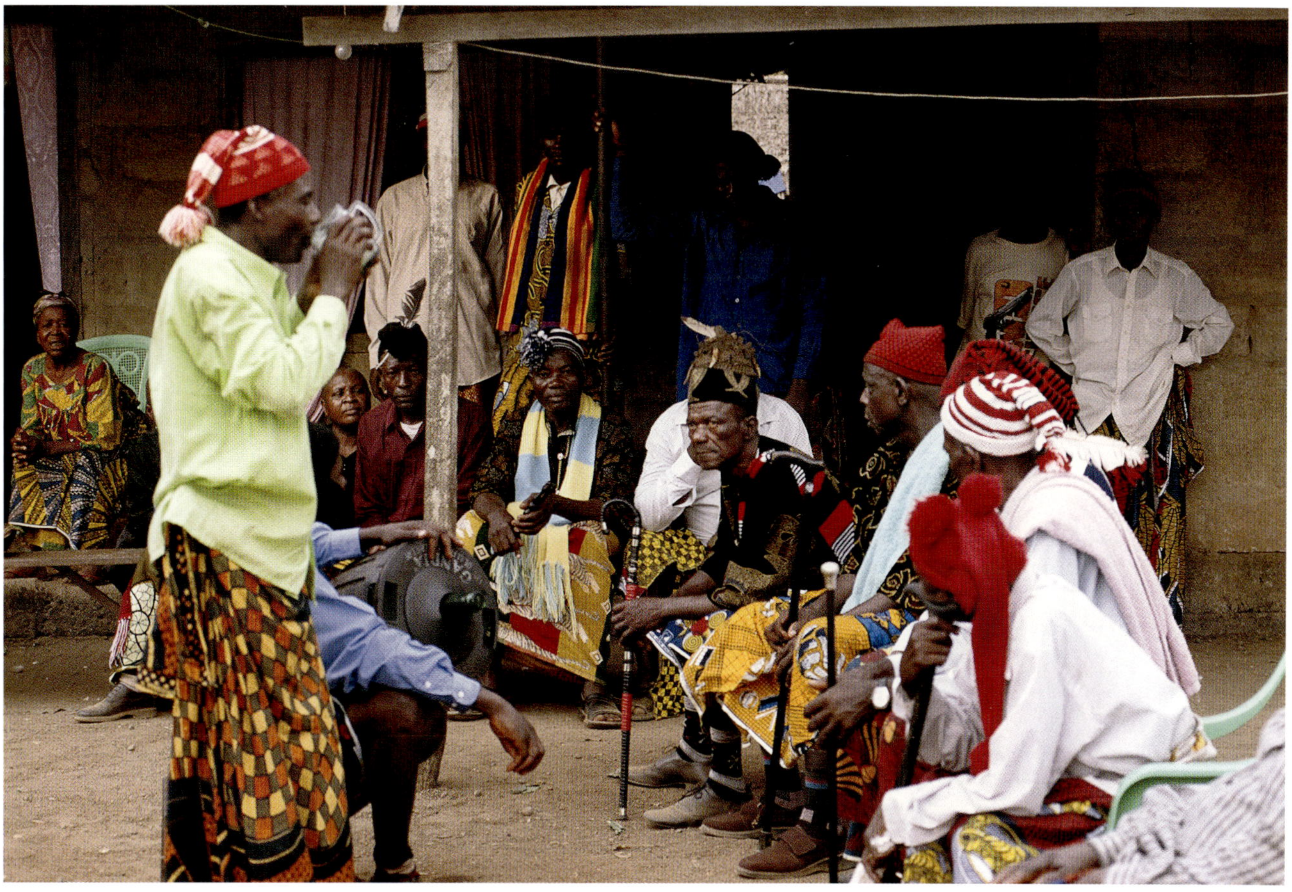

Fig. 94 Drinking palm wine. On the right some *boseseku* (Kembong, January 18, 2004).

Nchockandah, the mask of the young boys, in Kembong (figs. 95–96).

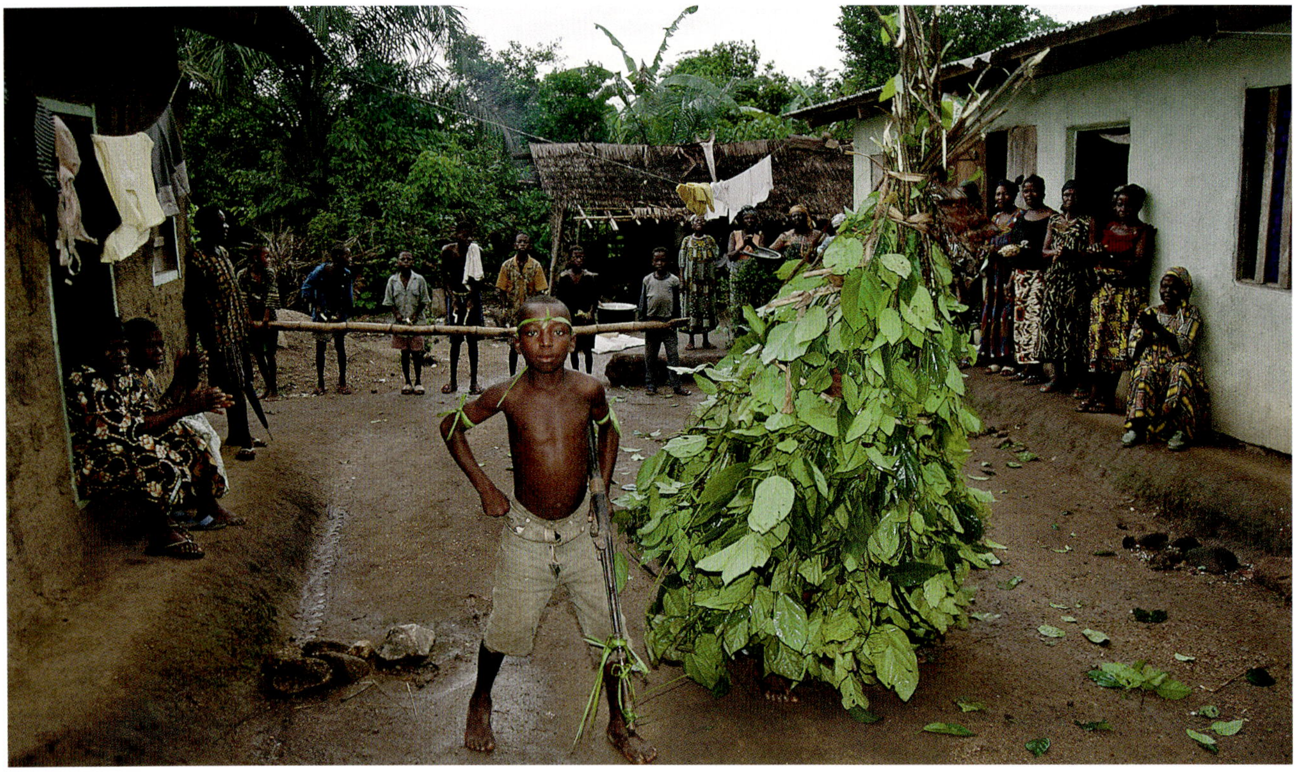

Fig. 95 Performance of *Nchockandah*, with *okina* (left) (Kembong, April 15, 2004).

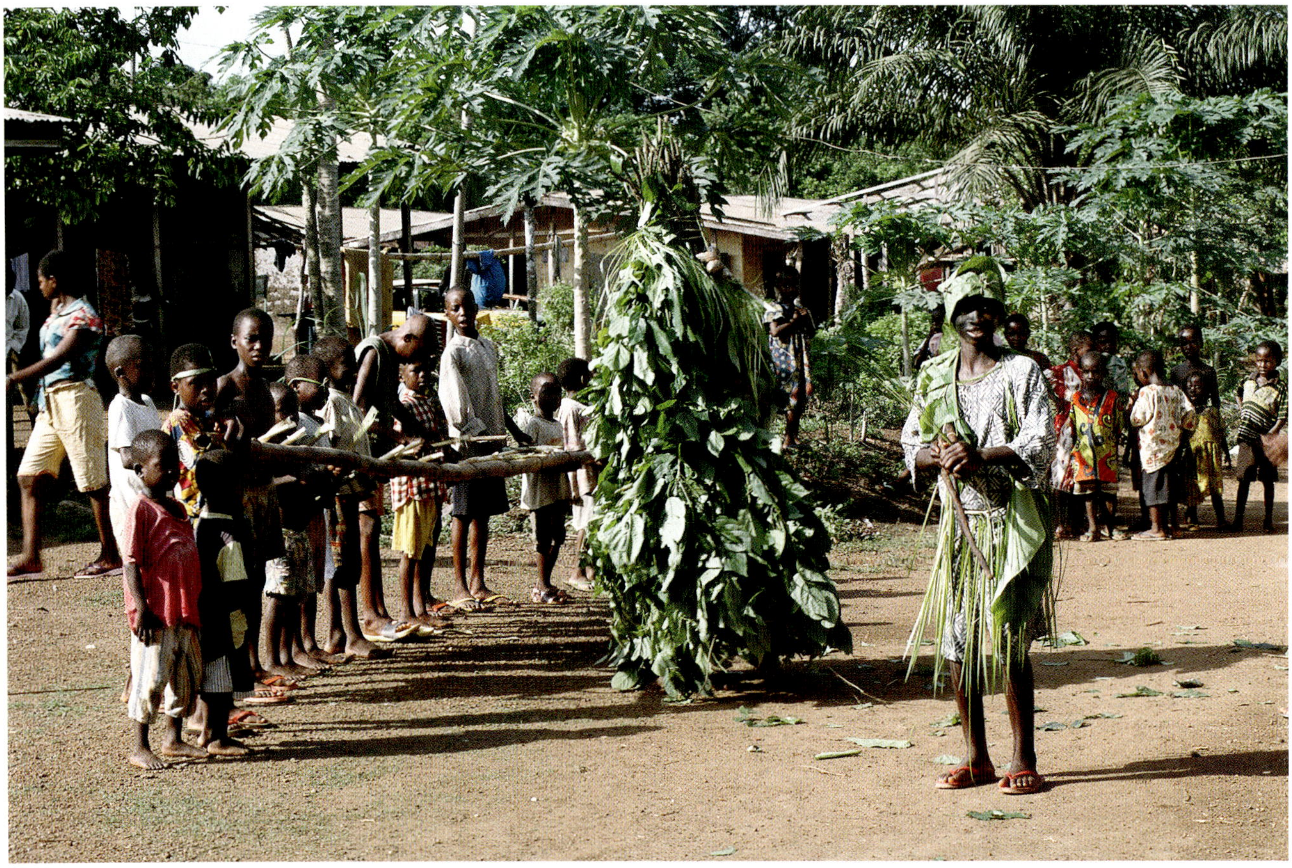

Fig. 96 Performance of *Nchockandah* in Okemebenem. The boys beat with sticks upon a long bamboo trunk (Kembong, April 20, 2004).

Performance of *Nchockandah* in Okemebenem (Kembong, November 18, 2005) (figs. 97–101).

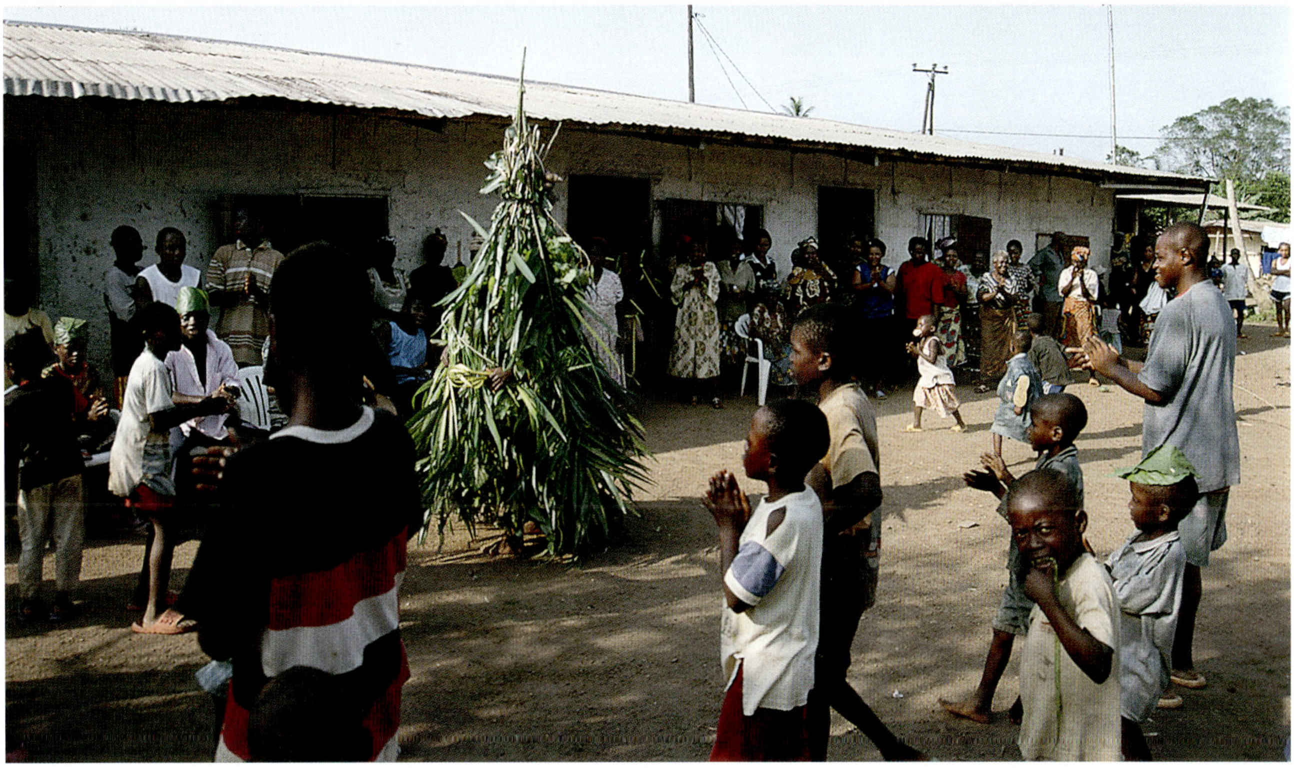

Fig. 97 Performance of the leaf-covered mask (Kembong, November 18, 2005).

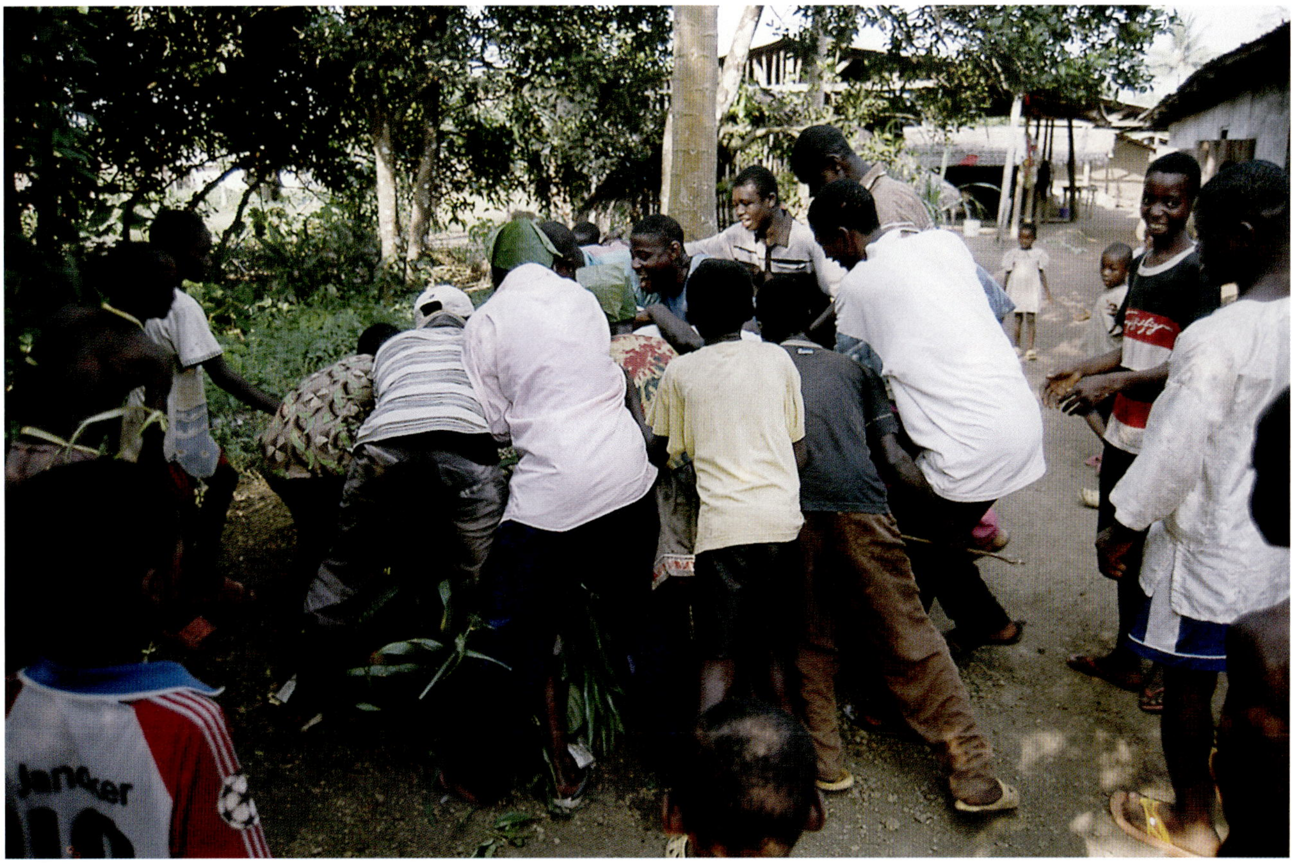

Fig. 98 The mask bearer leaves the mask "costume" upon the grave of the deceased. In doing so he is surrounded by other young men, in order that he remain unrecognised (Kembong, November 18, 2005).

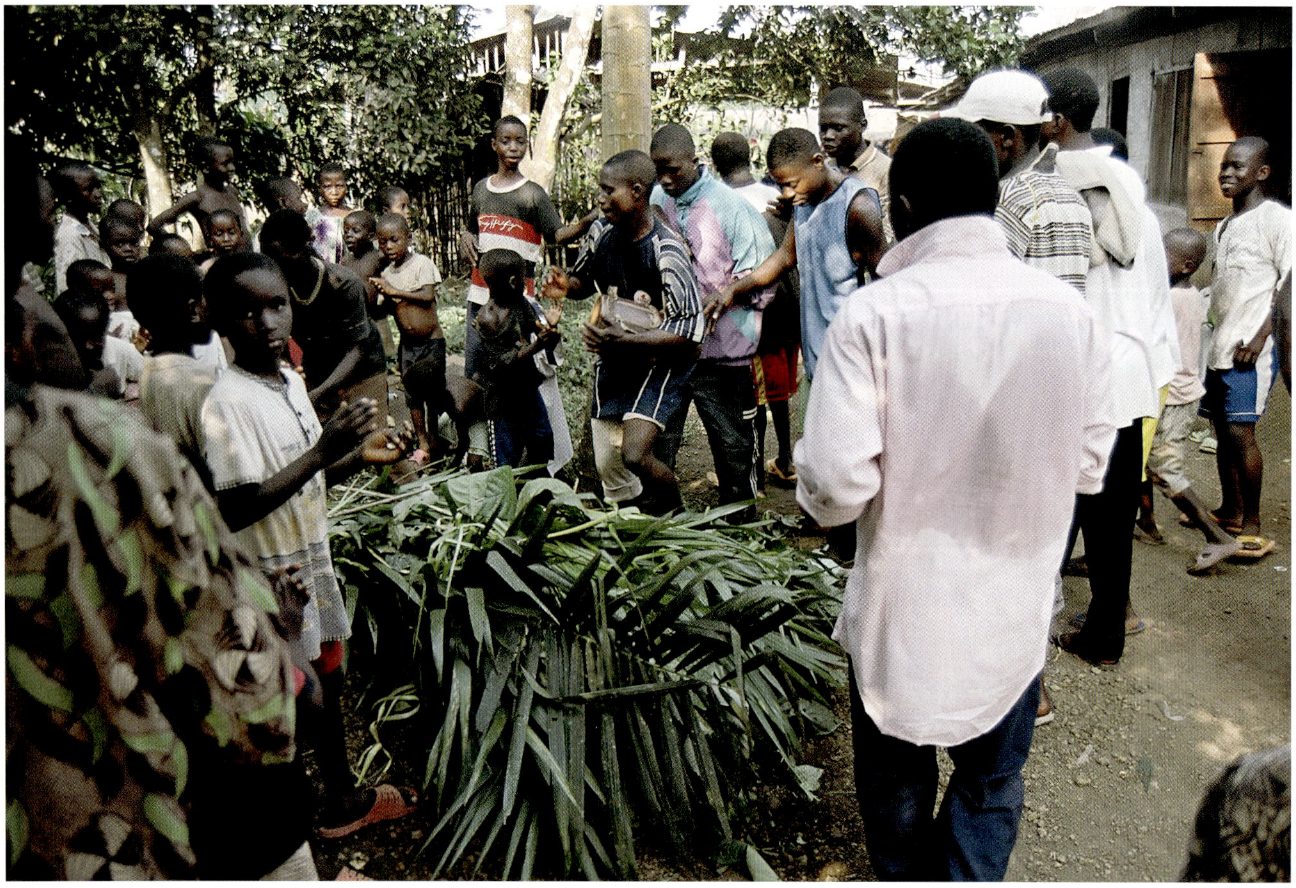

Fig. 99 The mask "costume" upon the grave of the deceased (Kembong, November 18, 2005).

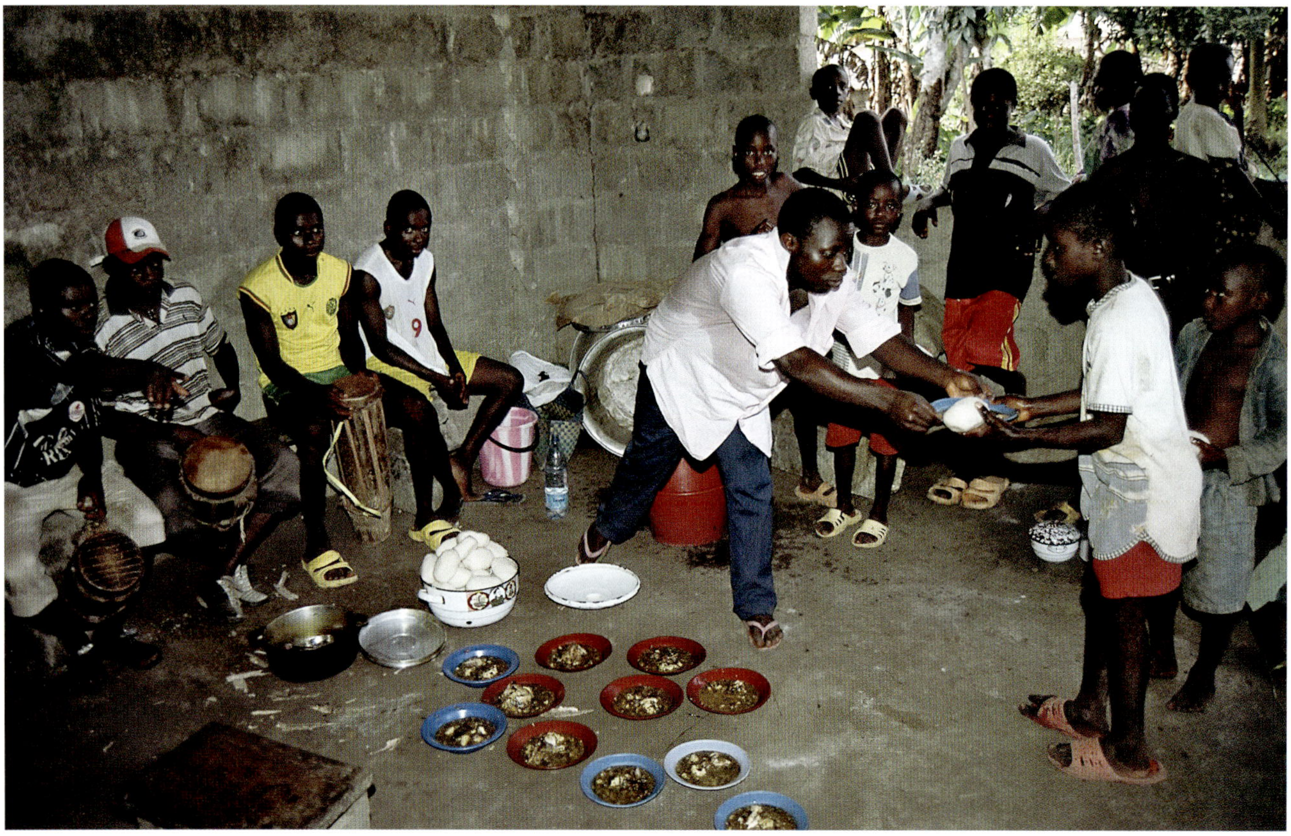

Fig. 100 Distribution of food to the young boys of *Nchockandah* (Kembong, November 18, 2005).

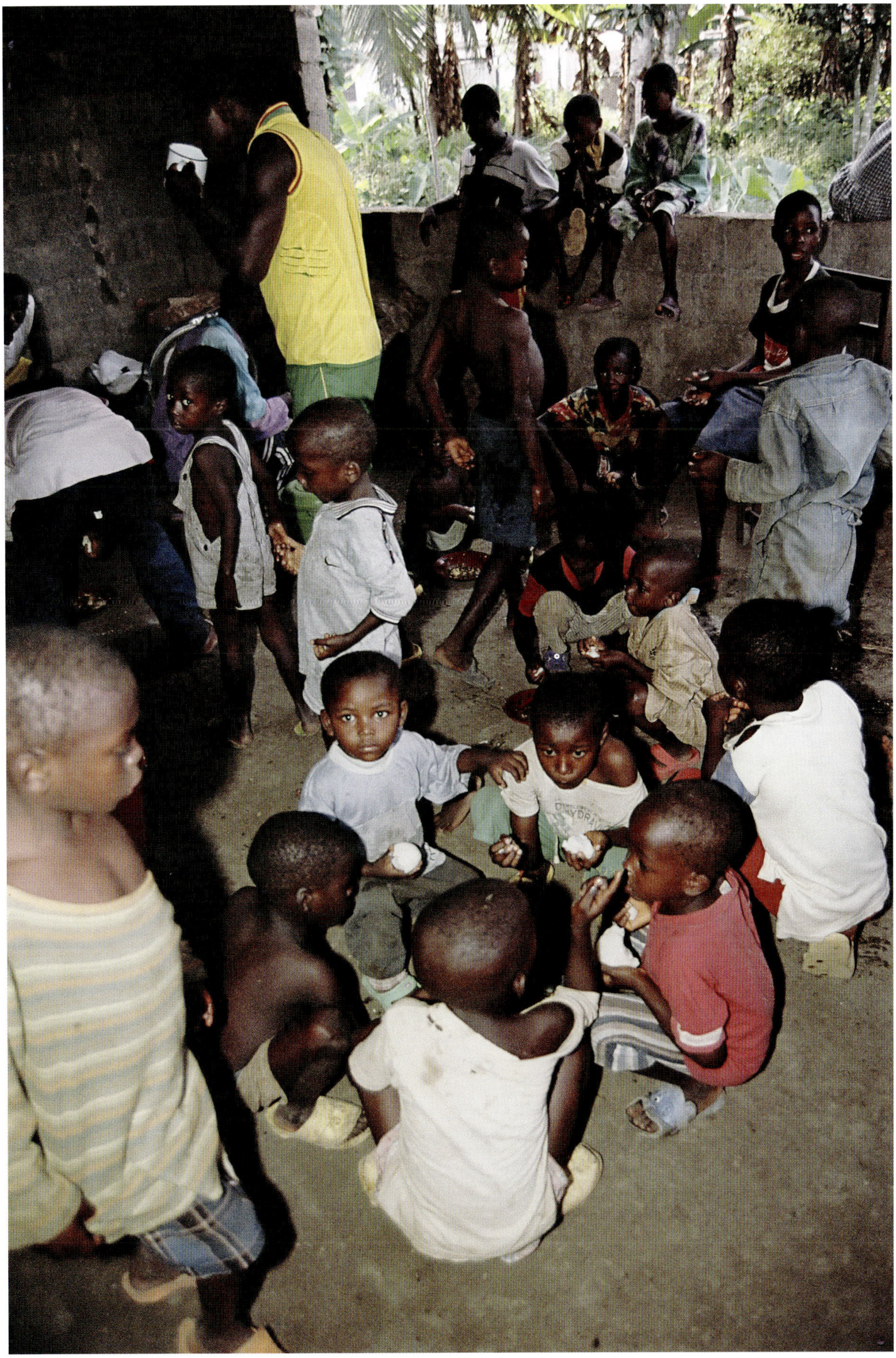

Fig. 101 Young boys of *Nchockandah* eating their festive meal (Kembong, November 18, 2005).

Following this other masks perform, such as *Ema* of *Mgbe* (figs. 85–94)[76] and *Nkanda* (figs. 102–109). The widows of the deceased also appear during the dance of *Ema*[77] and sweep clean the area in front of the deceased's house (fig. 93). In earlier times the widows were beaten by the mask with switches, to make sure that they destroy the possession of the deceased.[78] Yet, *Obasinjom* or other medicine societies do not appear on *aboku*; in fact, they do not participate at all in death celebrations held to honour their deceased members. After the masks *Ema* and *Nkanda* have finished their performances, dancing for the general public begins, and this usually lasts throughout the whole night until dawn. Then the dancing ends with the fourth and final appearance of *Ema*.

The last part of the death celebration is a festive meal (*etaah*), which comprises food for the dead, i. e. an offering to the ancestors – *etaah nji eyatek* ("food which is outside") (figs. 27–32, 74), as well as food for the living – *etaah nji ojyanju* ("food inside the house"). On this occasion it is the head of the family who carries out the offering. Holding the food for offering in both hands, he speaks: "*Ata Obasi ka oso, Akeku Kansi* (God in heaven and you ancestors below, i. e. in the earth), come and eat this food, which has been prepared for you." He places the food on the ground, then takes the vessel with palm wine in his left hand and addresses the ancestors: "*Ata Obasi ka oso, Akeku Kansi*, come and drink this wine. This wine is offered to you people. Take this wine and share it with the other ancestors whom I know and whom I do not know." Pouring some of the wine onto the ground for the ancestors, he now takes the vessel of palm wine in his right hand and turns to the living: "We who are living, the ancestors should give us blessings to have money in order to feed the children and the whole family." Taking a mug of water with his left hand, he addresses the ancestors anew: "If the ancestors have taken food and wine, they also take water to drink. This is the water. Take and drink it."

The death celebration concludes with an oracle (*ebanghaah*), which shows whether or not the ancestors have accepted the offerings. The oracle is made with two leaves, which the head of the family lets fall to the ground. The remaining food for offering to the ancestors is given as last to the children. With great interest the guests observe what happens to the food offered to the ancestors. Whereas it would be a very unfavourable sign if the food were taken by a dog, it would be – by contrast – a favourable sign if the chickens should devour it. Here, one could say, the hand of fate is influenced: dogs are chased away from the place of offering, while chickens are driven into its vicinity in order to attain a favourable omen. Following the offering to the ancestors the entertainment of the guests begins. Most of the guests are relatives and from the same community. Afterwards the members of the family gather – many of them are from other regions – to settle important family matters. If the dead person was a member of *Mgbe, Mgbe* would have left the compound in the meantime. So would the leopard – it would have fled back to the grove of *Mgbe*.

4.1.7 The *Mgbe* society today

To this day *Mgbe* still holds considerably great authority; moreover it is the institution that attends to proper customs and to peace and order in the community. Thus, upright and moral conduct is always expected of its members: they may not steal, deceive, commit adultery, use obscene words, become involved in fights, waste food, behave improperly towards women and – in former times – mistreat slaves. Nowadays *Mgbe* is seen in public primarily at death celebrations for its deceased members, which it determines more or less and also enhances with its impressive processions and dances accompanied by its spectacular masks. It is thus granted that the members of *Mgbe* are generously accommodated by the bereaved family for several days. In general, the members receive abundant food and drink, on the one hand, through the many death celebrations, and, on the other, through the many fines that are imposed. In this respect the high fees for admission into the society and for reaching numerous levels are good investments.[79] Occasionally, however, the remark is heard that the exceedingly strict enforcement of laws and the severe sentences are made in the interest of *Mgbe* members alone.[80] Yet, the strictly regimented behaviour undoubtedly also serves the purpose of emphasising and safeguarding the hierarchical distinctions that are nonetheless present in so-called egalitarian societies.

In any case, today *Mgbe* still holds a well acknowledged political standing in Kembong, although it has lost much of its former significance and power.[81] Most of the legal and criminal cases are administered by public courts and offices. Still the members of *Mgbe*, wearing their special caps and insignia, appear in public self-confident and proud. The secrets of *Mgbe* are preserved as ever in utmost silence, and its regulations are always followed. Besides, in the age of television and mobile telephones *Mgbe* is respected and feared as the "watchdog" of society: "*Mgbe* catches faster than medicine."

4.2 *Nkanda*

Nkanda is a secret society for men, which is widespread in the Cross River region.[82] Persons in *Nkanda* meet only when new members are admitted and at death celebrations for deceased members. In the latter case *Nkanda* honours the dead person with dances, the performance of its mask being the climax of the occasion. Also non-members can engage *Nkanda* to dance by paying an accordant fee, for instance, for a death celebration or a visit by a high-ranking personality. In all cases the performance of such a renowned society underscores the significance of the respective event. Meant as entertainment for those present, these dances represent the single purpose of *Nkanda* – it does not have any other duties. It does not possess medicines and, as explicitly stated, its mask has nothing to do with spirits.

Presumably in most communities *Nkanda* is a section of *Mgbe*.[83] In Kembong, by contrast, there were allegedly several independent *Nkanda* lodges, which, however, gradually dissolved following the deaths of their chiefs. Today *Nkanda* is present only in the quarter Okonyenge. Although it functions as an independent society, it does have ties to *Mgbe*; for example, its centre is the "*Ekpe* Hall" (the hall of *Mgbe*). According to my informants *Nkanda* became established in Kembong before World War I.

Nkanda in Kembong has four levels:
1. *Nsibiri Nkanda* – the first level for young members. None of my informants knew the reason for the curious designation *nsibiri*, which literally means "bad feelings and intentions".
2. *Eteme Nkanda*, "the grove of *Nkanda*", is the stage of full membership.
3. *Eboho Nkanda*, "the mud-bed of *Nkanda*", has two to three members who function as big men.
4. *Njoho Nkanda* is the chief of *Nkanda*, the "man who performs the sacrifices".

All public performances of *Nkanda* begin with a procession, in which the protagonists must maintain a spe-

Performance of *Nkanda* in Okonyenge (Kembong, January 27, 2004) (figs. 102–109).

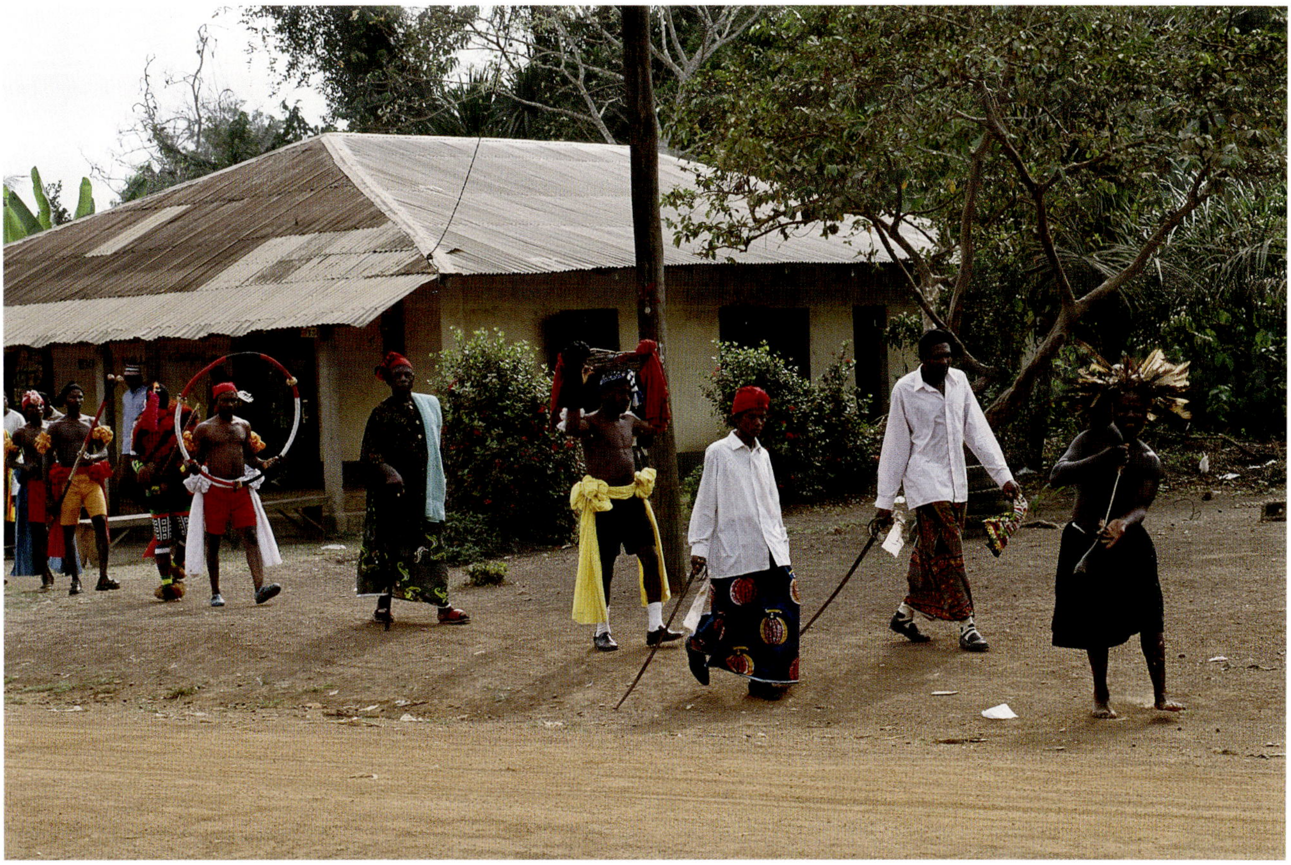

Fig. 102 *Nkanda* proceeds to the compound in which its mask will perform. At the head is *iroko*, followed by two men each carrying a cutlass, after them *ekpang Nkanda* with a basket upon his head, *ejoho Nkanda* (the chief of *Nkanda*, Elias Tanyi), *ekasi Nkanda* with a hoop and the mask itself; behind the mask are two men with special staffs. In the background the "*Ekpe* Hall" (the hall of *Mgbe*) in Okonyenge (Kembong, January 27, 2004).

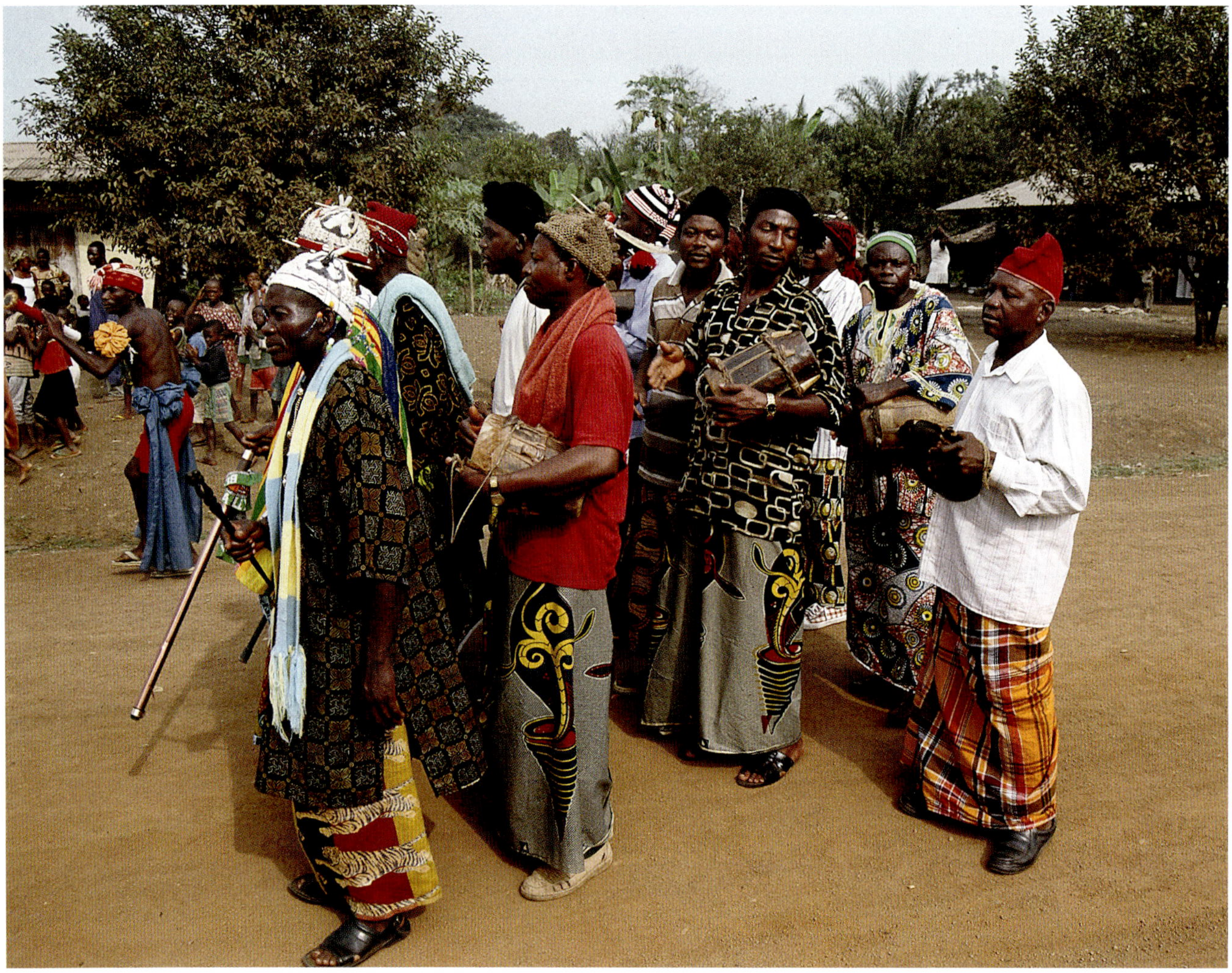

Fig. 103 *Nkanda*: in front, a few *boseseku*, behind them ordinary members with drums and other percussion instruments (Kembong, January 27, 2004).

cific sequence in actions (fig. 102).[84] The procession is led by the announcer, *iroko*, who informs the community of *Nkanda's* pending appearance, and who like *okina* of *Ebongu/Ema* also acts as a jester. Typical of *iroko* are the dark feathers, which he wears upon his head, and the dark skirt. In his hands he holds two buffalo horns, which are tied together with a string (figs. 103, 111, 114). *Iroko* is followed by two men, *anne akangkang*, armed with cutlasses, who clear the way for *Nkanda* and attend to keeping order. Next in the group is *ekpang Nkanda*, who bears a basket upon his head. The fifth position is reserved for the *njoho Nkanda*, the chief of *Nkanda*. Behind him dances *ekasi Nkanda*, an extremely agile figure, who holds a hoop. His role is to lead the mask, to show it the way and, thus, he always stays near the mask (figs. 104, 110, 112, 115). Accordingly, the mask, *okum Nkanda*, takes this place in line. It is followed by two men, *mfa Nkanda* ("fork of *Nkanda*") and *echakara ngomba* (no translation), each carrying a special staff. It is their task to protect the mask. The procession is completed by the rest of the members of *Nkanda*. When it reaches the festive square, the participants separate from the line and then begin to dance.

The mask, *okum Nkanda*, represents the central figure (figs. 104–108, 110, 112, 113, 115). It is similar to the mask of *Ebongu*: It does not wear a wooden headdress, and its dress is also knitted, but with bright and more colourful yarn. A ring of fibres hangs around its neck and around its feet, and it wears a stick with beautiful multi-coloured feathers tied loosely upon its head. Also like the mask of *Ebongu/Ema,* a big bell is attached to the back of the mask's garment (figs. 108, 112).[85]

Fig. 104 *Iroko*, the announcer of *Nkanda*, with his two buffalo horns (Kembong, January 27, 2004). ▸

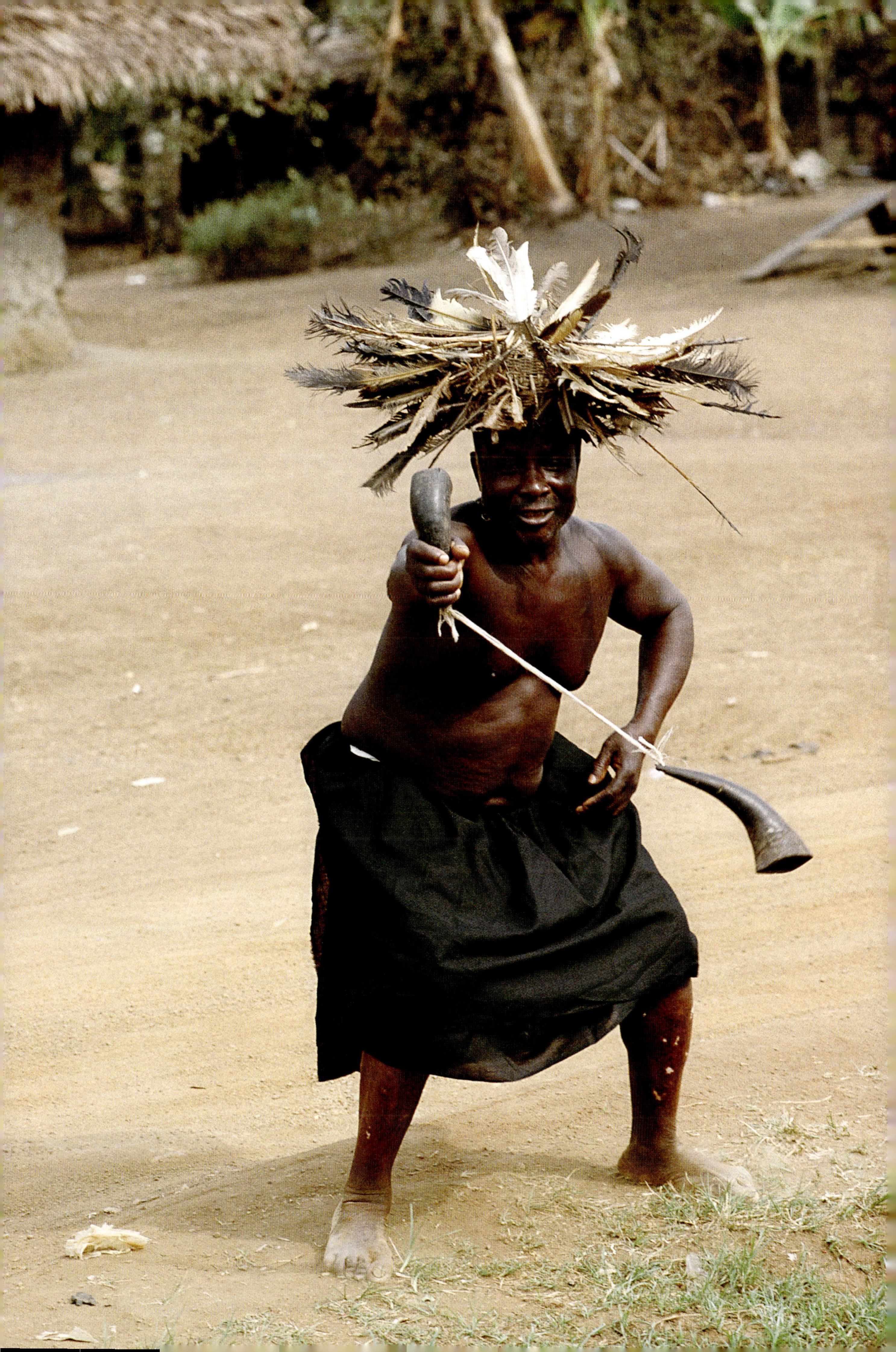

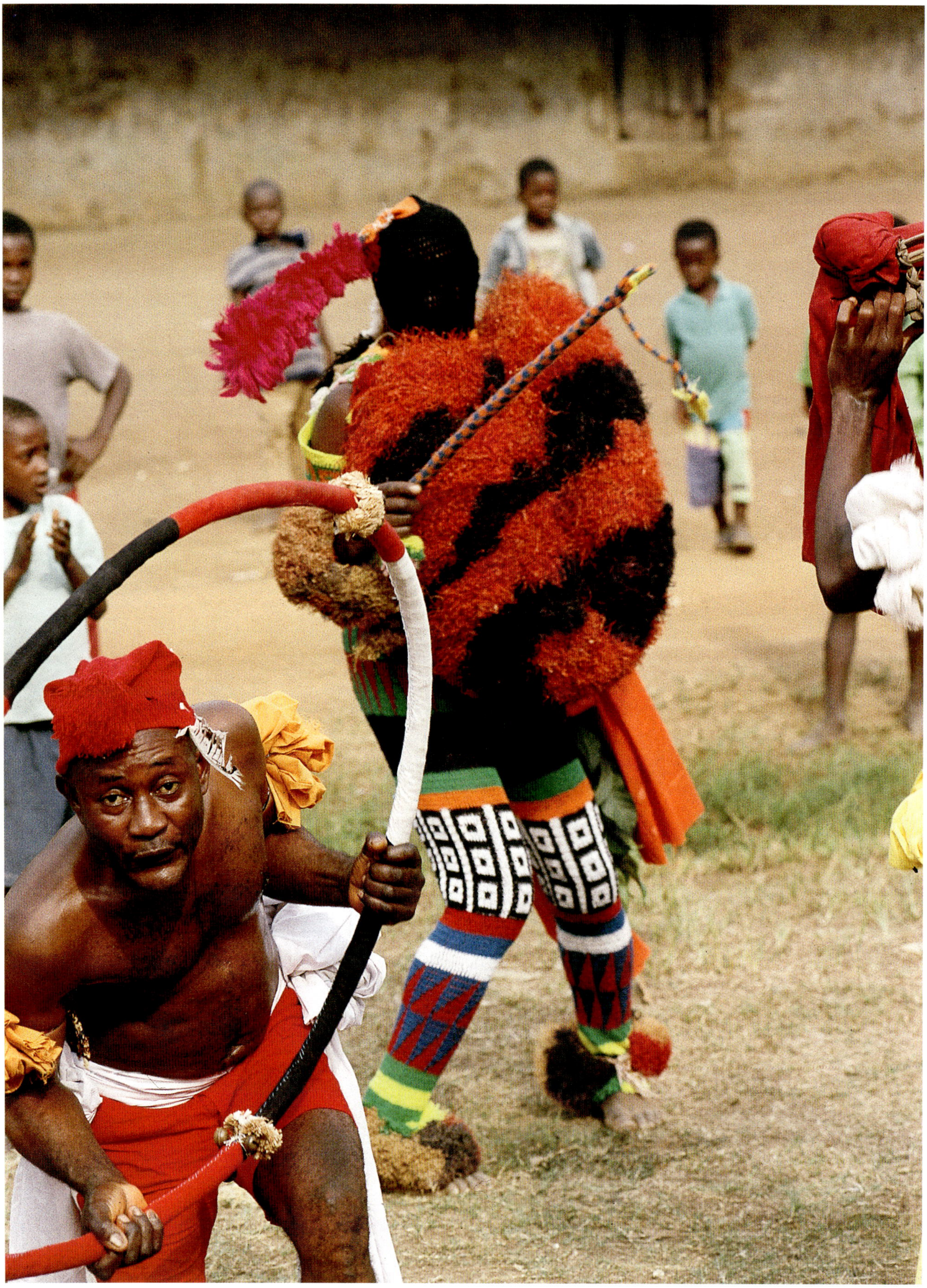

Fig. 105 The mask of *Nkanda* with *ekasi Nkanda*, an agile figure with his hoop (Kembong, January 27, 2004).

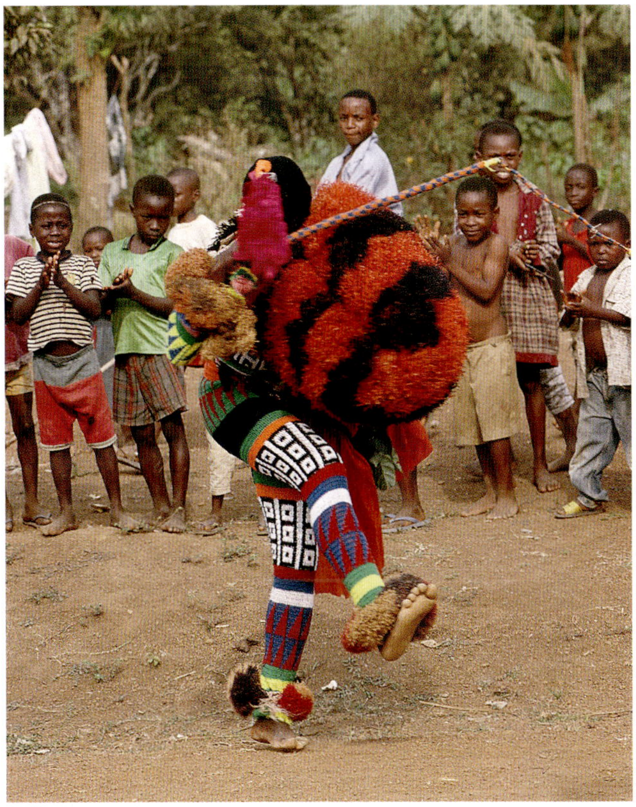

Fig. 106 Performance of the mask *Nkanda* (Kembong, January 27, 2004).

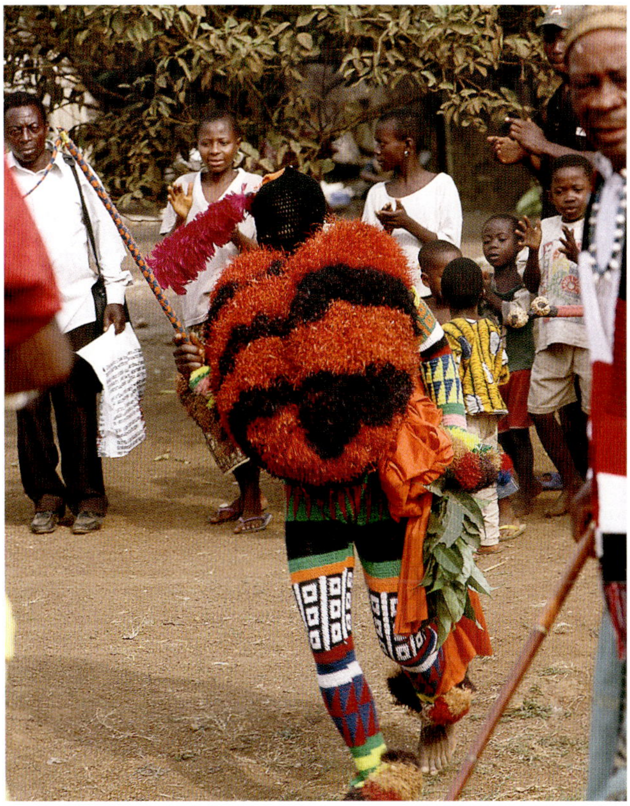

Fig. 107 *Nkanda* holds a stick in the right hand and medicine plants in the left (Kembong, January 27, 2004).

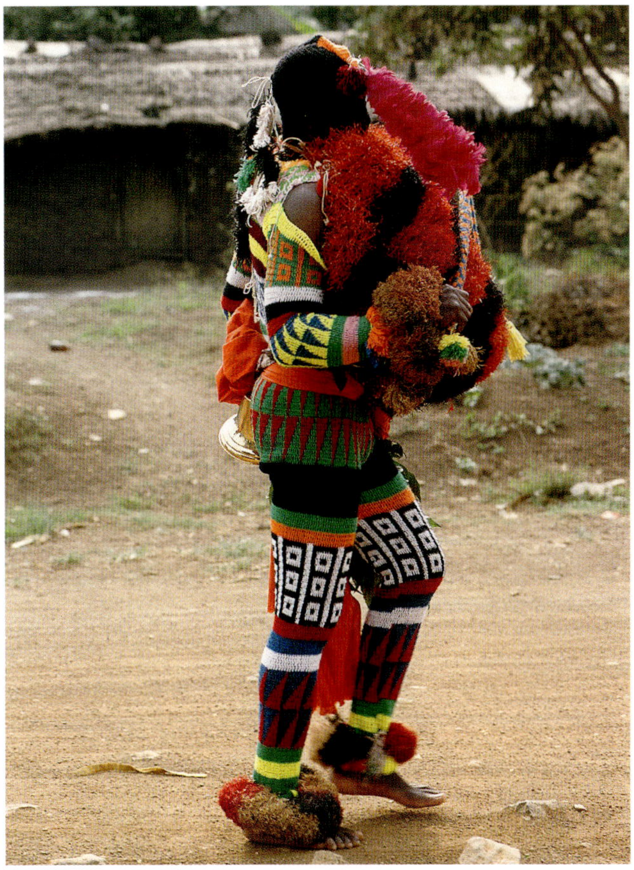

Fig. 108 *Nkanda* with its colourful dress (Kembong, January 27, 2004).

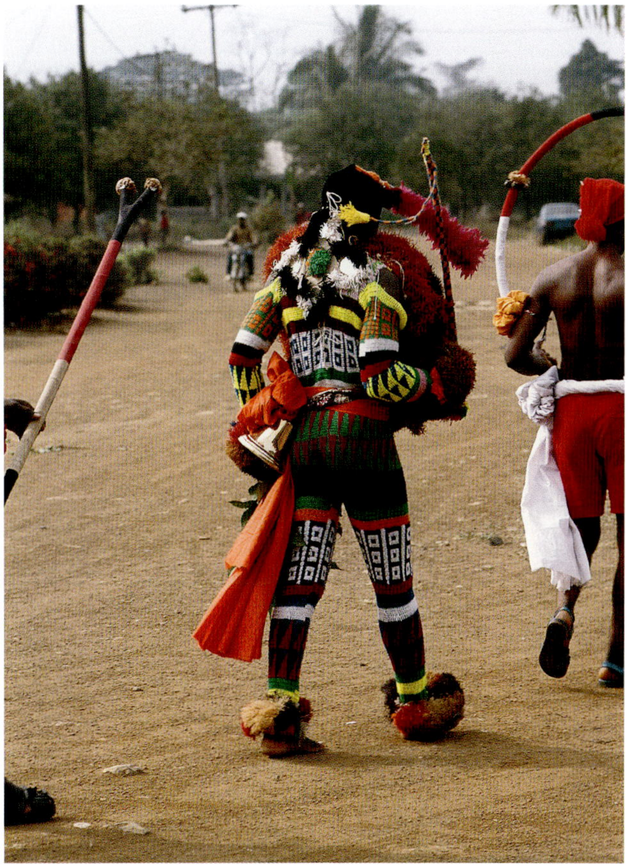

Fig. 109 Like *Ebongu/Ema*, *Nkanda* carries a bell on its back (Kembong, January 27, 2004).

Performance of *Nkanda* in Babong (February 20, 1980) (figs. 110–112).

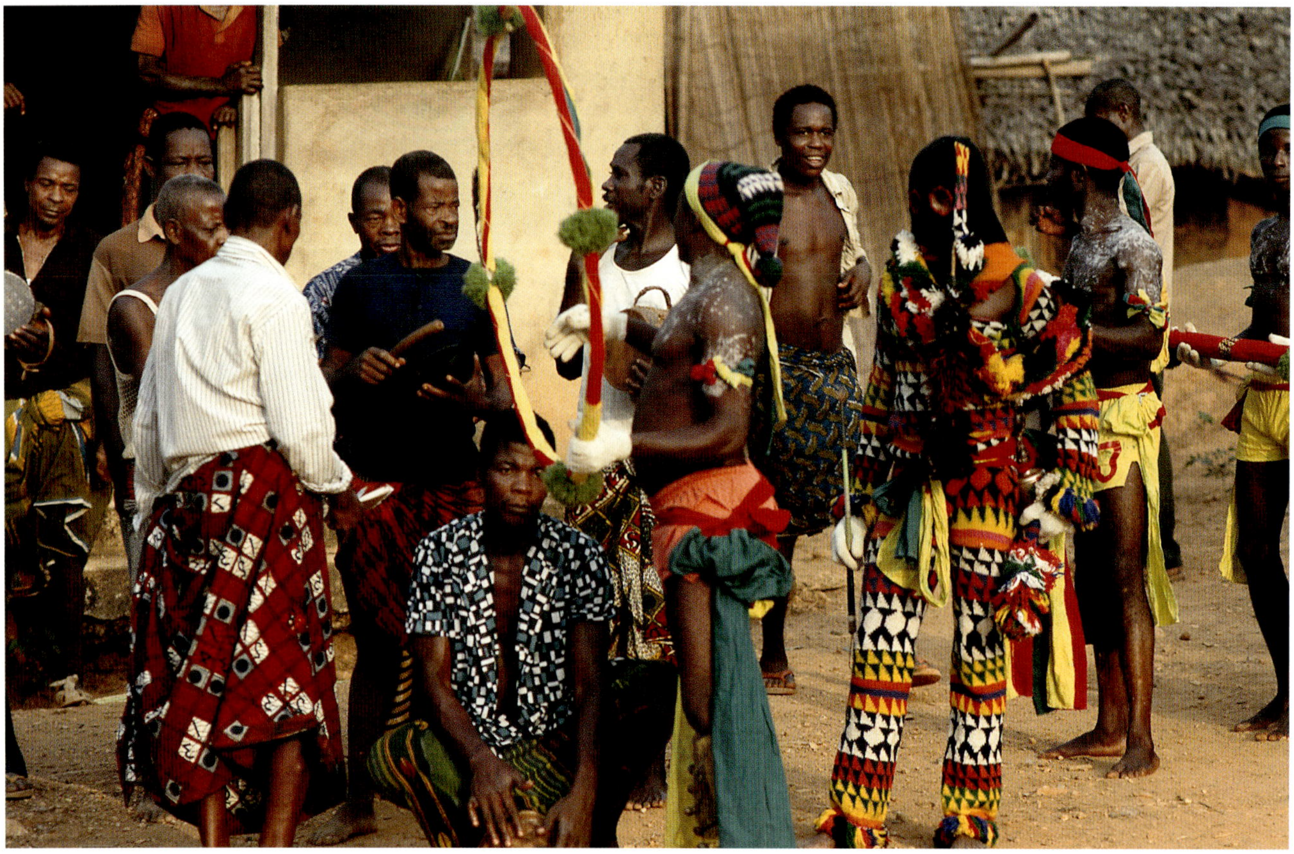

Fig. 110 Gathering of the members, among them the mask in the knitted outfit and *ekasi Nkanda* with his hoop (Babong, February 20, 1980).

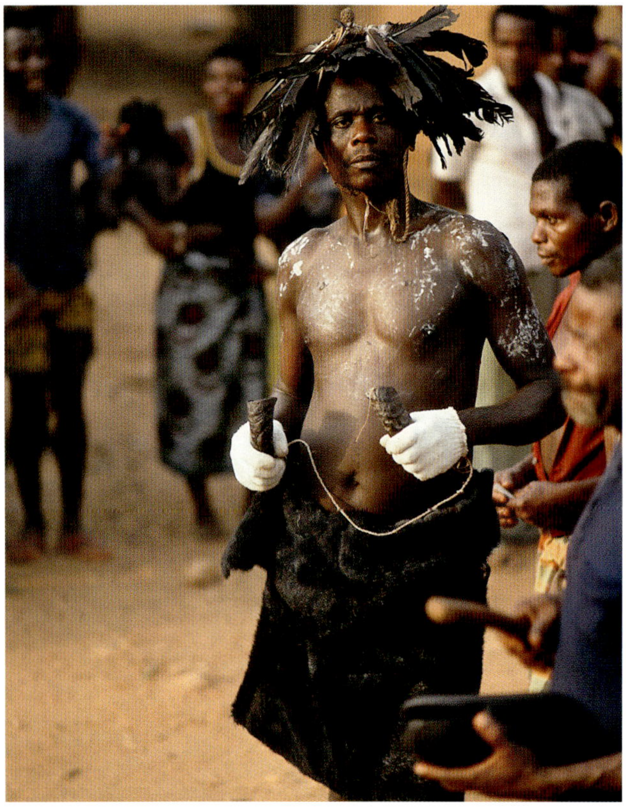

Fig. 111 *Iroko*, the announcer of *Nkanda*, with his two horns (Babong, February 20, 1980).

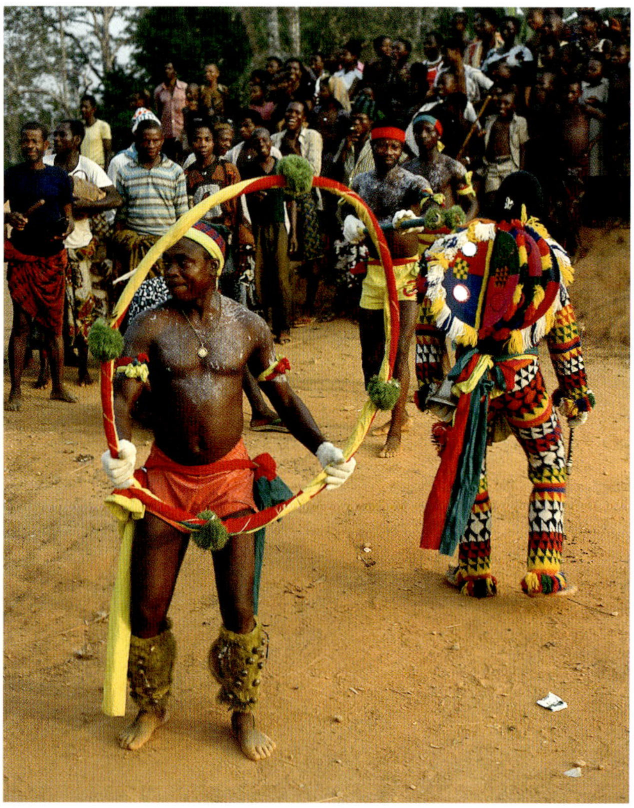

Fig. 112 *Ekasi Nkanda* (left) and the mask with a large bell (right, view from behind) (Babong, February 20, 1980).

Performance of *Nkanda* in Ewelle (March 26, 2005) (figs. 113–115).

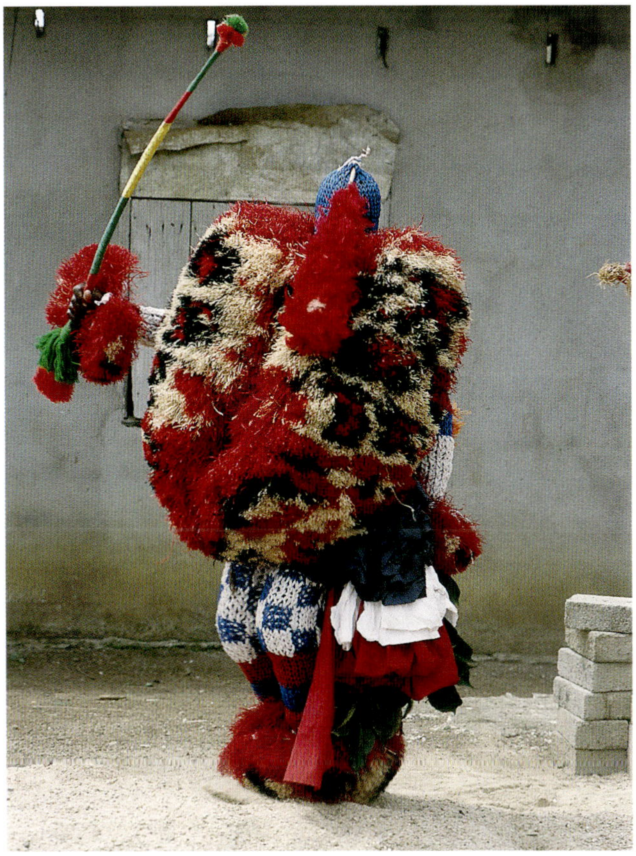

Fig. 113 The mask *Nkanda* itself (Ewelle, March 26, 2005).

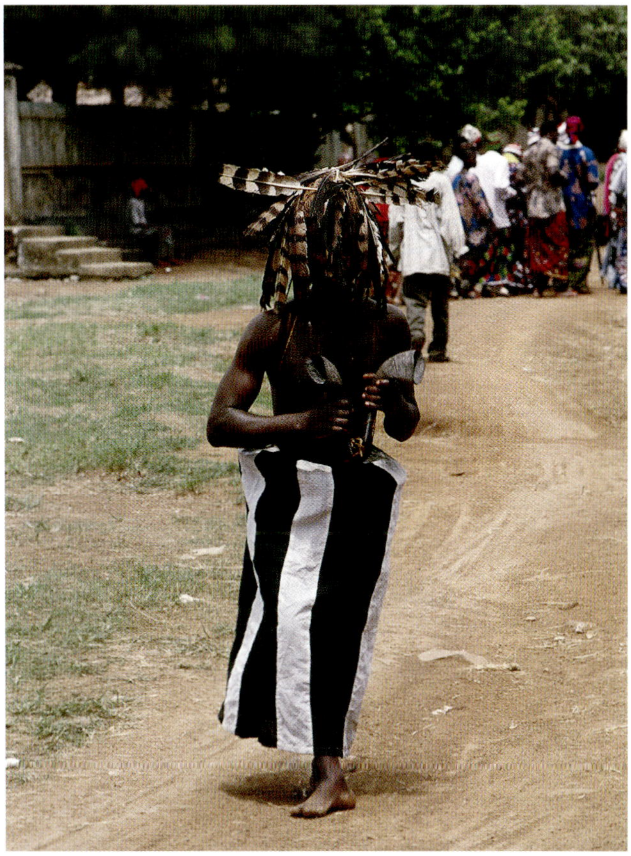

Fig. 114 *Iroko*, the announcer of *Nkanda* (Ewelle, March 26, 2005).

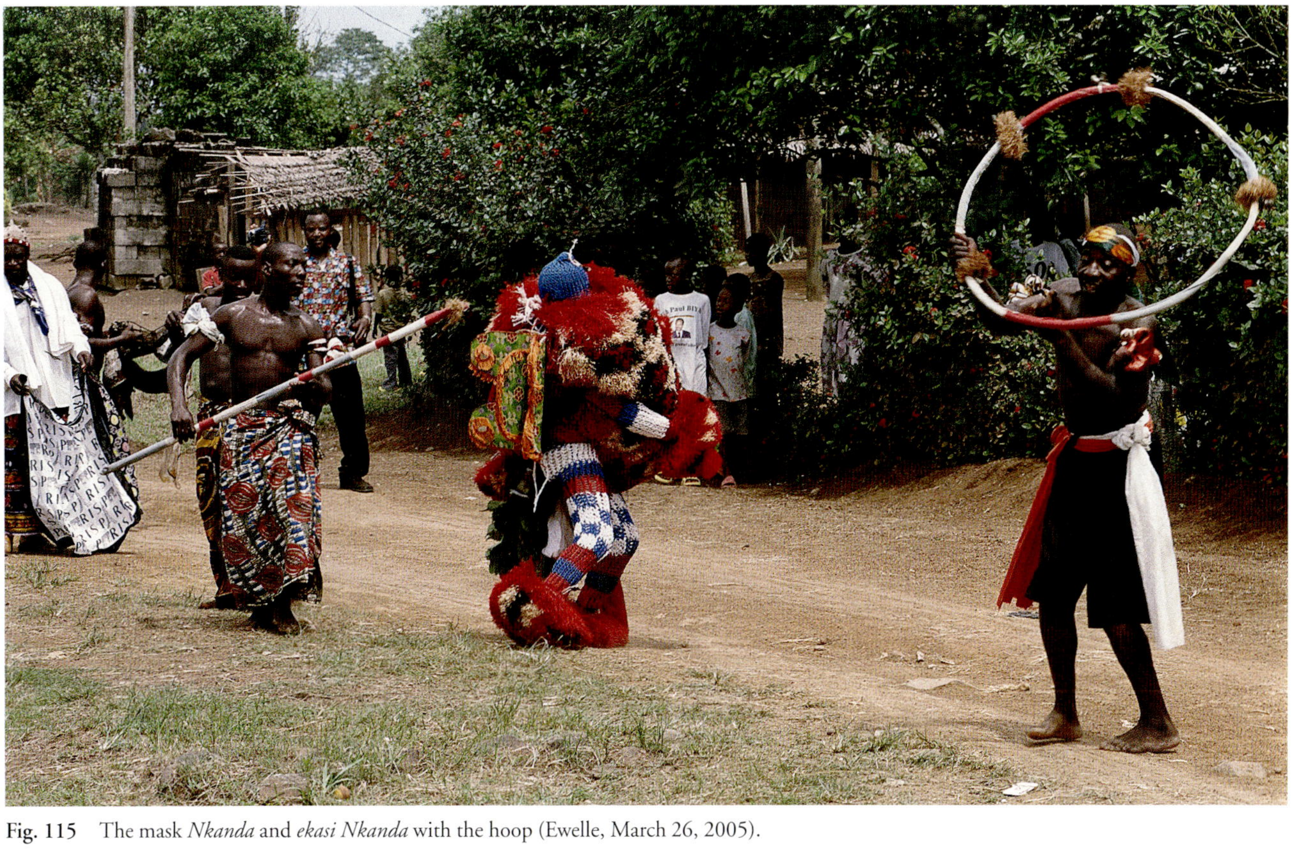

Fig. 115 The mask *Nkanda* and *ekasi Nkanda* with the hoop (Ewelle, March 26, 2005).

4.3 The skin-covered masks, *Nchebe* and *Mkpe*, and night dances

Among the most important and eminent works of traditional art in Africa are the skin-covered masks, which display human or animal form. Long known in the Cross River region, the masks are disseminated throughout the area between Calabar in the south and the Boki in the north, and between the Ibibio and Ibo in the west and the Widekum and Bangwa in the east (both in the Grasslands).[86] Surprisingly masks of this type are not found in any other part of Africa. Whereas almost one thousand examples of this strongly expressive and exceedingly realistic work are now in European and American museums and art collections,[87] skin-covered masks are seldom encountered in their homeland. Even in earlier times, these masks evidently appeared in public only on very special occasions, which might explain the paucity of available information about them.[88] Thus, there is neither detailed knowledge about the societies to which they belonged nor about the exact background of the ceremonies for which they were intended. Furthermore, even less can be stated with certainty about the meaning and importance that they possessed and whom or whatever they "represented".

It is, without doubt, the unusual construction of the mask with a skin-covered headdress that has led to speculations about their derivation as well as their special position in the respective social and religious systems. Thus, most of the anthropomorphic mask headgear is seen as representations of ancestors,[89] the covering of skin – some examples allegedly of human skin – having obviously been used as additional evidence for this assumption.[90] It has even been stated that formerly all masks of this kind were covered with human skin. Mansfeld already expressed that opinion, which he cautiously formulated: "Formerly, the masks were covered with the skin of slain enemies and then worn at dances in honour of the respective *juju*-society. It is of course difficult to say whether this explanation of the head-*juju*-masks is correct; in any case, it does hold great likelihood."[91] Additional arguments in favour of this theory – masks are representations of ancestors – resulted from the fact that the human skull was used as mask headgear, although rather rarely. Talbot noted several times that "wooden masks covered with skin (were) used, in lieu of the freshly killed heads of enemies formerly borne by the victors."[92] Yet, these theories still lack concrete evidence. And Nicklin was completely correct in his statement that, "The original inspiration for this art form must at present remain a matter for conjecture, ..."[93]

As has become clear in the course of this study, the theory that African masks are to be understood as representations of supernatural powers cannot be asserted for the masks of *Mgbe*, *Ebongu* and *Ema*, nor for the masks *Angbu* and *Obasinjom*, as will be discussed below. This applies as well to the skin-covered masks of the Central Ejagham. Aside from information received from my informants, to be discussed below, difficulties arise when attempting to expand the above theory to animal-shaped masks that are covered with skin.[94] According to Ekpo Eyo, such "animal masks" were "models of animals killed during hunting expeditions."[95] Even long ago Talbot was of the opinion that performances of such masks "were conducted for the purpose of fertility in animals."[96] Both attempts at an explanation are hardly convincing, for there are too few reports about hunting rituals in this region, in which masks played or still play a role.

As noted above, there is little information about these special masks. The few reports about them are scarcely sufficient, and even fewer photographs record the masks' performances.[97] In addition, scholarly documentation of the masks has become all the more difficult due to the apparent decline of this tradition since early colonial times. Thus, Mansfeld remarked that at his time only one single "producer of the *juju*-heads" still existed,[98] and in 1979 Nicklin noted concisely that "In Nigeria ... the carving of skin-covered masks is virtually extinct."[99] Mansfeld also described the intense trade in these masks, which had developed on the coast as early as the beginning of the 20th century. "White collectors of rarities" obviously had bought considerable numbers of "*juju*-heads", and also "the trading companies had a general order ... for the purchase of things which they in turn sold at a high price on the coast." It is noteworthy, too, as he pointed out, that masks were already produced specifically for sale to Europeans.[100]

I myself had the opportunity to make the acquaintance of a carver of these masks in the Ngunaya area in 1980. He was supposedly the last of his trade in this region. Augustine Etta was about thirty years of age at that time and lived in Mbakang. Following three years of training under a master carver, for which he had to pay one cock, a carton of tobacco and a new cutlass at the beginning and thirty English pounds at the end, Augustine Etta has worked independently as a carver since

Fig. 116 Close-up of the skin-covered headdress of *Nchebe* (Ewelle, February 26, 1980). ▸

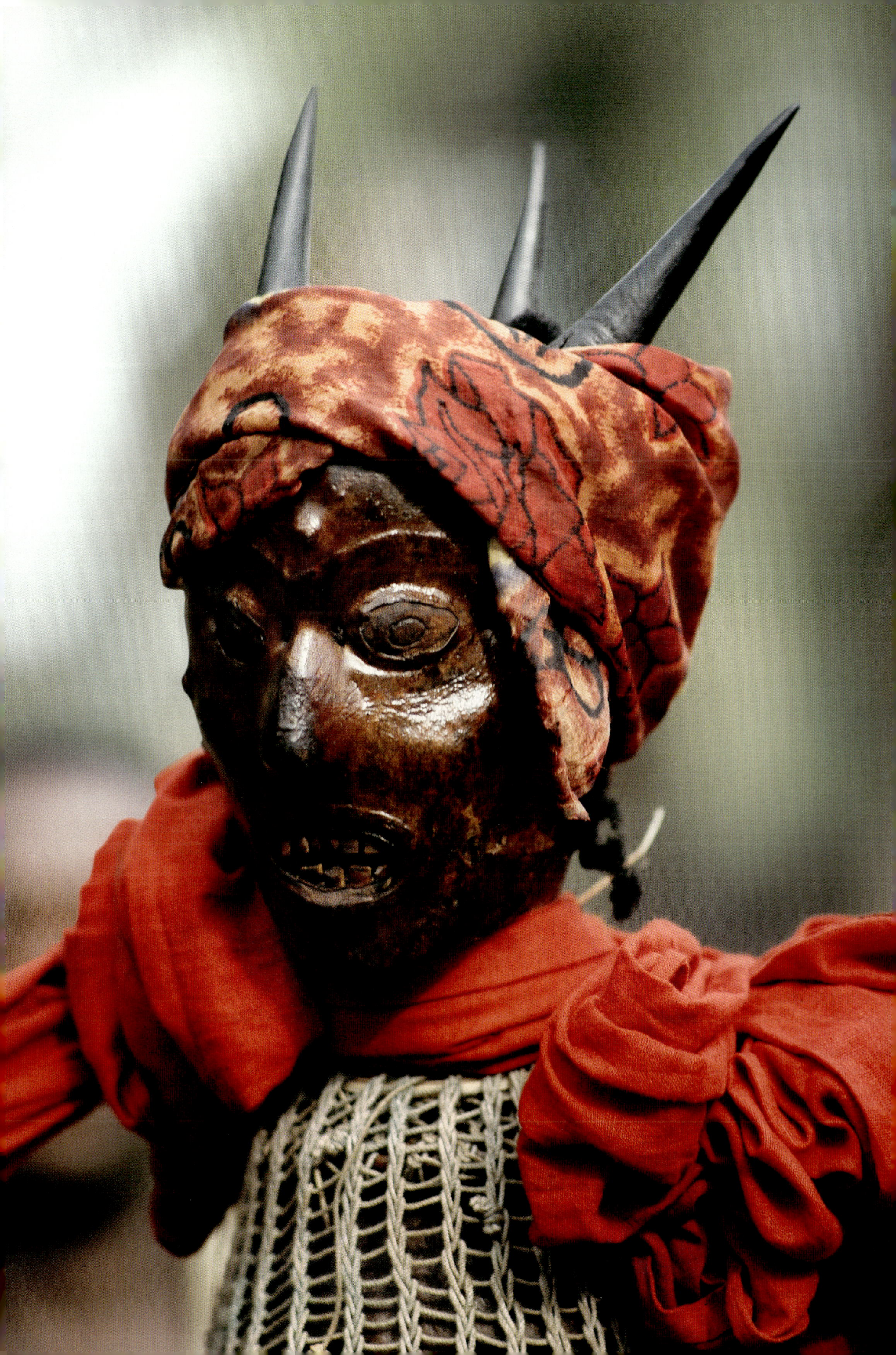

his twentieth year in life. He carried out orders from indigenous customers, but also kept contact with an art dealer in Douala. During my trip to the Cross River region in 2005, I learned that Augustine Etta still lives in Mbakang and occasionally makes carvings.

At that time (1980) most orders were for masks in human form; few customers wished to have animal masks. Augustine Etta made the core of the masks out of wood from the *ogbok* and *mbek* trees.[101] All of the masks were covered with skin, specifically skin of the "duiker", a dwarf antelope (*bese*), whose hide, as Augustine Etta emphasised, is especially thin. In order to soften it, the skin is soaked in water for twelve hours and then covered with hot ashes. When the ashes have cooled, the hair of the skin can be scraped off easily. Upon completion of the wooden core, generally black in colour, the soft skin, usually divided into three parts, is pressed upon the wood. Depressions and raised parts on the surface are formed through intensive work with the fingers.[102]

According to Augustine Etta, at that time there was at most one single skin-covered mask in each community, and it was usually in the possession of a family. When an order for a new mask was made, he received one jug of palm wine from the contractor as pre-payment; upon completion of the mask he received 20,000 Francs CFA (then equal to about 200 German Marks or 100 Euro), five more jugs of palm wine and a case of beer. Ritual dedication of new masks was not customary. Wrapped in a cloth, the masks were stored under the roof above the fireplace, where they were protected from insects and mold by the heat and smoke.[103] Their surface was rubbed with palm oil three times a year.

After meeting Augustine Etta I went to great efforts to contact the owners of such masks. But again and again I was told that these masks had been out of existence for a long time. A few weeks had passed, when I finally received the news that there was still a mask of the kind I was in search for in Ewelle, a neighbouring locality of Kembong. The mask belonged to Samuel Asy, one of the big men, and had long been in his family's possession. It soon became clear that the mask was *Nchebe*, a name that had been mentioned frequently in research on this region.[104] Samuel Asy informed me that *Nchebe* has no society, and therefore its dancers, drummers and singers are recruited from among those living in the village. Although they are not paid for their services, they are given food during the ceremonies. There are no secrets surrounding the mask. Women may watch and even help when the dancer dons the suit. Before a performance begins, the dancer wearing the mask, which is covered with a cloth, is led into the compound to stand before a large slit-drum. He as the leader conducts the offering to the ancestors, saying: "My father. I have been invited by Mr. X to bring *Nchebe.* As we move out, let nothing harmful happen. Let the celebration be peaceful. Let no one be hurt by gunpowder."[105]

The big man reacted positively to my question whether or not it was possible to see *Nchebe*; in fact, he suggested that it should dance. In those days the asking price for a mask performance was one goat, one "animal", one cock and one jug of palm wine. However, as this did not involve a ceremony, Samuel Asy thought that a lower price might be possible. On the same day the mask was supposed to appear. One of the young men went on his own to don the mask outfit, remarkably in the presence of two women who actually helped him to dress. At that time I could hardly believe my eyes. For from my experiences of many years in the Cameroon Grasslands, where even today women are still strictly forbidden to encounter the secrets of the masks, I could not imagine that there might be a place in Africa where women should have access to the sphere of masks. As the big man had announced, the mask – its head concealed by a red cloth – was led by him into the compound's yard, where the dance was to take place. After the big man had slowly and demonstratively removed the red cloth, the beating of the drums began; songs were sung and the mask *Nchebe* began to dance (figs. 116–118).

The mask wore a knitted suit beneath a light-coloured cotton skirt. The shirt-like upper garment with a large ruff of raphia had a hood, that concealed the head of the dancer. The hood was knitted in stitches large enough so that the dancer could see. Upon the hood was a remarkably beautiful anthropomorphic headdress, which was mounted upon a base of plaited reed. A long red cloth like a shawl, which the dancer held in his hands, was fastened to the mask. Although *Nchebe* had masculine features, it was not intended to be a portrait of a man. As Samuel Asy stressed several times, it did not represent any of the ancestors. The village of Ewelle once boasted possessing several other skin-covered masks – *Nküambok*,[106] *Ekpungyök*, and *Nkang*, but they had long since been sold to traders and were never substituted.

In the old days, Samuel Asy continued, it was quite normal that these skin-covered masks could be sold to other villages. *Nchebe* costs five fathoms of cloth; in addition, one chicken, one "animal" and palm wine were demanded at the preliminary negotiations. The buyers then invited the owner to come to their village to teach them about *Nchebe* and to give instructions for making their own mask. No special consecration of the mask took place, but at the first commemorative festivity in which the new mask participated, the seller would appear and address a short prayer to his ancestors: "My fathers, you taught us this *Nchebe,* and our friends have called us to tell everything to them. This is the wine and cloth we have received. *Nchebe* shall remain with them." At the next death celebration, it was the turn of the new owner to introduce the mask to his own ancestors: "My fathers, this is the mask we have bought, and now Mr. X has invited us to dance it. Let no gun go off and let no one be burned by gunpowder."

When I returned to Kembong 24 years later, in 2004, I learned to my great surprise that there had "always" been two skin-covered masks in the community, and that – as ever – they could be engaged for a performance at death celebrations. The masks present here were *Nchebe* (the same name as the mask I had seen in 1980 in Ewelle) and *Mkpe.*

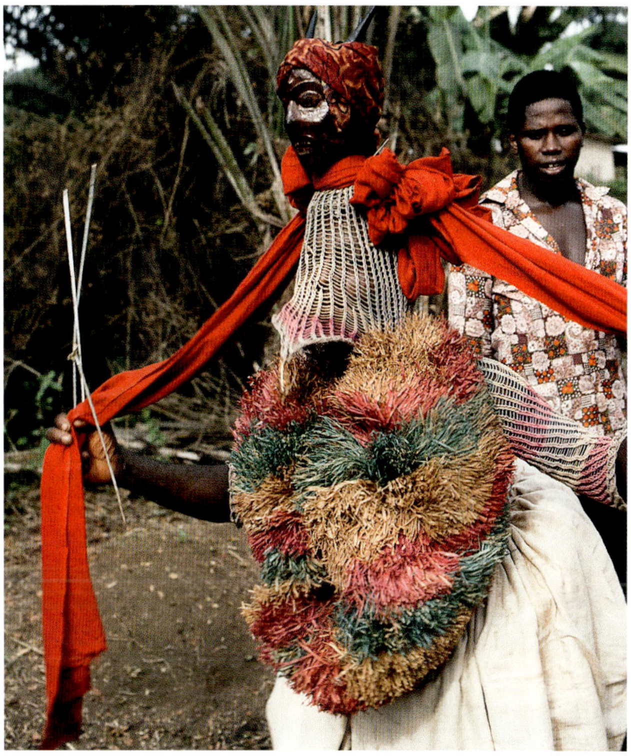

Fig. 117 *Nchebe* during its performance in Ewelle (February 26, 1980).

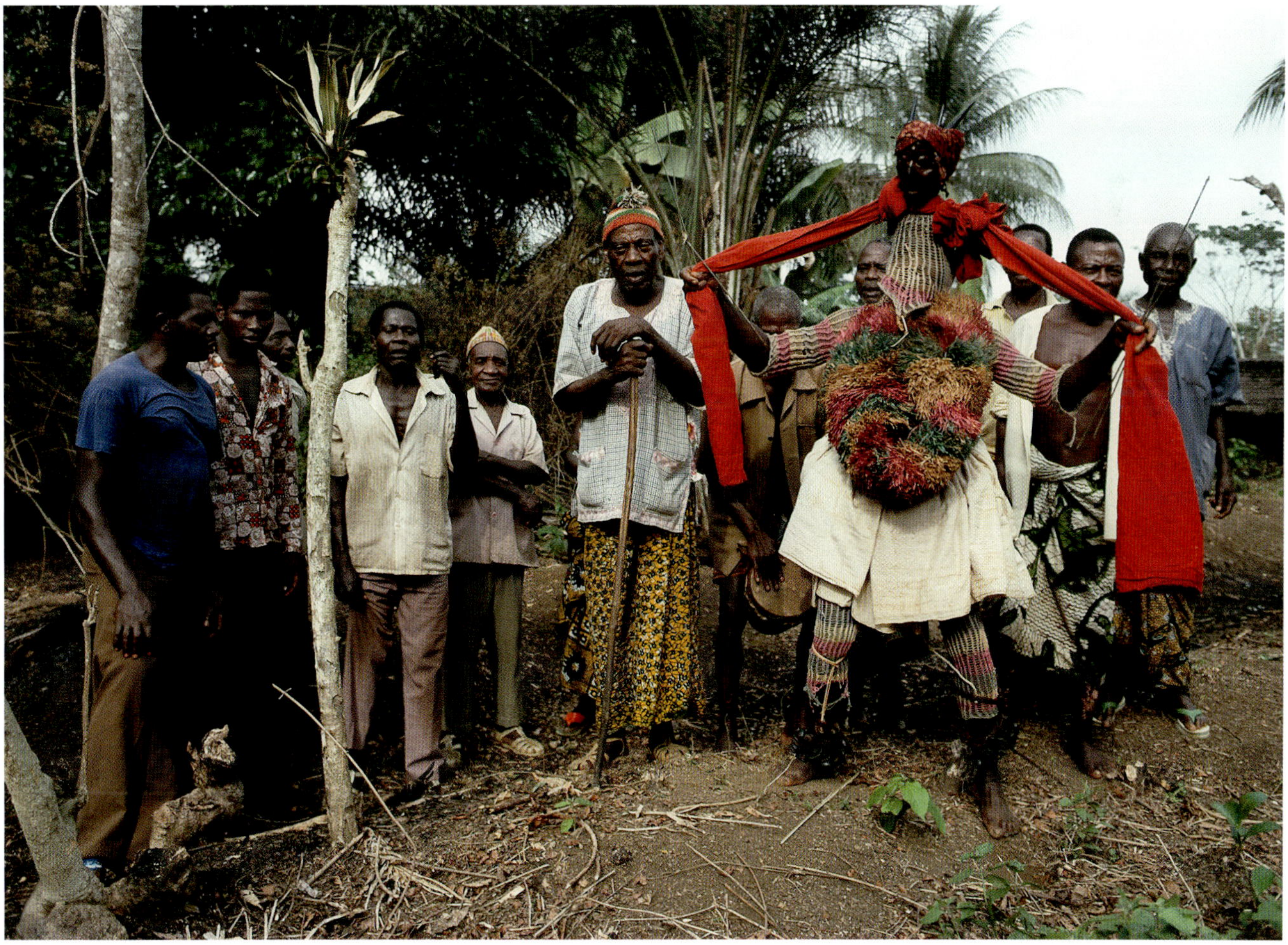

Fig. 118 The mask *Nchebe* and the members of its society in Ewelle (February 26, 1980).

Performance of *Nchebe* in Okonyenge (Kembong, January 27, 2004) (figs. 119–123).

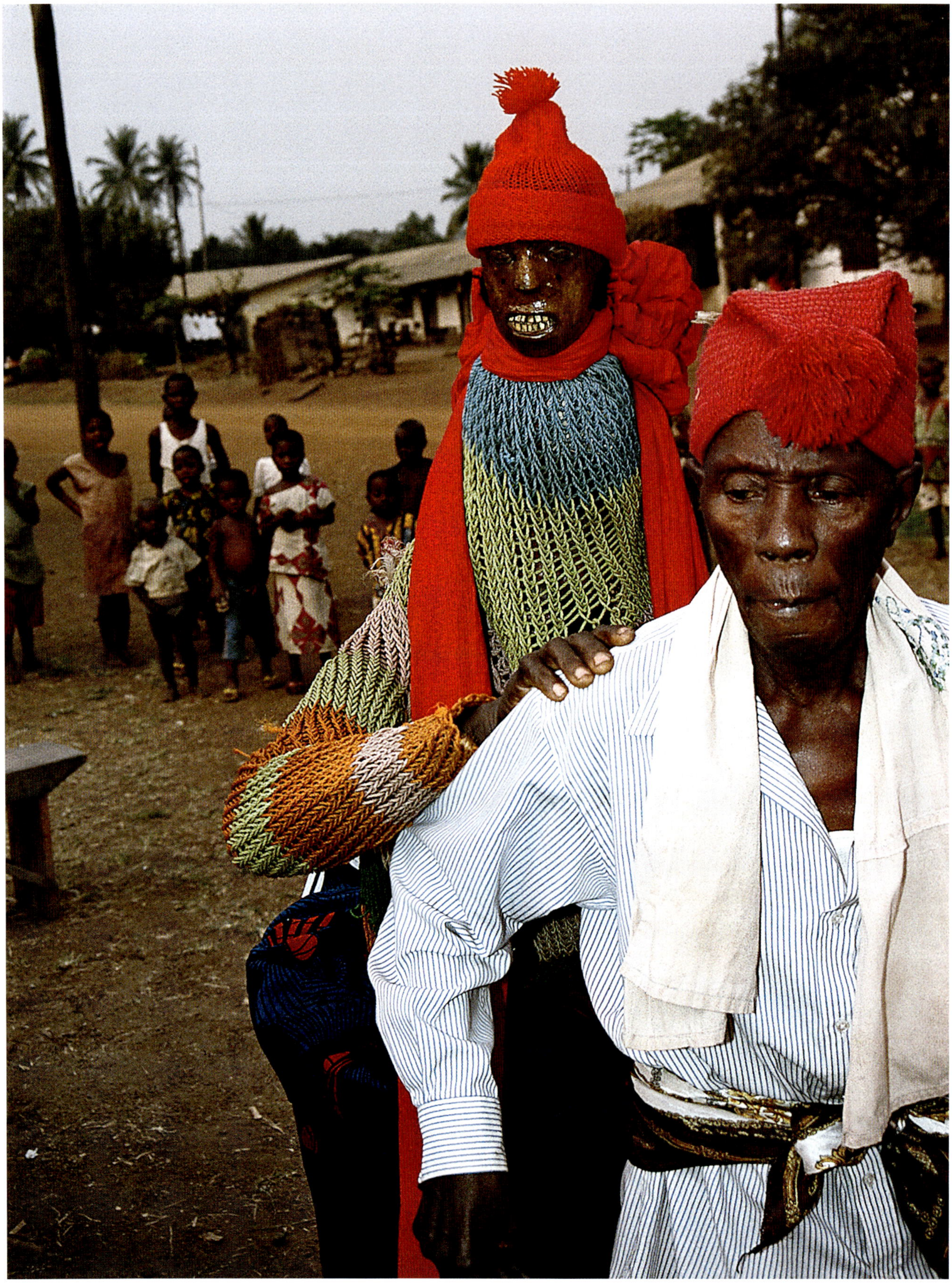

Fig. 119 *Nchebe* is led to the dancing place by its leader Samuel Tanyi Tambe (Kembong, January 27, 2004).

After an initial period of loose contact with some members of *Nchebe*, the opportunity later presented itself for extensive interviews. I learned that *Nchebe* appears exclusively in so-called night dances, which are the climax of the religious and social life in this region. It was noted somewhat with pride that *Nchebe* is not at disposal for the usual death celebrations. Night dances, which are extremely expensive, are only befitting for very few deceased men, men who had reached a very old age and were highly esteemed. Some families saved money for ten years in order to conduct such a festivity. Not only are sheep and goats slaughtered, but even a cow. Hence, night dances in this region are correspondingly seldom, mostly at intervals of several years.

The night dance encompasses rituals and dances that, however, are not only performed at night. Also after the actual night dance (*etokobi atu*), the day dance (*etokobi efe*) takes place. There is no translation for the word *etokobi*, which designates this special dance. The most important part is the night dance, and that is why people often refer to both parts of the ceremony as night dance. Corresponding to its name the night dance, which is only for men, indeed free men, begins at midnight. In earlier times it was strictly forbidden to slaves, and even today all those who are descendants of slaves are not allowed to participate. At the beginning an offering is made to the ancestors by the head of the family. It is the only ritual sacrifice offered to all ancestors not only of the locality, but of the whole clan. It consists of the customary items: grains of maize, meat, colanuts, palm wine and water, but in view of the special occasion of a sheep or a goat as well. In earlier times a slave was sacrificed. The slaying of the victim was carried out by a specialist, the *ntui oyim* or "chief of wickedness". It was expected of him that he sever the head from the trunk with a single blow of his cutlass.[107] Today the greater part of the sacrificial animal's blood is allowed to flow over the large slit-drum, the most important musical instrument of the respective community. The dances of the men follow the offering ceremony and last until dawn.

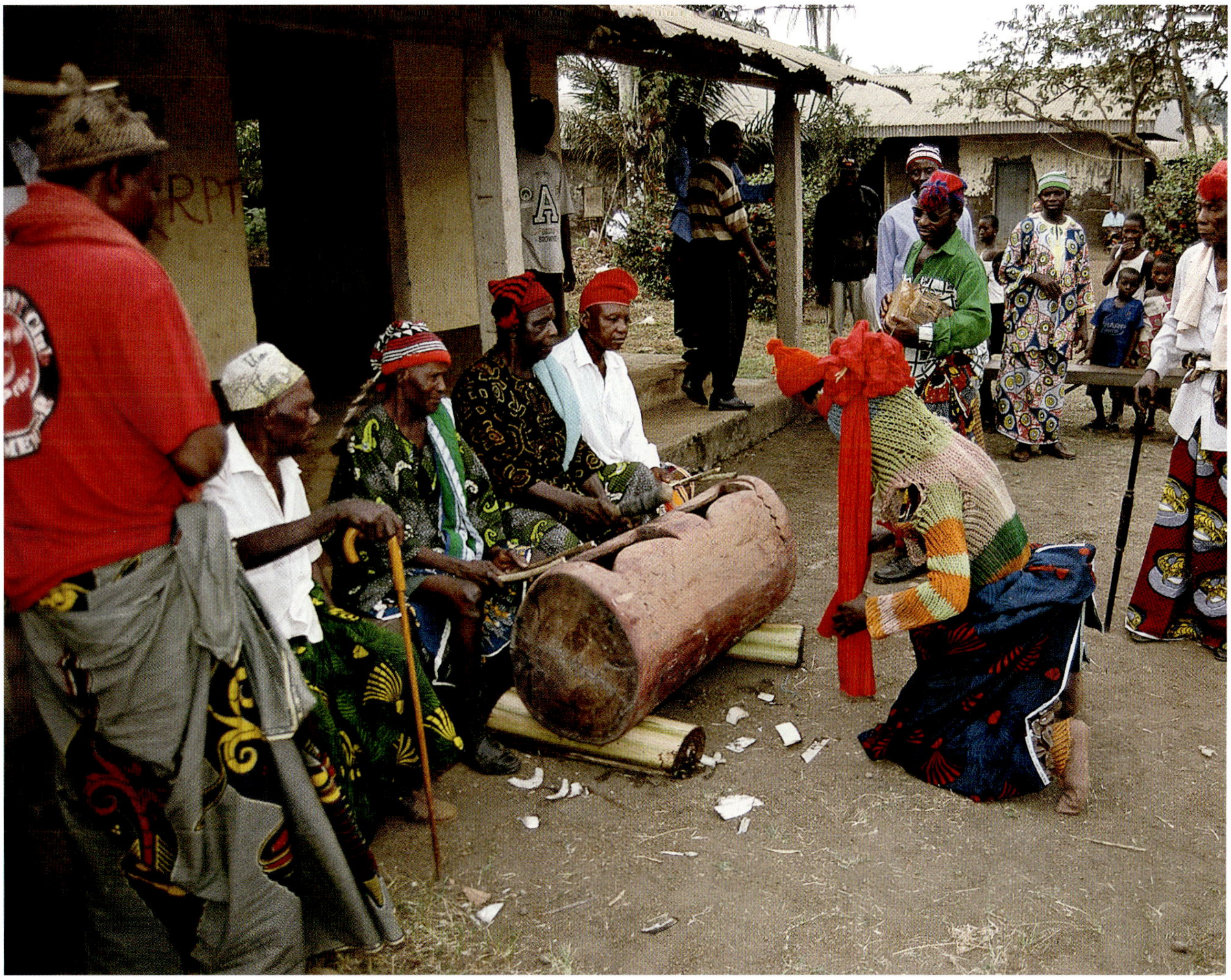

Fig. 120 *Nchebe* "greets" the slit-drum (Kembong, January 27, 2004).

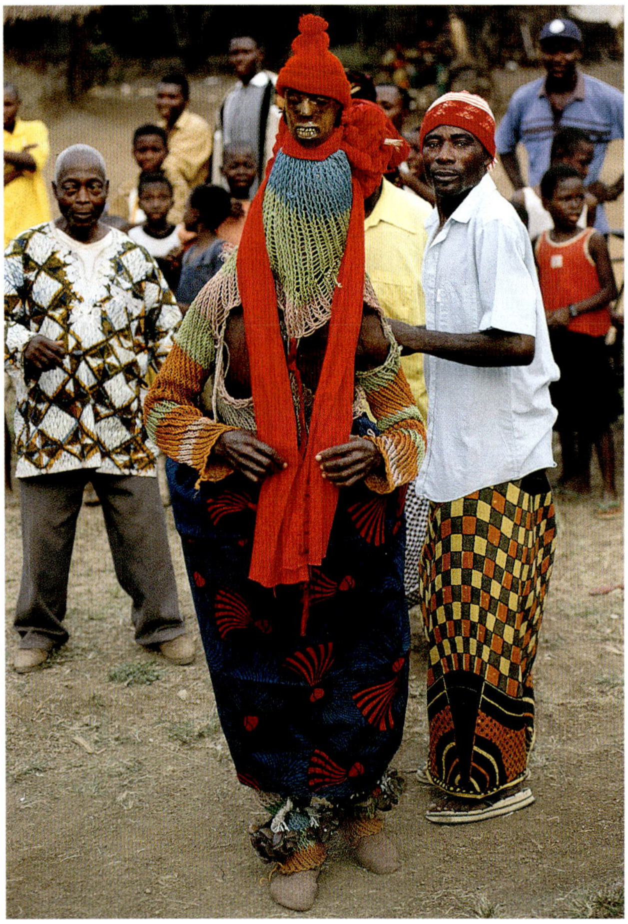

Fig. 121 *Nchebe* performs, wearing a red cap, a hoop under its skirt and rattles around its ankles (Kembong, January 27, 2004).

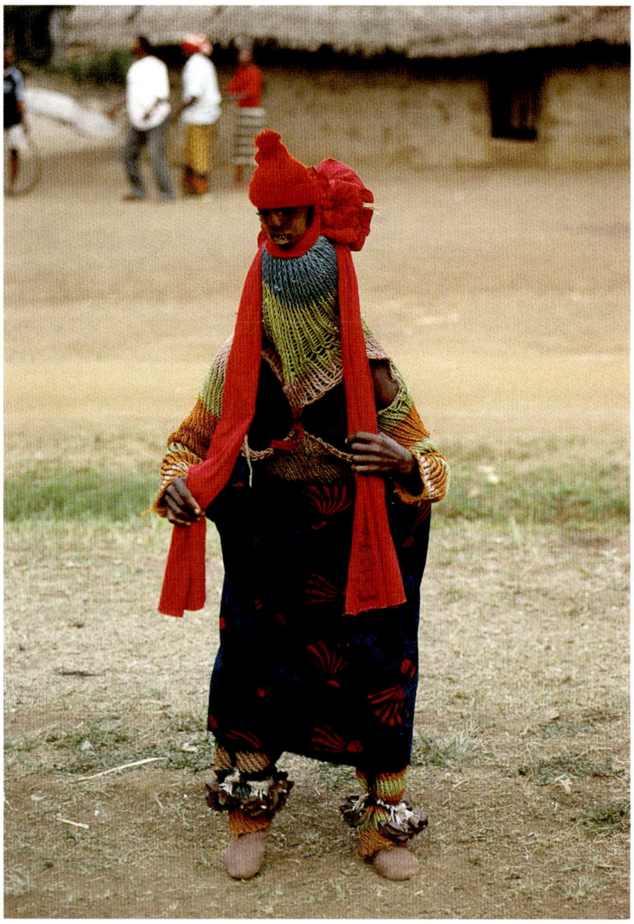

Fig. 122 *Nchebe* during its performance. The red knitted cap is a recent addition to the mask's outfit (Kembong, January 27, 2004).

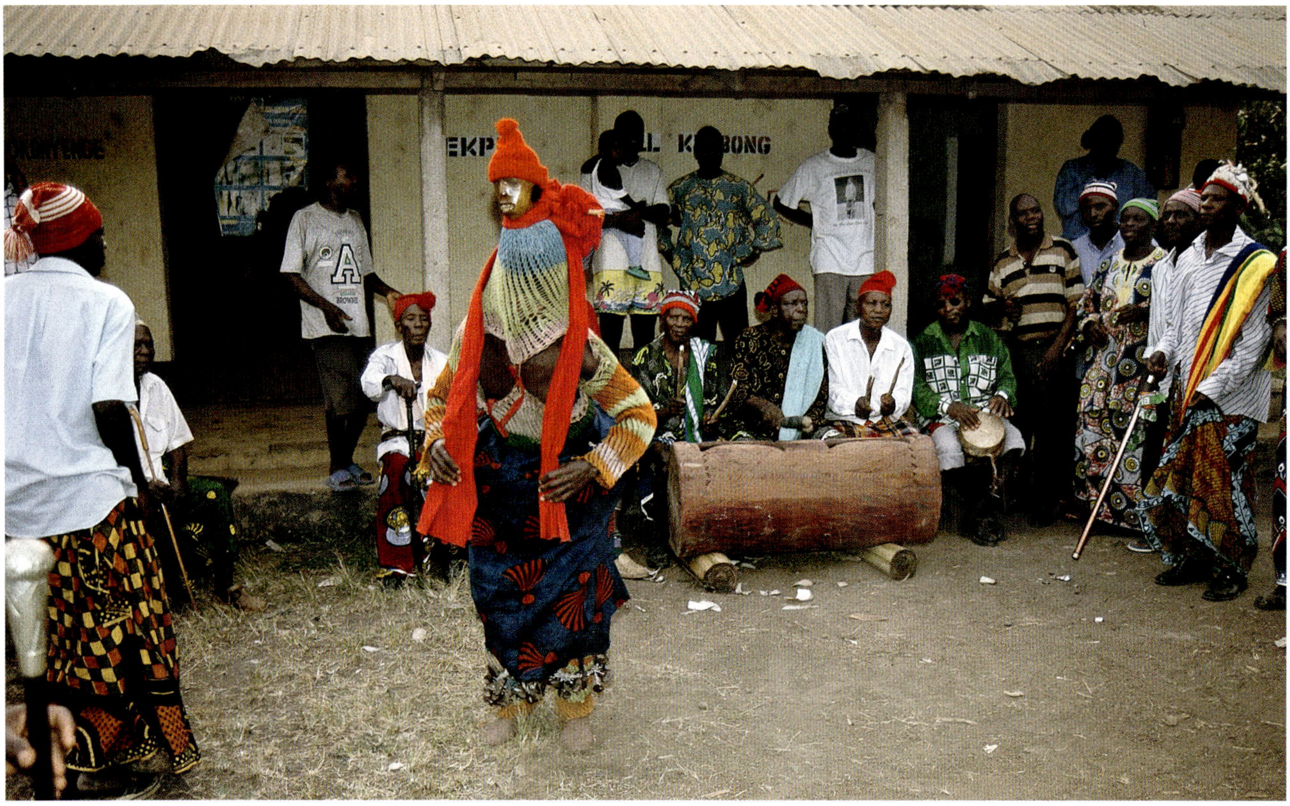

Fig. 123 *Nchebe* in front of the large slit-drum, which is placed before the "*Ekpe* Hall" (the hall of *Mgbe*) in Okonyenge (Kembong, January 27, 2004).

Night dance in Okonyenge, with the performance of *Nchebe* and *Mkpe* (Kembong, March 27, 2005) (figs. 124–135).

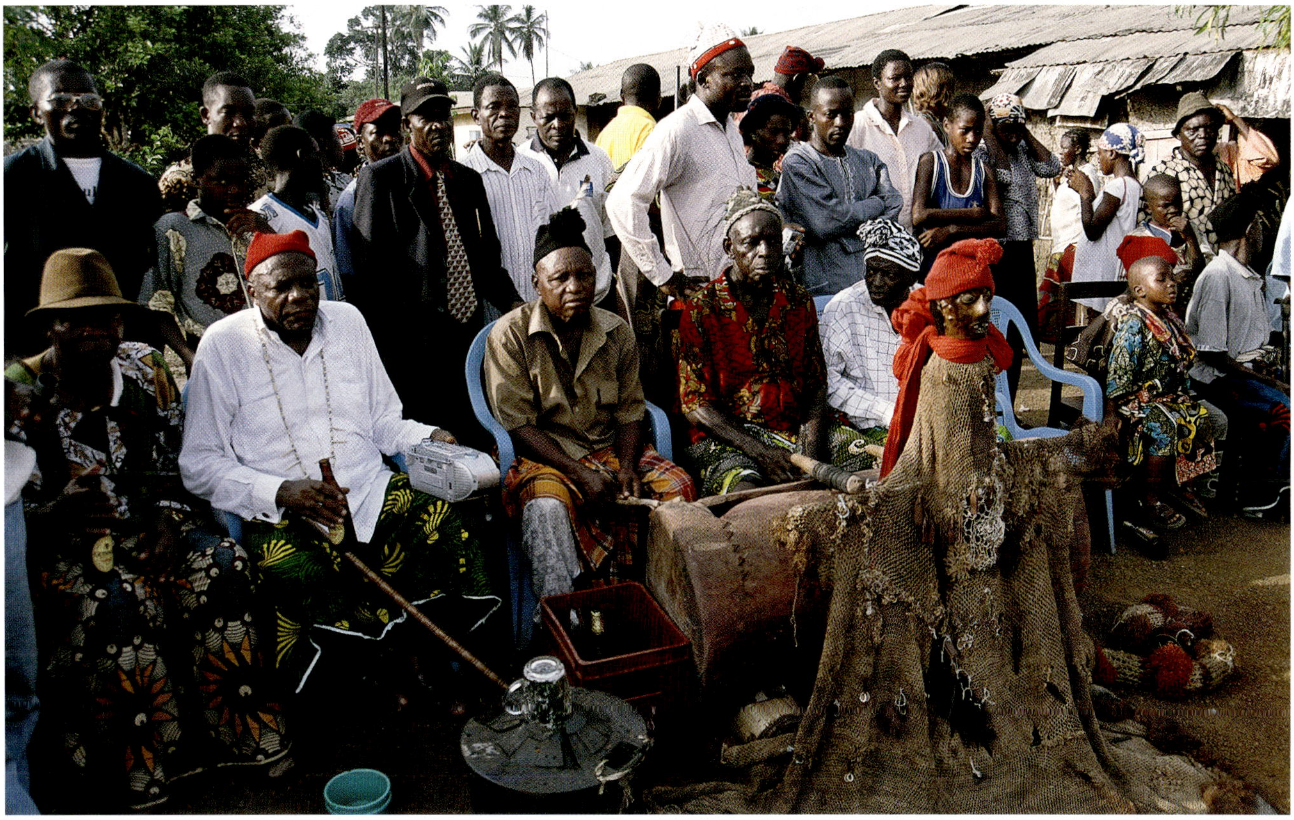

Fig. 124 The slit-drum as the most important instrument in the night dance; in the foreground, the mask garment of *Mkpe* (Kembong, March 27, 2005).

The day dance continues in the afternoon of the next day, which is called *aboku* just as the day of feasting after a burial (cp. p. 93 ff.). It is marked by the performance of masks with skin-covered headdresses, during which one mask appears alone or several masks, but one after the other. Although medicines do not play a role in this association, there is nevertheless a religious element present in the offering to the ancestors, which is carried out by the head of the family. *Nchebe* in Kembong has a repertoire of fourteen different dances, and the man playing the slit-drum directs the masked dancer; with the language of the drum he tells him which dance to perform. As the performances can last one or two hours and are strenuous and exhausting in the hot climate, there are several pauses. During these breaks the dancer removes the "hood" with the mask headdress, so that his face is visible. Astonishingly, it is the duty of women alone to fan fresh air into his face.[108] After the mask has departed, the slit-drum ceases to play and now the generous feasting begins for the numerous guests. This is followed by dancing for the public, which can last until dawn. The night dance concludes with an offering to the ancestors by the family head (*etaah nji eyatek*).

Needless to say, I was very interested in seeing the performance of a skin-covered mask, but no one knew when another night dance would ever take place. However, in order that I might see *Nchebe*, it was arranged with the big men to let the mask appear at a death celebration that took place on January 27, 2004, in Lower Kembong. It was a shorter performance, in which the *Nchebe* only performed six of its fourteen dances, but it was in complete accordance with tradition, as all of my informants assured (figs. 119–123).[109] Somewhat surprised I noticed that the mask headdress was donned with a red knitted cap, which is typically worn above all by members of *Mgbe*. Uncommon in the past, the red cap upon the headdress is a recent development.

In 2005 I was in Kembong again, and soon after my arrival I received the surprising news that after a lapse of many years of silence a night dance was to be conducted once more. It was to be held in honour of *Ata* Mbu Ashu, who had died five years before. He came from the family of Samuel Tanyi Tambe and was the elder brother of Elias Tanyi, one of the most influential big men in Kembong. After the deceased was "celebrated" by *Mgbe* on March 23–24, 2005, the night dance (*etokobi atu*) commenced on the night of March 26–27, 2005. Although this event was strictly taboo for outsiders, it did not remain a secret that the important ceremony of offering was made shortly after midnight. In earlier times a slave – often several slaves – was sacrificed. Aside from the usual offerings to the ancestors, including fried corn, meat, colanuts, water and palm wine, one cock and one sheep were sacrificed. The offering was conducted by Samuel Tanyi Tambe, the head of the family who arranged for the night dance. It was he as well who spoke prayers to the ancestors, while the slaying of animals was executed by a young man. However, the latter was not the *ntui oyim* or "chief of wickedness", the actual person whose duty it was. There was no *ntui oyim* anymore, and the family who was responsible for this position had died out. Samuel Tanyi Tambe held the severed head of the sheep over the slit-drum, so that the blood dripped into the drum. The drummer beat the drum while this went on, and after it was finished, the drummer praised the big man with the words, "You have done well." This together with the firing of a rifle was the signal that the dances could begin, which lasted until dawn.

In the early afternoon of March 27, 2005, preparations had already been completed for the day dance, *etokobi efe*. The large slit-drum that belonged to the quarter stood in the yard of the compound of the respective family in Okonyenge. The drum stood upon short trunks of banana trees. In front of it was the mask garment of *Mkpe*, hung upon a frame in full view of everyone (fig. 124). On the ground I saw the head of the cock with blood; it had been sacrificed the night before.

Mkpe was not from Kembong, but from Ndekwai.[110] Similarly, *Nchebe* in Kembong had not been engaged for this afternoon, but instead *Nchebe* from Ewelle. As mentioned above, I had already encountered *Nchebe* in Ewelle in 1980. However, it soon proved that the mask that appeared on this day was not the same mask that I had seen in 1980. *Nchebe* and *Mkpe* often dance at such celebrations, but it is not a rule that they must dance together. In earlier times many more societies danced during the *etokobi* dance, depending upon how wealthy the particular family was.

Around three o'clock in the afternoon the first visitors and spectators began to arrive, and after about half an hour the area was full of people, who awaited the first highlight of the day, the offering to the ancestors. The ceremony took place in front of the slit-drum. It was the role of the head of the family to conduct the offering (figs. 125–128). Samuel Tanyi Tambe took fried maize mixed with red palm oil (*ebore*) in his left hand and addressed the ancestors – those of his own family as well as those of all of Kembong and the Nchemti-Clan – in a long prayer: "*Ata* Ashu Eta, Bate Ojong Nchong, Tambe, Mbu, Ndip Tanyi, Tanyi Oben, Tambe Besong, Etchu, Tabot Ndip Arrah, Ndip Nchot, Manchang Ajbor, Nchemti, Mbeng Changaragbor, Tambe Ndip – this includes those I know and those I do not know. We are only children and so forgive us, if I forgot any name. Let us have money in this family, so that we can celebrate other deaths like this one. In this celebration, if anyone comes here with a bad mind or bad food or bad palm wine, let the person drop dead and let the dish with the food break and let the calabash of wine break, before anyone eats the food and drinks the wine. And now to all of you, the spirits of the living dead, I have called, here is your food." His prayer indicated that the celebration was not only meant for the deceased, but for all ancestors. Then Samuel Tanyi Tambe took maize in his right hand and said: "Here is our own food, for us the living." (fig. 125). Afterwards an offering of meat was made, in which three pieces were intended for the ancestors: "Here is your own meat." Four pieces of meat were meant for the living: "Here is our own meat; may you send us more of it." Colanuts were offered in the same manner: three nuts were offered to the ancestors ("After eating the food, here is your own colanut."), and four were meant for the living ("Here is the colanut for us the living."). Samuel Tanyi Tambe then took a glass of water in his left hand and poured some upon the ground, saying: "Once the spirits have eaten, they drink water first. Here is water for you." This was followed by the family head holding the water in his right hand and pouring some, saying: "Here is water for the living." Finally, he held the glass in both hands and offered it once more: "If what I have done is your wish, then let these colanuts show to us that you have accepted this sacrifice." He threw two colanuts to the ground. One landed with the upper side upwards, the other downwards: "They (the ancestors) have accepted."

The ceremony proceeded similarly with the offering of palm wine. First holding the glass in his left hand Samuel Tanyi Tambe addressed the ancestors: "Here is your own palm wine." And then holding it in his right hand, for the living: "Here is our own palm wine." He took a sip of the wine and poured the rest onto the ground for the ancestors (fig. 126). Next the cock had to be offered to the ancestors. Likewise, the family head first held the cock in his left hand, saying: "Here is your fowl." And then in the right hand, with: "Here is our own fowl." Following this he swung the cock around his head three times and then handed it over to

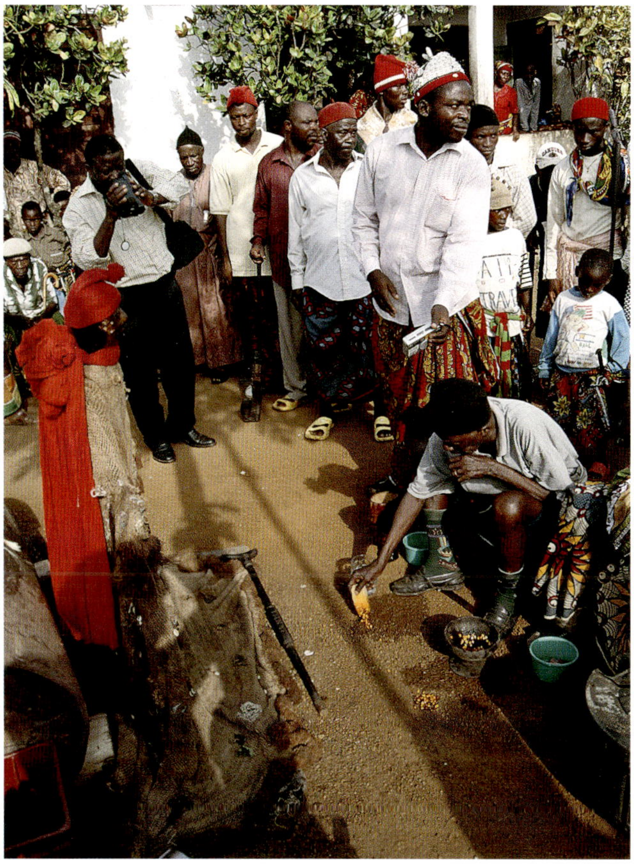

Fig. 125 Offering of maize (Kembong, March 27, 2005).

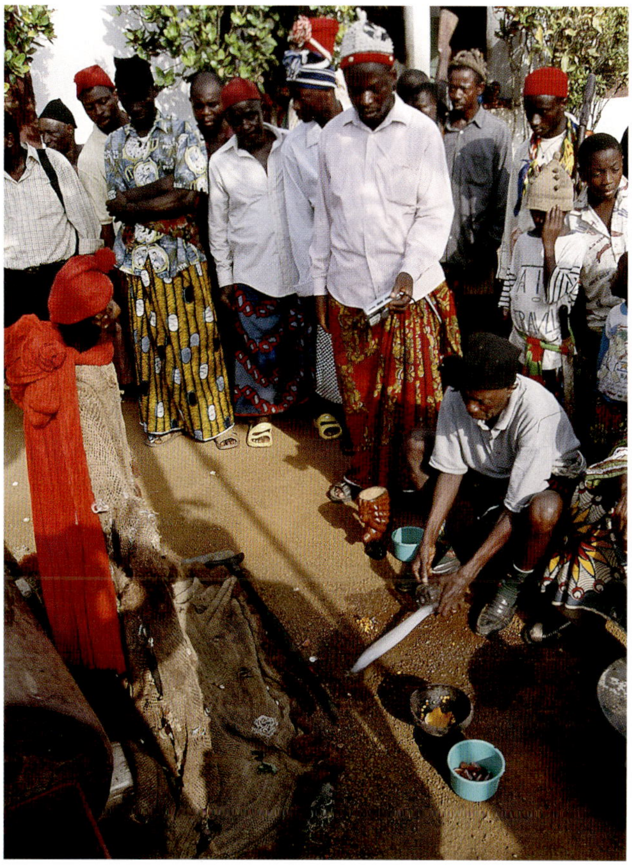

Fig. 126 Offering of palm wine (Kembong, March 27, 2005).

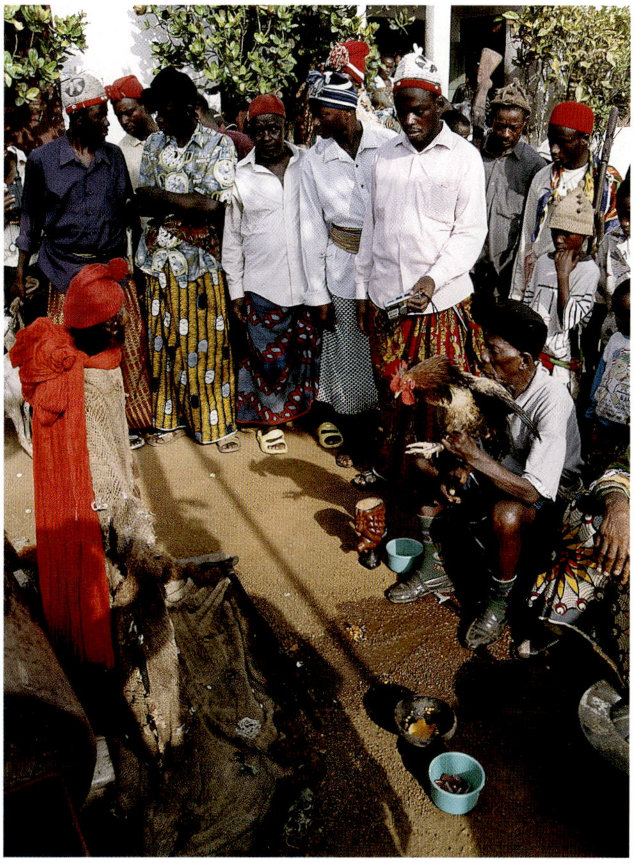

Fig. 127 Offering of a cock (Kembong, March 27, 2005).

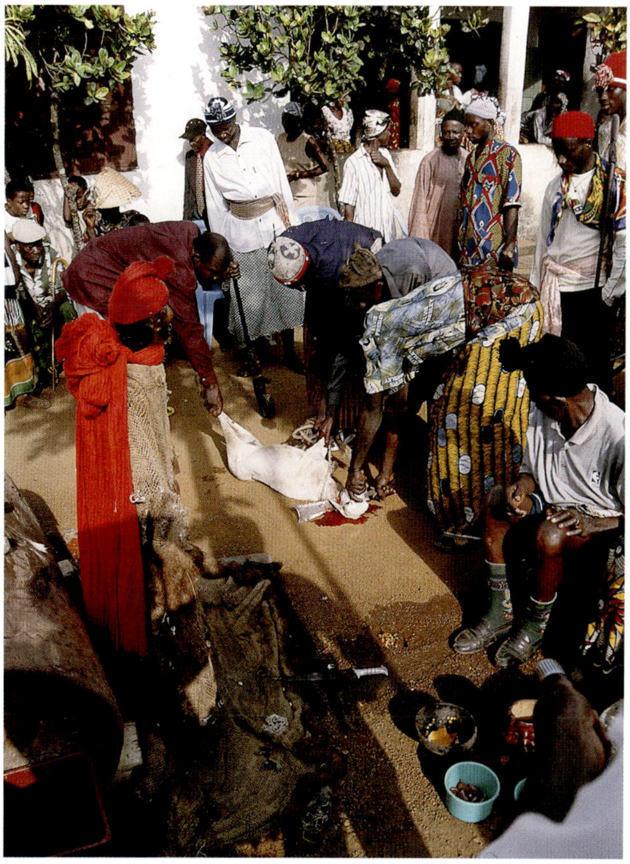

Fig. 128 Offering of a sheep (Kembong, March 27, 2005).

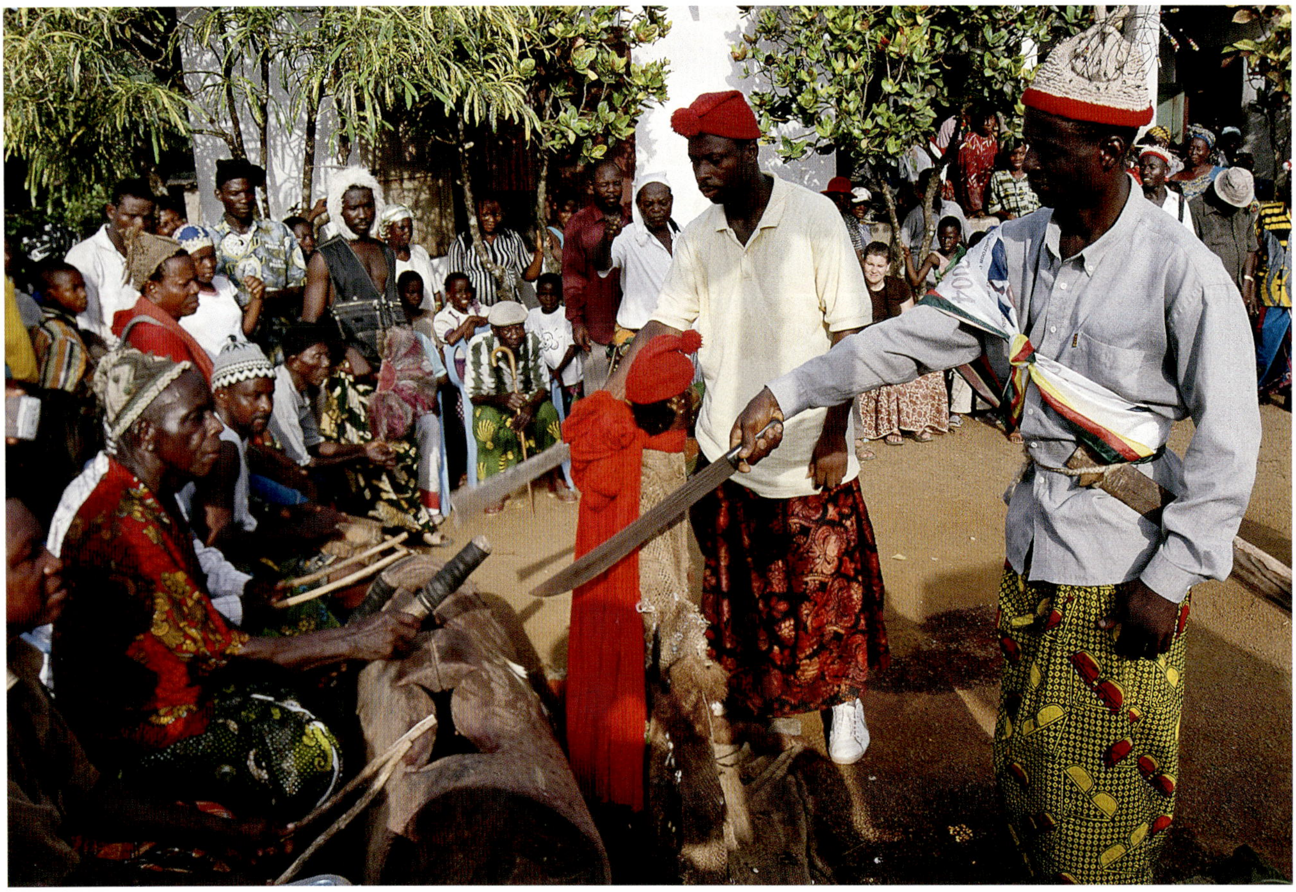

Fig. 129 Two members of *Nchebe*, each carrying a cutlass, in front of the slit-drum announce the appearance of the mask (Kembong, March 27, 2005).

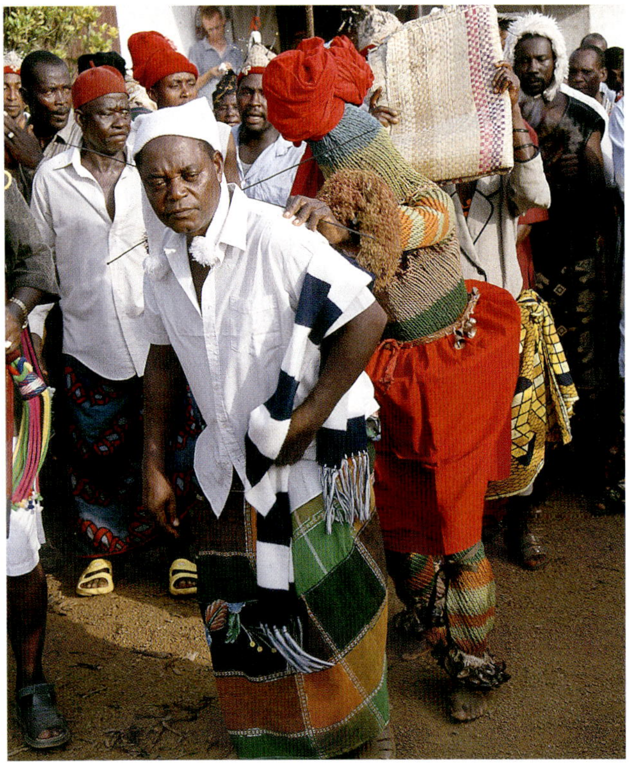

Fig. 130 The mask, its headpiece concealed, is led to the dancing place by a *seseku*; it wears a knitted suit, an additional skirt with a hoop underneath, bells at its waist and rattles around the ankles (Kembong, March 27, 2005).

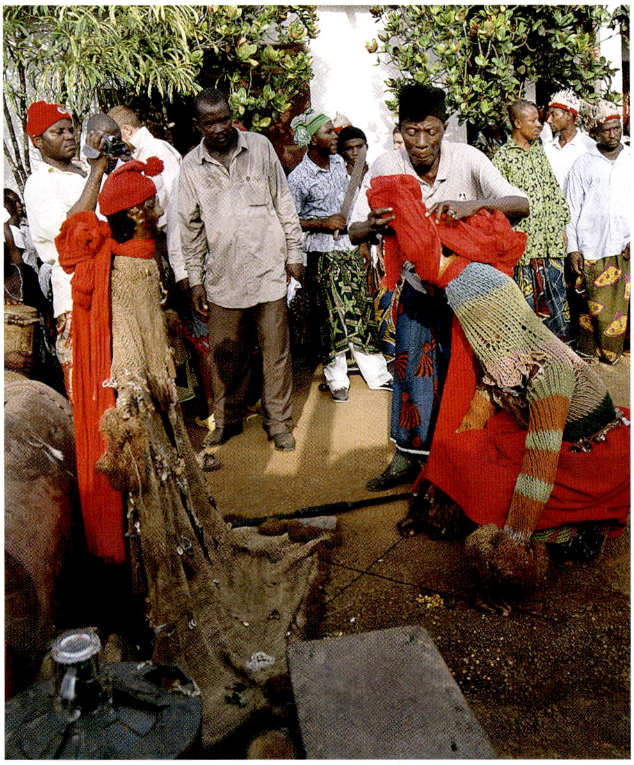

Fig. 131 Samuel Tanyi Tambe, head of the bereaved family, removes the covering from the headdress of the mask, while it is kneeling in front of the slit-drum (Kembong, March 27, 2005).

a young man who was to slay the animal and prepare it for the feast (fig. 127).

The final offering, and the most important at that, was that of a sheep. This, however, was announced to the ancestors in one single and very short sentence: "Here is your sheep." The head of the family did not carry out the slaying of the animal; this was taken over by another member of the family (fig. 128). In contrast to the offering during the night, the blood of the sheep was not allowed to flow into the slit-drum. It simply flowed onto the earth, as a share for the ancestors, while the meat was intended for the living alone.

Following the sacrifice, twenty litres of palm wine were consumed by the people around, and only after that did the forerunners of *Nchebe*, two men each equipped with a cutlass, appear. They bowed before the slit-drum – the centre of the dance activities – and pointed to it with their cutlasses, seven times in all, which signified their greetings and announced the arrival of the mask (fig. 129). Aside from the fact that the slit-drums are regarded as the most important gifts from the ancestors and are "strengthened" with sacrificial blood at intervals, it is the drummer who controls the drum's actions and the mode of dancing (cp. p. 131).[111] The appearance of the two forerunners signified at the same time that the occasion had started, and the crowd was now to wait for the *Nchebe* mask. It appeared soon, its head covered with a red cloth, in this way holding the attention of the crowd (fig. 130). The unveiling of the mask by the family head was already one stage of the dance (fig. 131). On this day *Nchebe* from Ewelle did not wear the red cap, like the mask of the *Nchebe* from Kembong that I had viewed one year before (cp. p. 116 ff). By contrast, at this night dance a red cap was worn by the mask *Mkpe*, which appeared after *Nchebe*.

During the dance of the mask there was frequent shooting, mostly with Dane-guns. One of the women was always near the mask and fanned it with a mat. On this particular occasion the masked dancer did not interrupt his dance, which would have followed tradition, and this was noted by some of the big men with displeasure. Therefore, I was unable to see how the masked dancer removed his mask outfit and thus exposed his face. *Nchebe* danced about one hour and then left the dancing area in the accompaniment of numerous, mostly young men (figs. 132, 133). This was succeeded by the performance of *Mkpe*, which likewise lasted about one hour. In contrast to *Nchebe*, *Mkpe* did not wear a suit, but instead a gown. The gar-

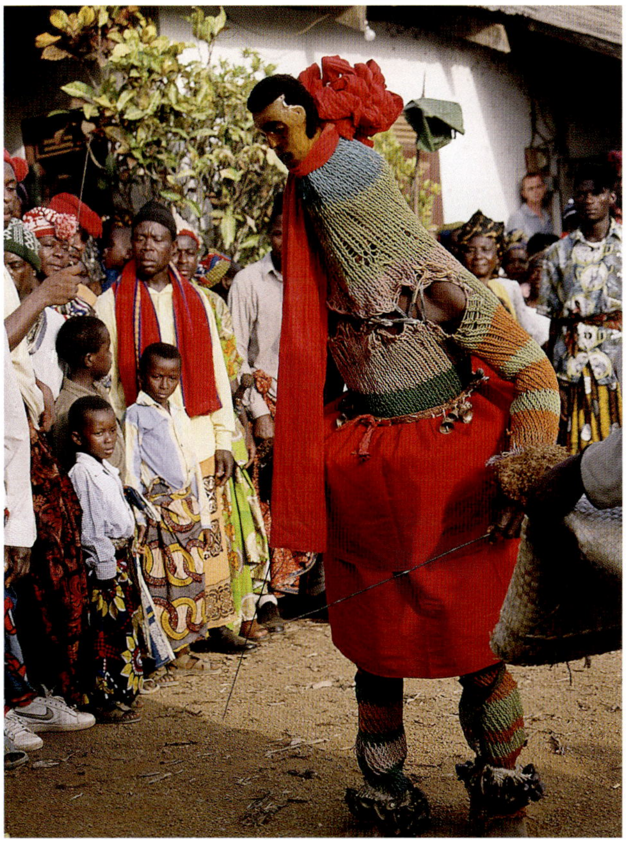

Fig. 132 The dance of *Nchebe* (Kembong, March 27, 2005).

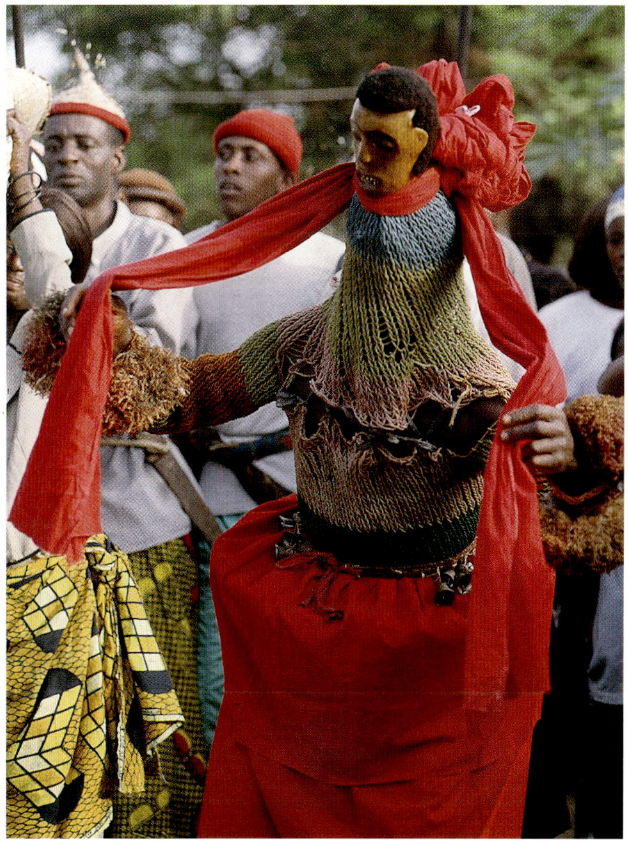

Fig. 133 Close-up of *Nchebe* (Kembong, March 27, 2005).

ment was not in very good condition; it had holes and other damages (figs. 134, 135). The mask performances were followed by the feast for the guests, and the festivities lasted well into the night.[112]

I was especially interested in obtaining information about what these masks represented or portrayed. Yet, not one of my informants mentioned any association or connection of the masks with the ancestors, nor were the masks seen as representing enemies, slaves or other people, which is quite contradictory to some theories in ethnographic literature. Furthermore, no one could remember ever hearing that such masks were covered with human skin or that headdresses were made out of human skulls. Moreover, there are no secrets about the masks. Everyone can see the dancer's arms and legs, my informants pointed out when I asked them about the mask's secrecy. However, there was no satisfactory or convincing answer to my question as to why it was necessary to conceal the face of the dancer, if his identity was known anyway. Nonetheless, the opinion was unanimous that these dances could only be carried out by a mask and not by ordinary humans: "But there is no spiritual attachment to these masks, they are only necessary to make a celebration serious and important."

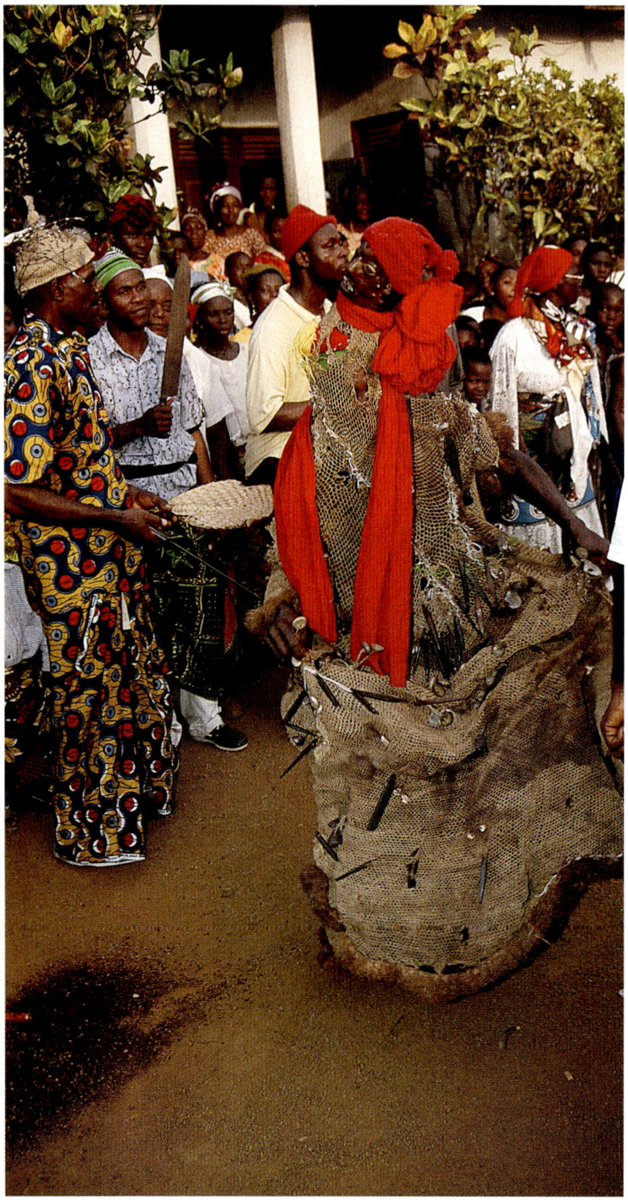

Fig. 134 The dance of *Mkpe*, wearing a net-like garment to which various small trinkets and other objects are attached (Kembong, March 27, 2005).

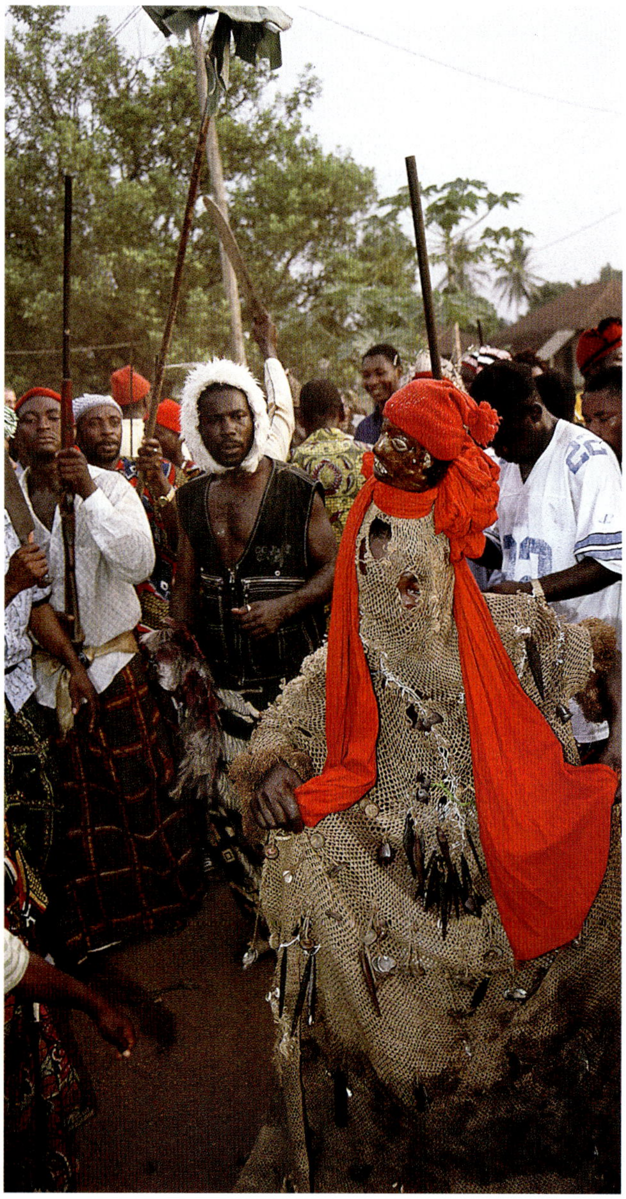

Fig. 135 Close-up of *Mkpe* with its red knitted cap, a recent addition to the mask outfit (Kembong, March 27, 2005).

Performance of *Angbu*, with a huge Janus-headpiece (Kembong, January 26, 2004) (figs. 136–143).

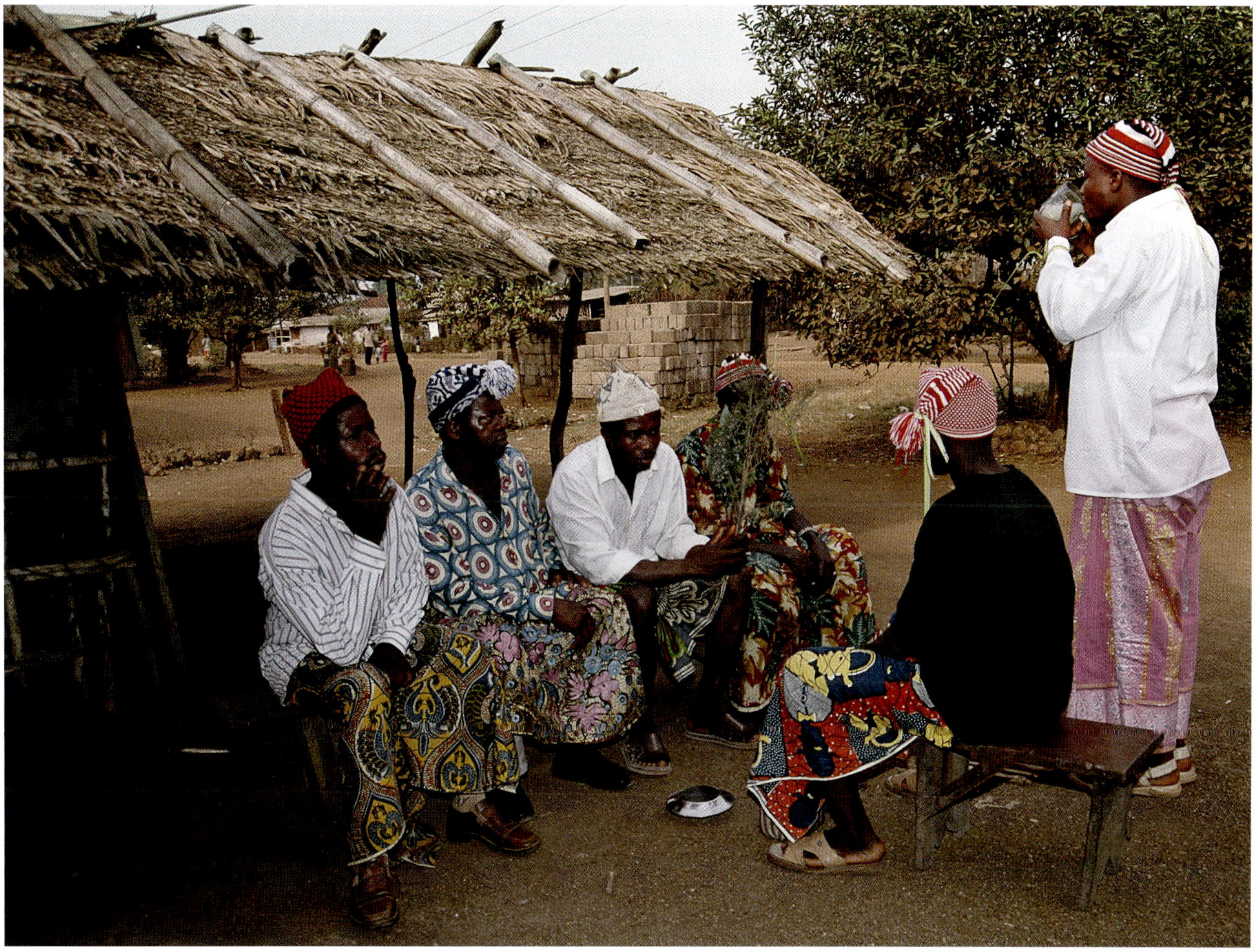

Fig. 136 Drinking palm wine. Seated on the bench (left) the big men of *Angbu* (Kembong, January 26, 2004).

4.4 *Angbu*

In Kembong it is said that *Angbu* is a "destructive" mask, a "bad *juju*".[113] Correspondingly, *Angbu* is associated with that which is "bad" and "ugly", and thus it protects and defends people from such things. The anthropomorphic and Janus-headed mask headpiece is made of wood and has a dark colour. The face in "front" signifies the male, the face in "back" the female. This position, it is said, accords with the greater importance and power of men. Attached to the gown of this powerful mask are twigs of the plant *oseleayong*, which if touched cause a burning sensation to the skin (figs. 138–142).[114]

Angbu is widespread in the forest area, but – in contrast to *Angbu* in Kembong – operates mostly with two masks, one male and the other female. I encountered *Angbu* in this form at a performance in Babong in 1980 (figs. 144–146). First the male mask named *Angbu* appeared alone; after a while it summoned the female mask. The latter is named *Mawu*, just as the above-mentioned society for women (cp. p. 191 ff.). In the course of their performance both masks met and embraced. They held the thorny remains of the fruit of the oil palm (*naob elemembhi*) in their hands, with which they attacked aggressive spectators at times.

As the designation "destructive mask" implies, the mask's help is sought when the community must be freed from anything that is evil, offensive and dangerous. *Angbu* is involved above all in contending against "devils" (*akeku*, sg. *nkeku*), those souls of the dead who return to earth and tyrannise their families. At first *Angbu* attempts to drive away the devils by making a mighty cry at night, for which it utilises a special instrument. If this is unsuccessful, the corpse of the suspected devil is exhumed by the villagers and cremated. Should the "devil" already have abandoned the grave, which in this case is empty, *Angbu* has a medicine that attracts it. When the devil appears, the mask "shoots" it

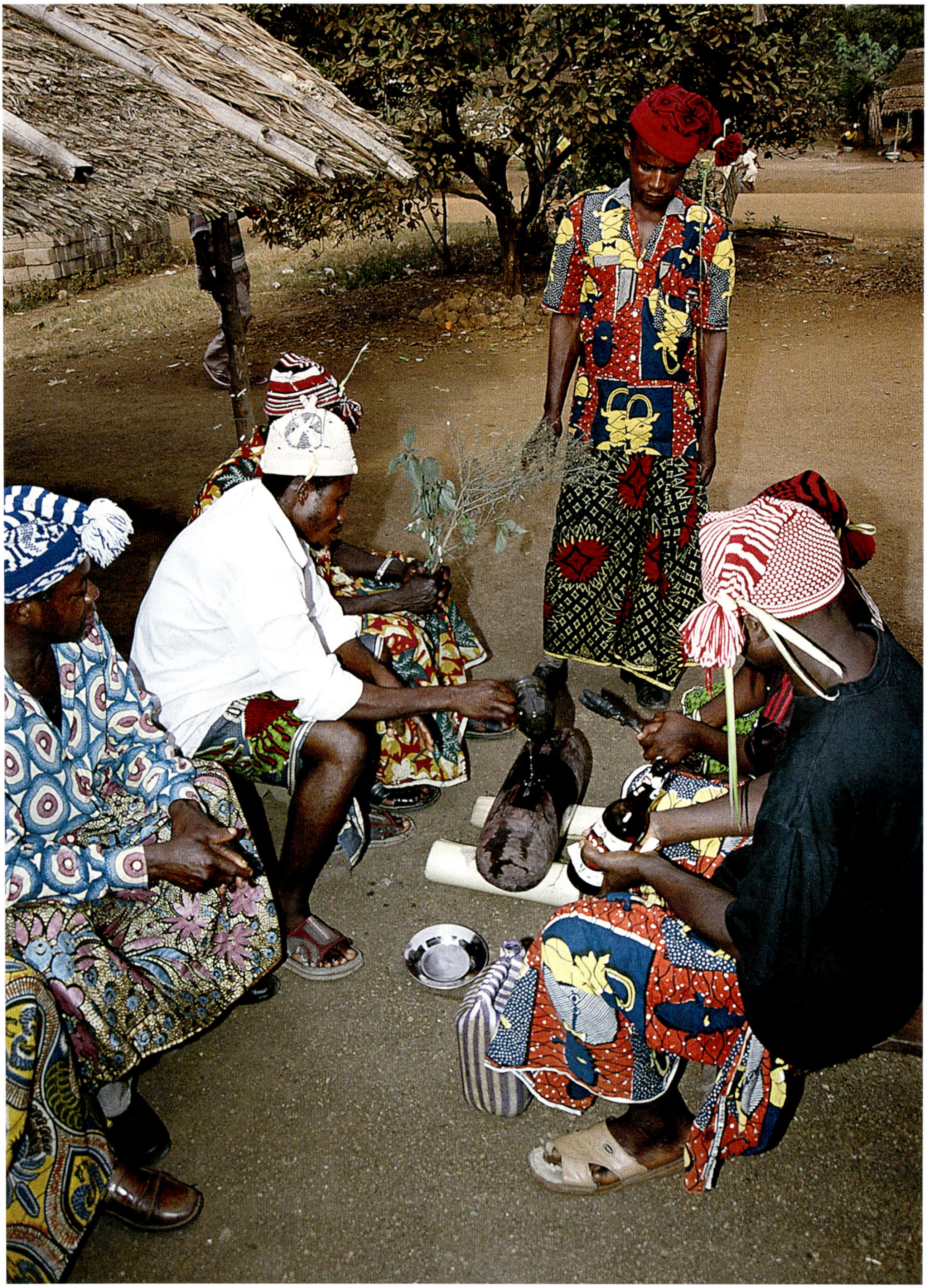

Fig. 137 Prior to the mask performance the "president" of *Angbu*, Agbor George, conducts the offering to the ancestors. He pours the portion of palm wine for the ancestors into the small slit-drum called "cripple" (Kembong, January 26, 2004).

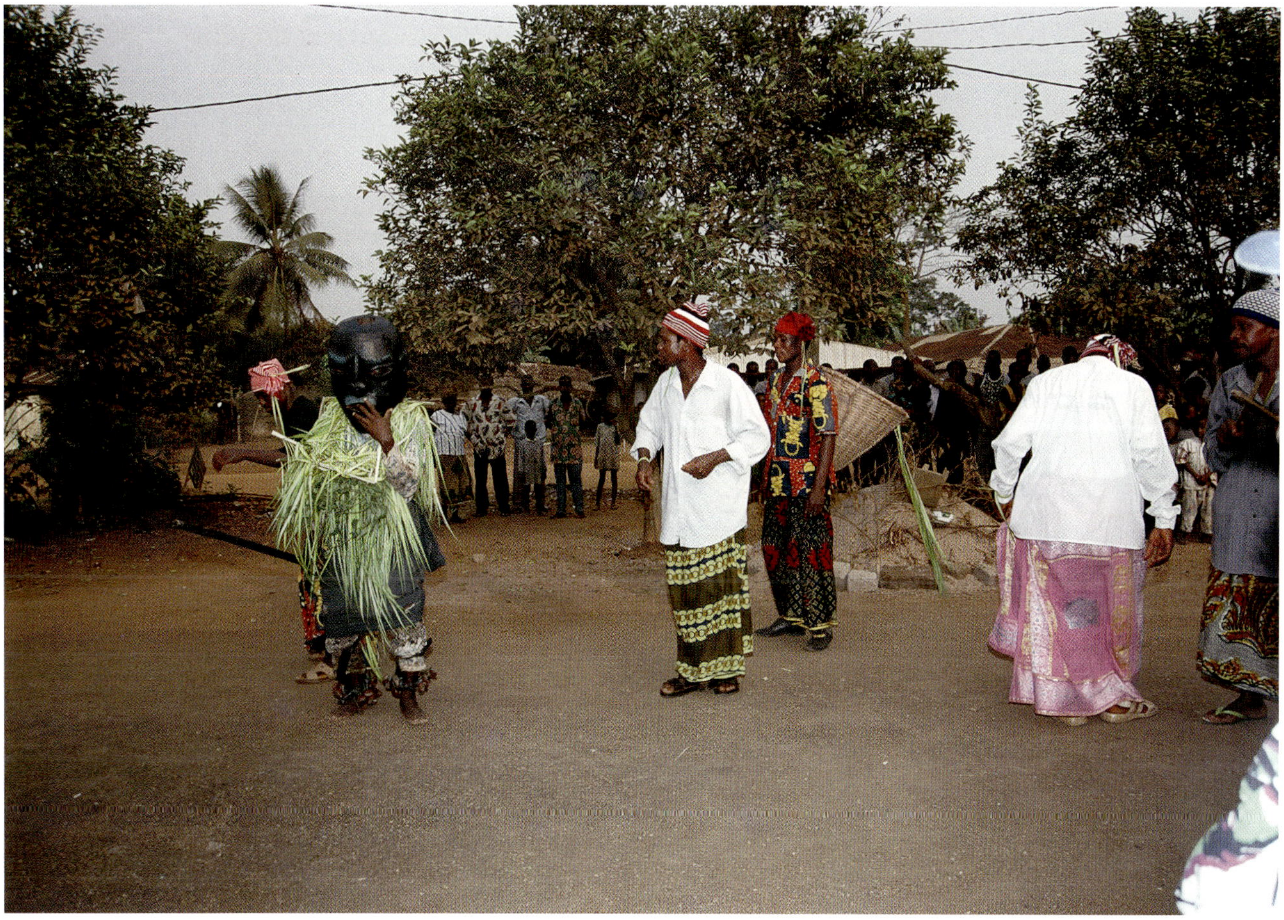

Fig. 138 In the right background a member of *Angbu* carries a large basket for the gifts, which the society expects to receive from the spectators (Kembong, January 26, 2004).

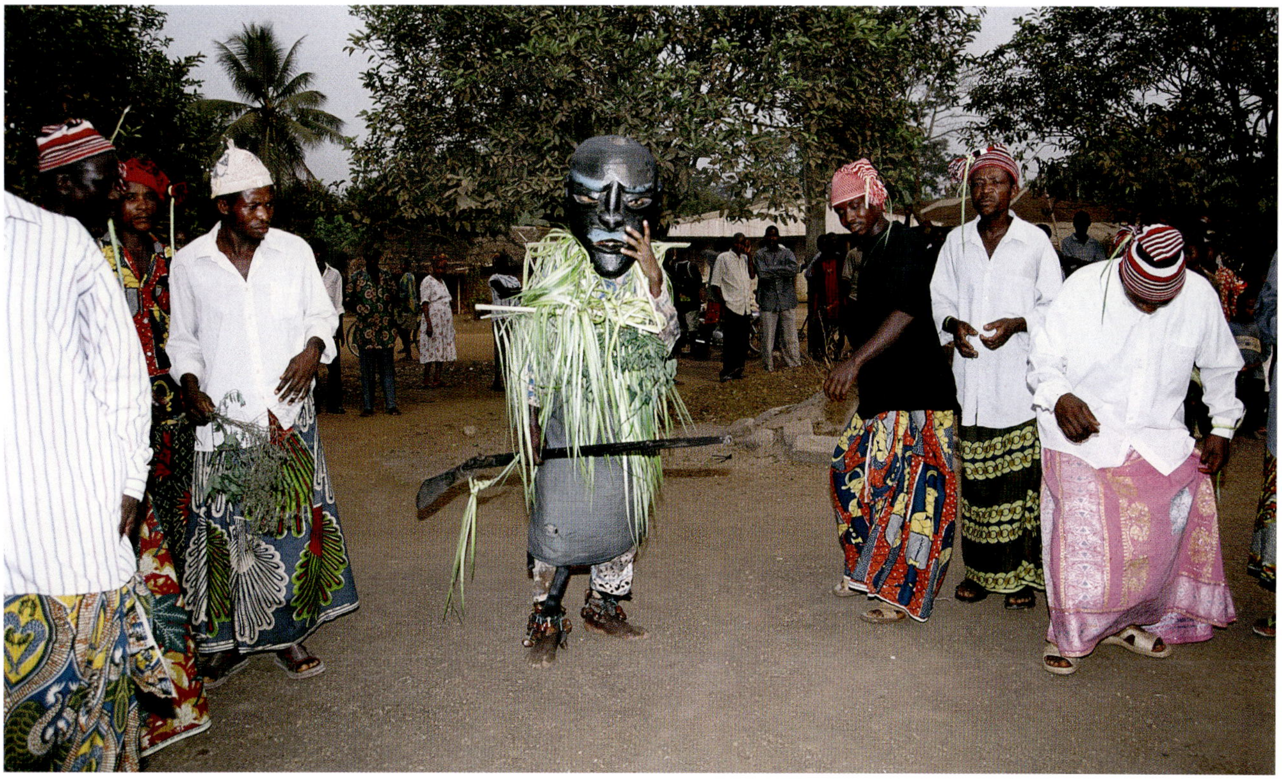

Fig. 139 *Angbu* with its rifle (Kembong, January 26, 2004).

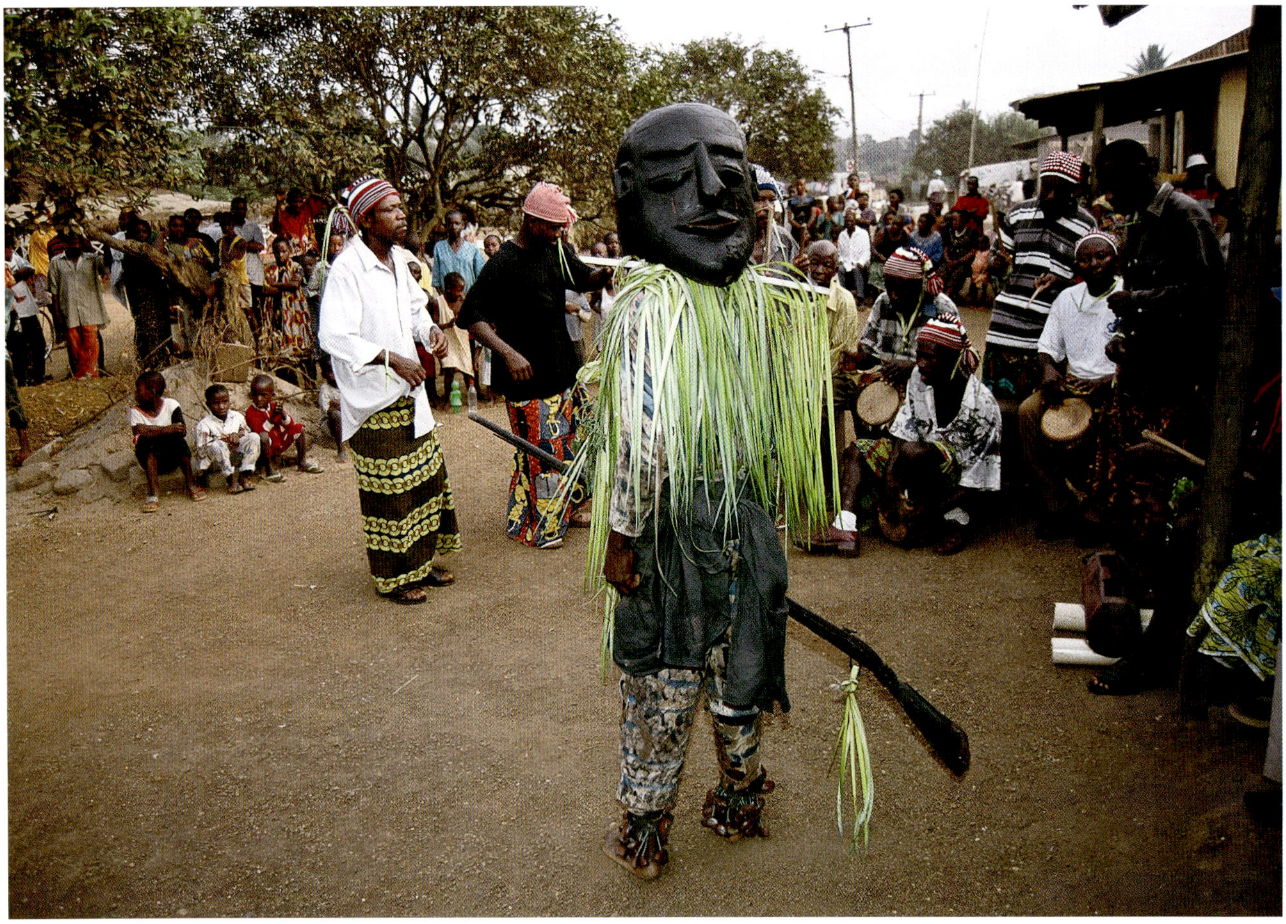

Fig. 140 The face on the reverse side is that of a woman (Kembong, January 26, 2004).

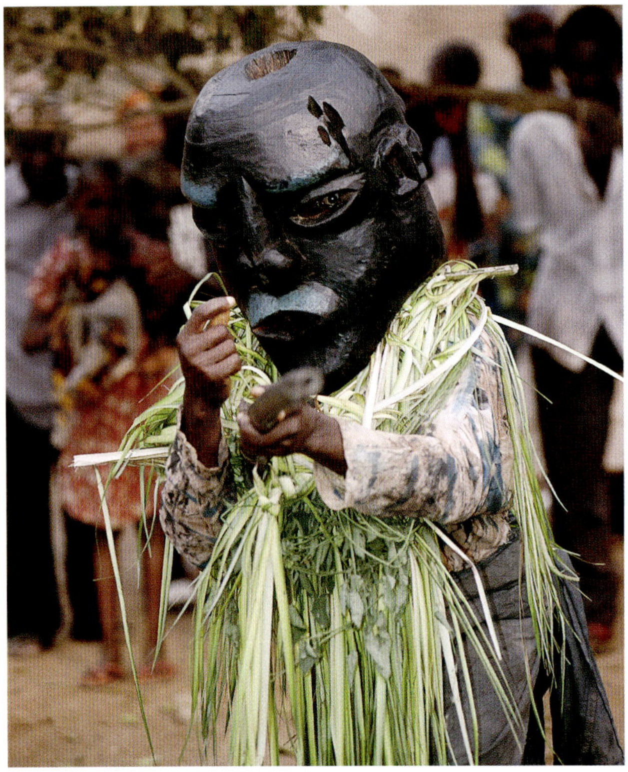

Fig. 141 Close-up of the front side of *Angbu* with the face of a man (Kembong, January 26, 2004).

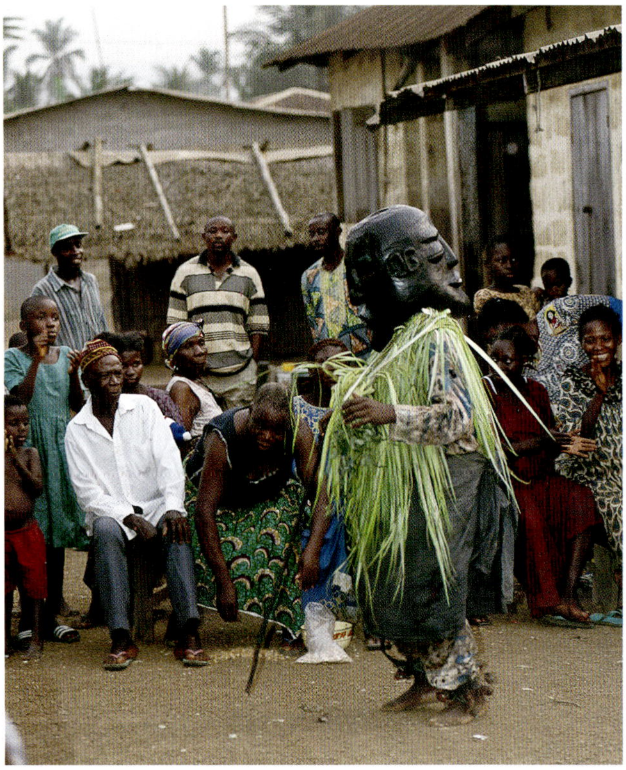

Fig. 142 Performance of *Angbu* (Kembong, January 26, 2004).

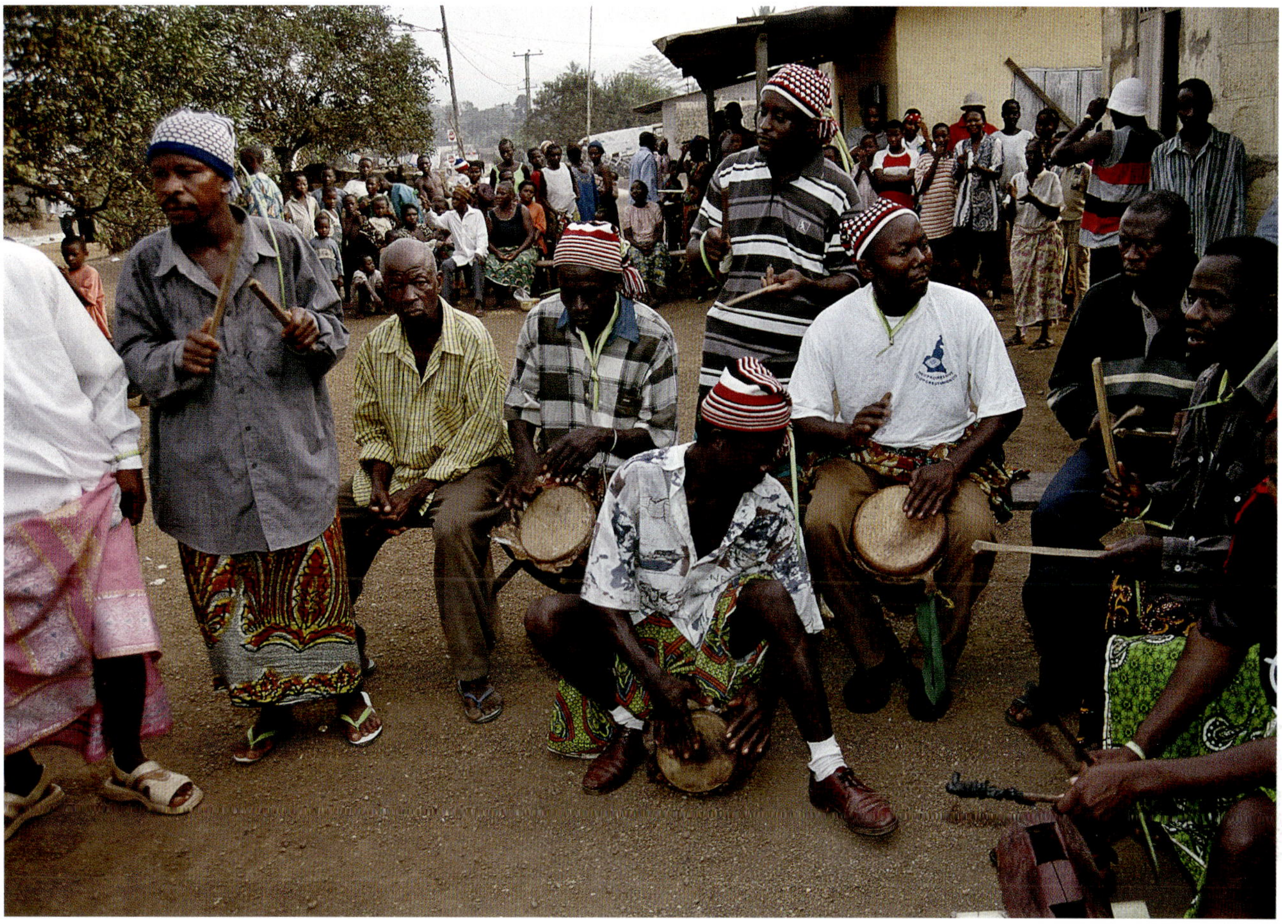

Fig. 143 Musicians and musical instruments of *Angbu*: a small slit-drum ("cripple"; right front), several drums and rattles (Kembong, January 26, 2004).

with a rifle, which in normal life does not function anymore (figs. 139, 140).

Angbu is engaged when a deceased man or woman, who suffered a "bad death", is to be buried. The mask is also contracted to collect debts or to aid in driving an unwanted visitor out of a community. The actual duty of *Angbu* is to carry out autopsies on the dead – one refers to the "heart of *Angbu*", a practise that obviously is still carried out occasionally (*ojahne*, meaning to operate on a man). The autopsy is supposed to determine whether or not the person's death was caused by a witch and, moreover, whether the deceased him- or herself was a witch.[115] *Angbu* is a "bad *juju*", yet at the same time it is a dancing mask and wears foot rattles at the dances. It appears above all after the burial of a deceased member to honour him in dance one last time. Sometimes the mask performs at the visit of a minister or other high ranking persons (figs. 136–143).

There are no set days on which members of *Angbu* come together. They meet only on important occasions. Every adult male may enter the society; women have no access. Each member must take an oath that he will preserve the secrets of *Angbu*, having the choice to swear upon a medicine (*njom*), for example *Okeboho*. This takes place in the presence of a medicine man of the respective medicine society. One may alternatively swear upon the Bible or the rifle of *Angbu*. When a person swears upon the rifle, he takes it into both hands and speaks the oath: "I swear on this very gun that – whatever the members of this society *Angbu* are going to show or to teach me – I will release the information to nobody privately besides the *Angbu* sitting. If I do this, let me become a victim of this gun." Then the new member licks the rifle with his tongue.

Persons aspiring to membership in *Angbu* have already paid some fees upon contacting the big men, consisting of colanuts, tobacco and one jug of palm wine. After taking the oath, the actual fees are due: one crate of beer, two "animals" and 30,000 Francs CFA (c. 50 Euros). The new members are not treated with medicine, as is the case in secret societies with "bad *jujus*" in the Cameroon Grasslands. There treatment with medicine is necessary in order to protect them from the dangerous medicines of their own society. Training and instruction take place first in the house of

Performance of *Angbu* in Babong (February 20, 1980) (figs. 144–146).

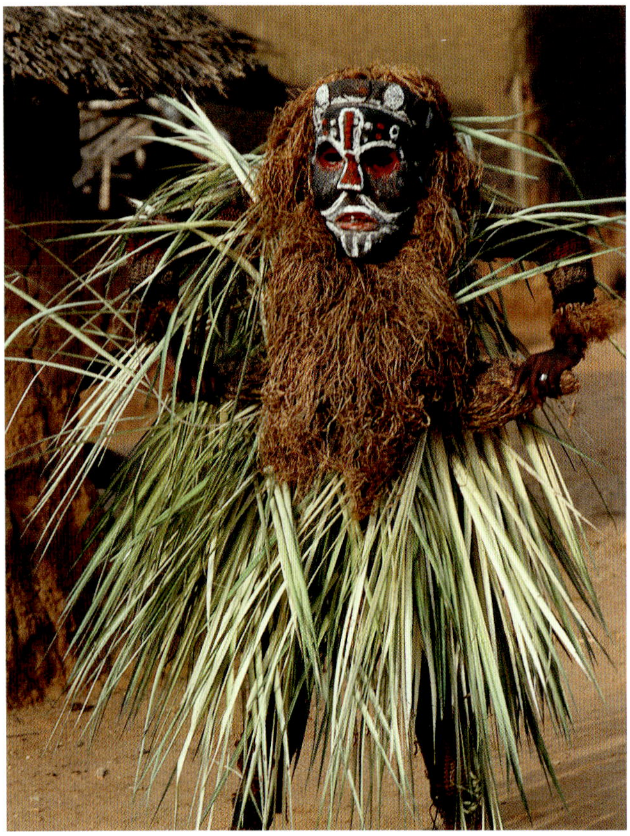

Fig. 144 The male mask of *Angbu* (Babong, February 20, 1980).

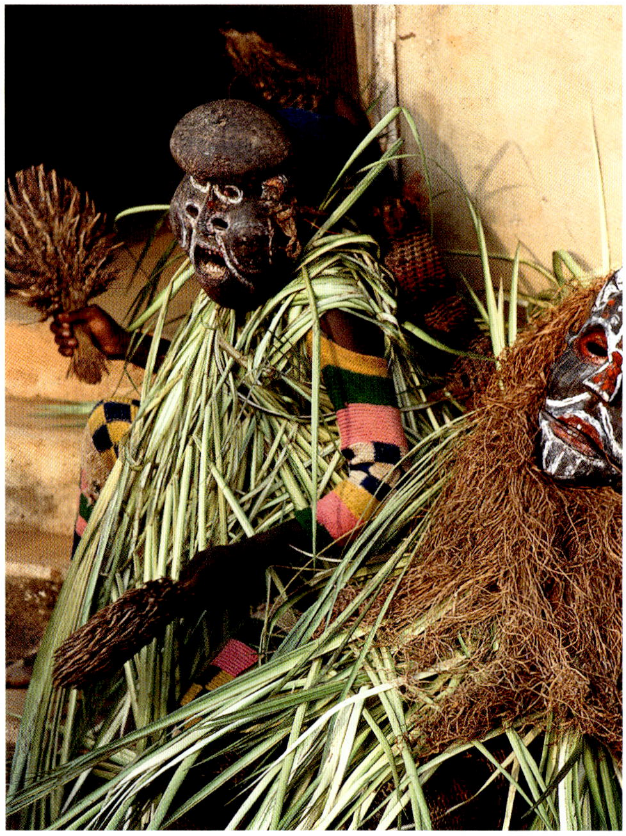

Fig. 145 The two masks of *Angbu*: the female mask holding the thorny fruit of the oil palm (left) and the male mask (right) (Babong, February 20, 1980).

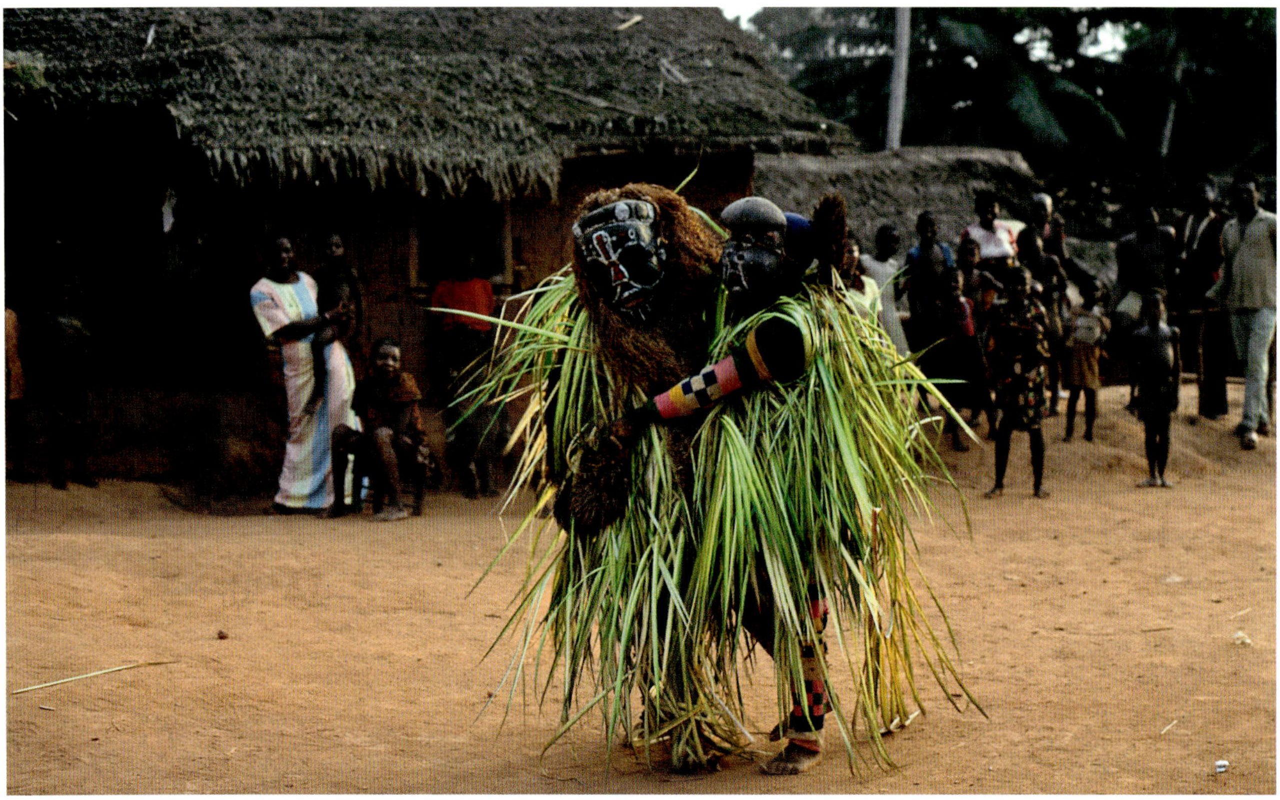

Fig. 146 At first the male mask dances alone; later it is joined by the female mask. In the course of the dance they embrace (Babong, February 20, 1980).

one of the two "speakers" of *Angbu* (see below). At this time the new members learn the songs and dances of the society and also to play the drum. All other secrets, such as conducting offerings to the ancestors, medicine rituals, post-mortem operations etc., are taught in the grove of *Angbu* (*ekot Angbu* or *ebaah Angbu*). However, the instruction may only occur when a group consists of four or five members, who are to be entrusted with the secrets.

As in all secret societies, in *Angbu* there are also several ranks. One of the higher positions is that of "president" of *Angbu*: *ntui mfam* (pl. *atui mfam*) or *njoho Angbu*, "the man who performs the sacrifice". Upon this person's death, his deputy (*etobe ntui*, pl. *betobe ntui*) automatically becomes president. His former position is, in turn, taken over by a second deputy, for whom a successor is chosen at the same time. Further, the society has two "speakers" (*achotekuble*, sg. *nchotekuble*). Besides instructing the new members, they purchase wine for the assemblies of members, direct discussions and announce the punishments decided in the assemblies. Sometimes they speak in public as well. The "operators" (*abosangito*, sg. *osangito*) are of special significance in that aside from other serious duties they are responsible for post-mortem operations. At the same time they are the bearers of the mask. It is expected that they are intelligent and courageous, and, hence, they receive special training. About three to five in number, the operators can be called to carry out all important and difficult tasks. On such occasions the mask usually appears as well, while the other operators have concealed their faces with a cloth. Those ugly and dangerous tasks are normally performed by middle-aged men.

Since it has the character of a "bad *juju*", *Angbu* is also associated with bad medicine (*njom*), which is kept in strict secrecy. In consequence this means that no outsider may witness the mask bearer donning the mask outfit. The treatment with medicine, which is rubbed on the arms, is intended to imbue the mask bearer with courage and additional strength and, moreover, to enable him to perceive things that are invisible to ordinary people. When the mask carries out dangerous actions, the persons accompanying it must protect themselves by using medicine, but of another kind.

In all activities, especially prior to the mask's performance, the ancestors are always invoked in order to secure their aid. Medicine derives from the ancestors, and they are the ones who make it effective again. Thus, in this respect *Angbu* has nothing to do with spirits and demons. Before an autopsy a prayer in the following sense is spoken: "*Ata Obasi* and *Mma Obasi* (Father God and Mother God) and Agborbelle Black (the person from whom *Angbu* was purchased originally and who has died in the meantime), we want to perform a post-mortem. One who is dead shall be brought to *Angbu* society, and *Angbu* should be enabled to do its business. While *Angbu* is doing its work, whether concerning witchcraft or any other bad thing, let nothing illegal happen to the operator. Through the powers of Almighty God, the creator of mankind, let no bad effect come to the people of this place. Let the ancestors help us to do this work peacefully."

The small slit-drum of *Angbu* is of special importance when communing with the ancestors. It is called "cripple" (*nkem*, pl. *akem*), as it is generally thought that the drum can move as little as a handicapped person. The instrument is placed upon the ground, i. e. the sphere of the ancestors. It is far more than merely a musical instrument, for it serves to communicate with the ancestors and, therefore, contains medicines (figs. 137, 143). The person who beats the drum is merely a medium for medicine and thus for the ancestors. Through him the ancestors direct the members as to what they should do. For example, if the rhythm of music changes during a mask performance, it is the wish of the ancestors. The drummer acts only upon the dictates of the ancestors and theoretically – following the conviction of *Angbu* members – even I, a European, could have played *nkem*. Yet, only members can understand messages from the ancestors, and only the "president" may answer the ancestors in normal speech. The extraordinary significance of this slit-drum is manifested prior to every dance performance of the mask: in all of the ancestral offerings, the drum *nkem* receives a share as well (fig. 137).

Angbu already existed in the region of Kembong prior to colonial times, when the population still lived in various separate hamlets. Interest in the society later declined, and around 1960 the society was dissolved. At the end of the 1990s none of the old members were alive. There were, however, efforts among young people at that time to revive *Angbu*, but they were not supported by the older generation. For the elders *Angbu* was a "bad society". Thus, the youths had to act on their own. They succeeded in gaining contact with the *Angbu* society in Bakut, a village about 25 km southwest of Kembong on the Munaya River. After discussing the matter a delegation of seven young men in Kembong was sent to Bakut at the beginning of 2000. The group stayed there for three days. During this time they learned the special songs, dances, techniques in playing the drum of *Angbu* as well as about carving the mask. The visit concluded with a celebration, which the delegation from Kembong organised for their hosts in Bakut. The festivity ended with a prayer by their "president", Agborbelle Black, addressed to the ancestors: "I am calling for God's blessings to bring the people from Kembong safely home, so that we can complete there our exercises of *Angbu*."

Two months later *Angbu* of Bakut visited Kembong in return; some twenty men stayed there for three days. Beforehand the preparations had been made as planned. An area had been searched out for the grove of *Angbu*, and drums had been carved. Only the mask itself was made in Bakut. During these three days the *Angbu*-initiators in Kembong received further instructions from their visitors from Bakut. Now spiritual aspects were the focus of attention, i. e. the special way in which *Angbu* secures the aid of the ancestors and uses medicine. Simultaneously, the Kembong group was taught techniques and rituals that are of special importance for *Angbu* and connected in particular with warding off witches and devils and conducting post-mortem operations. At the end of this period of instruction and founding, the first "president" of the newly established society *Angbu* in Kembong thanked his friends from Bakut: "Pa Black, you sold us *Angbu*. We are very happy about it, we received it with great gratitude. Your delegation, which was sent to Kembong to instruct us, was received with joy and happiness. We wish God's guidance and leadership over *Angbu* in Bakut and Kembong. May God bless you in Bakut." The visiting *Angbu* members from Bakut were later paid the purchase price of 370,000 Francs CFA (c. 600 Euro). Thereafter the mask of *Angbu* appeared in public for the first time on Sunday, April 30, 2000. The mask danced from Lower Kembong to Upper Kembong and back, and it was received by the population with great enthusiasm.

Since that time the *Angbu* societies in Kembong and Bakut have been in close contact. If laws of *Angbu* are seriously violated in Kembong, *Angbu* in Bakut is notified immediately. Immediate notification would also occur if *Angbu* in Kembong intended to sell the society with all of its secrets, in which case Bakut would have no influence upon the planned sale. The former big man of *Angbu* in Bakut, Agborbelle Black, was also chief of Bakut; after going blind, he became known as a "devilish" man. After his death, he was included among the ancestors of the new *Angbu* society and is always invoked in prayer. Meanwhile *Angbu* has become an integral part in the cultural life of Kembong again as an important and serious society.

4.5 *Obon*

Obon is a society, in which solidarity, reciprocal aid and entertainment play a central role.[116] It does not have any duties that are concerned with keeping peace in the community or fending off hostile powers. Consequently, *Obon* does not have any medicines. However, the society does possess a secret musical instrument (*nchokot Obon*). The instrument is played in public as well, but in such a way that it is concealed from view. The members of the various lodges of *Obon* that are present in Kembong usually assemble only when new members are admitted and when a death celebration is held for a deceased member (figs. 147, 148). The lodge members who do meet regularly – sometimes every week – are those who have organised a mutual savings account. In all cases of death it is the messenger of *Obon* who announces the death to the public by beating a tortoise shell, thus also summoning men from each quarter to help dig the grave pit.

There are three levels in *Obon*:
1. *Abo Obon* (children of *Obon*). Fees: 30 litres of palm wine, 3 bottles of whisky and 5,000 Francs CFA.
2. *Bechi Obon* (leaders of *Obon*). Fees for this level correspond with those of the first level.
3. *Atui amfa Obon*. This is the level of the two chiefs. Fees: 3 "animals", 30 litres of palm wine, one bunch of plantains, one bottle of palm oil, one cup of salt, one cup of pepper.

There are three groups of lodges of *Obon* in Kembong:
1. *Akaran Obon* (*akaran* = razor). The lodges in the quarters of Mbiofong, Takpang, Ndengane, Okangku, Obiola and the joint lodge in Nchofang and Okune belong to this group.
2. *Ndem Obon*. The lodges in the quarters Nkonghobe, Ebarensi, Okemebenem, Nserong and Abotabe.
3. This group is constituted by the lodge in Okonyenge alone.

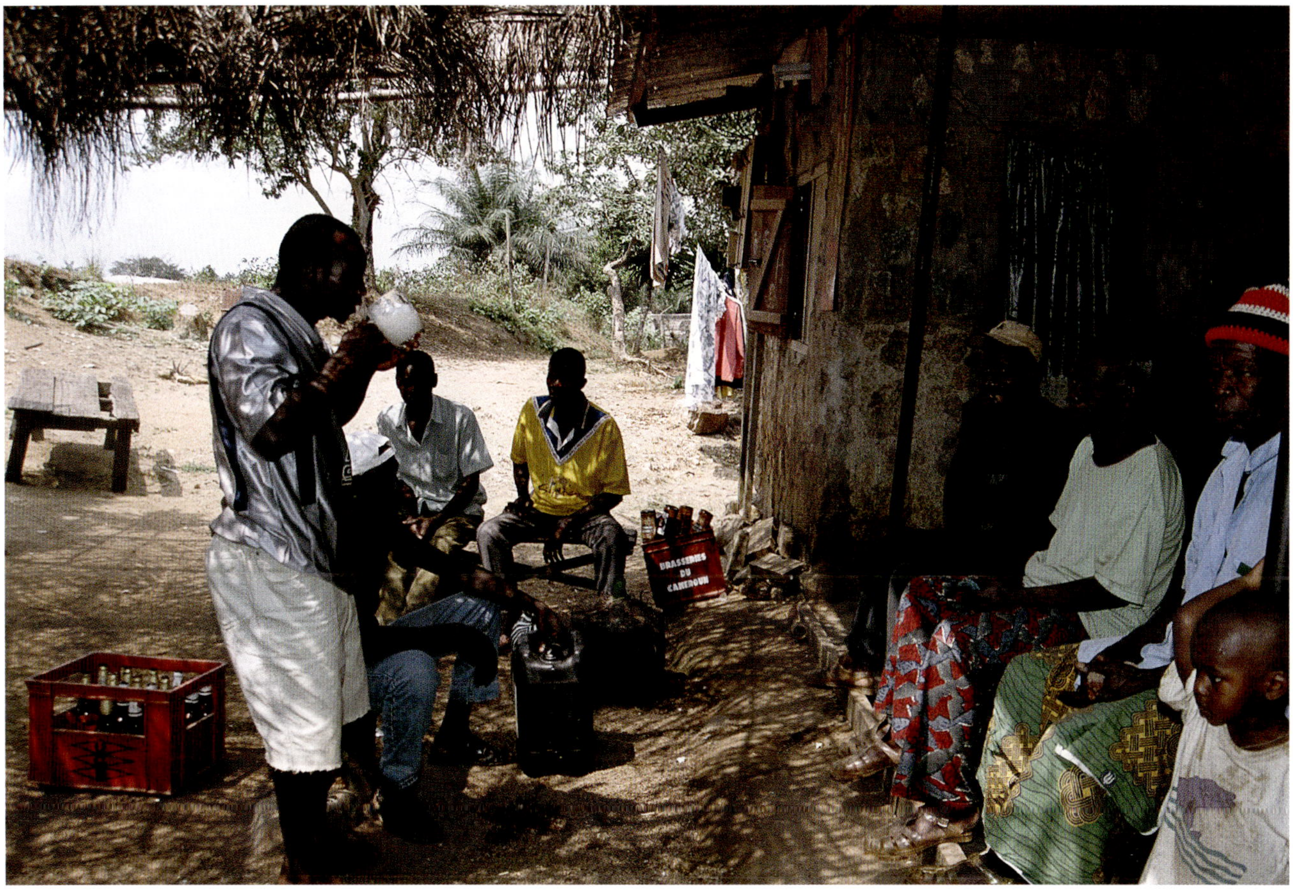

Fig. 147 Members of the men's society *Obon* in Takpang, drinking palm wine; three big men are seated on the right (Kembong, January 22, 2004).

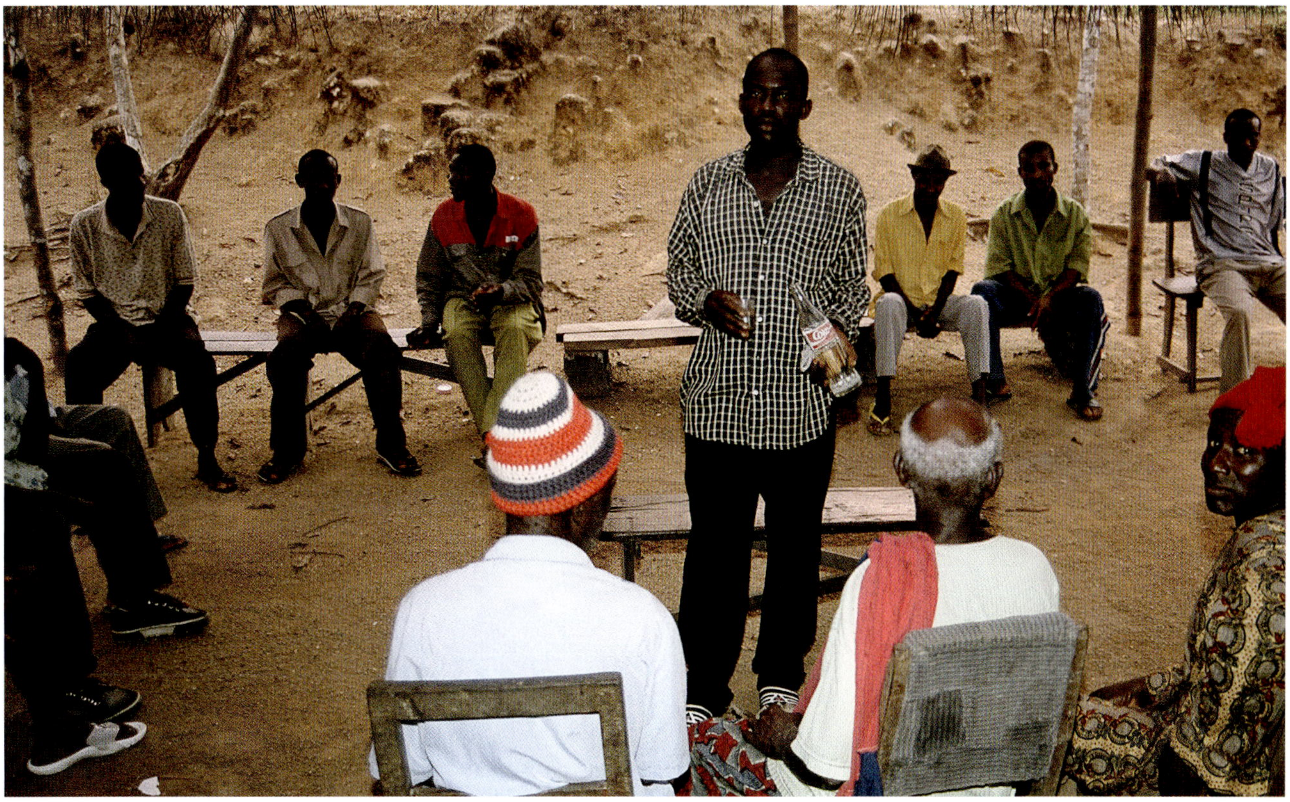

Fig. 148 A hearing is held by *Obon*. In the foreground three big men, in the background ordinary members and – standing – the person giving a report (Kembong, January 22, 2004).

Footnotes

1 Onor (1994:101 ff.) and Agbor (2001:11) also speak of *Mgbe*. Yet, during conversations in English the word "leopard" was seldom used, instead more often "tiger" (see also Nicklin 1991: 15). An earlier but only brief mention is made about this by Bastian (1884:9).

2 Talbot 1926: III:779, 782. Similar reference to the power and influence of *Ngbe/Ekpe* is made by Partridge 1905:34 f.; Parkinson 1907: 262; Mansfeld 1908:159 f.; Jones 1956:137 ff.; N'Idu 1959:747 ff.; Abalogu 1978:78.

3 In Old Calabar *Nyampkwe* was the highest rank in the secret society of *Ekpe* (Jones 1956:138 ff.; Latham 1973:39; Northrup 1978:109; Nicklin 1983:72). In other regions *Emanyankpe* is still the designation for the mask, which is called *Ebongu* or *Ema* in Kembong (Ruel 1969:233 f.; Thompson 1974:182; Leib and Romano 1984:54; Ottenberg and Knudsen 1985: 38). There is a mask in Bende (Igbo) with a rather similar name *nwainyankpe* (Abalogu 1978:83).

4 Partridge 1905:35 f. Later Talbot (1912:40) also remarked: "It is difficult to discover more than the merest fragments of the secrets of Egbo, as any known informant would meet with a speedy death". Parkinson (1907: 262) noted with reference to *Egbo* "that its members are under a strict pledge to reveal nothing". (Cp. N'Idu 1959:749; Ruel 1969: 244 f.; Ekpo 1978:73).

5 There are numerous reports on the origin and history of *Ngbe/Ekpe*: Talbot 1912:37 ff.; 1926:III:779 ff.; Jones 1956: 137 ff.; Ruel 1969: 250 f.; Abalogu 1978:78 ff.; Ekpo 1978:74; Northrup 1978:173, fn. 95; Nicklin 1983:72; Thompson 1984: 239 ff.; Ottenberg and Knudsen 1985:38 ff.; Hackett 1989:34 ff. All of these authors assume that the secret society first emerged in the area of the Ejagham in southwestern Cameroon.

6 During his research trip to southwestern Cameroon in 1988, Nicklin gained convincing information that *Ngbe/Ekpe* did not originate among the Ejagham, as assumed earlier (see fn. 5), but in the community of Isangele in the area of Balondo (Nicklin 1991:7 ff.).

7 Talbot 1923:162, 164, 170, 199; 1926:III:780; Thompson 1984:241 ff.; Leib and Romano 1984:48; Nicklin 1991:10 f.; Röschenthaler 1993:244, 248 ff.; Onor 1994:101 ff.

8 Nicklin 1991:11.

9 Early reports pertaining to this are found in Bastian 1884:9 ff. and Thormählen 1885:332 (cp. Frobenius 1898:83 ff.); further, Talbot 1926:III:784 ff.; Jones 1956:135 ff.; Nair 1972: 14 ff.; Latham 1973: 35 ff.; Northrup 1978: 108 ff.; Hackett 1989:35 f.

10 Ruel 1969:217 f.

11 Brain and Pollock 1971:107 ff.

12 These are likewise pointed out by Ruel 1969: 218, 228, 255; Ekpo 1978:74; Ottenberg and Knudsen 1985:103; Röschenthaler 1993:130 (fn. 8).

13 Cp. corresponding information in Parkinson 1907:264; Udo Ema 1938:314; Ruel 1969:229; Thompson 1974:181; Abalogu 1978:94 f.; Ukpong 1989:20.

14 There are numerous references to ranks in *Ngbe/Ekpe*, yet they differ greatly concerning individual societies. Solely the most important elements – for example, acceptance into the society and the special meaning of the rank of the "evil forest" or "grove of *Mgbe*" – are evidently the same: Bastian 1884:9; Frobenius 1898:88; Talbot 1912:40 ff.; Talbot 1926:III:786; Udo Ema 1938:315; Jones 1956:137; N'Idu 1959: 749; Ruel 1969: 223; Ekpo 1978:74; Abalogu 1978:88; Latham 1978: 39; Leib and Romano 1984:50 f.; Ottenberg and Knudsen 1985:37; Dike 1987:33 f.; Hackett 1989:36; Röschenthaler 1993:130.

15 The saying is also known among the Banyang (Ruel 1969:219, 244).

16 Mansfeld (1908:162 f.) noted, oppositely, that acceptance of new members into *Mgbe* depended essentially upon required qualities of the candidate's character.

17 The same is found in Old Calabar: there slaves could gain admission to *Ekpe*, but only in the lower ranks (Bastian 1884:14; Frobenius 1898: 90; Nair 1972:17 f.; Latham 1973:39; Northrup 1978:109; Hackett 1989:36). In other regions they were barred from *Ngbe/Ekpe* in general (Abalogu 1978:79; Nicklin 1991:6 f.).

18 A woman apparently with the same functions is also present among the neighbouring Banyang (Ruel 1969:226).

19 Most of the *Ngbe/Ekpe* societies are solely for men. If a woman is accepted, she may enter the lower ranks only (Talbot 1912:44; Udo Ema 1938:314; Ekpo 1978:75).

20 In many reports about *Ngbe/Ekpe*, the instrument with which the voice of the leopard is imitated is seen as the greatest secret (cp. Talbot 1912:221 f.; 1926:III:780; N'Idu 1959: 748; Ruel 1969:225; Ekpo 1978:75). There have been repeated conjectures as to how this fear-instilling cry is made. I am rather certain that Leib and Romano (1984:50) do not err in their assumption.

21 Talbot 1912:44.

22 *Afungbe* is a term also known among the Banyang (Thompson 1974:182).

23 Talbot already made reference to these masks (1912:44). In the meantime there are numerous and detailed reports about them: Ruel 1969:226, 233 f.; Abalogu 1978:81, 96; Leib and Romano 1984:54 ff.; Ottenberg and Knudsen 1985:38, 95; Nicklin 1983:67; Nicklin and Salmons 1984:32; Nicklin 1991:7. According to these reports the masks do not use the same mask garment as in Kembong; instead each has its own outfit, which, however, is generally quite similar. It should be noted that in Old Calabar *Ema* – one of the *Mgbe* masks in Kembong – was the name of one of "the two legendary founders of the original Creek Town" (Jones 1956:158 f.).

24 According to Thompson (1974:182) this disk-shaped element was present among the Banyang, which was "another head (*isun*), in the form of a disk. The disk, made of cloth over a circular cane frame, recenters us within the notion of Janus. The disk grants the spirit-dancer extra eyes, sometimes boldly rendered as appliqued mirrors. The mirrors guard his back, imparting magic vision."

25 According to many references, the masks of *Ngbe/Ekpe* served as an important means of asserting the society's interests, and, consequently, they were extremely aggressive and correspondingly dangerous for non-members: Talbot 1912:44; 1923:161; Udo Ema 1938: 314, 316; Jones 1956:140, 142; N'Idu 1959: 748; Nair 1972:15; Latham 1973: 37; Abalogu 1978:97; Leib and Romano 1984:54; Ottenberg and Knudsen 1985:38; Nicklin 1991:7.

26 Leib and Romano mention such taboos as well in Babong (1984:50 f.).

27 *Okina* is also known in *Ngbe* of the Banyang (Ruel 1969:226; Thompson 1974:184).

28 Talbot (1926:III:786) already pointed out the special meaningfulness of this level among the Ekoi: "Those who have passed through all the grades are allowed to take part in the celebration of the Bush Egbo, which is performed with the greatest ceremony in the depths of the bush; it is on this occasion that the final mysteries are unveiled. There is no doubt that human sacrifices were offered in connection with the rites" (cp. also Talbot 1912:43). Pertaining to the Banyang, Ruel (1969:221)

also mentions "some rather heightened accounts" that take place in the "*Ngbe* bush": "for example, that the initiant sees the dead ancestors as though they were living."
It is possible that musical instruments, which are viewed as important objects of cult by many African secret societies, were played at the ceremonies. According to some authors (Parkinson 1907:265; Talbot 1926:III:758 f., 780); Ekpo 1978:75), *Ngbe/Ekpe* makes use of bullroarers.

29 An extensive description of the sign-language called *nsibiri* or *nsibidi* is provided by Abalogu (1978:83, 92 ff.). See also Nicklin 1983:67 f.; Ottenberg and Knudsen 1985:103, fn. 5. Furthermore, *nsibiri* is also the designation for a system of pictographs, which was known primarily among the Ejagham, but also among other tribes. Thompson devoted a comprehensive and detailed work to the study of the *nsibidi*-signs (1983: 227–268). No information could be attained in Kembong about this pictographic sign-system; however, more was learned about the secret section of *Mgbe*, which carries the same name. In earlier times one of its duties was to carry out the execution of offenders (see corresponding details in Talbot 1912:305 f. and 1926:III:792) as well as to conduct post-mortem examinations. Correspondingly *nsibiri* can be translated with "bad feelings and intentions". According to Thompson (1983:227) *nsibidi* means "cruel letters". He learned this from an informant from Mamfe, the main town of the Manyu Division: "If you want to execute heavy things, dangerous matters, *nsibidi* takes the lead" (Thompson 1983:298, fn. 4).

30 A comprehensive description of initiation into this level of such importance in *Ngbe* in Babong – although called *bekundi* – is provided by Leib and Romano (1984:51 f.).

31 A special cap of *eteme Mgbe* is pictured in Mansfeld 1908:168 (Pl. XXII, no. 3).

32 Present everywhere in the Ngunaya area, the red cap is already noted in Staschewski (1917:16; cp. also Röschenthaler 1993: 162). There the red cap is not only worn by members of *Mgbe*, but also by those of other societies, as for instance *Nkanda* and *Obasinjom*. Individuals who own dangerous medicines may wear a red cap as well as men in part of formal dress. *Mgbe* members may wear the red cap with an eagle feather, members of *Obasinjom* and other medicine societies wear the red cap together with a feather from a parrot. In former times, the red caps were knitted locally. With the advent of industrialisation and influenced by the high demand, red caps were produced in Nigeria; besides, many ethnic groups in southern Nigeria use the red cap as well. No one knows exactly when red caps were introduced to the Central Ejagham. Obviously, they came with the introduction of *Mgbe, Obasinjom* and the other societies that use it. Certainly the red cap was in use before the coming of Europeans. Among the Bakossi the red cap was the privilege of the *Ahon* society (Balz 1984:184, 225).

33 Talbot (1923:165) describes a similar practice of *Egbo* among the Ibibio. The procession during the "long-tail dance" is led by a "man of high position ... His position was formerly one not only of honour but danger, for behind him follows a man holding the sword called Ika, which he keeps shaking close to the neck of the leader. According to old custom, should the latter stumble or let fall his sceptre before he could raise himself the blade fell and his head rolled in the dust."

34 As early as the times of Old Calabar the *eyamba* was already known as the "president of *Ekpe*" (Bastian 1884:9, 12, 16; Frobenius 1898:86, 88; Jones 1956:158; Nair 1972:15 f.; Latham 1973:36 f., 39; Northrup 1978: 88). The title of *eyamba* is reported in other regions as well: Talbot 1926:III:786; N'Idu 1959:749; Ekpo 1978:74; Abalogu 1978: 78; Leib and Romano 1984:50; Hackett 1989:35. Among the Aro, who belong to the eastern Igbo, *iyamba* is the "female equivalent" to *Ekpe,* which "looks after the affairs of married women, particularly those in trouble with their husband's kinsmen" (Dike 1987:34).

35 Ceremonial staffs, likewise called *monyo*, are also found among the Banyang (Thompson 1974:185) and in Babong (Leib and Romano 1984:50, 52).

36 A description of the "board of *Ngbe/Ekpe*" was already made by Parkinson (1907:262): "...on the wall at the back of the dais is hung a large plaited mat; on this are fastened three pig-skulls in the centre and an edging of kids' skulls surrounding all." The indigenous designation was first mentioned by Mansfeld (1908: 219) in his report on the dedication of a house of *Ngbe/Ekpe*: "As soon as the granite block (the *eteh Mgbe*, i. e. the "stone of *Mgbe*", H.-J. K.) was set in place, a kind of plaque, the so-called *orongbe*, was hung above it, upon which the skulls of cows and goats that had been slaughtered on the day of consecration were attached." Talbot makes no mention of the "board of *Ngbe/Ekpe*"; however, a "board of *Ngbe/Ekpe*" is pictured in the illustrations of the "sacred stone and pillar" from the *Egbo*-house in Ojokk (Talbot 1926: II:346) and in Ndebbiji (Talbot 1926: III:783) (both of the Ejagham Ekoi). This is in complete correspondence with Mansfeld's report (see above) that they hang from the house posts above the "stone of *Ngbe/Ekpe*". Ruel mentions this meaningful cult object as well (1969: 220 f.): "Bekundi (among the Banyang, H.-J. K.) also has its own form of shield (*nkpa*), a woven mat, with a raphia surround, on which are fixed certain leaves, animal bones, skulls, and horns, and which is usually hung from the central post of its leader or owner's *aca*." A special study on the "board of *Ngbe/Ekpe*" was presented by Nicklin (1991:3–5), together with his own research material and a field survey (cp. also Nicklin 1983:72).

37 Rubin 1984:68; Forkl 1989:67; Nicklin 1995:372; Poynor 2001:334.

38 Essential information about the "stone of *Ngbe/Ekpe*" together with a sketch was already provided by Parkinson (1907:263 f.). Mansfeld (1908:218) included a photograph of the stone in his study. For him the stone was the "most important part" of the *Ngbe* house. Many interesting notes can be found in Talbot (1912:40, 141, 172, 219, 263, 265; 1926:II:345 ff.; 1926:III: 782 ff.). He also provides photographs (1912:172) and drawings (1926:II:346 und III:783) of the stone. Staschewski (1917:4) and Nicklin (1991:6) also make mention of the stone. Ruel (1969:222 f.) offers an extensive analysis of the stone as found among the Banyang.

39 Talbot (1926:II:345, see also 1926:III:782 ff.) supplies similar information: The stone "is as a rule set up before one of the pillars supporting the roof and projects out of a small clay mould, in a hole in which are kept sacred 'medicines', together with some small round pebbles ...".

40 Mansfeld (1908:218) designated the stone as an "altar, that is, a place for prayer and offerings". Similarly, Talbot (1926:III: 783 f.) called it "the most important part of the club-house", in front of which offerings are made and prayers are spoken. See also Ekpo 1978:74.

41 The same principle of rotation is also practised in Babong (Leib u. Romano 1984:50).

42 The house of *Ngbe/Ekpe*, the centre of every settlement, soon attracted the interest of the first Europeans, which is evident in the detailed descriptions: Partridge 1905:208 ff.; Parkinson 1907:262 f.; Mansfeld 1908:218 f.; Talbot 1912:262 ff.; 1926: III:786 ff.; Ruel 1969:224 f.; Ekpo 1978:74.

43 For ceremonial drinking, see also Ruel 1969:225 and Leib and Romano 1984:50.

44 "Ekpe became synonymous with good and orderly government. Its decisions were based on equality and justice" (Abalogu 1978: 89). "Ngbe is responsible for maintaining the well-being of the community" (Leib and Romano 1984:48). See also Onor 1994:103.
45 Jones 1956:157.
46 Jones 1956:141; Latham 1973:36 f.; Hackett 1989:35 f.; Onor 1994:104.
47 Jones 1956:140 f.; Nair 1972:19 ; Northrup 1978:109; Hackett 1989:36.
48 Jones 1956:141 f.
49 For example, in Bende (Igbo) *Ekpe* had legislative duties: "It became the local government of the people. All important policy matters affecting the people were usually taken at the meeting of the club" (Abalogu 1978:79). Likewise, among the eastern and northern Ibibio groups *Ekpe* was "the governing power" (Talbot 1926:III:782).
50 Nicklin (1983:67) in accordance also notes that it is generally the duty of *Ngbe/Ekpe*, "to enforce judicial and legislative decisions." (See also Onor 1994:101, 103). *Ngbe* acts entirely in this sense among the Banyang, the eastern neighbours of the Central Ejagham: "The rights which Ngbe protects are not Ngbe rights, but the rights of any individual member of a community: 'Ngbe laws' are laws which originate from decisions of a community council but which are given the added formality of being announced through Ngbe" (Ruel 1969:235). Mansfeld (1908:161) already rendered due respect to *Ngbe* when he noted that the government may dress an order in a pleasing form, but "it will never impress the indigenous as much as when proclaimed as paragraph so-and-so by *Ewi-Ngbe*."
51 See corresponding findings in Bastian 1884:10; Frobenius 1898:86; Parkinson 1907:264; Ruel 1969:235; Abalogu 1978: 89; Northrup 1978:109.
52 Koloss 2000:306.
53 Jones (1956:142) makes mention of such signs as do Ruel (1969: 235); Latham (1978:38); Abalogu (1978:90) and Ukpong (1989:21).
54 For an overview of judgements and punishments made by *Ngbe/Ekpe* in the past and still today, see Mansfeld 1908:173 f.; Jones 1956:142 ff.; Latham 1973:38; Abalogu 1978:90; Ukpong 1989:20 f.
55 Several authors have reported social isolation: Talbot 1926:III:784; Jones 1956:143; Ruel 1969:152, 236, 249; Latham 1973:38; Abalogu 1978:90; Ukpong 1989:21.
56 This arrangement is also customary among the Banyang (Ruel 1969:229).
57 Talbot 1912:38. In the last decades this theory was presented in nearly all research studies, which made reference to the "leopard spirit": Jones 1956:136 f.; Nair 1972:15; Wirz 1972: 44; Thompson 1974:173 ff.; Nicklin 1983:67; Leib and Romano 1984:52 ff.; Ottenberg and Knudsen 1985:37 f., 94 f.; Dike 1987:30; Hackett 1989:35; Nicklin 1991:6.
58 Secret societies in the Cameroon Grasslands act towards non-members with implications, rumours and threats, thereby creating uncertainty and fear. However, there is no ambiguity as far as the effectiveness of medicines, on the basis of the *jujus*, is concerned; they are feared by all, by the initiated as well as non-initiates (Koloss 2000:101).
59 Koloss 2000:150, 179.
60 Talbot 1912: 39 f.; see also Jeffreys 1939:96. The ceremonies in the house of *Ngbe/Ekpe*, on which Mansfeld (1908:217 ff.) also reported extensively, are dedicated exclusively to the ancestors – and thus to God – and not to a leopard spirit. Unfortunately, there are only few reports on the religious sphere of *Ngbe/Ekpe*, yet from the little known it can be deduced that God and the ancestors are the sole entities to whom *Ngbe/ Ekpe* is obligated. Cp. e.g. Ekpo 1978:74 and Abalogu 1978:89, 96.
61 Mansfeld 1908:148; Jones 1956:140; 1963:19; Latham 1973: 37; Ekpo 1978:73; Ukpong 1989:19.
62 Talbot 1926:III:785.
63 Ruel 1969:241.
64 The same obligation exists in the Grasslands (Koloss 2000: 331).
65 Talbot (1926:III:526) noted similarly: "If it (the "second burial") is not given, the family would not only be ridiculed by their age-classes, but the dead man would trouble his people and would say, 'I have left plenty property. Why should not some be spent on my second burial?'"
66 There is a similar regulation among the Banyang: "Finally, at the death of a member of Ngbe, other dues, proportionate to those originally paid by him, are required by the association from his relatives" (Ruel 1969:228).
67 Sound recordings of *Ebongu's* performance, made in Kembong on April 10, 2004, are preserved in the Department of Ethnomusicology in the Ethnological Museum, Berlin (Inv. No. VII OA 0739.001).
68 Leib and Romano (1984:52) note that participants in a funeral procession hold a *nje iren* leaf in the mouth, which is seen as an "oath of secrecy". Thompson (1983:237) reports on a "sign of silence" in Calabar, which is a feather "sealing" the lips of a dancer (see also Anonymous 1957:160, 161, 169).
69 Cp. Talbot (1926:III:524) and Abalogu (1978:96) for a description of this ritual as well.
70 Cp. Udo Ema 1938:314; Ruel 1969:50; Röschenthaler 1993: 247. For the Cameroon Grasslands, see Koloss 2000:326, fn. 5.
71 The same ritual in Babong is mentioned by Leib and Romano (1984:52, 95, fn. 25). See also Talbot 1912:44.
72 In Bende (Igbo) as well it is said that "... no one cries until *Ekpe* has been officially informed and cries first" (Abalogu 1978:95).
73 Ruel (1969:234, 246) reports the same about the Banyang, and Onor (1994:103) for the Ejagham as a whole.
74 A photograph of a mask of the Banyang that belongs to the boys is presented in Ruel (1969:235, plate 10). As is the case with *Nchockandah*, the mask's "garment" is composed of branches and leaves, but – unlike *Nchockandah* – wears a face mask.
75 Sound recordings of *Nchokandah* in Kembong are preserved in the Department of Ethnomusicology in the Ethnological Museum, Berlin: April 15, 2004 (Inv. No. VII OA 0739.001) and April 20, 2004 (Inv. No. VII OA 00739.003).
76 A detailed description of a performance by *Emanyankpe* of the Banyang is offered by Thompson (1974:182).
77 Sound recordings made during the performances of *Ema* in Kembong are preserved in the Department of Ethnomusicology in the Ethnological Museum, Berlin: January 18, 2004 (Inv. No. VII OA 0430.001) and April 10, 2004 (Inv. No. VII OA 0739.001).
78 For the same ritual among the Banyang, see Ruel 1969:233. There it is *Ebongu* "who is expected to chastise [the widows] if their mourning is insufficient." See also Thompson 1974:182. A similar ritual in Babong is described by Leib and Romano 1984:54. Mansfeld (1908:202) also mentions "the custom that the widow is beaten upon the death of the husband..."
79 Nair 1972:17; Ekpo 1978:75 and Abalogu 1978:95.
80 Cp. N'Idu 1959:748; Leib and Romano 1984:50. I heard an equally critical opinion in Oku: "*Jujus* (i. e. secret societies) are only hunting for food and wine, nothing else. If anybody tells another thing, it is a lie" (Koloss 2000:266). Similarly by the

Bakossi it was said: "The juju people … are those who make the belly to be their god; through egoistic feasting and idling they waste what the hard labour of others, who cannot join them in their privileges, has produced" (Balz 1984:281; s.a. 215, 225, 354).

81 This has been emphasised repeatedly by other authors as well: Jones 1956:157; Abalogu 1978:97; Ekpo 1978:75; Leib and Romano 1984:57; Ottenberg and Knudsen 1985:40.

82 Probably the first reference to *Nkanda* is found in Mansfeld (1908: 149). The "renowned mural" from the "palaver house" in Okuri (Ekoi) illustrated in his publication could be that of a performance of the mask of *Nkanda*, i.e., if the figure to the left of whom a hoop is characteristic does indeed represent the mask's accompaniment. Mansfeld designates the mask as "*Ngbe-Juju*"; presumably the name *Nkanda* was unknown to him. This name first appears in Talbot's studies, and likely the first photographs of the mask as well (Talbot 1912:42; 1923: 167; 1926:III:786). Since then several reports have been made on the mask and the section of *Ngbe/Ekpe* that bears the same name: Ruel 1969:223; Leib and Romano 1984:49, 56 f.; Nicklin 1991:16 f.; Röschenthaler 1993:130. For photographs of *Nkanda* performances, see Röschenthaler 1998:40 and 1999: 43.

83 See the following references: Talbot 1912:42; 1926:III:786 (Ejagham); 1923:167 (Ibibio); Leib and Romano 1984: 51 (Babong); Nicklin 1991:16 (Balondo); Röschenthaler 1993: 130 (Ejagham). According to Ruel (1969:223) among the Banyang *Nkanda* is "a linked association partly separate, partly dependent upon *Ngbe*."

84 Leib and Romano (1984:57) provide a detailed description of such a procession in Babong.

85 A sound recording was made at the performance of *Nkanda* in Kembong on January 27, 2004, which is preserved in the Department of Ethnomusicology in the Ethnological Museum, Berlin (Inv. No. VII OA 0430.004).

86 Nicklin 1974:8; 1979:54, 59.

87 Campbell 1983:36 f.

88 Mansfeld, in: Tunis 1985:501; Nicklin 1974:8, 14; 1979: 54 ff.; Röschenthaler 1998:47.

89 Mansfeld 1908:211; Talbot 1926:III:755; Nicklin 1974:8; 1979:56; Röschenthaler 1993:229 f.; 1998:47 f.

90 Mansfeld 1924:26 f.; Talbot 1912:272; Brain and Pollock 1971:54; Nicklin 1974:8; Thompson 1974:175; Eyo 1981: 167; Röschenthaler 1993:219.

91 Mansfeld, in: Tunis 1985:513.

92 Talbot 1912:261, s. a. 223 f., 272; 1926:III:850. Likewise in Talbot there are photographs of masks, for which human skulls served as a headdress (Talbot 1912:223 and 1923:258). References to the use of human skulls as masks are also found in Cole (1970:50), Zwernemann 1972; Nicklin (1974:8; 1979: 56), Eyo (1981:167) and Tunis (1985: 514). Prior to this Frobenius (1898:180) proposed that "African face masks ... evolved from masks made of skulls." Later Schädler (1982:8) came to the same conclusion.

93 Nicklin 1974:8.

94 For photographs of animal masks, see for example Mansfeld (1908: 152, Tafel XVIII) and Blier 1980, Cat No. 17.

95 Eyo 1981:167.

96 Talbot 1926:III:754 f.

97 Some of the first photographs showing skin-covered masks are found in Mansfeld (1908:211; 1924:71) and Talbot (1912:38, 222 f.; 1926: III:754); see also the photograph by R. Raikes, presumably made at the beginning of the 20th century, in Nicklin 1981:168.

98 Mansfeld, in: Tunis 1985:502, 510.

99 Nicklin 1979:57; see also 1974:13, 68.

100 Mansfeld, in: Tunis 1985:501, 506, 512; see also 1924:47. Important references pertaining to the role of the art market in the Cross River region are found in Nicklin (1979:54, 57).

101 Mansfeld (in: Tunis 1985:510) likewise reports the use of wood of the "Mbeg tree" for carving.

102 Cp. Mansfeld's description of covering the mask with skin, in: Tunis 1985:510 f.; see also Nicklin (1974:13; 1979: 59) and among the Bangwa, Brain and Pollock (1971:54 f).

103 See also Nicklin 1974:68.

104 Mansfeld 1908:213; Talbot 1912:412; Tunis 1985:505 f. *Nchebe* is found foremost to the east of the Ngunaya area: among the Banyang (Talbot 1926:II:133 and III:792: "In old days the Banyangi were mainly ruled by the Nchebbi Society..."), in Widekum (Nicklin 1979:57 f.) and in Mogamo (Migeod 1925:82).

105 Mansfeld (1908:207) mentions a similar prayer.

106 Mention of this society is also made by Mansfeld (1908:213 and in: Tunis 1985:505).

107 Nicklin (1979:56) mentions a human sacrifice, at which a slave "was beheaded at one blow".

108 A corresponding note is made by Mansfeld 1908:207.

109 A sound recording of this performance made on January 27, 2004, is preserved in the Department of Ethnomusicology in the Ethnological Museum, Berlin (Inv. No. VII OA 0430.004).

110 Talbot mentioned a mask by the name of *Nkpe* among the Banyang (1926:II:133).

111 Widespread in southwestern Cameroon and southern Nigeria, slit-drums are one of the most important objects of a community and, thus, usually in the possession of the village chieftain. They are played on special occasions, for example at performances of important secret societies (in the Ngunaya area, the appearances of *Mgbe, Nkanda, Nchebe, Obasinjom*, among others), in cases of death and in earlier times in connection with wars and conflicts. Slit-drums generally are of religious significance, and, therefore, offerings must be made to them; in former times even human sacrifices were made. Indeed, slit-drums were and are still indispensable for mask performances, as one report on the northeastern Igbo demonstrates: "The entire masquerade is 'owned' and activated by the zoomorphic slit-drum, also called *Okperegede*... (It) governs the *Okperegede* spectacle, directs its action, defines its character, and summons its masks. Prior to a performance the drum, not the masks, receives sacrifices to ensure its successful performance and that the spirit display will be peaceful and productive. When the drumming begins at a festival, people know the spirits are preparing to dance, and they gather at the common" (Weston 1984:147).

112 Sound recordings made of the night dance, the offering ceremonies and the performance of *Nchebe* and *Mkpe* made on March 27, 2005, are preserved in the Department of Ethnomusicology in the Ethnological Museum, Berlin (Inv. No. VII OA 0739.006).

113 Talbot (1912:413) made first mention of *Angbu*: "'*Angbo*'. It is impossible to learn the meaning of this word. Every town has a lodge. In many none but adults are allowed to join. Dances are always given at night, and no woman may be present." Further information about *Angbu* is found in Röschenthaler (1993:37, 181 f., 239, Fig. XVII) and Onor (1994:108 f.). *Angbu* has been attested among the Tali and in Besongabang as well (Ruel 1969:202, 223). According to Brain and Pollock (1971:109 f., Col. Pl. 18) among the Bangwa *Angbu* was a section of *Ngbe*. Both of its masks – one male, the other female – wore large anthropomorphic masks of wood.

114 Sound recordings made of the performance of *Angbu* in Kembong on January 26, 2004, are preserved in the Department of Ethnomusicology in the Ethnological Museum, Berlin (Inv. No. VII OA 0430.003). An illustration of an *Angbu* mask from Akwa, which is remarkably similar, can be viewed in Röschenthaler (2004[a]:200). For further photographs of *Angbu* masks, see Röschenthaler 1998:49 and 1999:44.

115 A report on an autopsy in the west Cameroon coastal area is found in Ittmann (1957:173). Post-mortem examinations were not commonly practised in the Cameroon Grasslands (Koloss 2000:326, fn. 13).

116 A society with the name of *Obon* was once present among the Efik. Nair (1972:14) reckons it to the societies which were "of lesser importance ..., which possessed five grades and functioned primarily as a burial society and honoured deceased members with memorial services." According to another source, among the Efik *Obon* was a dance of *Ekpe* (Anonymous 1957:166 f.). Among the Ibibio *Obon* is considered the "twin-brother" of *Ekpe*. Special note is made of its dances, at which the "sacred" musical instruments are used that are concealed from non-members. The night performances are taboo for non-members. Aside from the dances, "Obon performed other functions such as the collection of debts and the enforcement of the laws of the community" (Ukpong 1989:21).

5 *Ajom* – magic medicines

Magic medicines, known among the Ejagham as *ajom* (sg. *njom*), hold the utmost importance in the battle against all evil, wickedness and offences and thus represent important elements of the traditional judicial system. If a severe illness or serious accident has been attributed by a diviner to the much feared witchcraft, the person affected is left with the only hope that with the help of medicine, witches can be forced to leave the victim. In a special ritual, the "swearing of medicine" (*sure njom*), the medicine or *juju* is activated against the witch. This can also be directed against thieves, adulterers and other criminals.[1] In general it is believed that the medicine punishes the evildoers with a severe illness, indeed, not just any affliction, but with a specific one that is solely at the disposal of the particular *juju*. When the medicine has "captured" a witch in this way, the witch can save her life only if she no longer pursues any more victims. But at the same time the medicine must be appeased. This is accomplished in a special ritual, for which the witch or her family have to pay unusually high fees. Yet, however expensive such a ritual may be for the witch, she may make use of it only one time. For if the person continues exercising witchcraft and is discovered by a medicine a second time, she or he will not be shown any leniency, but mercilessly put to death.

The objects of *ajom* can differ considerably in form and appearance. For example, a small anthropomorphic figure can serve as a *juju* or a "fetish", or a pair of buffalo horns, a seemingly nondescript lump of clay or small bags can have this function, just to name those which I observed in the region around Kembong in 1980 and which will be discussed in the following. The outward appearance of *ajom* is apparently of less significance, whereas the strength and power of the medicine are most important. Yet the "champion" of all medicines is not a stationary fetish, but a mask: *Obasinjom*, the "God of medicine". *Ajom* are seldom the property of individuals alone, instead they usually belong to a secret society. Indeed, it is also said that their strength rests upon the knowledge and experience of many people and generations and that *ajom* manifest their trust and cooperation in impressive ways.

As I shall explain in detail (cp. p. 183 ff.), the significance of *ajom* in the Ngunaya area has diminished considerably in recent years. The medicines that I was able to study in 1980 – *Enok Ateng*, *Mfam*, *Amok* and *Okeboho* – are now rarely employed or they no longer exist at all. Furthermore, since I was unable to acquire any essential additional information during my stay there in 2004/2005, in the present contribution excerpts from my text published in "African Arts" (1984) will be used to great extent. [2] The present tense will be retained, even though today the "swearing of medicine" is seldom practised in this area; at any rate it has not disappeared altogether.

5.1 *Enok Ateng*

Ayuk Tambla lives in Afap, a small village near Kembong, and is a native healer who specialises in rheumatism and broken bones. He was born in 1928; his father was a bricklayer from Calabar. As Ayuk Tambla has no family, he lives in his small hut alone (1980). Besides a healer, he is also well-known for his medicine *Enok Ateng* ("fighting alone"), being bound to an anthropomorphic figural carving, and for his faculty as a diviner (figs. 149–150). The medicine or *juju* was passed on to him, as the first-born son, by his father around 1960, who also taught him the art of healing. Since a healer must also be able to deal with witchcraft, Ayuk Tambla is believed to have special endowments that only God can give him. Ayuk Tambla's father had shown the medicine to his other sons as well, but they proved to be unsuited to this difficult profession and were unable to learn to identify and use the medicinal plants. Therefore, shortly before his death, the father transferred all of the medicine to his eldest son, Ayuk Tambla. He took the figure in his hands one last time, taking his leave: "I am going. I do not carry this with me. I empower you. If you wear this medicine, it should do its work. And if you treat a victim who has been attacked by it, and he has confessed, may he or she be well. I have given you food." As during all of the ceremonies, he faced the sun, the source of light, power and life.

According to Ayuk Tambla the figure has no gender, although he designates its face as male and its hairstyle as female. The tooth of a wild pig is suspended from the neck, and several feathers are attached to the head. It was explained that in this human form the medicine is able to detect and approach invisible witches without arousing their suspicions. The feathers allow the medicine to follow witches even in flight. With the tooth of

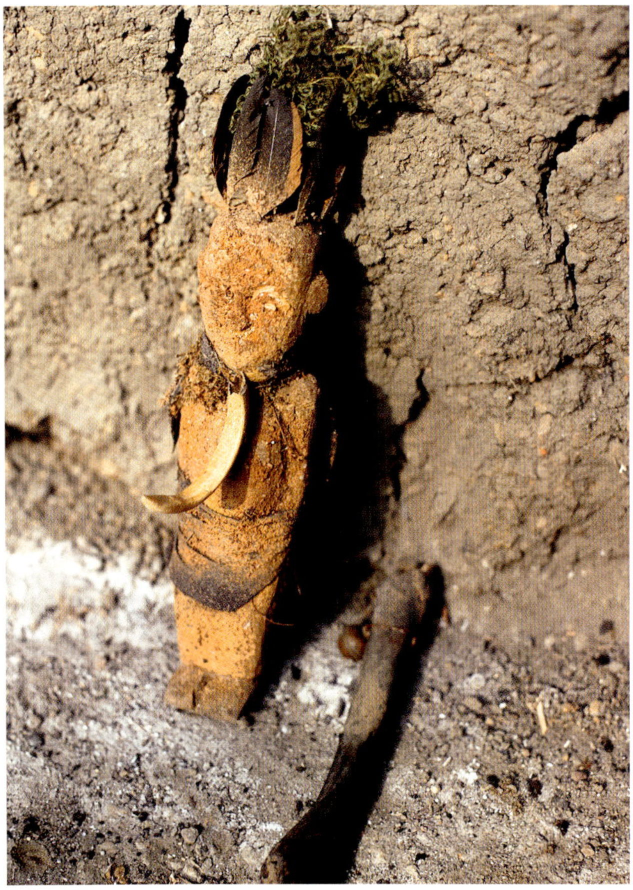

Fig. 149 *Enok Ateng*, a magic medicine (*njom*) in the form of a small human figure, rubbed with yellow camwood; the tooth of a wild pig is suspended from the neck and feathers are attached to the head. Next to the figure is an animal bone with a small bell, used as a rattle (Afap, February 1, 1980).

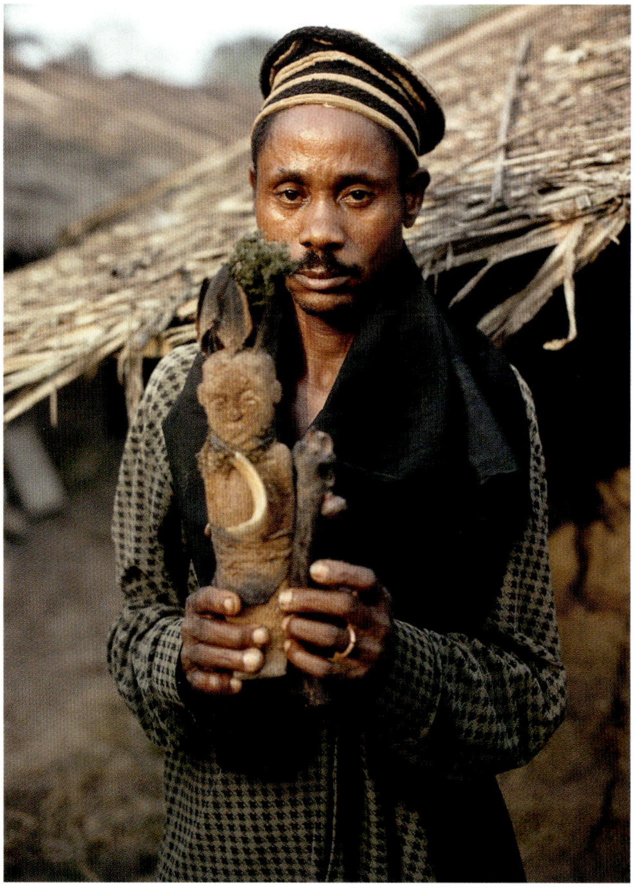

Fig. 150 Ayuk Tambla holding *Enok Ateng* and the rattle (Afap, February 1, 1980).

the wild pig, a very aggressive animal, *Enok Ateng* can strike at these supernatural creatures. Its equipment includes a black cloth used to create darkness and capture witches by throwing it over them like a net.

Unlike many other medicines, *Enok Ateng* has no special society and therefore no "evil forest", for instance, like *Mgbe*, *Angbu* and *Obasinjom*. Anyone may see or touch the figure, but menstruating women must keep their distance so as not to weaken the *njom*. Whenever Ayuk Tambla, as medicine specialist, activates the figure, he must have abstained from sexual relations with women the night before. He must also take care that *Enok Ateng* is "fed" occasionally, or it will turn against him. Approximately every two months, if the medicine has remained unused, he spits upon the figure with alligator pepper and pours palm wine on it, saying: "Father God, Mother God, you made us all. Let there be no trouble. This is your food. Take and eat." In case he should ever wish to give up his *njom* – a question that would never have arisen in the old days – he would kill *Enok Ateng*, or rather, its power, with a special medicine.

Every time Ayuk Tambla begins treatment of a patient, he makes an offering to his deceased father and his other ancestors. He takes a sip of palm wine and, holding the glass in his left hand, addresses a prayer to his father and his ancestors: "Father, you taught me this medicine. And all that I do, I learned from you. I want to start treatment. If anyone, through witchcraft or by any other means, tries to hinder this treatment, let this medicine fight such a person. But (and now he takes the glass in his right hand) if it is true that I got these powers from you, let what I do bring success. May the patient and myself be in peace." Taking the glass in both hands, he pours the rest of the palm wine – the portion for the ancestors – onto the ground.

When it is to be activated against witches and criminals, *Enok Ateng* asks for one jug of palm wine, one cock, one "animal" (meaning the leg or joint of a deer), 3,500 Francs CFA (a worker earned about 300 Francs CFA a day in 1980) and pepper. Payment must be made in full, with each item shown to the medicine before it can be activated. Ayuk Tambla spits upon the figure with palm wine and then shows it the cock ("Here is the cock. I have taken it."), then the meat ("Here is the 'animal'. I have taken it.") and finally the money ("Here is the money, 3,500 Francs CFA. I have taken it."). Then he chews the alligator pepper and spits it upon the figure: "If the witch sets him (this patient) free, you also set the witch free. But if she persists and kills the patient, then also kill the witch." Leaving the figure in the patient's room, Ayuk Tambla goes home.

If the afflicted person, who receives no further medical treatment of any kind, recovers, that is the end of the affair. The medicine specialist has received his fees. If, however, the patient dies, the *njom* will not be satisfied until it has killed not only the witch but the witch's whole family, unless the *njom* is reconciled in a special ceremony. The payment for reconciliation is particularly high: one goat, one cock, one new cutlass, one bottle of liquor, alligator pepper and one raphia bag. The conciliatory process involves the following: One of the members of the witch's family officially approaches the medicine specialist: "Father, this, my illness, is the result of the medicine you swore last time. I have gone to the diviner and have been told that it is because my late sister did such a bad thing. So we have come to appease your medicine." Facing west, the medicine specialist rubs magical plants between his hands, saying: "Father God, Mother God, I sent out a soldier to war. I now know the victim, the witch. And now I want to appease you." The figure is then rubbed with the medicine: "I have told Father God and Mother God. From this moment do not go again against this family." He spits upon the figure once more, and the curse is lifted from the family of the witch. Together the participants in the ceremony eat the meat.

Enok Ateng is used not only against witches, but against all those who break the law, including adulterers, murderers and thieves. The prayers that the *njom* specialist addresses to the medicine in these situations are basically the same. In the case of theft, for example, he might say: "*Enok Ateng,* I want to send you to war. That man who has stolen this article, hunt him. If he brings back the article and puts it behind the house, set him free. But if he hardens his heart and refuses to return the stolen article, catch him. Do not kill him, but make him confess."

As mentioned, Ayuk Tambla is also respected as a diviner. His method of divining is unusual, in that he employs the assistance of a virgin boy. In a glass of water containing some dissolved medicine, the boy is able to discern a spirit who questions the criminal. During this interrogation, Ayuk Tambla places his hand upon the boy's head. These sessions take place only in the morning or in the evening, when the sun is not at its zenith. According to the *njom* specialist, criminals caught in this manner have never denied their crimes.

Ayuk Tambla offered to sell the figure (which was not very old) containing *Enok Ateng* to the Linden-Museum, Stuttgart (Germany), where I was curator of the Africa department at the time.[3] Before relinquishing it, he held it in both his hands saying: "*Enok Ateng,* I have sold your object to the white man, but not your power. You leave this object now and come back to me. This is the money I have received. May the object go without anger from you." He concluded by spitting upon the carving.

Ayuk Tambla alleged – but in actuality never did, as we shall see later (p. 184) – that he would give the following instructions to the carver for a new figure for *Enok Ateng*: The figure must be able to stand without help; it must be straight and have natural proportions; and it must have eyes and ears to be able to see and hear. It need not be beautiful; instead, it should look fearsome. The finished figure would be introduced to God in the early morning according to the following procedure: "Oh Father, I am going to the bush to look for the various herbs to empower this figure. Help me not to forget any." Before cutting the most important and at the same time most dangerous herbs, Ayuk Tambla spit upon them with alligator pepper and apologised for having to kill them: "I have come in the name of God and my father to get you. I am not taking you for harm but to serve mankind." Back in his compound, he would grind and mix the herbs, rub the figure with the medicine, and then kill a cock, letting its blood flow over the carving: "God, give power to this figure, because all power in life comes from you. Let things be good and not bad."

According to tradition, Ayuk Tambla has the right to sell the medicine – not only the figure, but also all of the knowledge and the utensils that go with it – at a high price. With the sale, however, he would create additional competition to himself, a drawback outweighing any momentary profit. He also refuses to make *Enok Ateng* into a medicine society, in which strangers, for a fee, can become members and acquire certain rights. This would be profitable, too, but he prefers to remain alone and independent. Probably most medicine societies developed when formerly independent *njom* specialists decided to take on partners in such a way.

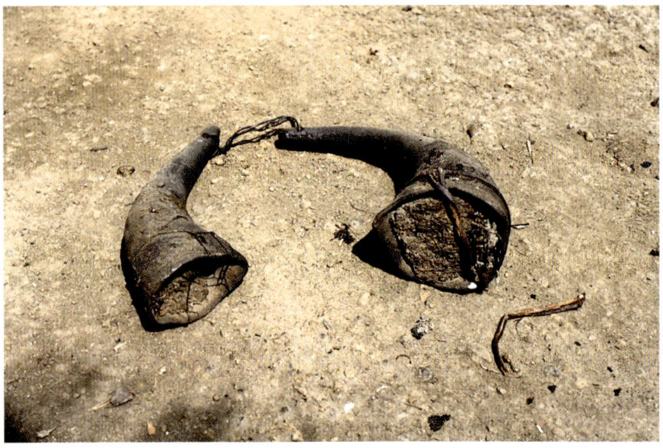

Fig. 151 *Mfam*, a magic medicine (*njom*), in the form of two buffalo horns filled with medicine (Kembong, February 10, 1980).

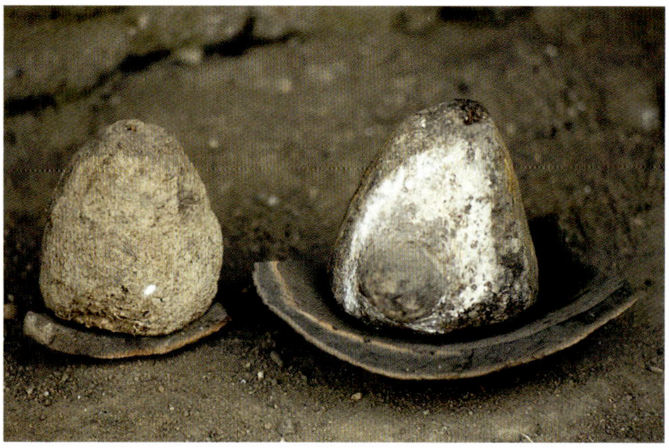

Fig. 152 *Amok*, a magic medicine (*njom*), in the form of a lump of earthen material from a termite mound, set upon a pottery sherd (here two examples) (Kembong, February 13, 1980).

5.2 *Mfam*

Unlike *Enok Ateng, Mfam,* the second *njom* to be discussed here, represents a medicine society (fig. 151). *Mfam* ("community") belongs to the most powerful and best-known magic medicines in the Cross River region and was already mentioned in early reports.[4] In Kembong its former membership of fifteen has dwindled to four, and its use, frequent in the old days, has likewise diminished to only two or three times a year (1980). The power of *Mfam* resides in two bushcow horns filled with medicine.[5] The reason for this form and its exact beginnings are unknown. It is said to have originated in Kesham (Mamfe-Overside region) and probably reached Kembong via nearby Afap during the 19th century. *Mfam* societies can be found in a number of villages, but these do not maintain connections with one another. Talbot also mentioned *Mfam* and classified it as one of the most important "Ekoi medicines", but he described it as consisting of six horns.[6]

In Kembong the members of *Mfam* do not meet on any particular day. They simply get together for ceremonies in the house of the society's leader. At present (1980) the society is led by Hollford Ndip, who says he was born in 1905. Anyone may look at the medicine, but the uninitiated are sent away if they get too close to it. A person who deliberately touches the medicine will fall ill. *Mfam* has a grove or "evil forest", where the most important magic trees and herbs of *Mfam* are to be found and where important ceremonies are conducted.

The society is structured in three levels. The first is called *abang Mfam* ("horns of *Mfam*"). Whenever new members have paid the required initiation fees – one "animal", one cock, one bunch of plantains, one jug of palm wine and one bottle of oil – a feast is held, but no religious ceremonies take place. Participation in the eating and drinking revelries of the society and the use of *Mfam* free of charge are the only privileges enjoyed by the members of this rank.

The second level, called *eteme Njom* ("grove of medicine"), is reserved for full members who know the magic plants. The fees for this rank are the same as for *abang Mfam*, but also include two fathoms of loincloth for the leader. Whoever has belonged to this level the longest will automatically become Hollford Ndip's successor after his death.

The third level is that of the leader himself. Upon being installed in office, he pays the following fees: one goat, one cock, one "animal", one bunch of plantains and one jug of palm wine. No religious rites are performed. However, during the next ceremony that takes place in the grove or "evil forest", the new leader embraces the sacred magical tree and calls out "Oh *Mfam!*" seven times.

Whenever *Mfam's* help is sought out, Hollford Ndip takes the medicine horns to the patient's compound during the early morning. They are laid on the ground, and he addresses them: "You have been brought here because of Mr. X's illness. It has become known that he is being bewitched. If the witch allows Mr. X to recover, set her free. But if she continues to hunt the sick person and kills him, follow the witch. If the witch replaces a child or an adult for the killed one, set her free. But if there is no replacement, kill the witch and also enter her family until the last member is dead." The family of the stricken person is obliged to give *Mfam* merely one gourd of palm wine for this treatment.

The "swearing of medicine" (*sure njom*) among the Ejagham is normally carried out in public, and, therefore, the witch can be sure of being forewarned. If she leaves her victim in peace to recover, the matter is considered settled. No further ceremonies or fees are required. If, however, the witch should continue her attacks and the patient dies, she herself will fall seriously ill – the affliction brought on by *Mfam* are kidney problems with swollen legs, and a diviner will tell her that she is being persecuted by *Mfam*. There is no escaping unless the medicine is appeased. In this case, the fees are one cock, one "animal", one bunch of plantains and one jug of palm wine. In such a case, Hollford Ndip speaks to the medicine under the tree of *Mfam*: "*Mfam*, we have come. Some weeks ago you were sent to war against those who killed Mr. X, and now you have done your work. The victim was caught by you. She has confessed and fulfilled all your conditions. Now we want to start treating her. Tell us if you accept the treatment or not." Should the medicine reject the ceremony because certain requirements were not fulfilled, preparations for it must begin anew. Only after the offerings have been accepted and *Mfam* has been appeased, may the stricken witch be treated with the usual curatives. Should she dare attack a human being again, she will not be spared by *Mfam*.

This medicine cannot be put to an end or "killed". If there is no one left who knows how to use *Mfam*, it will turn against the descendants of its owners, who will have to propitiate it. The *njom* is not altered or reconsecrated unless the horns, or the medicine in them, are damaged. Should this occur, a cock is sacrificed, and its blood is allowed to flow into the horns.

Unlike other *ajom*, *Mfam* does not demand regular sacrifices, yet in his morning prayers Hollford Ndip always mentions *Mfam*, too: "My father, I am washing my face this morning, and I remember you are the one who taught me *Mfam*. *Mfam* has been sworn for many purposes. It seems as if you are sleeping. As I pray to you, wake up and do the jobs that you are called to do. Father God, Mother God, you are the giver of all things. You made the leaves and taught our ancestors how to use them. If the prayer I make is true, let success follow. But if I am unfair, bring any ill to me."

5.3 *Amok*

The power of *Amok*, another *njom*, rests in rather nondescript amorphous lumps, which are made from the earthen material of a termite mound. The *njom* is composed of one large lump (approximately 9 cm high) called *nse Amok* ("father of *Amok*"), which must never leave the compound, and fourteen smaller lumps (about 8 cm high), which are simply called *Amok* (fig. 152).[7] These objects are placed upon pottery shards to avoid their contact with the ground. Women are forbidden to touch them. *Amok* has no grove. It does not even belong to a society, in the strict sense of the word, where the leader may be descended from any of the various families in the town. Instead, it is the particular property of a single family and not for sale. In Kembong the current chief is Moses Ojong (1980), who took over this office from his father, *Ata* Ogomarreje, around 1968. The chief of the family is also the leader of *Amok*.

Amok was founded by an ancestor named *Ata* Enowekuku, when there were allegedly large numbers of witches and consequently many leopards, the preferred guise of witches. At that time, the family lived in the small hamlet of Abaresire Otop, which no longer exists.[8] The magical herbs, the details of the equipment and the rituals were revealed to *Ata* Enowekuku by God in a dream. The revelation of such knowledge in dreams is common in both the Cross River region and the Grasslands, as well as in other parts of Africa.[9] God explained to him that magical herbs have power and would protect the family. The name *Amok* ("to push away") derives from *Ata* Enowekuku. Since his time, no detail connected with the medicine has been altered; *Amok* is the same today as when God and the ancestors created it. In the past, it had a good many more members and was used much more frequently. Today its services are needed only about ten times a year (1980).

All of *Amok's* important functions must remain within the domain of family members. Only they may know its secrets, especially those of the magical plants. At about four years of age, the boys of the family begin their education in the medicine. When they are older, they are taught the magical herbs, a process called *osuamet* (the "washing of eyes") in many secret societies (cp. p. 157 f.).

Neither special initiation into *Amok* nor initiation fees are obligatory for members of the family. These requirements for membership are demanded only of outsiders, who may come from any of the different quarters in the community. The initiation fees consist of one "animal", one cock, plantains and palm wine. When the food has been prepared, *nse Amok* is brought into the yard, and Moses Ojong takes a little of it into his left hand, with which the ancestors are always given their share of food: "*Ata* Enowekuku, come here, take this food and meet your sons and grandsons *Ata* Tabengombo, *Ata* Enowugombo, *Ata* Agbormungui, and *Ata* Ogomarreje." He sets the food in front of the medicine and adds a little meat: "This is your own share of the meat." He also pours a little water onto the ground: "This is to remove particles of plantains and meat from your teeth." Last, he offers the ancestors palm wine: "And now here is wine; take and drink." When this is done, he fetches the food for the members of *Amok* and explains the reason for the gathering: "This is our own food, meat and wine, brought by Mr. X to become a member of *Amok.* We want to eat it now. May no one suffer from headache and neck pains." Everyone receives the same food, except the bones which are reserved for the leader. It is important that no leftovers be taken home. In the end, Moses Ojong takes the glass in both his hands and pours the rest of the wine on the ground, saying, "*Amok fem*" ("cause the person to swell"; *Amok* punishes its victims by making their bodies swell, in connection with liver problems), and the others answer, "*fem kput*" ("swell very large").

Anyone who wishes to make an appeal to *Amok* has to bring a jug of palm wine. The leader may grant the person's request to take an *Amok* clay object to his compound to be sworn there, on the condition that *Amok* never come into contact with water and that the supplicant has abstained from sexual intercourse with a woman the night before. If the leader himself is asked to activate the medicine, he must be paid one cock. Moses Ojong "awakens" *Amok* by rubbing the lump of clay with yellow camwood, throwing a pebble at it with his left hand, and finally spitting upon it with alligator pepper: "*Amok,* you are listening. If the one who entered Mr. X's house and carried away the money from Mr. X brings the money back, let him be free from your attack. But if he persists and will not bring back the money, then catch him. When he comes for treatment, set him free only if he returns the money." Should the thief secretly return the money to the compound of the robbed man, the latter must take it to Moses Ojong, who in turn shows it to *Amok*: "This is the money that was stolen. After your swearing, the thief feared you and threw the money into the owner's compound. As the owner brought it to me to show it to you, now I hand it back to him. If he uses it, let his head and neck not be pained." Returning the money to its rightful owner, Moses Ojong turns once more to *Amok*: " I still send you to war against the thief. Catch him. Catch him until he brings the necessary things for the sacrifice." The medicine must thus be reconciled even after the thief has contritely returned the stolen money to its owner: "The thief has shown fear and has accepted his guilt. He has brought the stolen money, and he has also brought the necessary things for your sacrifice. Don't go to war against him any longer."

Should the thief try to keep the money, *Amok* will cause him to fall ill, and eventually he will be forced to pay the prescribed fees: one goat, one "animal", one cock, one egg, one bunch of plantains, one jug of palm wine, one bottle of palm wine from a standing palm tree, one bottle of palm oil, alligator pepper, yellow camwood, indigenous salt, one fathom of cloth, tobacco and one piece of chalk. All of these things are taken behind the house. In the presence of the leader the thief must then confess: "I have stolen the money", and at the same time hand the money over to the leader. The leader then asks: "Have you finished?" The reply is: "Yes, I have finished." The leader says: "*Amok,* he has finished." Subsequently, the usual offerings of food are made, accompanied by prayers ending with the words "This food has been brought by Mr. X for the pacification of *Amok* against him and his family."

Only the members of *Amok* are allowed to partake of the meal that follows. The patient – the thief stricken by *Amok* – and his family are excluded. Then the egg and the cock are sacrificed and the contents of the egg and the blood of the cock poured over the lumps of clay: "I give you this egg and blood. When you catch somebody, let the person shine (the body swells up and the skin begins to shine), if he bathes or not." Finally, the testicles of the sacrificial cock have to be examined. If they indicate that *Amok* has accepted the offerings, the treatment of the patient (the thief) stricken by *Amok,* who always exhibits the symptoms of a swollen body and shiny skin, can begin. First, the patient is given a room of his own in *Amok's* compound. Then a diviner must determine which of the *Amok* members should administer the treatment. That person must procure the necessary herbs and prepare the curative medicine that the afflicted person will receive orally and in the form of an enema. During the healing process, he is given only plantains and salt to eat. If it appears that the *njom* has not accepted the offering, which would occur, for example, if the thief had not returned all of the loot, *Amok* keeps the fee. Consequently, the thief will have to pay again to free himself of his illness.

All cases of this kind conclude with the leader's returning the stolen money to its rightful owner. The latter will turn to the medicine saying: "*Amok,* I have taken all my money which was stolen, and then I sent you to war against the thief. May now the sacrifice be good and also the treatment that follows. Give back health to the victim." He then hands about ten percent of the stolen money to the leader, who may either keep it for himself or divide it among the *Amok* members in this family.

In order not to warn the witch unduly, prayers are sometimes dispensed with when *Amok* is activated. Ordinarily, however, Moses Ojong spits upon the lump of clay with alligator pepper and gives very detailed instructions: "*Amok*, I give you food. This man has invited you to guard and protect his house. Do the job for which you have been invited." *Amok* remains in the patient's house until he has recovered. No medical treatment is given, so his recovery indicates that the witch has ceased her attacks out of fear of the *njom*. It is assumed that at this point the medicine also ceases to pursue the witch any further, but this is not known exactly. The patient thus saved by *Amok* is not required to pay any additional fees.

If the victim dies, *Amok* will persecute the witch mercilessly until she is destroyed, unless the family of the witch is willing to replace the victim with one of its own children. After paying the customary high fees to the medicine *Amok*, the witch must deliver the child: "I replace the bewitched person with this my own child. If I do this with two hearts, let the sacrifice not be effective. But if I give this child with one heart, let me go free from this medicine."

An unusual situation occurred to the society in 1979, when the leader's house had to be torn down and rebuilt. That meant that the *Amok* objects also had to be renewed. During the initial phase of rebuilding, the magical herbs were collected and the lumps of clay were made. On that day the members were forbidden to eat and allowed to drink only palm wine. During the preceding night they were required to abstain from sexual activity. Seven days later, when the clay had hardened, the objects were consecrated by the leader: "*Ata* Enowekuku and other fathers, I have made with my brothers these various lumps. I invite you now to give power to them. This is the food, which I have brought for you, and this is the water and wine." After another seven days this ceremony was repeated, and the lumps were rubbed with yellow camwood: "*Amok,* I am inviting you. A wicked man, who does not want the other people to prosper – hunt such a person. If he spoils the blood of other persons, then spoil his own." *Amok* does not demand regular sacrifices and there is no way of "killing" it. If the family should cease to care for it, it will turn upon them. However, as things turned out, *Amok* was later destroyed by its owner (cp. p. 185).

5.4 *Okeboho*

The last kind of static *ajom* to be discussed here is *Okeboho*, a society whose medicine consists of small bags (about 8 cm high) woven of raphia fibres (fig. 208). *Okeboho* originated in Bali in the Cameroon Grasslands and probably reached Kembong during the 19th century. Medicine societies of the same name are also found in Besongabang (near Mamfe airport) and in Ajayukndip, a village west of Kembong. Allegedly *Okeboho* was purchased at the price of one woman and seven pounds, five shillings. A person selling medicine may only demand the sum that he himself once paid for *njom*, or else he will incur the wrath of the medicine.

Formerly *Okeboho* had many members, not only from Kembong but also from the surrounding villages. Now headed by Agbor Enow, the society currently numbers only nine men (1980). Some of the rituals can no longer be performed, because the members who knew the herbs and the exact procedures of the ceremonies have died since then. *Okeboho* requires no regular sacrifices, and it is impossible to destroy it. If all the members should die, the medicine would turn against their descendants. Their only recourse then would be to turn for help to other *Okeboho* societies outside the Kembong area who know the medicine and how to appease it.

The society has two levels. At the first level, initiation fees for new members consist of one "animal", one cock, one bottle of oil, one bunch of plantains, palm wine and food. At the second level, which requires the same initiation fees, the members are taught the magical herbs and all of the secrets associated with them. Upon the death of the leader, a diviner determines a successor from among the members of the second level.

Not only does *Okeboho* have a grove, but among the Kembong medicines it alone also possesses a considerable "part of the night"; i. e. important ceremonies that take place under the cover of night, which is also the temporal realm of witches. The ceremonies include the most diverse mystical elements, whose secrets remain inaccessible to the uninitiated even today. The ceremony performed by the leader of *Okeboho*, when he sold one of the small medicine bags to the Linden-Museum in Stuttgart (Germany),[10] could be regarded as an example of these mysterious rituals. The head of the society later gave me the following account. After selling the bag, he went to the grove at night and, as is customary at all important events, played one of the four *Okeboho* pipes made from a crab claw. Subsequently, a python appeared and, after some moments, it coiled. The leader, who had laid the payment for the bag on the ground even before the serpent had arrived, explained: "This is the money obtained from the white man who wants to take away one of your bags. He is not going to swear, but to keep it only. If you want me to take the money, pick it up and throw it in front of me. But if you don't want me to use it, take it and go away with it." After the python had shown its agreement, he addressed the medicine directly: "*Okeboho*, I am sending you on a journey. It is as if you were dead. So travel in peace. Let his (the white man's) neck or head never be painful. He has done as you wanted."

At important ceremonies there are always four medicine specialists, each playing one of the pipes. The leader then swings the sacrificial cock and begins the prayer: "Father of *Okeboho*, we have come to give you your own food, brought by Mr. X as we sacrificed in the day." Again the python appears and coils itself. The leader throws the cock to the serpent, and the medicine specialists leave the grove without turning or speaking.

Ceremonies are also necessary whenever the raphia bags or the medicines in them are renewed. In both cases, a goat is sacrificed and its blood is allowed to flow over the bags. The medicine specialist spits upon the bags with alligator pepper and sprinkles them with yellow camwood. Then the leader of *Okeboho* intones a prayer, such as: "If the man of the night (i. e. witch), who comes to the house where you, *Okeboho*, are, brings an ill intention, any member in that household must go to war with him. But if he comes with no bad intention, leave him in peace."

The swearing of this *njom* is similar to that in other medicine societies. Whoever requests *Okeboho's* aid, must pay the society a jug of palm wine. Again, it is the society's leader who activates the medicine: "This is the person who has come to hire you for a thing that has happened. And now I want to send you with him." The leader then gives instructions to the person seeking help. Should he need to urinate on his way home, he must deposit the bag on the right side of the path and then urinate on the left side. At his compound he must place the bag on the ground and appeal to the medicine: "The thief, the thief, the thief who has stolen my money. If he brings the money back, as I have sworn this *Okeboho* against him, he shall be set free. But if he hardens his heart and does not return the money, *Okeboho* shall go to war against him. His hand and leg shall be paralysed." *Okeboho* normally afflicts his victim with a stroke. If the thief secretly returns the money to the compound of the person robbed, the latter must contact the head of *Okeboho,* so that the medicine can be reconciled: "You were sent to war against the thief who stole this man's money. Now the thief has feared your powers and has returned it. This is the money that I show you now. If the owner uses it now, whether for marrying or for buying an article, let nothing happen to him." *Okeboho* is then given as much of the money as is needed to buy the ingredients for a meal that will be prepared in the grove: one goat, one cock, one "animal", one bottle of oil, pepper, salt, one bunch of plantains and one jug of palm wine. Before pepper and salt are added, *Okeboho* receives its share. A part of the food is placed in front of the large palm wine pot: "*Okeboho*, this is your food we have come to give to you. It has been given to Mr. X, whose money was stolen and which has now been returned. We now come to consult and inform you not to go to war again." The meal may not be eaten in the grove, but at a remote farm.

If, however, the thief does not return the money and is stricken with illness by *Okeboho*, he will be forced to capitulate anyway, and the medicine will have to be appeased: "Mr. X, who has been caught by you, has confessed to us that he did such a bad thing, and now we want to undertake treatment. If you want us to carry out the treatment, let the oracle tell us." Should *Okeboho* reject the offering, all of the fees are left behind in the bush, and the thief is told to consult a diviner, who must determine which of *Okeboho's* demands was not complied with. The ceremony is repeated in the hope that it will be accepted so that treatment can begin: "*Okeboho*, you caught this man, because he had stolen Mr. X's money. He has confessed and has paid back the money. And now he wants to be healed. So come out of him and let him recover." Medicinal herbs and palm kernel oil are mixed in a coconut shell. The medicine is rubbed into the cuts on the repentant thief's hand as well as on his cheekbones, for those persecuted by *Okeboho* often lose the power of speech. This treatment is repeated seven times every other day for a period of seven weeks. Should the thief fail to confess, *Okeboho* will eventually kill him. If the crime is murder, *Okeboho* will unquestionably punish the culprit with death; that is the law of this particular medicine.

5.5 *Obasinjom*, the "God of medicine"

5.5.1 First encounter with *Obasinjom* and an initial orientation: its house and grove

In the preceding chapters I discussed four types of medicines (*ajom*) found in the community of Kembong. These medicines are located in specific objects: a carved figure (*Enok Ateng*), a pair of horns (*Mfam*), lumps of clay (*Amok*) and raphia bags (*Okeboho*). In the case of the fifth medicine, *Obasinjom,* whose importance and characteristics I shall discuss in this chapter, the object is a mask, a speaking mask that has the gift of prophecy. This is the reason why the dancers of *Obasinjom* are believed to have supernatural faculties, i. e. to be witches – however, the kind of beings who use their special capabilities for the well-being of the community and not towards its destruction, as is the aim of usual witches. It is believed that with the help of *Obasinjom*, God can show man what man cannot know by himself and how to fight evil and dangerous powers. This mask demonstrates most tellingly the multifarious relationships between masks and medicines in Africa.

My first encounter with *Obasinjom* was on March 19, 1975, in Ashum, a locality in the southern Banyang area, located about 45 km southeast of Mamfe on the road to Kumba (figs. 153–158). To my great surprise, the mask bearer, wearing a red knitted wool cap, donned the mask garment that had been hung upon a frame at the side of the road, in full public view (figs. 153–154). While drums and a large slit-drum were played in the background and incited by numerous men and women, the mask moved back and forth about the street and in between the houses (at that time still built in the traditional style, but today mostly made of brick). The mask was accompanied by two men with rifles and by other members of the society. Also present – as I discovered years later when studying

Performance of *Obasinjom* in Ashum (southern Banyang) (March 19, 1975) (figs. 153–158).

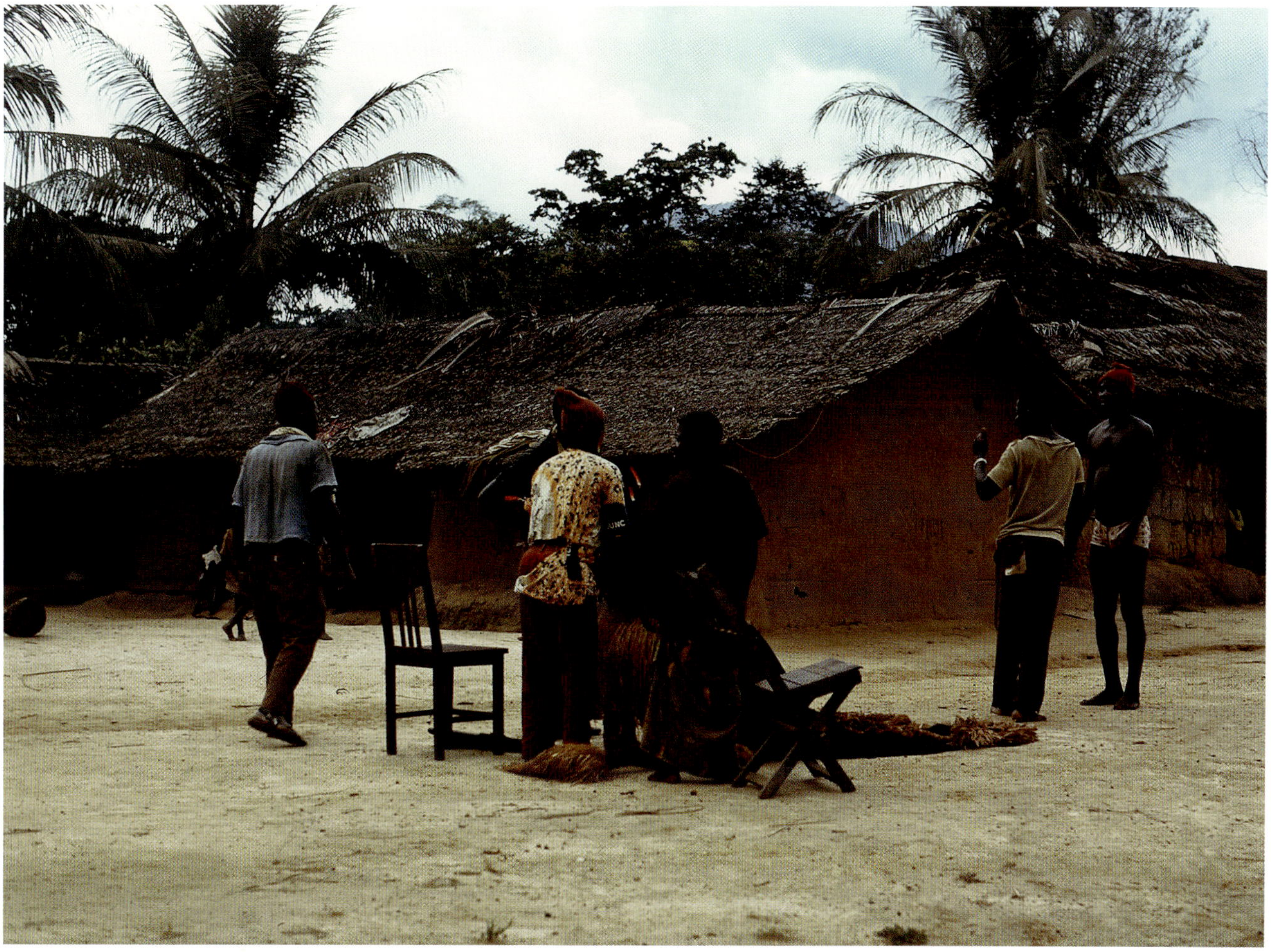

Fig. 153 The mask-bearer with a red cap in front of the mask outfit, lying on the ground (Ashum, March 19, 1975).

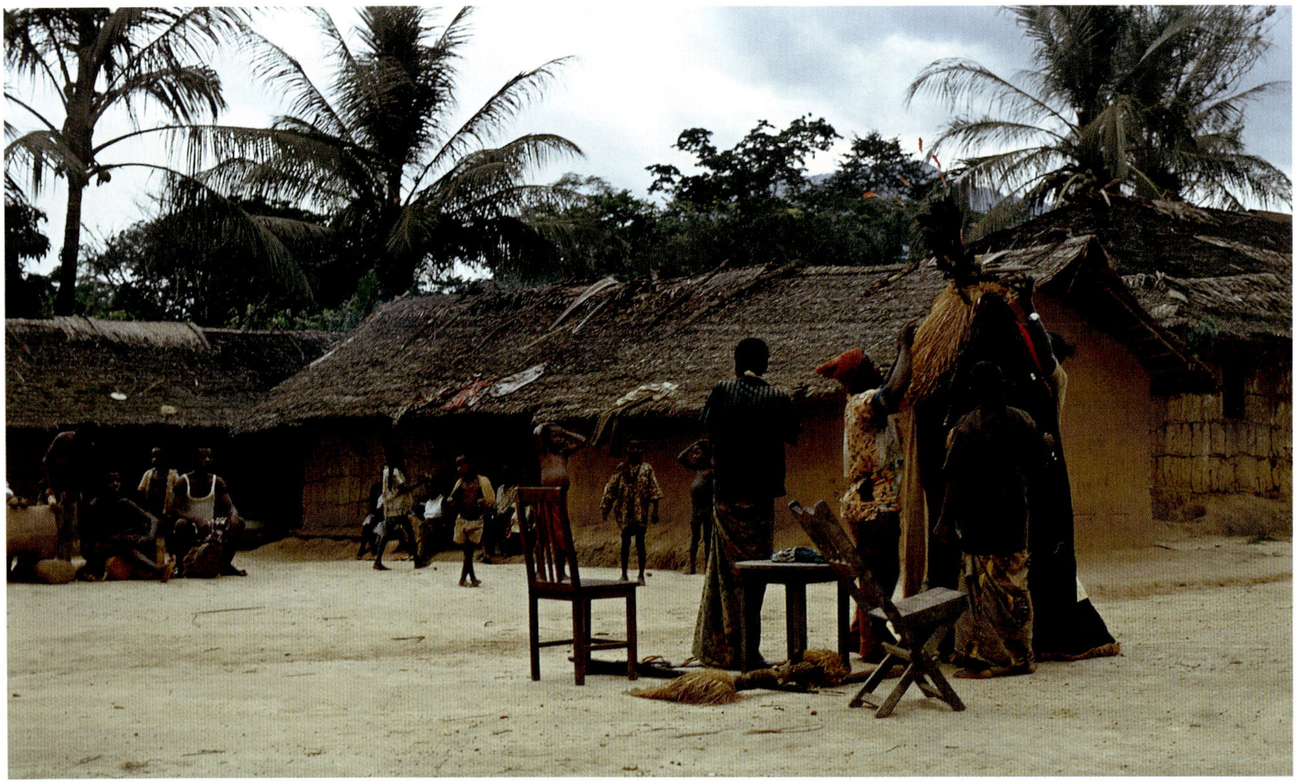

Fig. 154 The mask bearer dons the mask garment, assisted by members of the society *Obasinjom*. The traditional houses visible in the background no longer exist (Ashum, March 19, 1975).

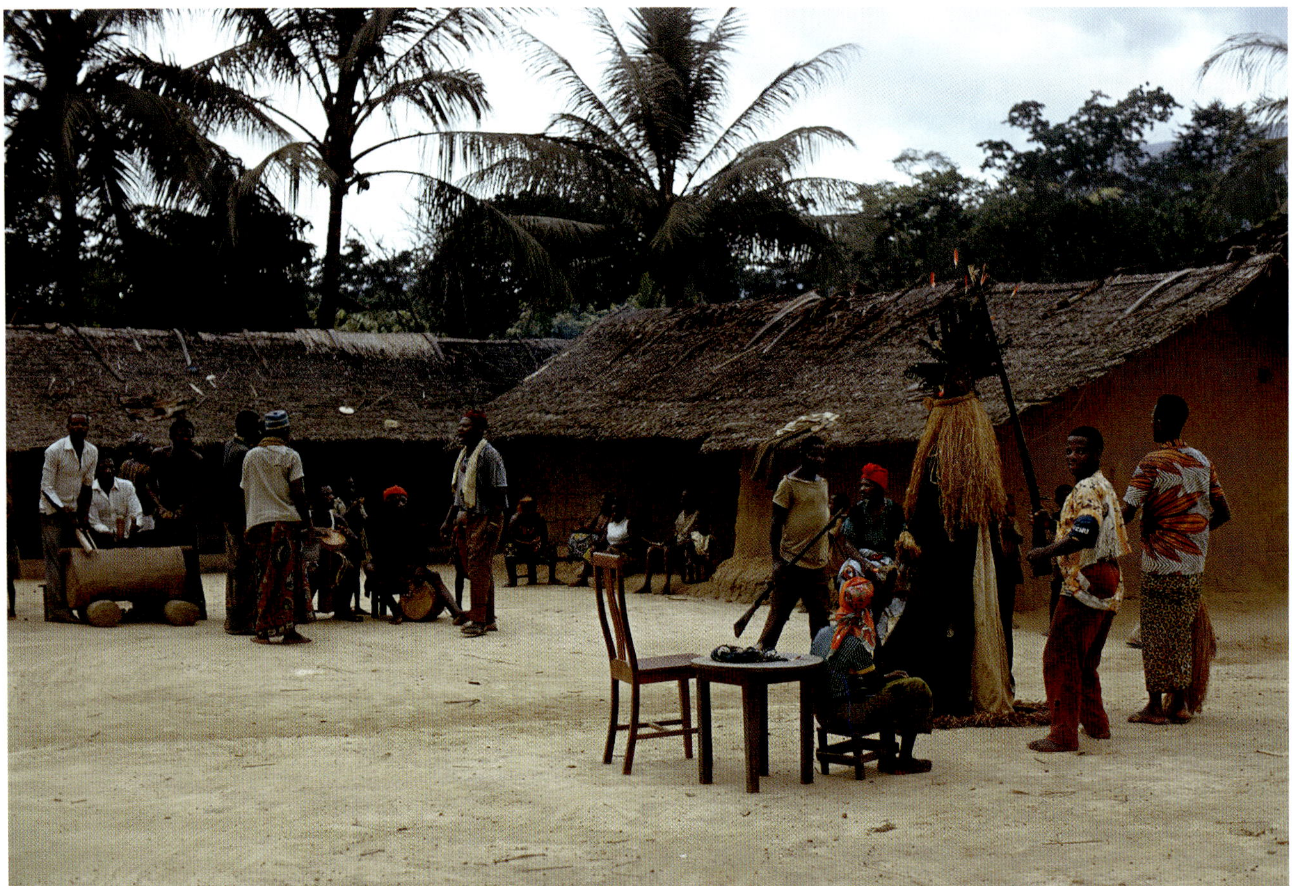

Fig. 155 Performance of *Obasinjom*. In the left background, a slit-drum; on the right, *mma Njom*, the wife of *Obasinjom*, seated upon a stool (Ashum, March 19, 1975).

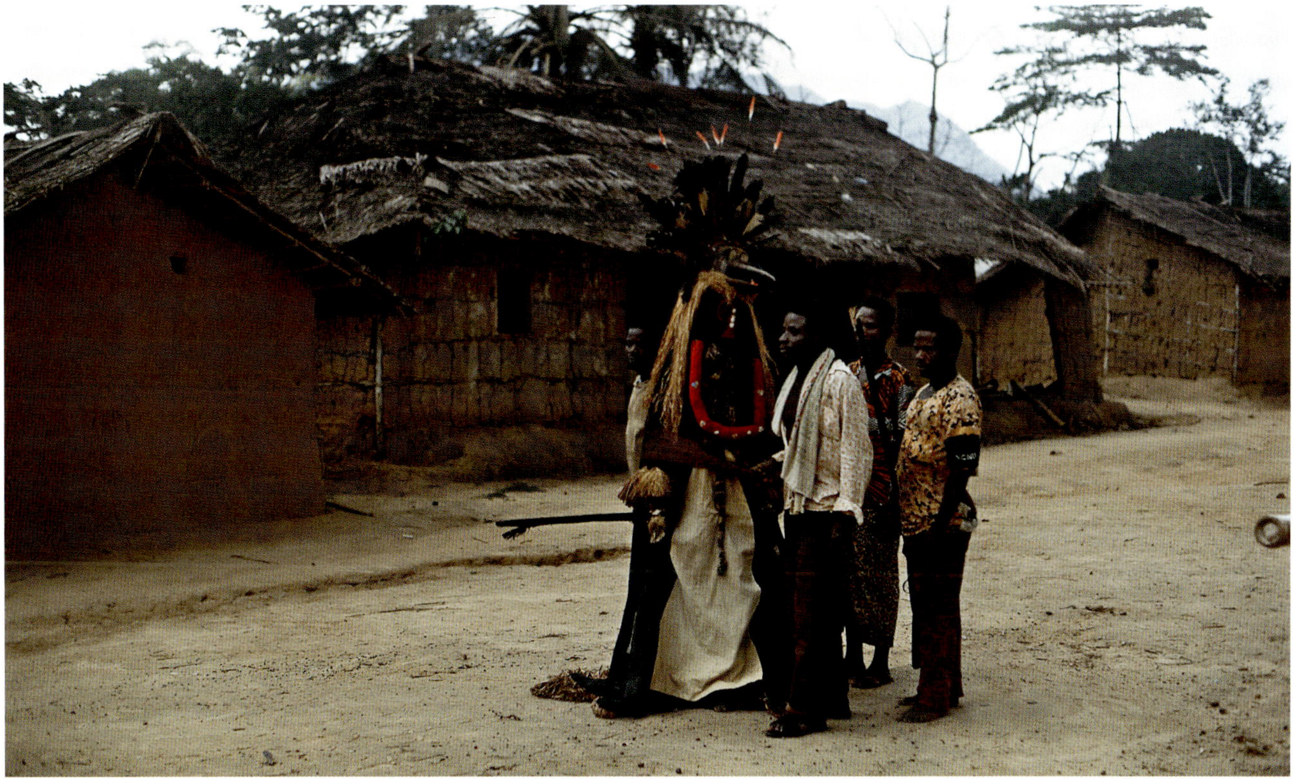

Fig. 156 The mask *Obasinjom* surrounded by members (Ashum, March 19, 1975).

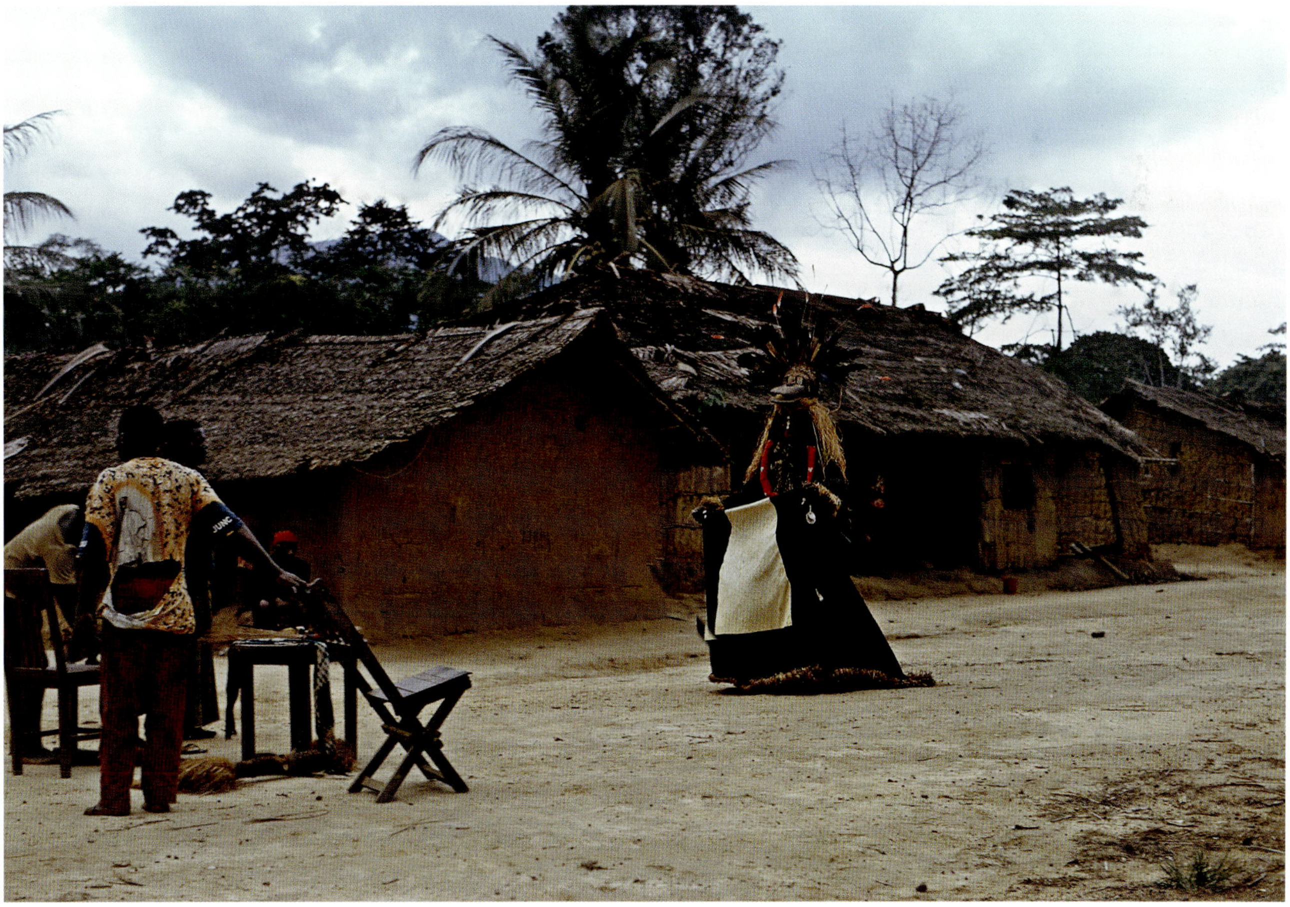

Fig. 157 The mask *Obasinjom*, holding up the garment so that it can run quickly (Ashum, March 19, 1975).

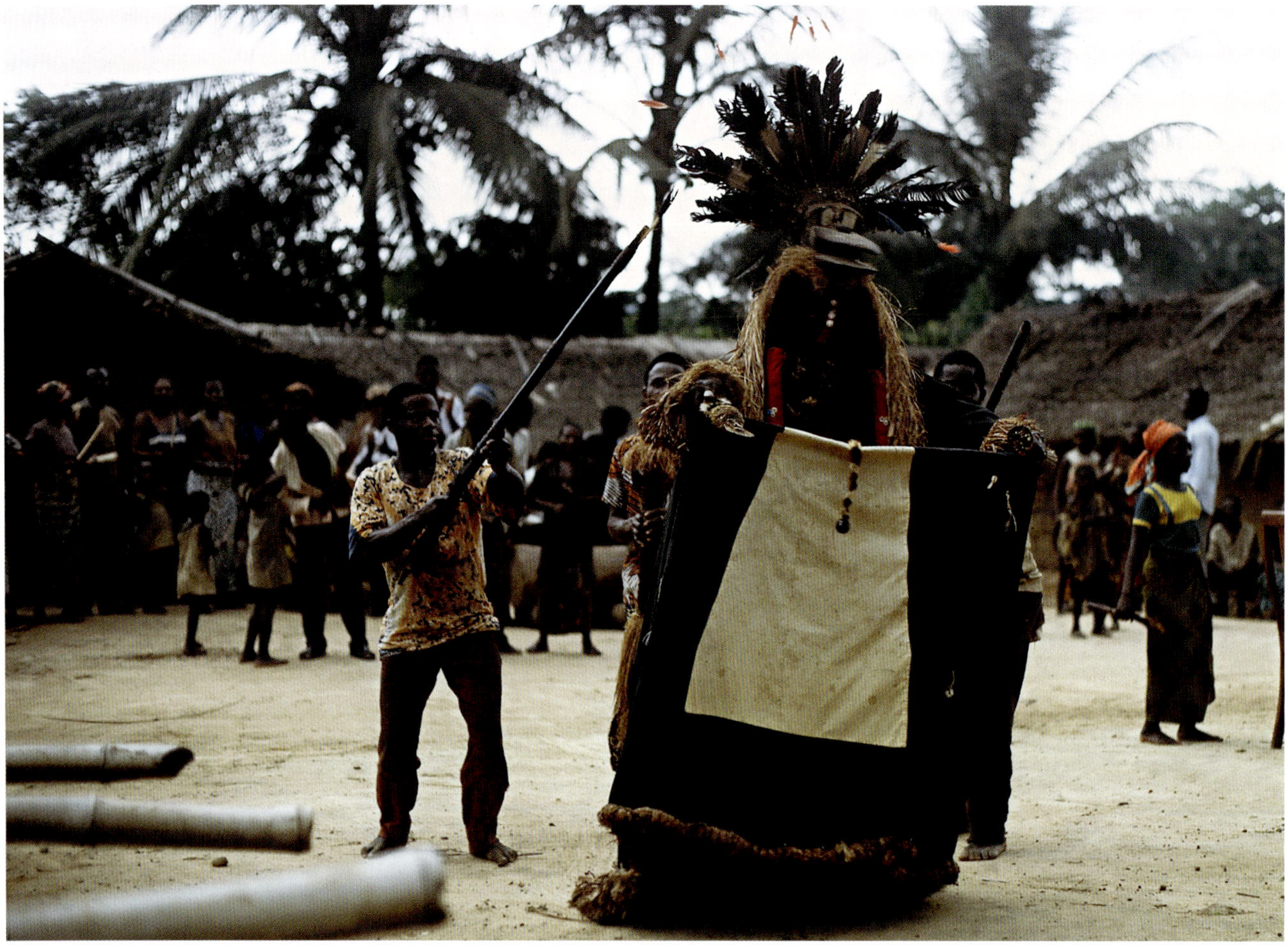

Fig. 158 The mask *Obasinjom*, accompanied by two members bearing rifles (Ashum, March 19, 1975).

the photographs and after gaining more knowledge about *Obasinjom* – was *mma Njom*, the wife of the mask (fig. 155). The performance of *Obasinjom* was a fascinating and exciting event for me, but at that time I had no opportunity to obtain further information about the mask. Later during my research sojourns in Kembong in 1980, 2004 and 2005, I witnessed several performances of *Obasinjom*, specifically the *Obasinjom* of Upper Kembong. The present chief of the society is Adolf Ojong Agbor (Okune). In the course of time, again and again I had the chance to carry on detailed and intensive interviews concerning the mask with the big men as well as with other members of the society.

In Lower Kembong, i. e. Okonyenge, there is another *Obasinjom* society, whose residence is in the compound of the current leader Samuel Tanyi Tambe. There the meetings of the society's members are held, and in one of the rooms, accessible to all, is an open box containing the mask equipment (figs. 159–160). At present the society has sixteen members, among them two leaders and nine other members who know the most important medicines. In 2005 *Obasinjom* in Okonyenge made seven performances, three of which were in Kembong and four in Muyuka, a coastal town. *Obasinjom* was so successful in detecting witches that it can probably reckon with more invitations in the future. Both *Obasinjom* societies in Upper and Lower Kembong work in close cooperation, especially since their medicines, ranks, rituals and mask equipment are almost the same. Thus, it is customary to invite at least the big men of other societies to ceremonies and likewise to help each other out. During my research in Kembong I spent considerable time in studying the *Obasinjom* of Upper Kembong. Hence, the following information stems to a great extent from this particular society.[11]

The society of *Obasinjom* in Upper Kembong had formerly numbered about forty members; in 1980 only eight remained. In recent years *Obasinjom* has gained in popularity once again, and at present (2005) the society consists of about 22 members, including five senior members. Currently the mask gives performances not more than about two or three times a year. This is quite a reduction compared to the former times.

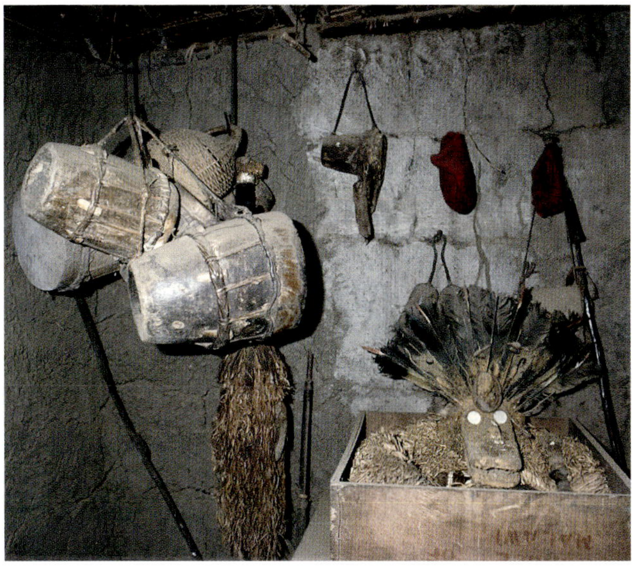

Fig. 159 The mask equipment of *Obasinjom* from Lower Kembong in the leader's house; the room with the mask is in principle accessible to all. (February 24, 1980).

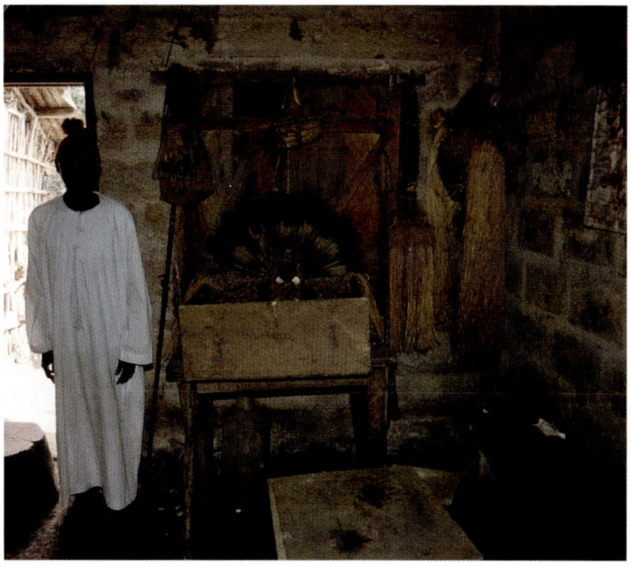

Fig. 160 The mask equipment of *Obasinjom* and the leader Samuel Tanyi Tambe (Lower Kembong, November 19, 2005).

Nevertheless, *Obasinjom* looks exactly the same today as it did then, as my informants repeatedly emphasised. Not the slightest detail of the mask's equipment or of the rituals has been altered.

The *Obasinjom* society does not possess its own house. The mask and its equipment are kept – as stated above – in the leader's compound. Whenever the mask garment is spread out in the sun to dry (fig. 161) or when the mantlebearer puts it on (figs. 185–187, 201, 202; cp. figs. 164, 166), the mask can be viewed by anyone, including women. The society does not hold regular drinking days. Members meet only for activities and ceremonies that are performed in connection with their fight against crime or when initiations take place. At these meetings (*ocha Njom*, "assembly of *Obasinjom*"), everyone eats and drinks, and the ancestors are commemorated with a libation of palm wine.

Like many other medicine societies, *Obasinjom* has a grove (*ebaah Njom)*, which is located in a dense and rather inaccessible forest, in which otherwise only the grove of *Mgbe* is located. The proximity of the two groves accentuates all the more the high rank that *Obasinjom* holds in Kembong. The grove may not be entered by non-members without special permission. *Ebaah Njom* is, as was explained to me in detail, a grove of about 3,000 square meters, the centre of which is a grassy area where all important and secret ceremonies are conducted. There is a rock for the leader to sit upon; temporary benches are set up for other members as needed. The grass, which is kept short with a cutlass, is edged with bushes and trees, underneath which the most important magic and medicinal herbs are grown. Most of these herbs are planted by members, in order to avoid having to gather them painstakingly in the bush. Kembong's grove contains neither buildings nor shrines, in contrast to some *Obasinjom* societies in eastern Nigeria who have shrines with anthropomorphic figures.[12] Generally, ceremonies that involve small fees are held in the house of the leader, whereas those requiring the sacrifice of a goat are held in the *ebaah Njom.*

5.5.2 Ranks of *Obasinjom* and special positions

Members of *Obasinjom* fall into three ranks or levels associated with different tasks, rights and duties.[13] Common to societies in this region is the first rank of the "young people" (*abo Njom*), who are prepared and educated for full membership, which is achieved with acceptance into the second level. The corresponding initiation takes place in the *ebaah Njom*, where the initiates are taught the most important medicines and at the same time treated with medicines. Afterwards they become *anne atemambi*, i. e. full members of *Obasinjom.* The third rank is that of the big men; they include the leader (*ebanghaah Njom*) and his deputies. They control the medicines and make all essential decisions.

As *Obasinjom* has the most important and powerful medicines, its members are considered to possess supernatural powers. On the one hand, they possess the gift of foresight and with that the faculty to see the realm of the dead and witches; on the other, it is said that they appear after death as a wandering soul and represent a

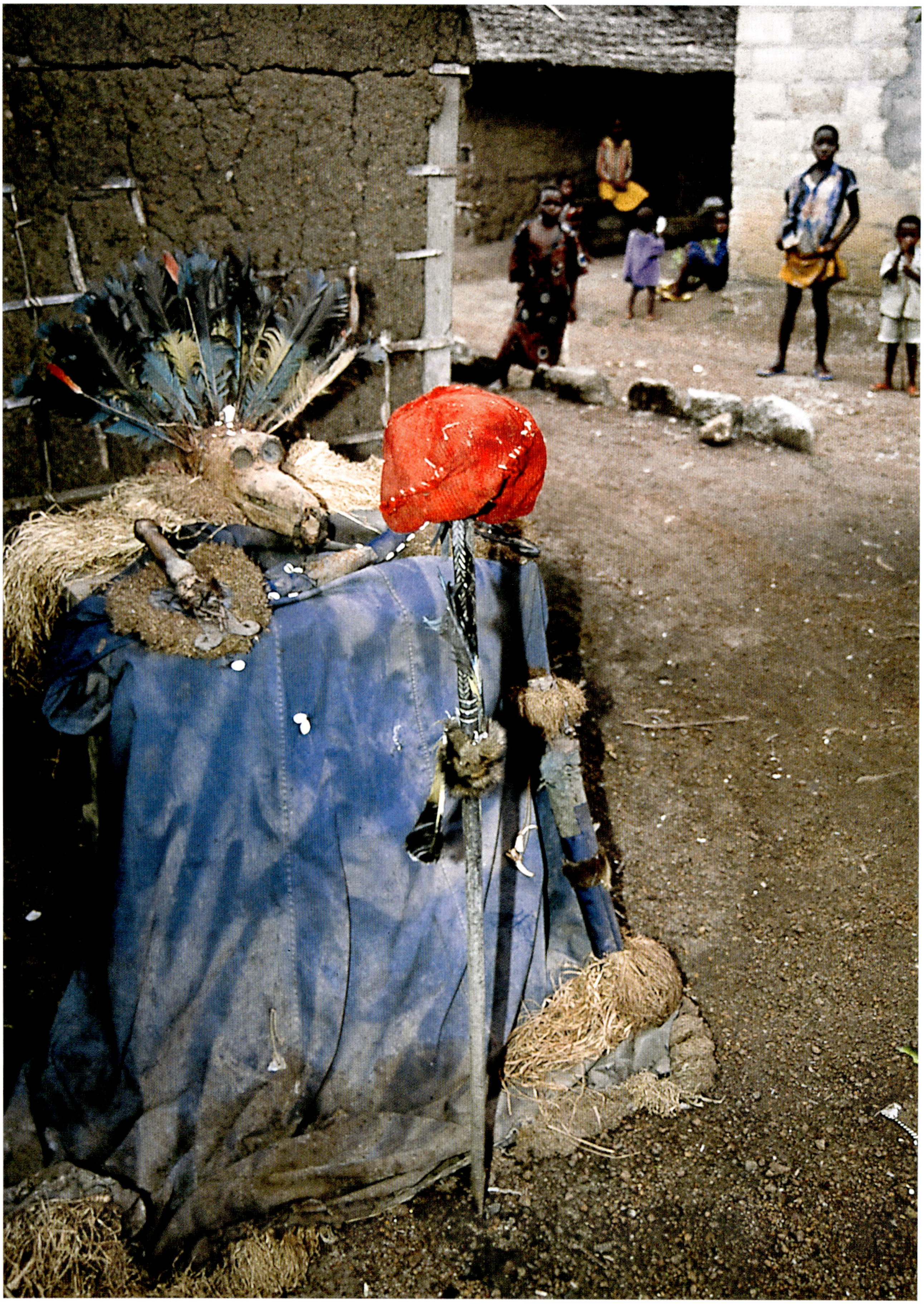

Fig. 161 The garment and accessories of *Obasinjom* spread out to dry in full public view (Kembong, April 9, 2004).

danger for the living. At death ceremonies for members *Obasinjom* has to confront this danger with a special medicine ritual. However, unlike other societies such as *Mgbe* and *Angbu*, on this occasion the mask itself does not appear to honour the deceased with a last performance.

5.5.2.1 *Abo Njom*, the young members of *Obasinjom*

Abo Njom ("children of *Obasinjom*", sg. *mo Njom*) designates the rank of the new members. Whoever wishes to enter the society must pay the members 10 litres of palm wine first, and then the society investigates whether the person is honest and trustworthy. If this is the case, the person is required to provide the following goods, which are mandatory for acceptance: one cock, two "animals", 30 litres of palm wine, one bottle of locally made whisky, one bunch of plantains, one bottle of palm oil, one cup of salt and one cup of pepper. The big man leads the new member in front of the mask. He spits upon the mask with alligator pepper and pours whisky over it, saying: "I have awakened you by giving you this whisky. Now you have a new member, whose name is Mr. X. From now on guide him and protect him, wherever he is." Thereupon the new member must swear that he will preserve the secrets of *Obasinjom*: "I, who am to become a new member of *Obasinjom*, if I should have the intention to show the leaves of *Obasinjom* to other people or to sell them outside to make money for myself without involving the whole *Obasinjom* society, let *Obasinjom* do away with my life and that of my family."

The new members must listen and learn their duties and responsibilities in the society. They may already act as drummers and singers (fig. 189), and one of their duties is to prepare food and distribute beverages at meetings. The new members are expected to acquire knowledge about the different medicines in order to become a "strong" member. The decision as to when a new member should go through the ritual in the grove of *Obasinjom* and attain full membership is left up to the person himself. When a member of this level dies, no special medicine ritual is necessary: "children of *Njom*" rarely come into contact with medicine; therefore they are not dangerous.

5.5.2.2 *Atemambi,* "heart of *Obasinjom*"

Atemambi is the level of full membership, the "heart of *Obasinjom*". Its members (*anne atemambi,* sg. *nne atemambi)* understand *njom*, i. e. the medicine, and may participate in the most important activities of the society. They have exceedingly strong medicines at their disposal, with which – it is said – they can destroy anything at any time. If a member of this group swears upon *atemambi* to carry out an action in any case, for example to kill an enemy, he must then follow through with his deed. There is no turning back, or else he himself must die.

The fees for this level are: one cock, two "animals", one cutlass, one bottle of locally made whisky, 30 litres of palm wine, one bunch of plantains, one bottle of palm oil, one cup of salt and one cup of pepper. Initiation into this level takes place in the grove of *Njom* and lasts for three days, the most important ritual the aspirants must achieve being to pass through seven "gates" made of palm fronds in an arch-like construction. When the aspirants pass through each gate, they receive cuts on different parts of the body: shoulders, elbows, wrists, buttocks, knees, ankles and big toes. Medicine is rubbed into the cuts, and medicine is also dripped into their eyes. Through these medicines the aspirants are protected against all hostile powers; they are, as is said, "well-cooked". When passing through each gate the person must swear an oath, each time on a different medicine (*Mfam, Amok, Okeboho* etc.): "All the leaves and bark of trees that they are going to show me, if I have one day the intention to destroy human lives with them, I myself should be destroyed by you." When a member of this level dies, the corpse must be treated with a special medicine. For it is feared that otherwise those who have constantly dealt with dangerous medicines would not find peace upon death and would return to the survivors and terrorise them.

To this group belong the positions of the mantlebearer, the interpreter and the player of the "trumpet" as well as *mma Njom*, which will be described in the following.

5.5.2.3 Special positions in *Obasinjom*

5.5.2.3.1 *Bebu Njom*, the mantlebearers of *Obasinjom*

The member of *Obasinjom* who bears the mask – the person is not a "dancer" in the real sense of the word – is called *ebu Njom* (pl. *bebu Njom*). Each society has several such persons. They are chosen personally by *Obasinjom,* and then each is prepared by treatment with medicine for this responsible position. Whenever a new mantlebearer is needed, *Obasinjom* invites young men to participate in a trial (*engeh Njom*, to try), which is always held in public. I had the opportunity to observe such a test twice, on January 28, 1980

Testing mantlebearers for *Obasinjom* (Kembong, January 28, 1980) (figs.162–163).

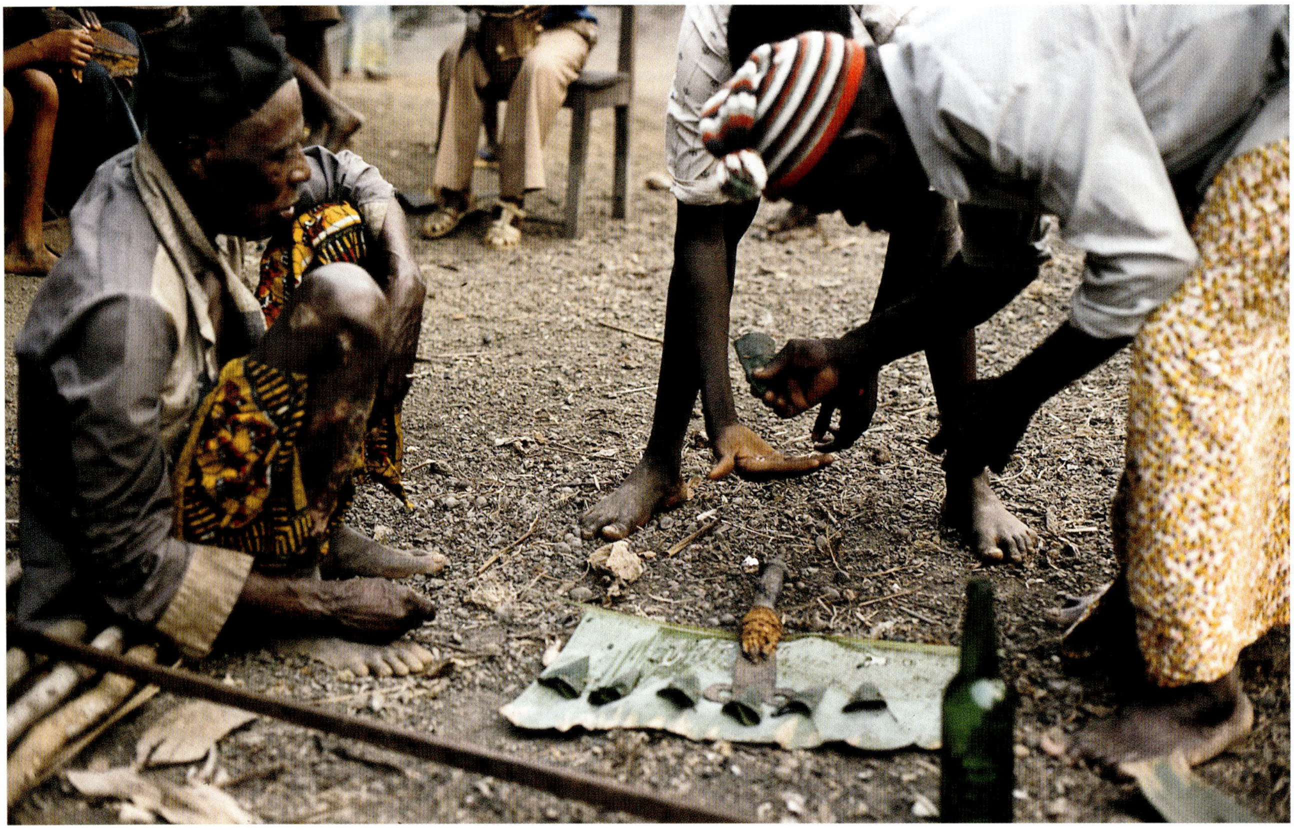

Fig. 162 A member drops medicine into the hand of the candidate; on the ground below lie the filters with medicine and *besom Njom*, which the mask always holds in the right hand. Tanyiashuh, the leader of *Obasinjom* (*ebanghaah Njom*), views from the left (Kembong, January 28, 1980).

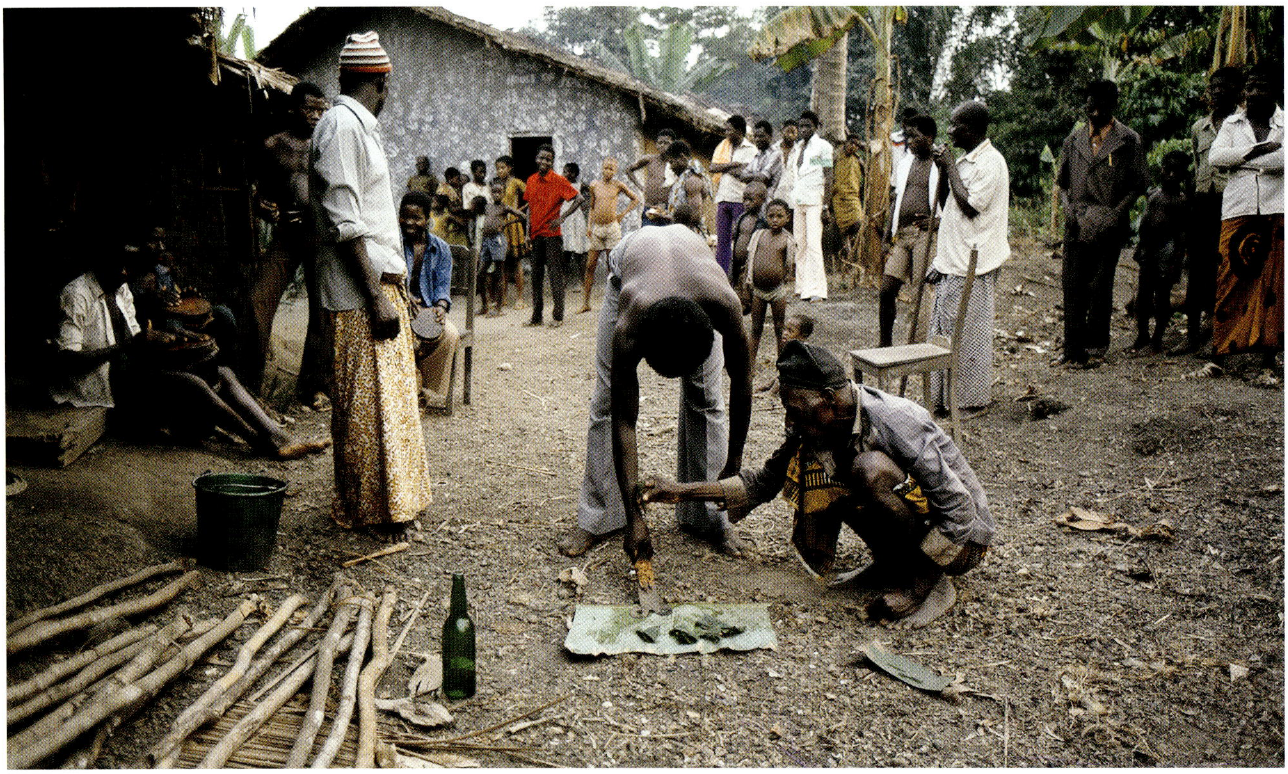

Fig. 163 The candidate takes hold of *besom Njom* with the assistance of Tanyiashuh (Kembong, January 28, 1980).

(figs. 162, 163) and April 29, 2004 (figs. 164–168).[14] A great number of people were present on both occasions, who did not want to miss this exciting and sometimes dramatic event, which only seldom takes place, about once every three years.

On that occasion the drums of *Obasinjom* beat wildly and then the candidates appeared. They were stripped to the waist and barefoot. Each test was held for one candidate alone, and before each test the candidate washed his hands. Then came the decisive moment: the candidate stood with widespread legs in front of the cutlass-shaped *besom Njom* (pl. *asom Njom),* which played the main role in the trial and lay upon the ground in the centre of the empty area. The "cutlass" is the most important object of the mask and contains powerful medicines (figs. 162, 165–167). During its performances the mask holds the *besom Njom* in the right hand. During the test in 2004 the *besom Njom* lay some three meters in front of the mask's garment, which was spread upon a wooden frame (figs. 164, 166). During the trial that I observed in 1980, by contrast, the mask garment was not present. While the candidate bent over in order to take the dangerous, indeed mysterious object in his right hand, one of the leading men of *Obasinjom* sprinkled a liquid on his head and right hand by pressing a liquid substance made of medicinal plants through a filter (figs. 162, 164). Most candidates – in 1980 there were about six young men who went through the test; in 2004, about one dozen – reached hesitantly, indeed fearfully, towards the *besom Njom*. The spectators encouraged the candidates with deafening shouts and cries, and the leader of the test invoked *Obasinjom* with loud cries: "Father, hold him, hold him, hold him, if you want him to be your mantlebearer."

When *Obasinjom* accepts a candidate, the young man falls into a trance, and the arm holding the *besom Njom* begins to tremble. If a candidate is especially gifted, the *besom Njom*, according to the reassurances of my informants, may practically fly at him before he has even touched it. If a candidate falls into a trance, this is considered proof of his calling for the supernatural. With *Obasinjom's* help, he can now perform the most unusual tasks, like climbing tall trees and buildings. Most importantly, he is now able to run to *ebaah Njom* and touch the powerful magic tree there (the "tree of medicine", *eti Njom*), which he has never seen before, further proof that he is under the influence of the medicine. Afterwards everyone returns to the leader's compound, where the initiate places the *besom Njom* on the

Testing mantlebearers for *Obasinjom* (Kembong, April 29, 2004) (figs. 164–168).

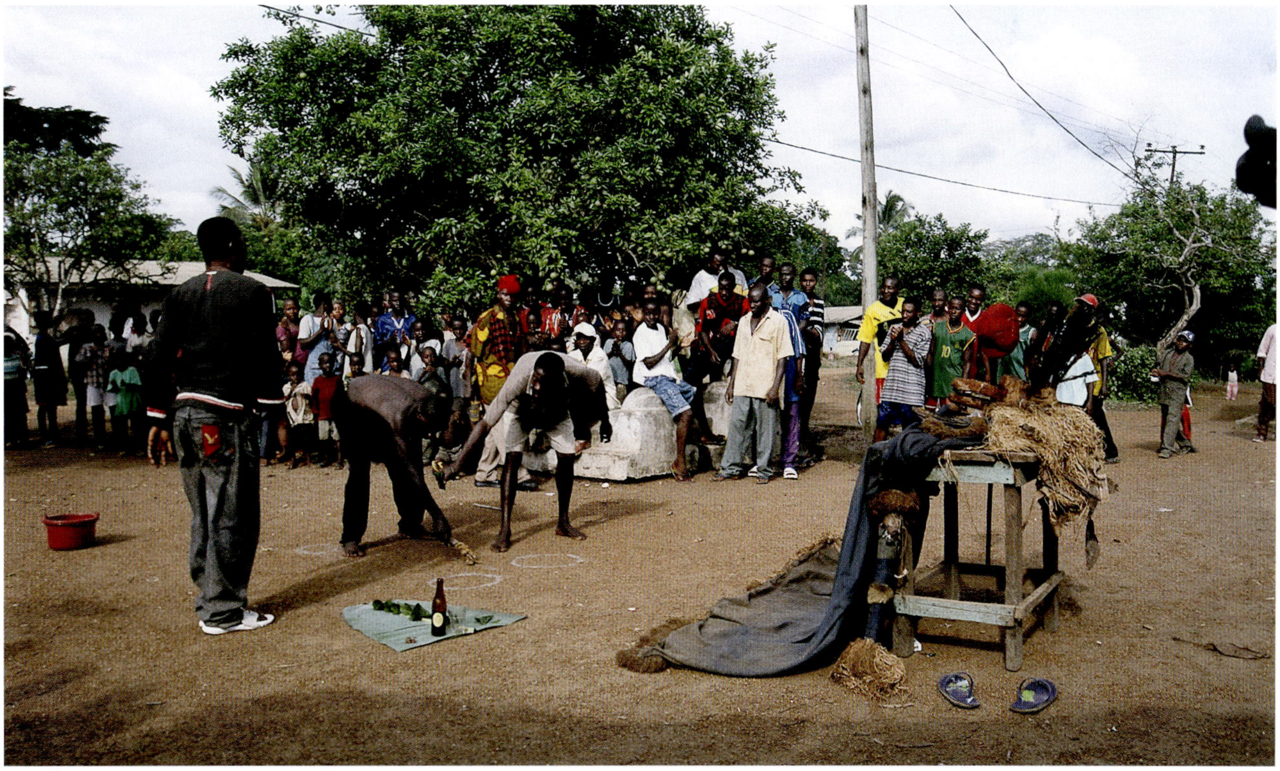

Fig. 164 The candidate takes hold of *besom Njom* with his right hand, while a member of *Obasinjom* lets medicine drip on that hand; the mask garment of *Obasinjom* is in full public view (right foreground) (Kembong, April 29, 2004).

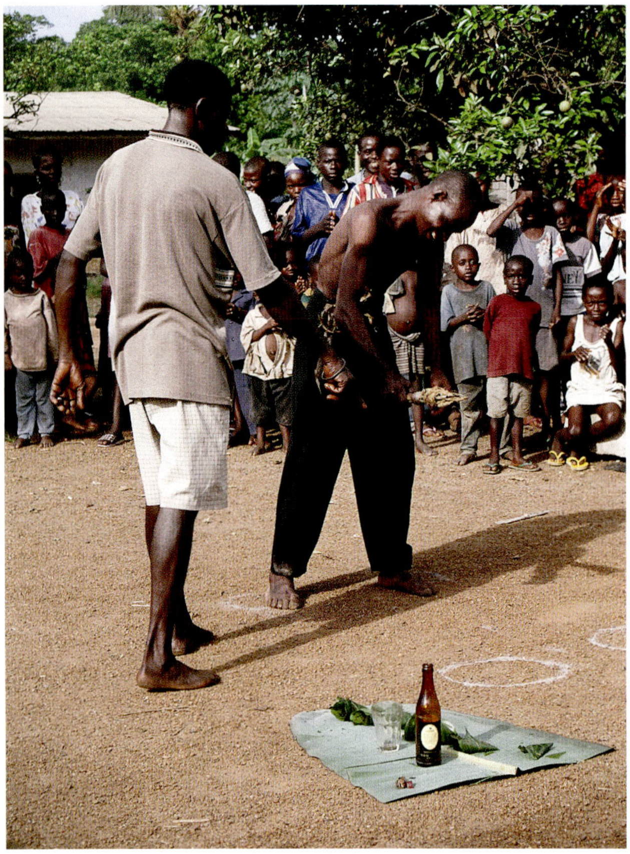

Fig. 165 The candidate holds *besom Njom* in his right hand and "struggles" to fall into a trance, i. e. to be seized by *Obasinjom* (Kembong, April 29, 2004).

ground. He is then given a special medicine that usually brings him back to consciousness at once.

During the trial in 2004 only one person of all the candidates passed the test, that is to say, only one was accepted by *Obasinjom*. This particular candidate had scarcely touched the *besom Njom*, when his right arm and hand, which gripped the mysterious object, began to swing upwards and downwards with increasing speed. The young man slowly stood up; his eyes were glassy and stared straight ahead, seeming to bulge (fig. 168). With unsteady, clumsy steps he ran through the shouting, uproarious crowd and disappeared behind the houses, followed by many children. After a time during which the drumming continued and even the spectators seemed to have fallen into a trance, the young man possessed by *Obasinjom* returned; allegedly he had been in the grove, *ebaah Njom*, which is expected in such an event. Then some members of *Obasinjom* surrounded him and took him to the house of the big man. After about a quarter of an hour the spectators were still roaring and the drums beaten. One of the *Obasinjom* members appeared and ordered the drummers to cease playing, as it was very difficult to bring the young man back to consciousness.

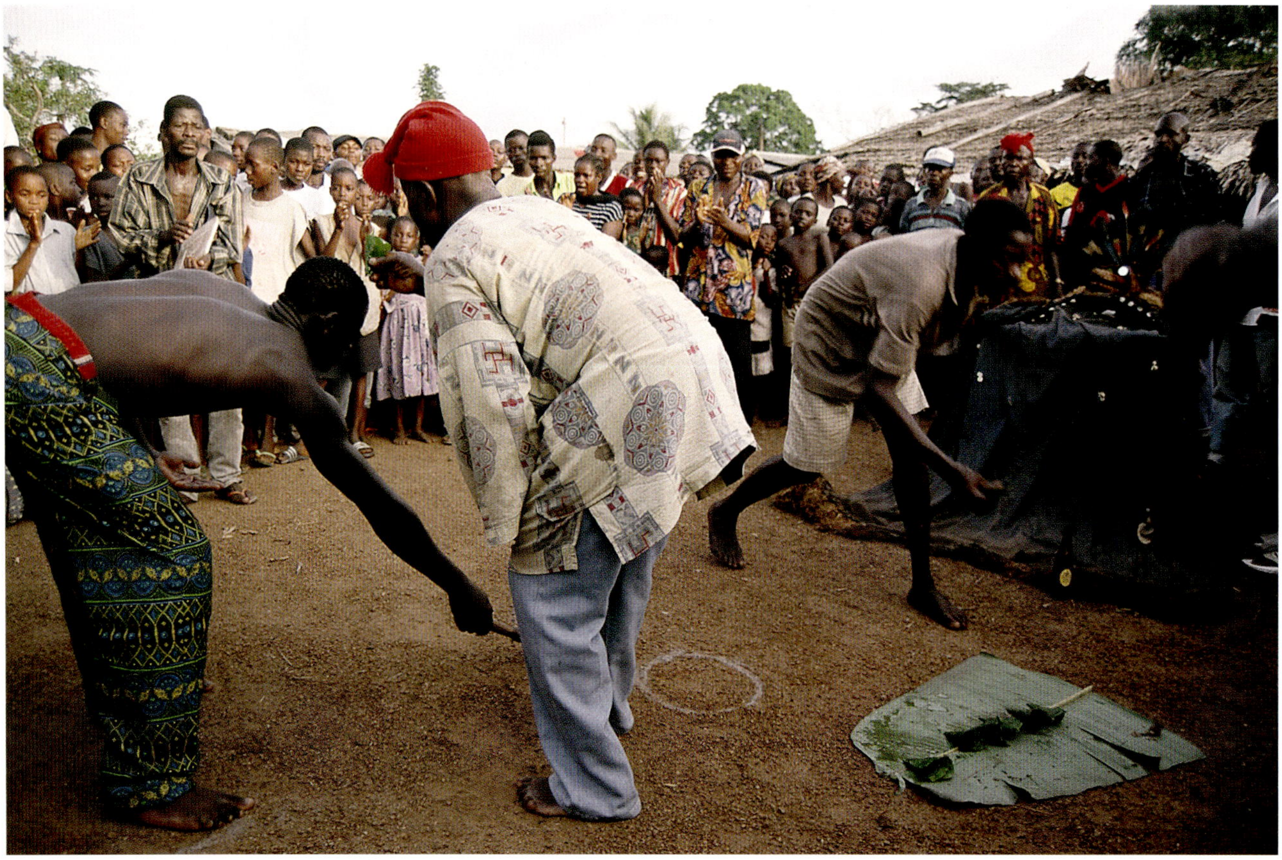

Fig. 166 Incited by the onlookers, the candidate holds *besom Njom* and attempts to reach the state of trance (Kembong, April 29, 2004).

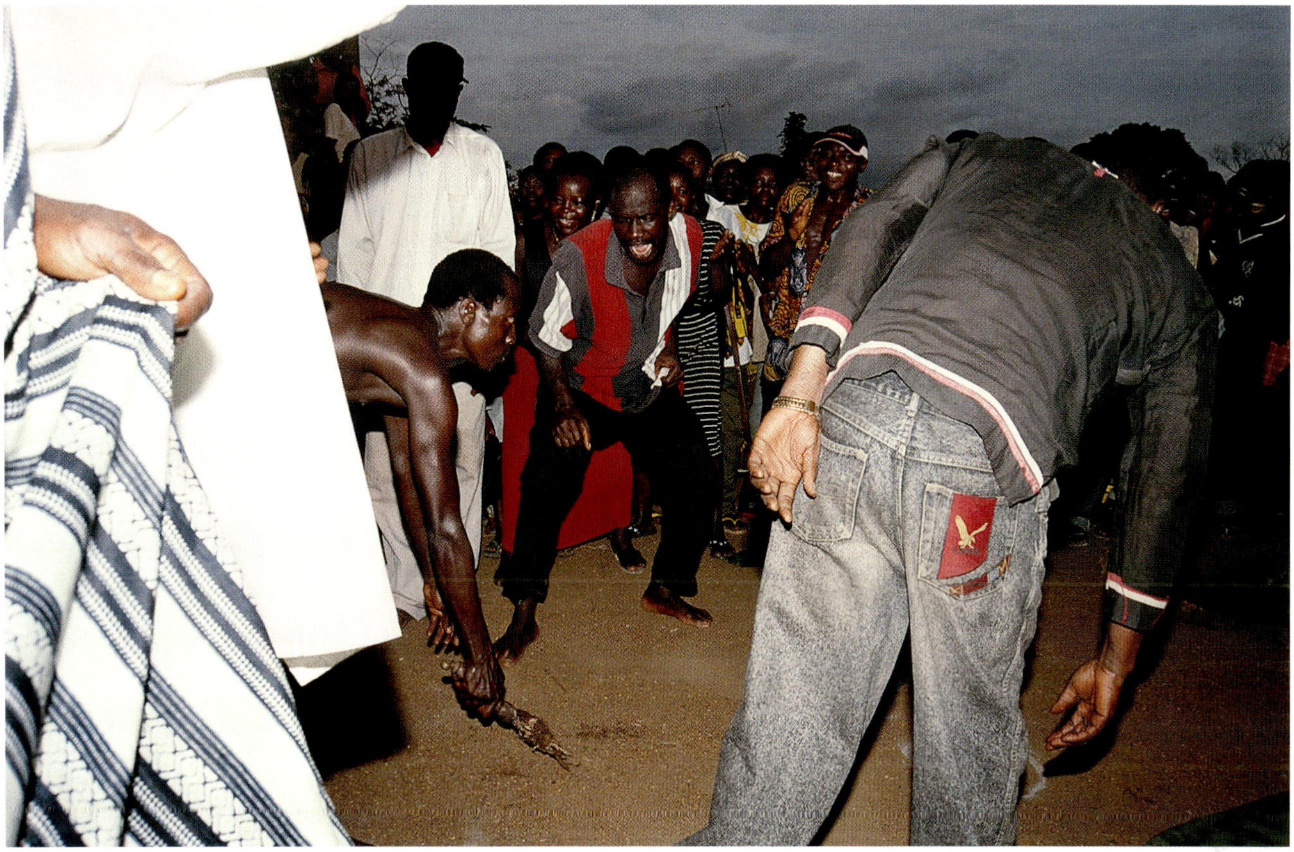

Fig. 167 A member of *Obasinjom* incites the candidate, who stares at the mask garment (Kembong, April 29, 2004).

If the family of the candidate agrees to assume the responsibility as mantlebearer for *Obasinjom*, then the initiation into *Obasinjom* follows, just as that which every new member has to go trough. Only thereafter can the initiation as mantlebearer take place. Additional fees are obligatory: three "animals", one bottle of locally made whisky, 20 litres of palm wine, one bunch of plantains and one cutlass.

The initiation as mantlebearer takes place in the house of the chief of *Obasinjom* and lasts seven days. During this time the initiate is treated with various medicines; among other things, cuts are made on his body and medicine is rubbed into the wounds. Every day medicine is dripped into his eyes, an action called "washing the eyes" (*osuamet*). The initiation of a mantlebearer ends when on the seventh day the chief sticks a small wooden pin into the mask headpiece, where other pins are already present. They belong to the mantlebearers of the respective society. By pulling out a wooden pin slightly, the chief can order the particular mantlebearer at any time to come and take over the mask garment. We shall return to this obligation later (cp. p. 158).

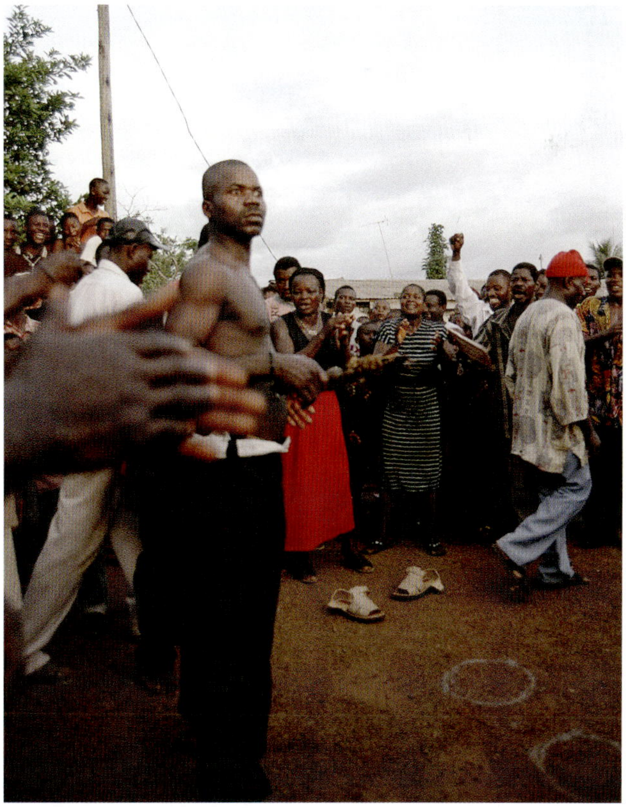

Fig. 168 The single candidate who passed the test is in a trance, with staring glassy eyes. He has been accepted as a mantlebearer by *Obasinjom* (Kembong, April 29, 2004).

If, on the contrary, the test was unsuccessful, *Obasinjom* must continue to search for a young man in the community, who might qualify for this important and responsible duty. Having found a suitable candidate whose family is in agreement, initiation can commence. The procedure is mostly like that described above for candidates in the public test. However, the medicines used in this initiation are more powerful, and therefore the usual duration of seven days is extended to ten days. During this time the candidate receives other medicines, in particular those that are dripped into the eyes. "Washing the eyes" is the most important part of initiation for every new mantlebearer and is to transfer additional powers to him. It is supposed to assist him in his future duty of detecting dangerous powers and other things in time.

Only after this period of initiation is he conclusively considered qualified to be a mantlebearer of *Obasinjom*. In other words, "*Obasinjom* has caught him to be its prophet". With the initiation as mantlebearer the process of acceptance into the circle of full members, the *anne atemambi,* follows. The new mantlebearer is not required to partake in this particular initiation in the grove of *Njom*; his initiation already includes full membership. Important and singular as the position of a mantlebearer of *Obasinjom* may be one aim – provided the person ever aspired towards it – is now forever unattainable for him: he may never become chief of *Obasinjom*.

At present (2005) there is only one mantlebearer left in *Obasinjom*, as two former mantlebearers have died in recent times. Principally all mantlebearers carry out the same duties, and all are equally worthy; there are no differences among them. Even a European could assume the mask outfit, if he were to be possessed by *Obasinjom* – at least this was the statement of the *Obasinjom* members. When mantlebearers assume the mask costume, they have already lost consciousness; they are not aware of their actions (figs. 185, 201– 202). Also after the end of their performance they cannot remember their actions. When the mask is to appear, *Obasinjom's* mantlebearers are summoned either by the medicine itself or by the society's leader or by *mma Njom*, the wife of *Obasinjom*. If the leader needs a mantlebearer, he pulls out one of the small wooden pins inserted next to the feathers in the headpiece. Each stands for a particular dancer.[15] At the same time he commands the medicine: "Call your dog to come." Dogs are considered to be strong, active, intelligent, obedient, and therefore indispensable in the hunt – in this case, for witches. Wherever the person may happen to be – even hundreds of kilometres from Kembong –, when summoned the mantlebearer falls into a trance instantly, with his only goal being to reach the mask. No one will be able to stop him as he crosses farms, forests, rivers, and lakes if need be, undeterred by thorns, shards and other obstacles. Mantlebearers, however, usually keep the leader informed of their travel plans, so that he can call on dancers he knows to be nearby. After the mask has performed, the leader inserts the pin again into its original position on the headpiece.

5.5.2.3.2 *Osam Njom,* the interpreter of *Obasinjom*

Another important figure in *Obasinjom* is the interpreter *osam Njom*, which is also the designation for his staff. *Obasinjom* is one of the few African masks that speak, and it is the duty of the interpreter to announce what *Obasinjom* has to say to the community. Conversely, those who have something to say to the mask must turn to the interpreter, for they are unable to address the mask personally.

The fees for the interpreter are the same as those for a mantlebearer. In order to fulfil his duties optimally, he is treated with the appropriate medicine. Medicine is put in his ears in order to improve his hearing. Another medicine is rubbed into cuts made on the cheeks in order to facilitate his speech.

During the performances the interpreter carries a spear-like staff (*osam Njom*, "staff of the medicine"), which bears medicine lodged in feathers of the peacock, a bird considered vital and active (figs. 161, 173–176, 182, 191, 196, 206). Feathers like these are also found on the headpiece of the mask. Occasionally the interpreter implants the staff in the ground in order to dance or to define the performance area of the mask, which may not dance beyond the limits delineated by the staff. Sometimes *Obasinjom* grabs the staff and raises it against witches (fig. 206). Before each performance the interpreter must announce his loyalty: "*Obasi*, what I am saying is true; I swear in the name of God."

5.5.2.3.3 *Eturu Njom,* the trumpet of *Obasinjom*

Further components of the equipment of *Obasinjom* are a wind instrument (*eturu*, pl. *beturu*) made of wood that is usually referred to as a "trumpet", and a pipe made from a crab's claw (*ekeneyamojeh*).[16] These instruments are essential at performances of the mask and are played by one single man. With their aid, he has the ability to direct the mask, for example, to force the mask to move in a certain direction (fig. 176). The man who plays the "trumpet" does not need any special education. He simply must be able to play the instruments. Therefore, lesser fees are required by him, amounting to 30 litres of palm wine.

5.5.2.3.4 *Mma Njom,* the wife of *Obasinjom*

In principle, women in the Cross River region have no access to the men's secret societies, for among other reasons their sexual organs would weaken the medicine. Nonetheless, women may become members of such a society, albeit with limited rights, if they cannot bear children anymore, and this usually means when they are of old age. In fact *Obasinjom* is dependent upon a woman: He needs a "wife", *mma Njom* (fig. 155).[17] She is the only person, whom *Obasinjom* never disobeys and who as a deputy of the big man can activate the mask at any time. Therefore *Obasinjom* "weds" a prepubescent virgin of five to ten in age. Girls at this age are said to possess the power to control and even stop the mask – to "cool it down" – should it go wild. During performances *mma Njom* repeatedly spits alligator pepper upon the mask, so that it will tell the truth and conceal nothing. If the mask lets itself speak about things that should not be said, the *mma Njom* can silence it by saying: "My husband, stop, what you are saying." If the mask has not performed in a long time, the *mma Njom* can take the initiative herself: "Husband, where is your dog? Send your dog to come." In this way the *mma Njom* fulfils her task, but she is nevertheless excluded from all important ceremonies, in particular from those that take place in the grove. Also, she is not entrusted with any secrets of the mask society.

Long before the girl reaches puberty, *Obasinjom* sends *mma Njom* away. The dismissal is perfunctory, requiring only a ritual purification. Medicine and palm wine are mixed on a large leaf and sprinkled on the girl: "*Obasinjom,* you had been married to this wife. Today she leaves you to meet her parents. Forget about her. As she goes away, let her stay in peace. Let her head and her stomach not have trouble. Let her not place her foot on a thorn, or dash her toe against a stone." Soon after, *Obasinjom* chooses a new wife, whose parents invariably agree to the choice. At the "wedding", neither religious ceremonies nor medicine rituals or prayers are required.

Since my stay in 2004/2005 *mma Njom* of *Obasinjom* has seldom appeared in Upper Kembong, because – it was said – she often stayed in the city of Limbe. In the meantime she has become engaged to a man, which means that *Obasinjom* needs a new wife.

5.5.2.4 *Anne eboho Njom*, the leaders of *Obasinjom*

Anne eboho Njom ("the people who sit on the mud-bed of *Njom*") is the level of the three big men or chiefs of *Obasinjom*. The highest ranking chief is the *ebanghaah Njom,* without whom important decisions pertaining to the society may not be made. The designation *ebanghaah Njom* already indicates that he is also in charge of conducting the oracle with two leaves (*ebanghaah*). He conducts ceremonies of offering as well, and aside from the mask he is the only person in *Obasinjom* who knows all of the medicines – something that the mask bearer does not. At official meetings the highest chief always sits in the middle of the bench; the place to his right is that of *ntui mfam Njom,* to his left that of another deputy. The fees for all three *anne eboho Njom* are the same: one goat, four "animals", one cock, one bottle of local or imported whisky, 30 litres of palm wine, one bunch of plantains, one bottle of palm oil, one cup of salt and one cup of pepper.

When an *ebanghaah Njom* dies, he is customarily succeeded by the *ntui mfam Njom.* When the present chief Adolf Ojong Agbor (Okune) assumed this office in 1997, he was not one of the *anne eboho Njom* and, thus, could not reckon with becoming chief of *Obasinjom.* The fact that he was awarded this office was due alone to the mediation of the medicine, meaning the intervention of the mask. When the society was discussing who was to be the successor to the deceased *ebanghaah Njom,* one of the mask bearers fell into a trance and donned the mask garment. The mask demanded that the assembled members choose Adolf Ojong Agbor as chief of the society, as he possessed all the characteristics and spiritual properties required for this position; above all he had the greatest knowledge about medicines.

The installation of the new *ebanghaah Njom* takes place in the grove of *Obasinjom.* The most important part of the ceremony are the offerings to the ancestors; this is followed by eating and drinking palm wine. On this occasion additional fees, including one crate of beer, 30 litres of palm wine, one "animal" and plantains, are given to *Mgbe*, whose grove is next to that of *Obasinjom.* When *Mgbe* has received the fees, a confirmation follows immediately: the cry of the leopard. As in all ceremonies of offering, at the installation of the *ebanghaah Njom* the oracle manifests the final act and the decisive climax. If the oracle is negative seven times, it is the sign that the ancestors reject the candidate as big man. He may never become leader of *Obasinjom*; his fees are lost and not replaced.

The previous leaders of *Obasinjom* in Kembong were Tabot, Nyang, Etap and Nkongho; in 1980 the leader was Tanyiashu, who died in 1985 (cp. figs. 162, 184). He was succeeded by John Etchu, who died in 1996 (cp. figs. 53, 183). John Etchu's successor in 1997 is, as mentioned above, Adolf Ojong Agbor, the present chief of *Obasinjom* (cp. figs. 170, 171, 200).

When a *nne eboho Njom* dies, his corpse is not treated with medicine as in the case of the *anne atemambi*. Instead, with respect to the upright character of the deceased during life, he is simply "warned" that he should depart from the work of the living: "You are dead. It is we, the *Obasinjom* people, who are on your corpse now. We know that you will not remain in the ground, but come out. When you come out, do not make people be afraid of you and do not make us ashamed. We know that where you are going, all of us will follow. Bye-bye and safe journey."

5.5.3 The mask and its medicines

The absolute centre of *Obasinjom* is its mask, which derives from God and the ancestors. Without the mask *Obasinjom* would not exist. It is a matter-of-fact that the different components of the mask equipment correspond with its special purposes: The mask should be dangerous and terrifying, so that it can destroy witches and other hostile forces. At the same time *Obasinjom* acts as a diviner, being able to foresee events in the future as well as to explain and interpret happenings in the past. Both properties of the mask equipment – physical power and the faculty of foresight – are possible through the use of medicines and certain body parts of animals that possess the corresponding properties, foremost from strong, aggressive animals. These body parts intimate the particular characteristics of the respective animal and, hence, are of symbolic significance.[18]

Consequently, *Obasinjom* does not have a colourful mask garment, as is typical of mask traditions in the Cross River region, but instead a dark, heavy material with the lower part interwoven with raphia. The mask headpiece is made of wood and its piercing eyes of mirror-glass, which are indicative of the mask's ability to recognise things that are normally invisible to ordinary people. It depicts the head of a crocodile, an animal that is strong and dangerous, on the one hand, and, on the other, abides in two elements: land and water (figs. 172, 183, 195). Correspondingly, *Obasinjom* is able to fight against its enemies on earth as well as in water. *Obasinjom* can also pursue its enemies in flight thanks to the feathers in the headpiece. They not only signify flight, but also imply other properties of birds. The black and white feathers are from the peacock, which is considered proud and self-confident, and the mask appears in a similar manner. The white feathers of the eagle, that powerful and dangerous bird of prey that also has extraordinarily far sight, point out that *Obasinjom* has similar remarkable powers and abilities. The red feathers are from the parrot, considered an especially clever bird. When *Obasinjom* sees a parrot, it can command the bird to fly to distant lands, such as Europe or the Americas, to learn about certain things. As I was told by members of *Obasinjom*, people are always surprised at how the mask can report in detail on foreign countries. Its extraordinary ability to see and to be informed about things that are normally closed to ordinary persons, is also exhibited when – for instance – afflicted and sick persons seek the mask's help. Their malady and illness often correlate with those of the deceased, who have been neglected or forgotten; *Obasinjom*, however, can recognise and name them.

Obasinjom draws its most important and strongest powers from the medicines that are attached to an unusually large number of places on the mask equipment, but foremost on the headpiece (*echi Njom*, "head of *Njom*"). Substances containing medicine are applied to the top of the skull and forehead, behind the eyes and in the holes into which the feathers are inserted. A particularly strong medicine is on the back of the head (*efe Njom*). It is considered the "brain-box", because there it is decided how the mask should act in different situations. The mask garment (*ngok Njom*) also holds medicine. The lower part of the garment (*esene Njom*) is important, for the medicine located there is capable of destroying any other kind of medicine or at least render it harmless, especially when the mask moves. This could even happen with *Obasinjom's* own medicines, should they come into contact with *esene Njom*.

The most outstanding object of the mask is the aforementioned cutlass-shaped *besom Njom* (pl. *asom Njom*), which the mask holds in its right hand during performances (figs. 174, 182, 190, 203–204). *Besom Njom* contains a specially potent medicine, which is repeatedly treated with new medicine. With *besom Njom* the mask can beat and kill invisible witches. Above all, *besom Njom* works like an antenna, providing the mask with information (this was the comparison made by my informants).[19] Therefore, when *Obasinjom* is in action, it intermittently holds *besom Njom* to the ground, the abode of the ancestors, and then raises the object to its ear to listen to the instructions of the ancestors.

The mask also passes *besom Njom* over the body of a sick person to ascertain what must be done to heal him/her. A further important medicinal aid is *efune*

Njom, a special wood from the bush, which the mask holds in its left hand. With *efune Njom* the mask can verify the information that it receives, in particular from *besom Njom*; it receives confirmation that the information is true and applicable. With *efune Njom* the mask can also destroy inimical medicines. The "heart of *Obasinjom*" (*mbenghe Njom*) is a band made of thick textile that the mask wears around its neck (figs. 156, 173, 182, 183). Decorated with cowry shells, the band contains all the medicines that *Obasinjom* has at its disposal. Like magic medicine (*njom*), *mbenghe Njom* can be activated against enemies.

There are members of the society who are specialists on the various medicines and responsible for their production. The medicines are renewed every one to five years. The most important components are vegetal, like leaves, grasses and tree bark, in addition to minerals and parts of animals. Special significance is ascribed to "dogs with four eyes", who are said to possess witch-like powers, above all the ability of foresight.[20] "Dogs with four eyes" are those that have two spots in the hair colour above the eyes, which can be seen as two additional eyes (fig. 169). During all important medicine rituals the sacrifice of such a dog is essential, as dogs are considered in general as animals that hunt and that are intelligent as well as dangerous. The flesh of the sacrificed animal is eaten by the participants of the ceremony, which is very uncommon, as dogs are not normally consumed as food among the Central Ejagham. The head, heart, tongue and paws of dogs are particularly powerful and are reserved for the mask bearers and the interpreter. These parts as well as the piece of dog skin with the two spots (the two additional "eyes") are also indispensable components of medicine.

Besides the medicines that belong to the mask equipment, *Obasinjom* also possesses other medicines, which it uses as a safeguard against dangerous and hostile powers as well as for healing purposes. Thus, *Obasinjom* also has the potential to heal all afflictions that were caused by the activation of magic medicines, such as *Mfam*, *Amok* and *Okeboho*. The most important medicine for defence against threats, danger and calamity of any kind is *nchip Njom*. It has the consistency of an oily paste, which is rubbed upon the body, especially on the arms and legs (fig. 205). This medicine is obtained in a special medicine ritual called *oje ba kpang*, which is conducted very seldom. Only three such rituals have been carried out by *Obasinjom* in Upper Kembong during the past 40 years. The production of *nchip Njom* is not the task of *Obasinjom* alone, but involves the entire community. First a man suited for searching for the medicinal plants must be sought in the community. The person chosen is then given a cutlass that has been treated with special medicines and in this way becomes rather like a substitute for *besom Njom*. Due to the cutlass's power, the man immediately falls into a trance. In this condition the person goes into the forest, where he cuts and collects diverse medicinal plants. Later in the house of *Obasinjom* the plants are first sorted out that are essential for healing medicines against the afflictions caused by the magic medicines *Mfam*, *Amok*, *Okeboho* etc., mentioned above. Yet the intent here is not only the production of the respective healing medicines; *Obasinjom* also takes the opportunity to instruct its members. They are to have the chance to study the plants and take careful note of them for the future.

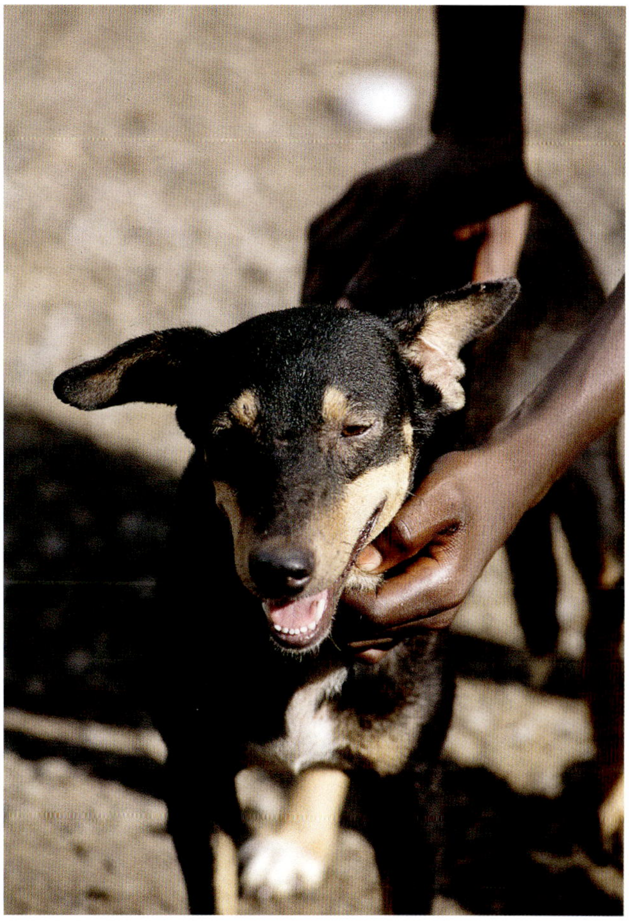

Fig. 169 A dog with "four eyes" (Kembong, April 14, 2004).

The rest of the gathered plants, leaves and tree bark are mixed with minerals and other things and then pulverised in a mortar; finally the substance is mixed with palm oil. The container with the *nchip Njom* is kept underneath the mask garment. The *ebanghaah Njom* may use it at any time, and high ranking members receive some of this medicine as well, which they may use for private purposes.

Performance of *Obasinjom* (Kembong, January 29–30, 2004) (figs. 170–180).

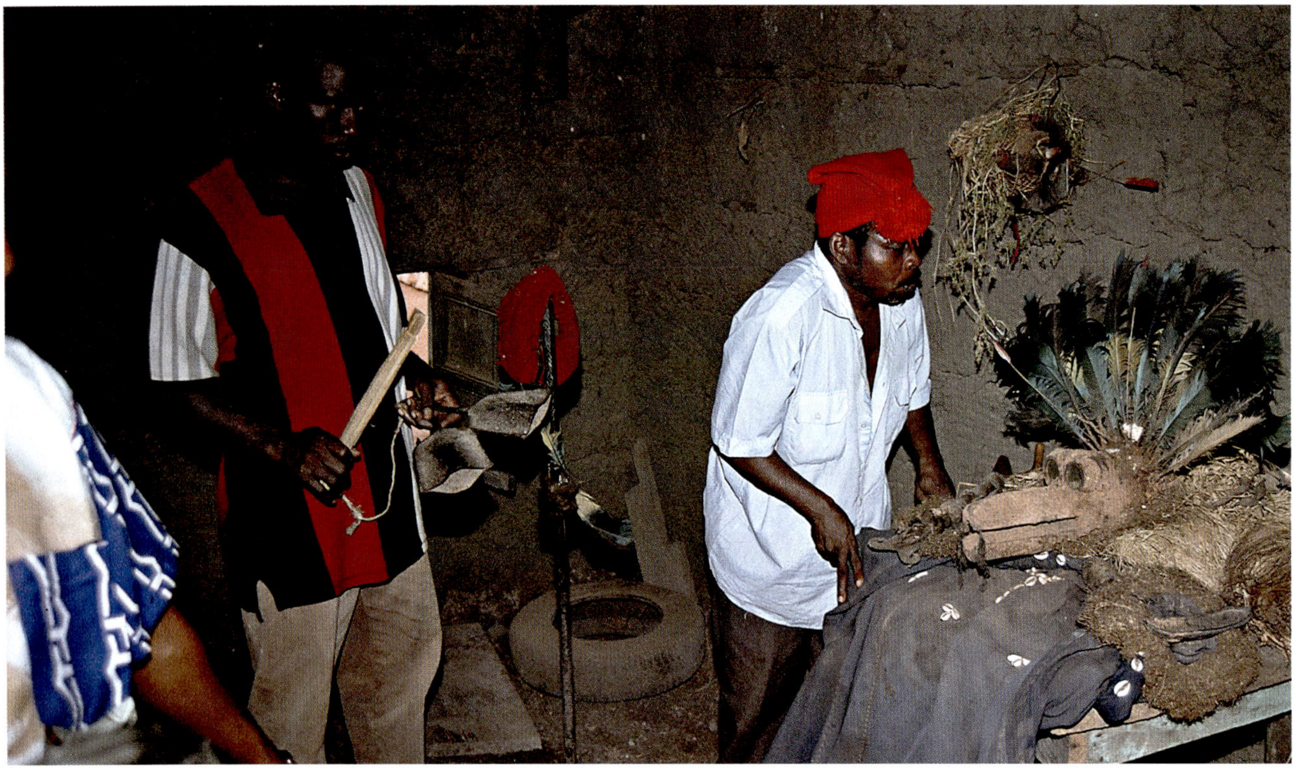

Fig. 170 Activating *Obasinjom* on the evening before the performance. The leader of *Obasinjom* (*ebanghaah Njom*), Adolf Ojong Agbor, spits alligator pepper onto the mask headdress, while a member plays the double bell (left) (Kembong, January 29, 2004).

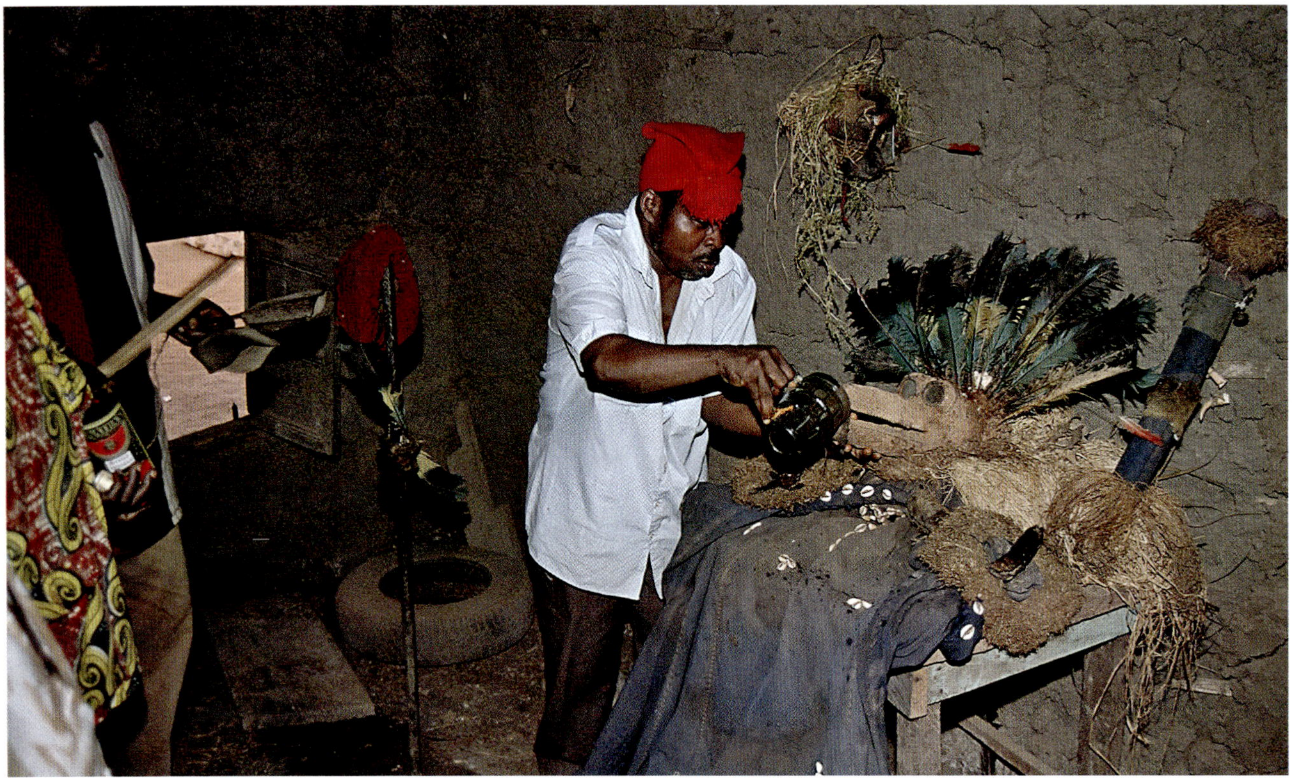

Fig. 171 Activating *Obasinjom*. The leader pours "whisky" into the mouth of the mask headdress (Kembong, January 29, 2004).

Fig. 172 The headdress of *Obasinjom* in the form of a crocodile head, carved out of wood and rubbed with yellow camwood, with eyes made of a mirror, a ruff of raphia at the neck and feathers inserted into the head. The mask bearer looks through the two holes encircled by cowrie shells (Kembong, January 30, 2004). ▸

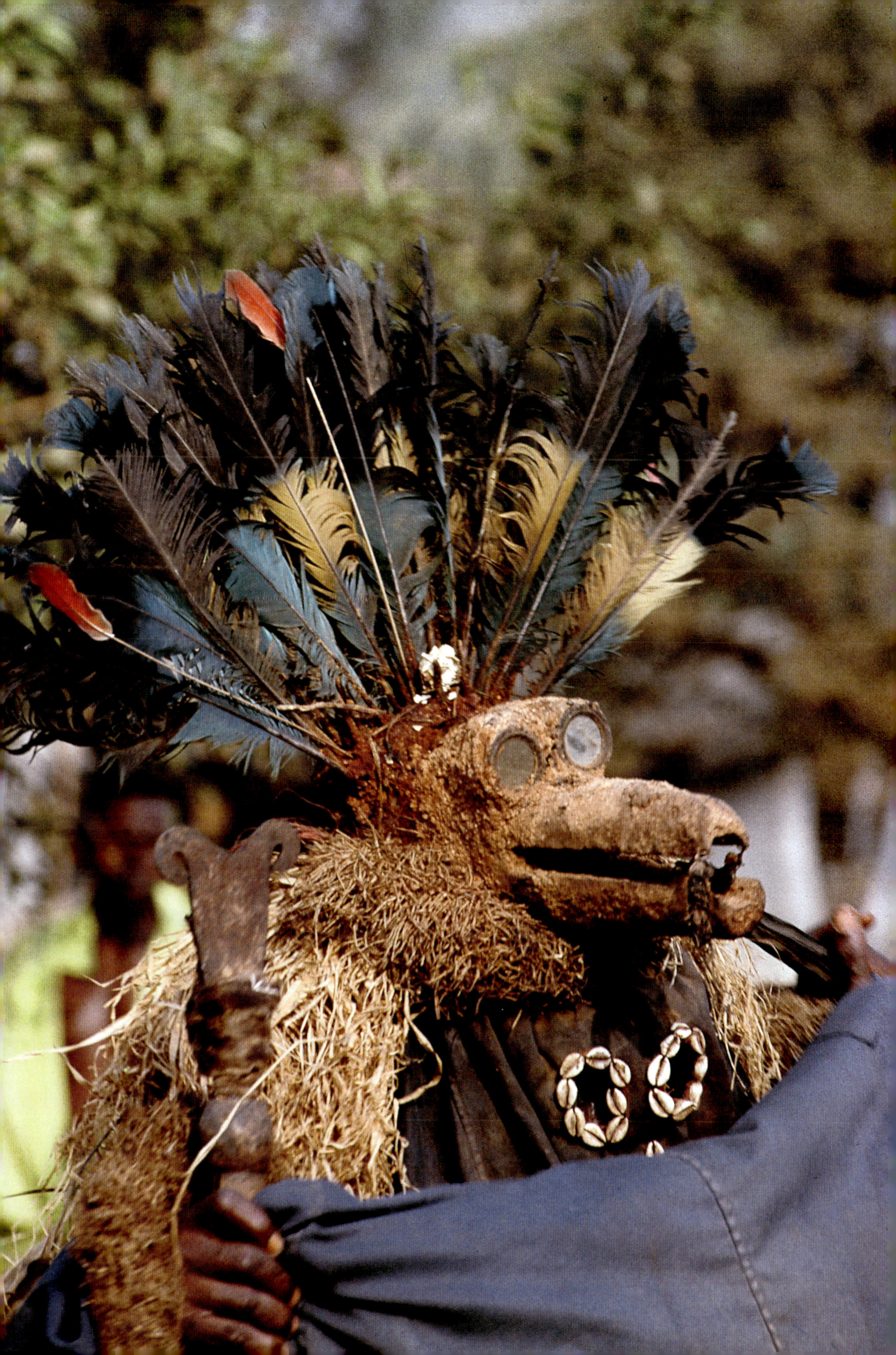

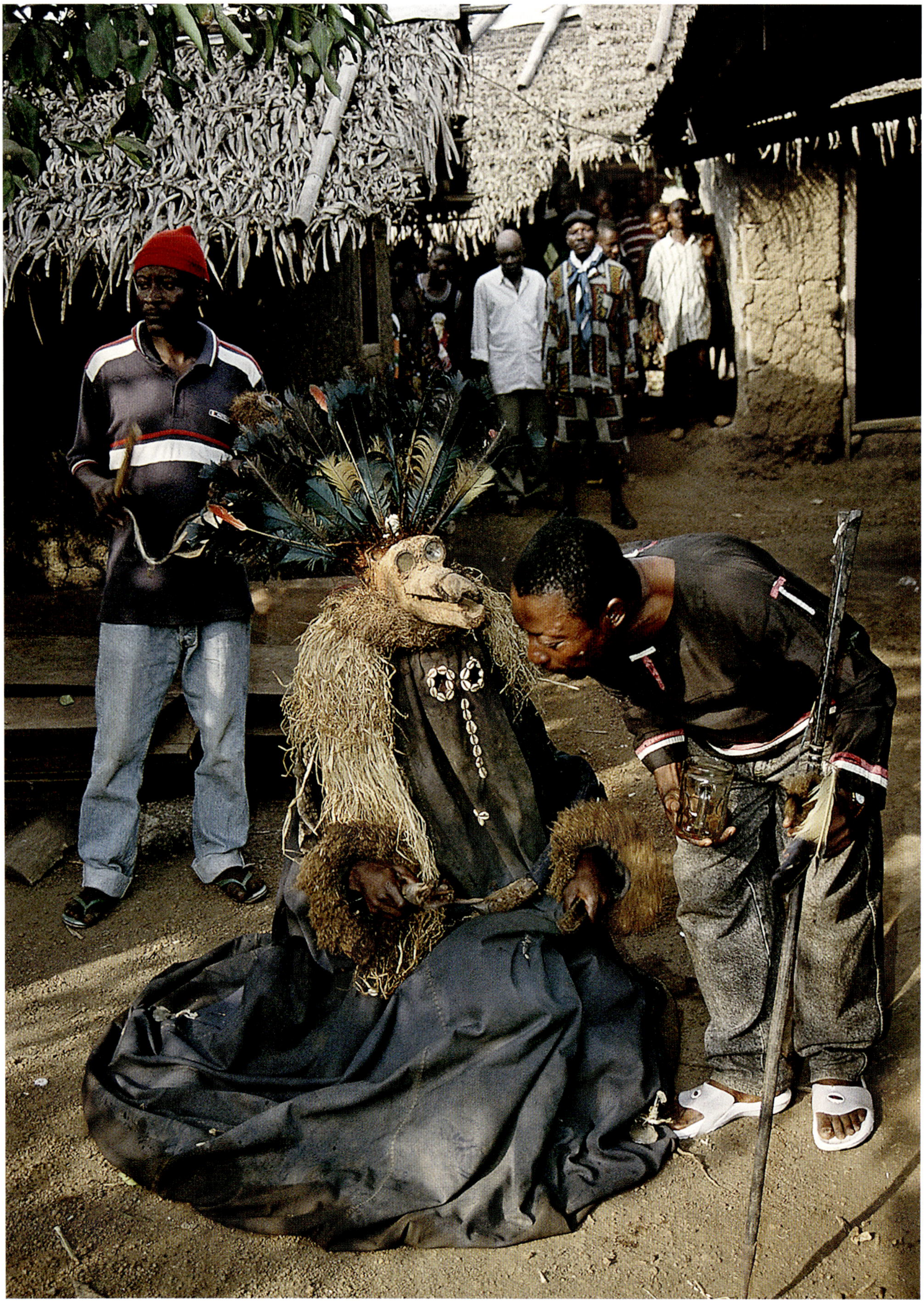

Fig. 173 The interpreter, *osam Njom*, receives information from the mask (Kembong, January 30, 2004).

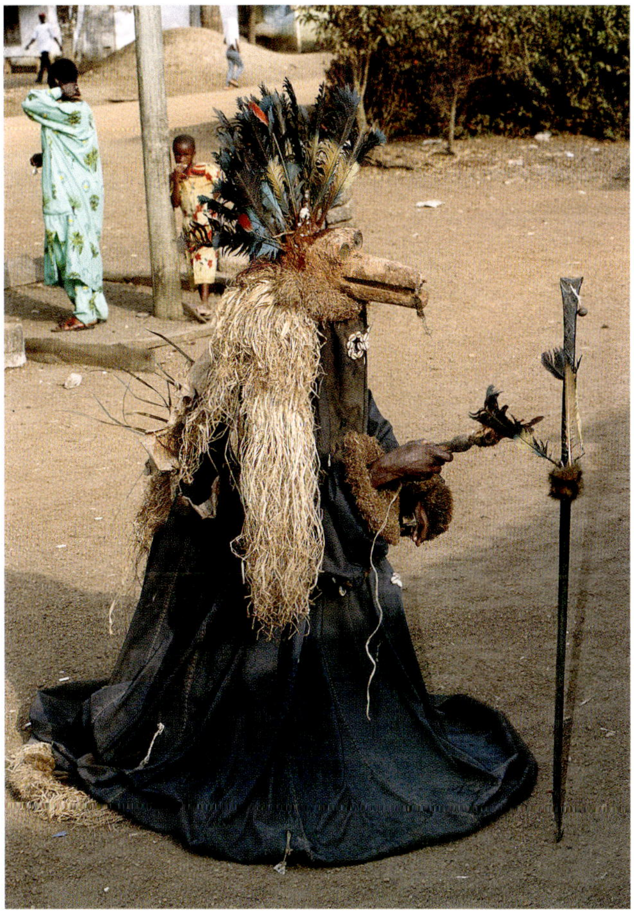

Fig. 174 *Obasinjom* holding *besom Njom* in the right hand; in front of the mask, *osam Njom*, the staff of *Obasinjom* (Kembong, January 30, 2004).

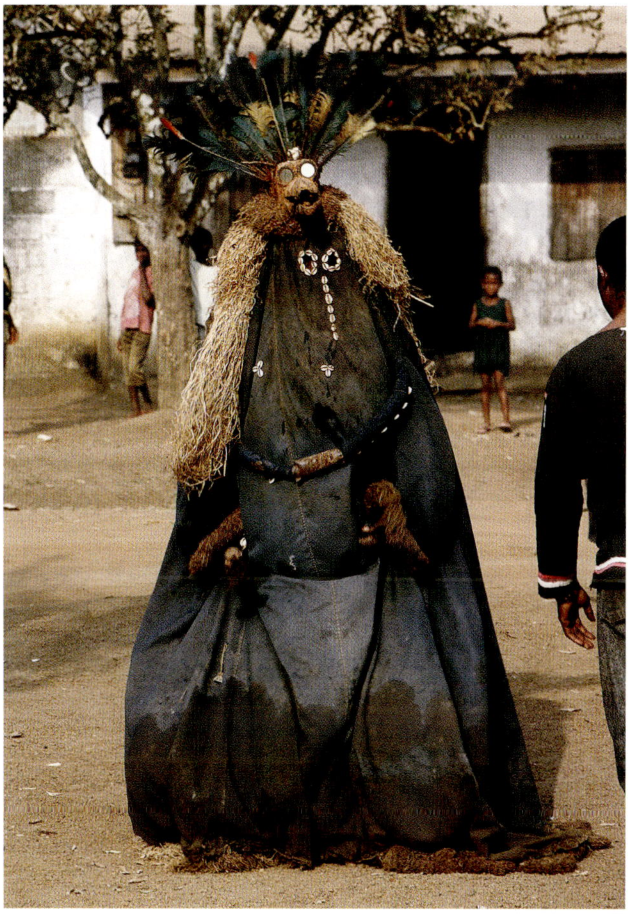

Fig. 175 The mask *Obasinjom* in full dress. The band around the neck is *mbenghe Njom*, the "heart of *Obasinjom*" (Kembong, January 30, 2004).

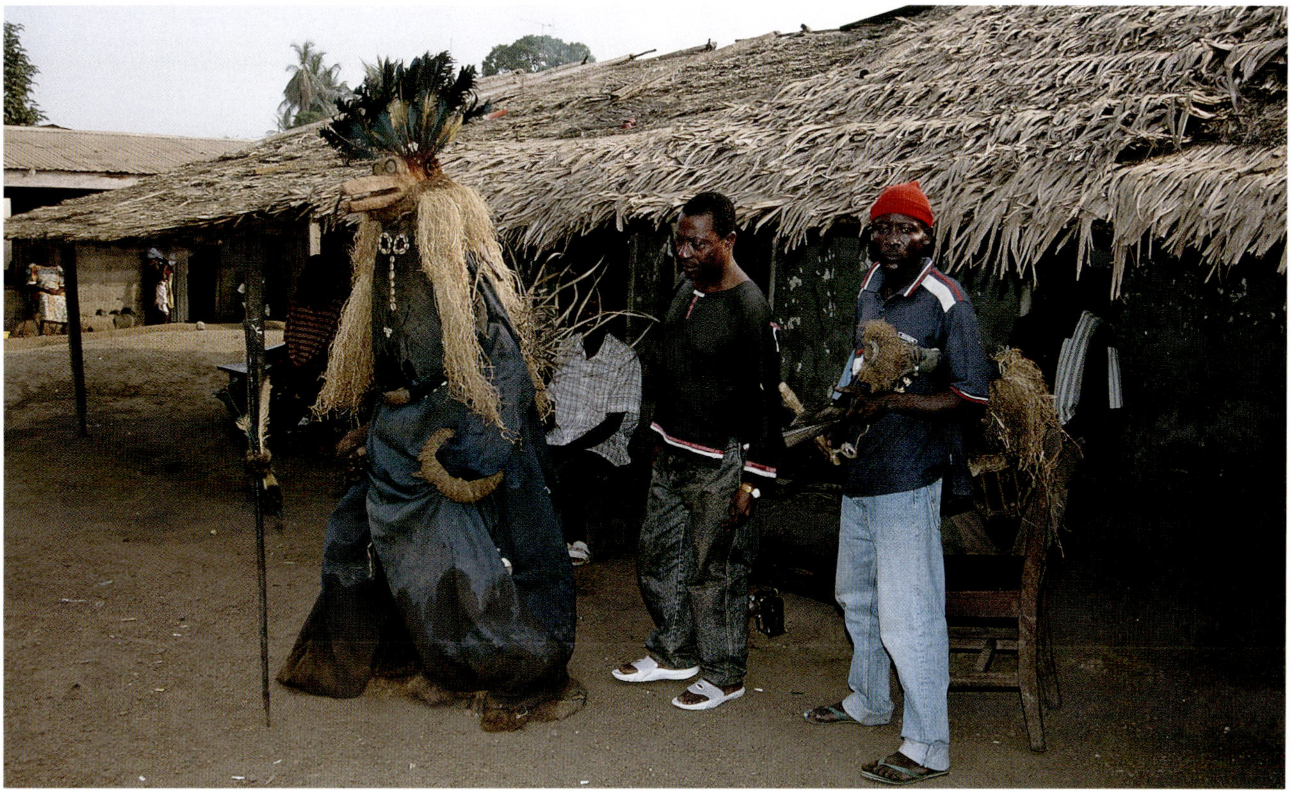

Fig. 176 *Obasinjom* with the interpreter and a person holding the *eturu Njom*, "trumpet" of *Obasinjom* (Kembong, January 30, 2004).

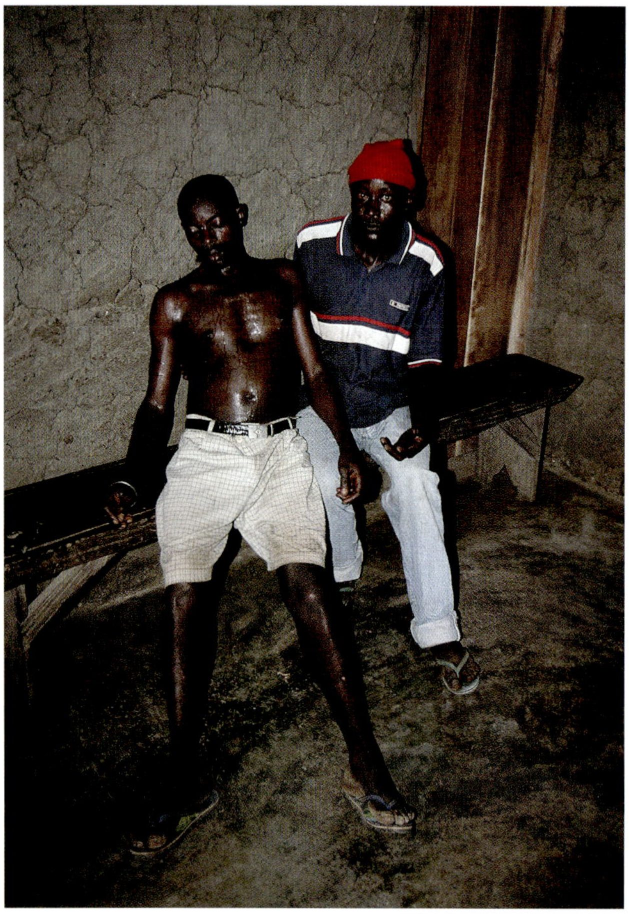

Figs. 177 The mantlebearer of *Obasinjom* immediately after the performance. He is attended to by members of the society (Kembong, January 30, 2004).

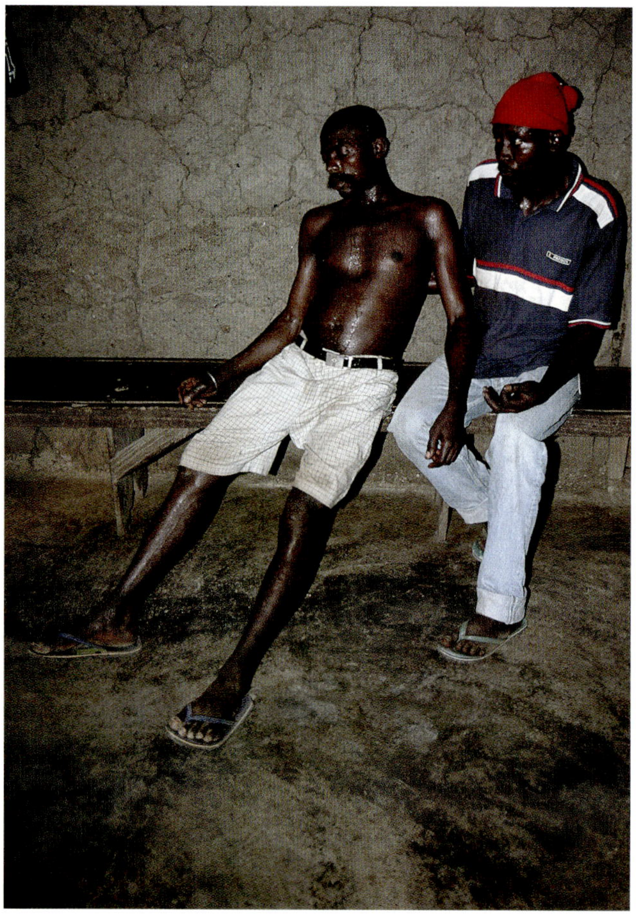

Fig. 178 In a state of exhaustion, he is still in a trance (Kembong, January 30, 2004).

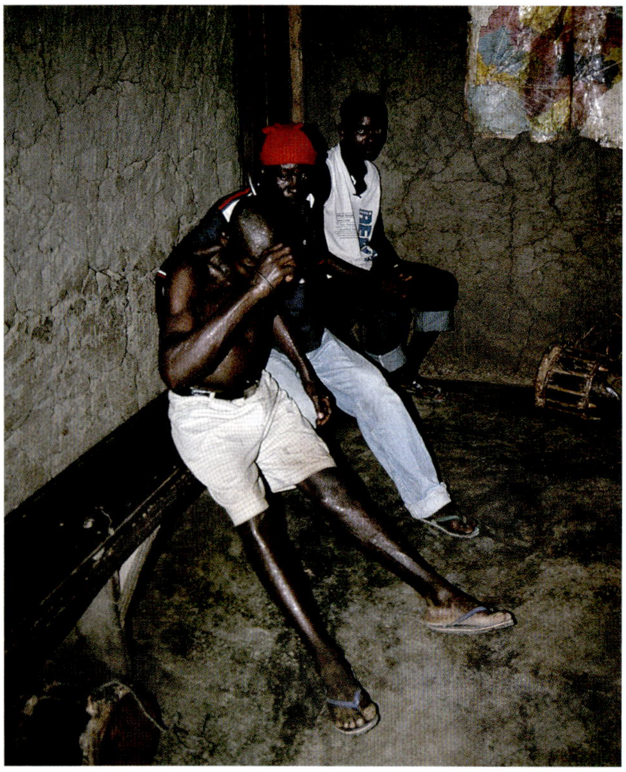

Fig. 179 Gradually, he regains consciousness (Kembong, January 30, 2004).

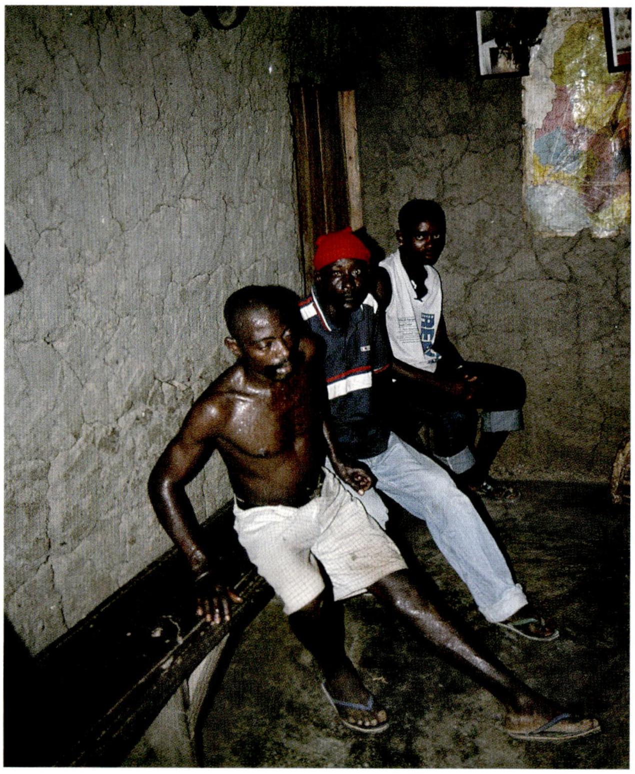

Fig. 180 About five minutes after leaving the mask garment, the mantlebearer of *Obasinjom* finally opens his eyes (Kembong, January 30, 2004).

5.5.4 Mask performances

Obasinjom fights evil powers directly with the help of its medicine or by activating the mask ("calling his dog"). In this way, humans are informed of the dangers threatening them, from which they can be saved only through *Obasinjom's* power. In principle, the mask can start action at any time; however, it may not come into contact with water, and for that reason its operations are limited during the rainy season. When the mask is to appear, it must first be activated, a procedure that sometimes commences one day before and, specifically, in the room in which the mask equipment is preserved. At that time the big man chews alligator pepper and spits it upon the mask headpiece (fig. 170). While stamping his right foot on the ground, he addresses *Obasinjom*: "Father, wake up. This family has come for you. Wake up and look what is wrong with them." Then he directs the client to rub his body with an egg, but without breaking it. When this is finished, the big man takes the egg into both hands and addresses the mask anew: "Mr. X has brought this egg for you, he has taken all his problems to it. So you can show him what is wrong with him."[21] The big man breaks the egg and spreads the contents over the mask headpiece and the mask garment as well as the *besom Njom* and the *efune Njom* . He pushes the egg shell down the mouth of the mask (fig. 199). The ritual concludes with an offering of whisky. The big man fills a glass with whisky and holds it in both hands. He takes a sip and then pours the major part on the ground in offering to the ancestors, or he pours it into the mask's mouth: "We have taken our own drinks. This is your own. Take it and drink it in order to follow up this matter" (fig. 171). He then pours the remaining whisky on *besom Njom*, *efune Njom* and the back of the mask's head, the so-called brain-box. The corresponding prayer made in 1980 was as follows: "Father, something has come that needs your attention. I invite you to speak the truth. Tell us what you see. Don't sleep, fight evil."

Aside from the "trumpet" (*eturu*), which is a part of all mask performances, every appearance of the mask is accompanied by music, for which the society keeps special instruments: two larger drums (*mpkile*, sg. *ekpile*), a short drum, a few woven rattles (*akachak*) and an iron double bell (*nkankang*). The most important instrument is the big slit-drum (*eyok*), which belongs to the general public. The slit-drum is played only on special occasions, and these include the performances of *Obasinjom*. These instruments may be played by non-members as well, because – and this was emphasised to me – *Obasinjom* belongs to the whole community. Songs are sung during performances to praise and to please *Obasinjom*.

The following description of a performance of *Obasinjom* is largely based on the appearance of the mask, which I witnessed in Kembong on January 25, 1980 (figs. 181–194). In the strict sense of the word the performance is not a "dance". I have seen other performances of Obasinjom, for example, in Ashum in the southern Banyang area on March 19, 1975, and again in Kembong on January 30, 2004 (figs. 170–180), but the experience in 1980 was probably the most interesting and impressive.[22]

In the early afternoon the mask equipment was already spread out neatly upon a table in the compound of the leader for all to see (figs. 181–182).[23] Music-making had long since commenced (fig. 189), but the mantlebearer had still not appeared. The two big men, Tanyiashu and John Etchu, gradually became uneasy, indeed angry, and several times they commanded *Obasinjom* to call its dog (figs. 183–184). Daylight started to wane and twilight descended, when the mantlebearer finally appeared, in a deep trance, his eyes glassy and fixed on the ground, his hands trembling (fig. 185). Although it is conceivable that he could have taken some sort of drugs between the time that he heard the music and his actual entrance, my informants denied this vehemently. Oblivious to his surroundings, the mantlebearer rushed toward the mask and mantle, which seemed to attract him like a magnet. Some members of *Obasinjom* held the mantle open and the mantlebearer sprang inside, as if to save himself (fig. 186). In full view of the public they assisted him in dressing (fig. 187); then he picked up *besom Njom* and *efune Njom*. And with that the actual performance began.

Obasinjom left the compound, running out into the broad village street where the people had congregated, their expressions showing respect rather than fear (figs. 188–191). In the old days, said the elders, the villagers would not have dared to approach the mask as closely as they commonly do today. Nevertheless, it is still strictly taboo to touch the mantle. Nor are spectators permitted to touch the low-hanging eaves of the roofs of the surrounding houses, for that would interfere with *Obasinjom*'s work. Accompanied by the interpreter and the "trumpet" player (the wife of *Obasinjom*, *mma Njom*, was absent on that day), the mask moved with quick steps towards the spectators. Frequently it stopped, throwing back its head as if listening, then bending down and pressing an ear to the ground as though receiving important information. The mask assumed the latter position too, when it held the *besom Njom* to its ear. Crossing the village square several times, it returned to the music makers and, with a downward and sideways motion, interrupted the music: *Obasinjom* had something to say.

Performance of *Obasinjom* (Kembong, January 25, 1980) (figs. 181–194).

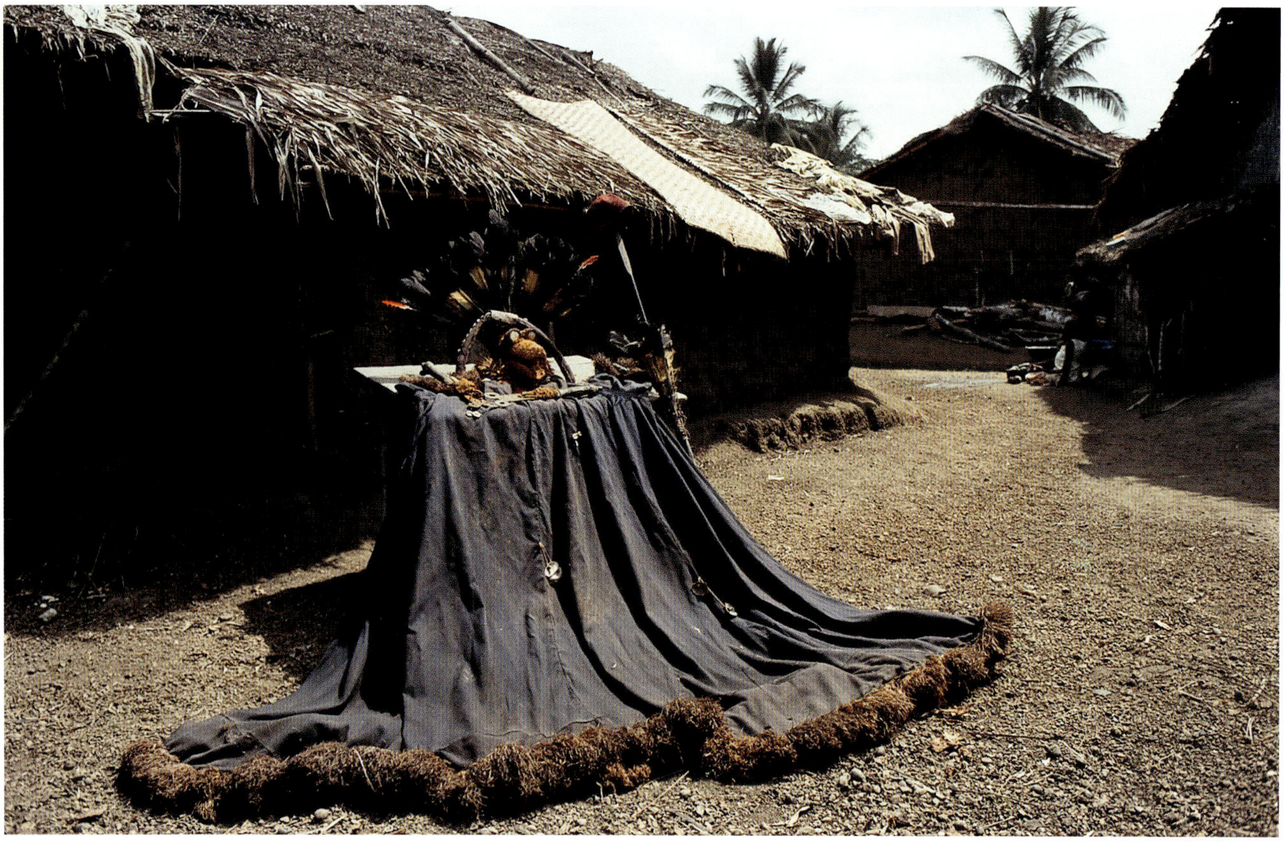

Fig. 181 The mask on display in public, in anticipation of the mantlebearer (Kembong, January 25, 1980).

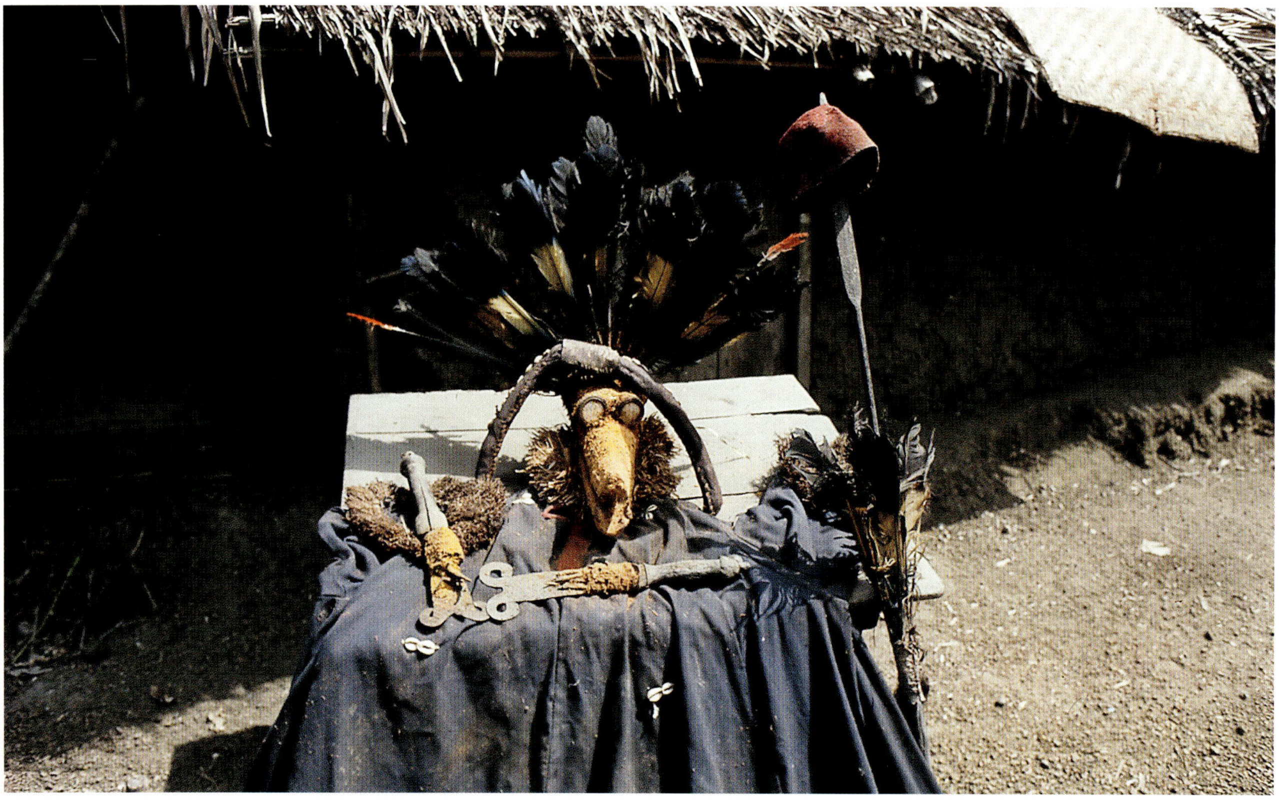

Fig. 182 Two *asom Njom* lying in front of and to the left of the mask headdress; above the headdress, *mbenghe Njom*, the "heart of *Obasinjom*"; on the right implanted in the earth is the staff of *Obasinjom* with the red cap for the mantlebearer (Kembong, January 25, 1980).

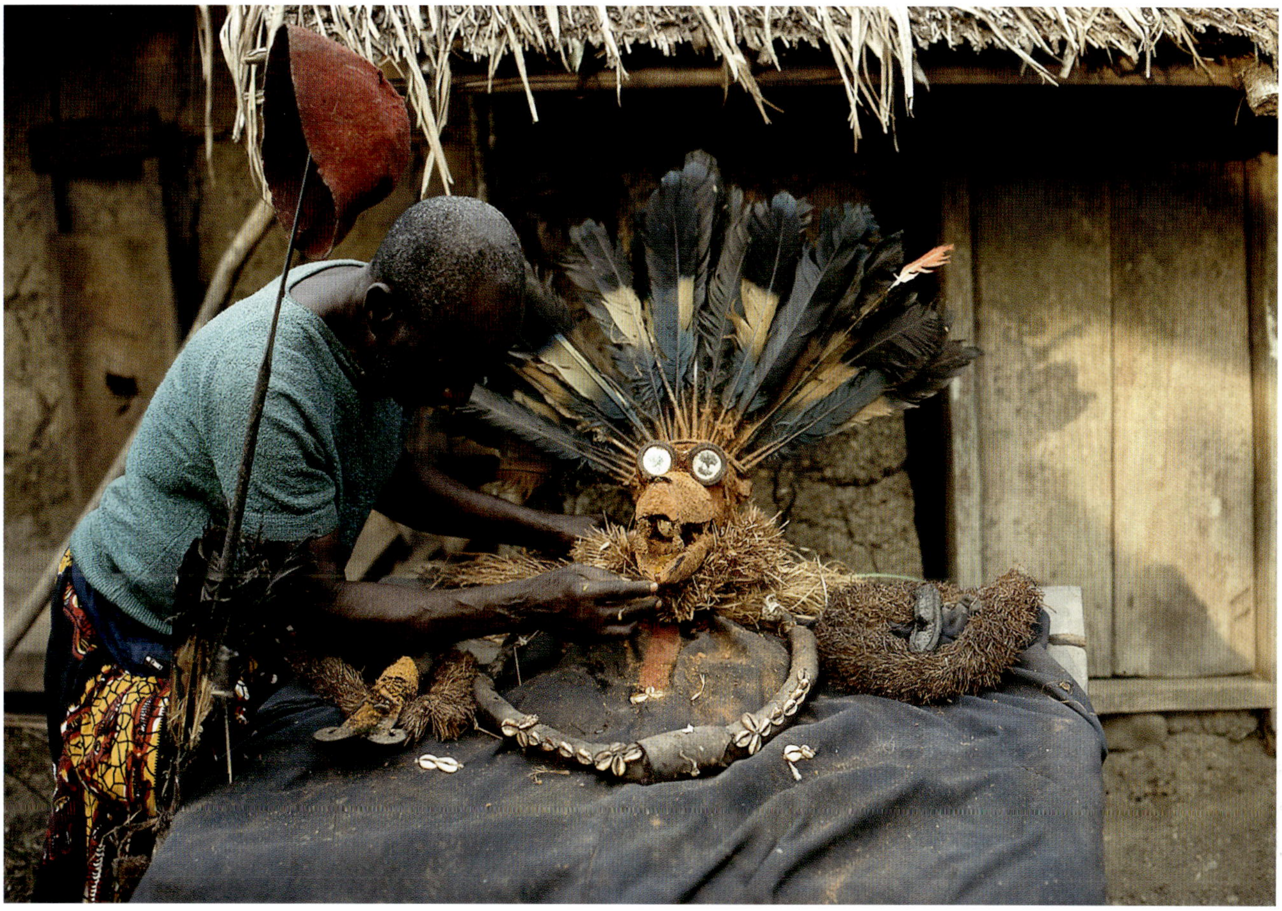

Fig. 183 John Etchu, one of the leaders of *Obasinjom*, exhorting the mask to look for its mantlebearer (Kembong, January 25, 1980).

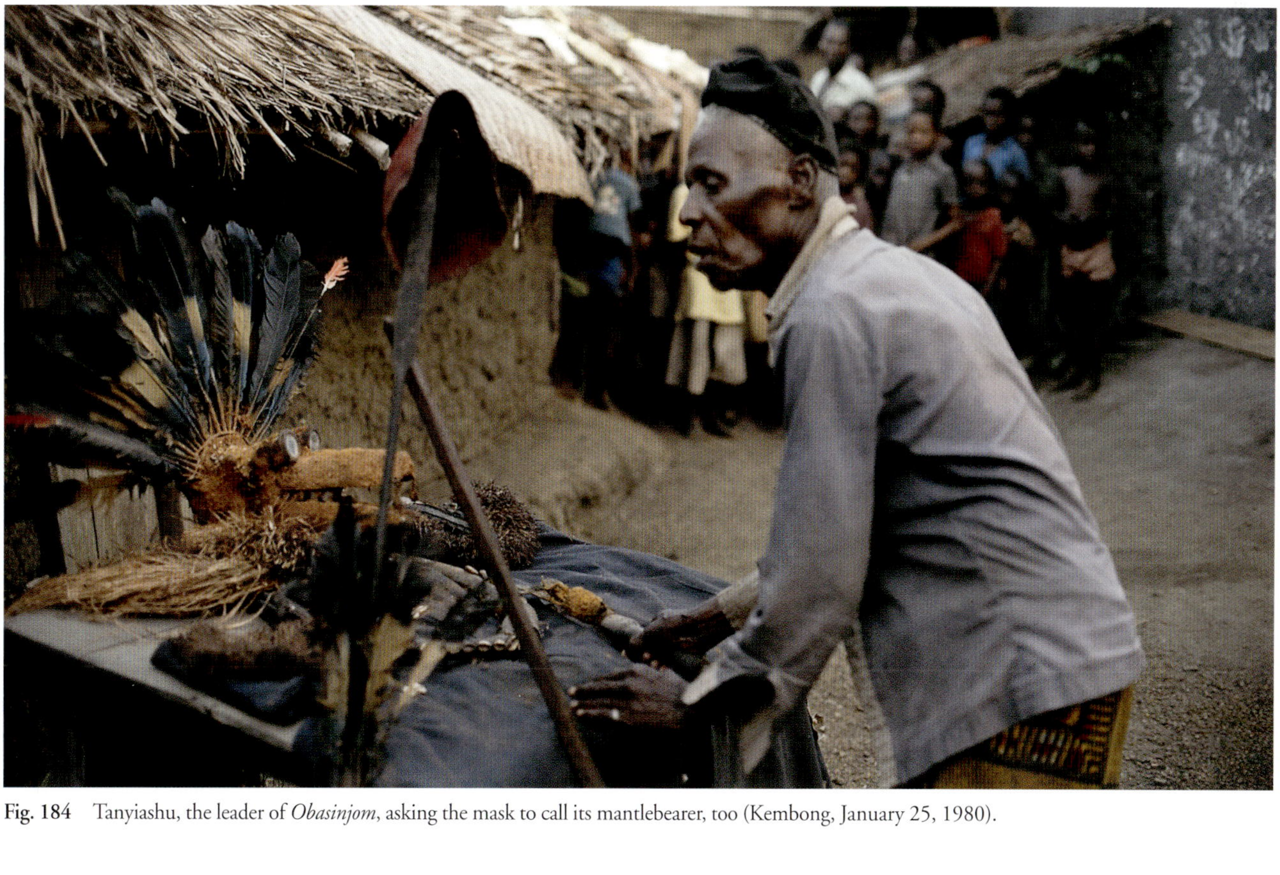

Fig. 184 Tanyiashu, the leader of *Obasinjom*, asking the mask to call its mantlebearer, too (Kembong, January 25, 1980).

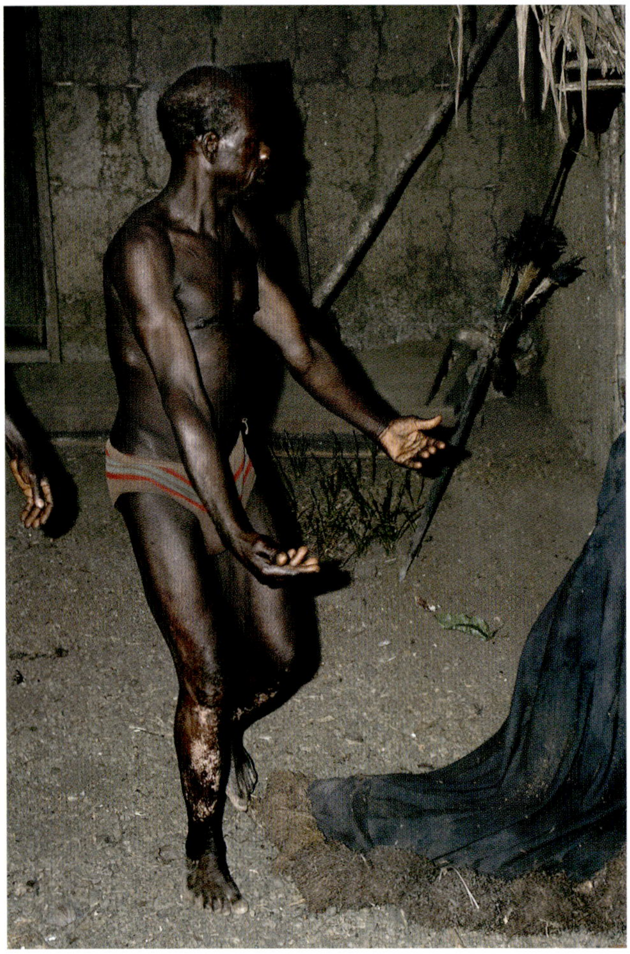

Fig. 185 The arrival of the mantlebearer – Johnson Ateke – in the evening. He is in a trance (Kembong, January 25, 1980).

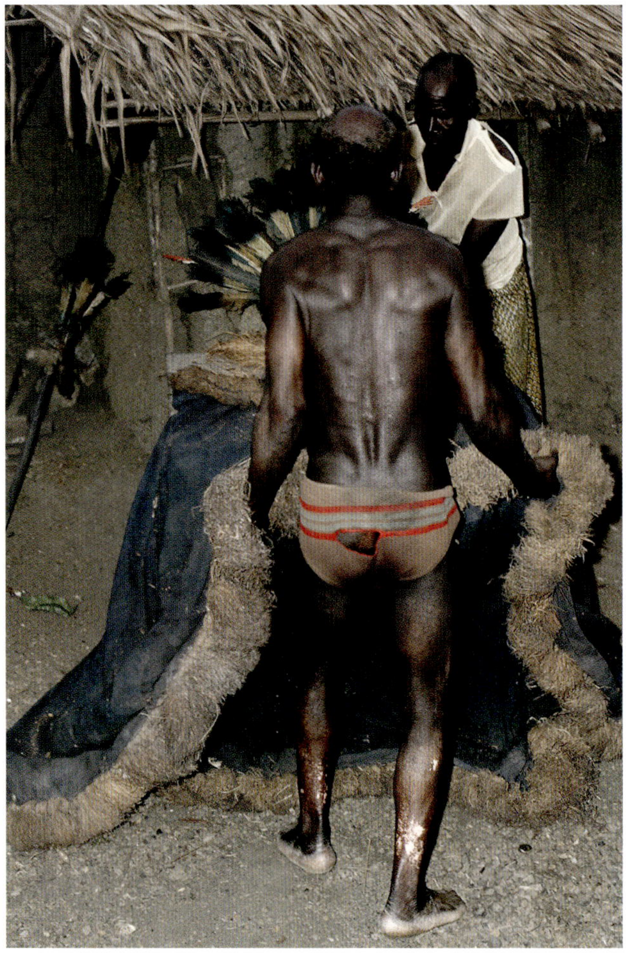

Fig. 186 The mantlebearer rushes towards the mask headdress and garment, which seem to attract him like a magnet (Kembong, January 25, 1980).

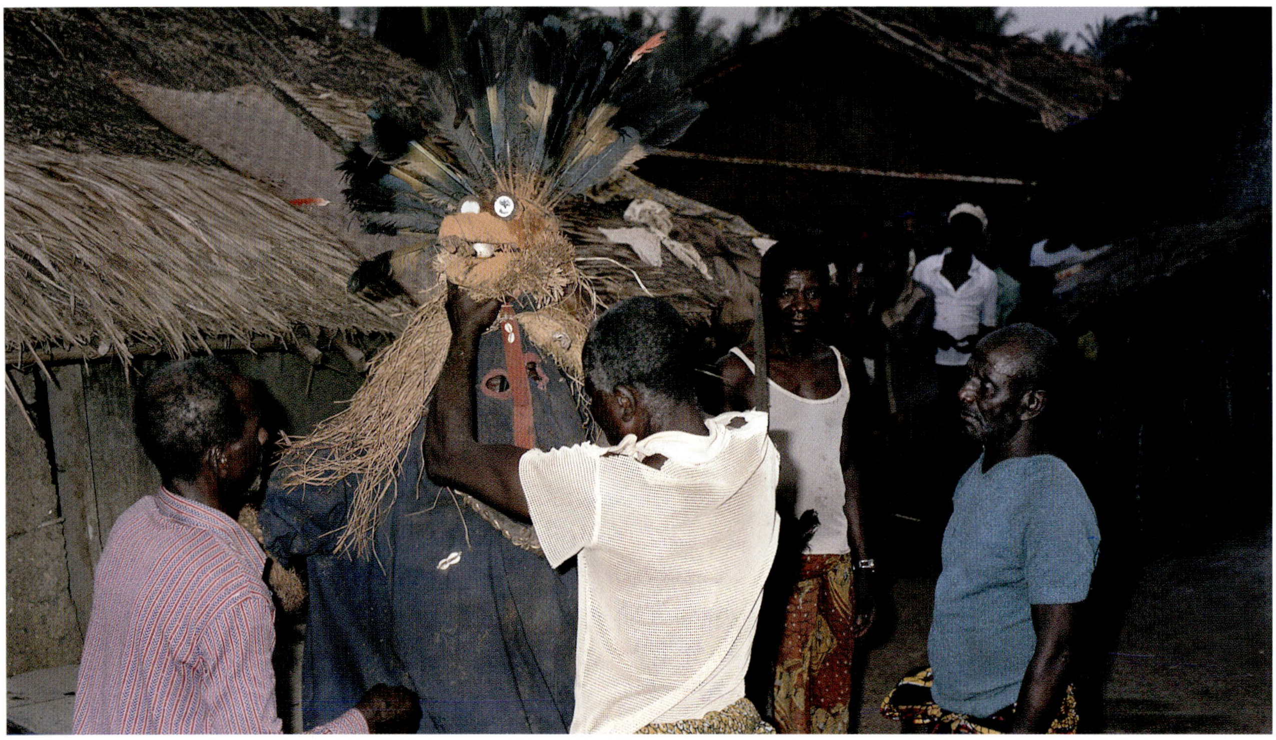

Fig. 187 The mantlebearer dons the garment hastily, assisted by some members (Kembong, January 25, 1980).

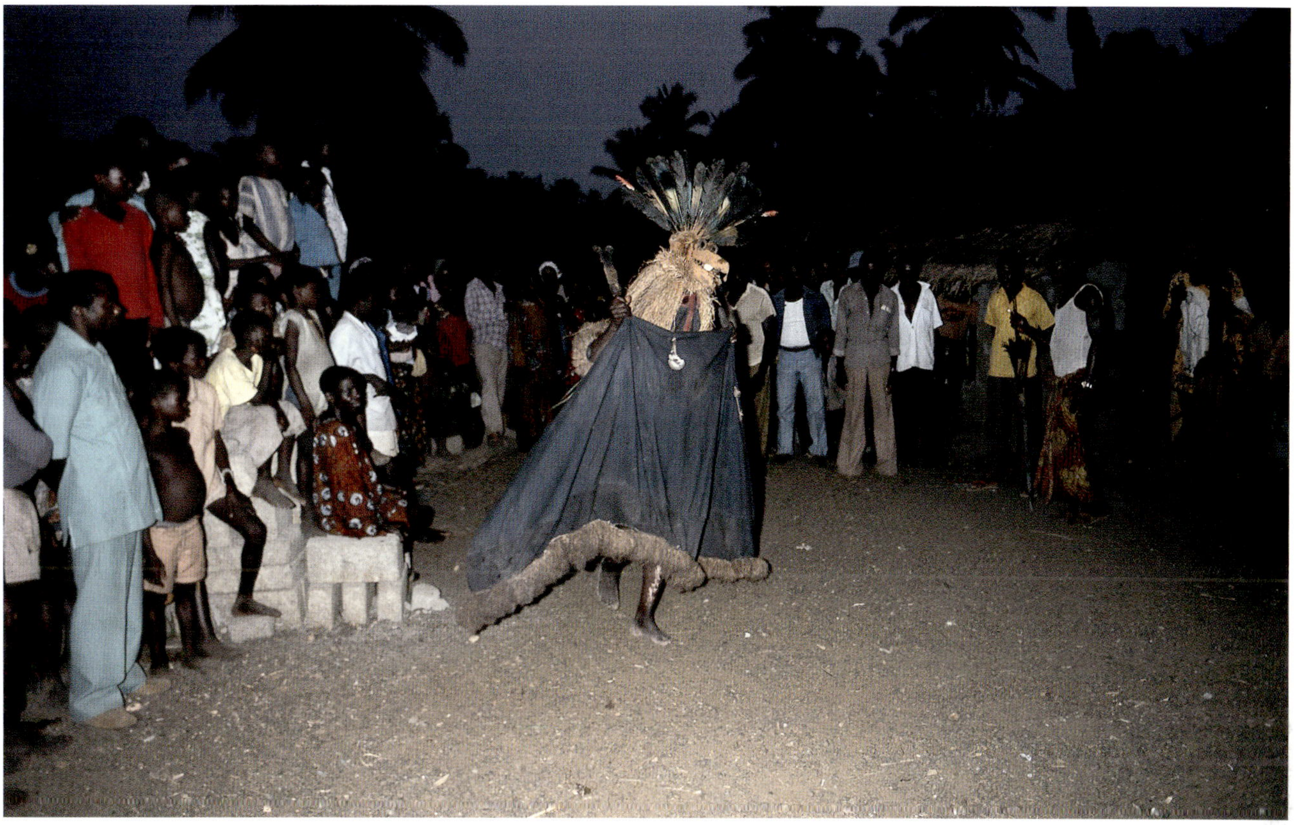

Fig. 188 Performance of *Obasinjom* in the main street of Kembong in the evening (Kembong, January 25, 1980).

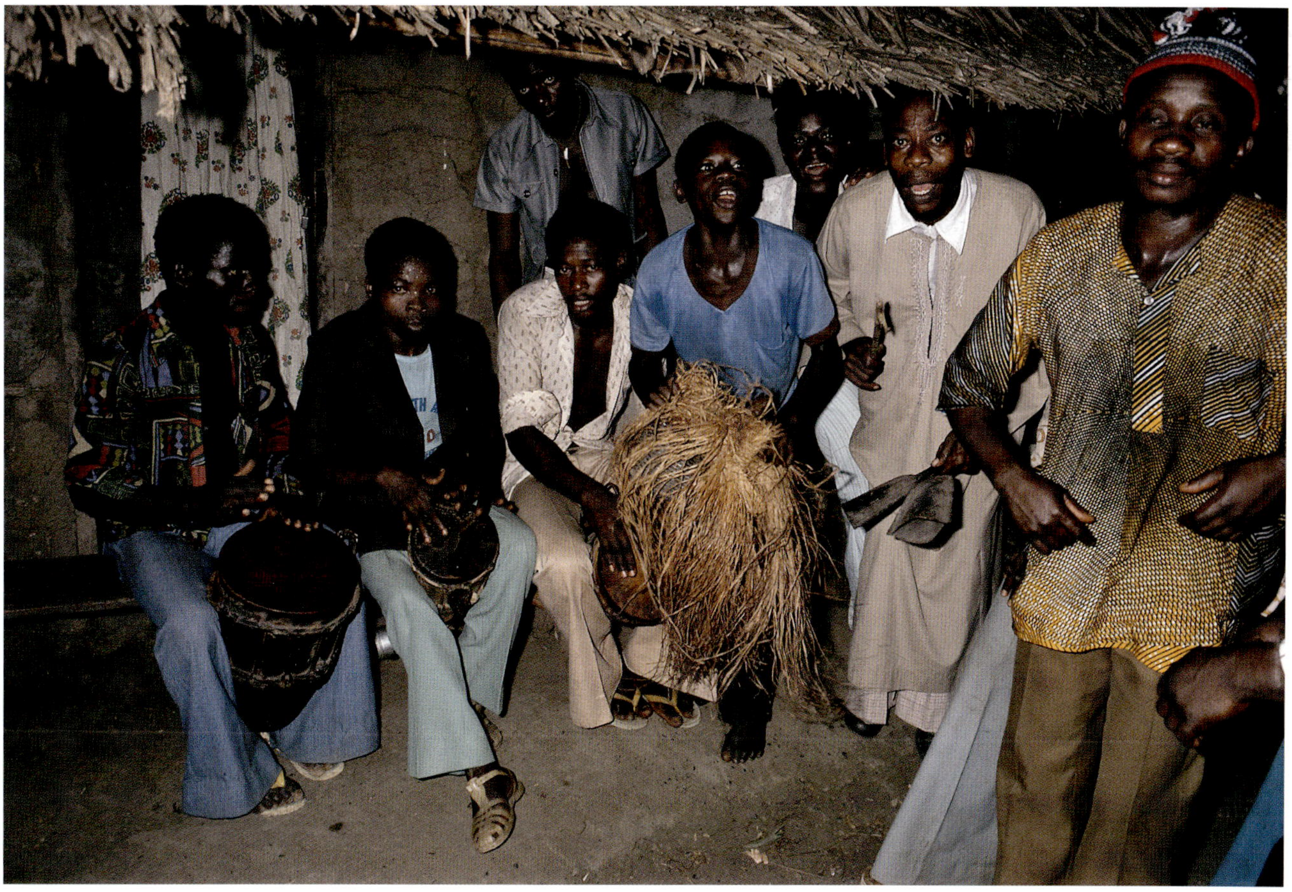

Fig. 189 Musicians with their drums and with the double bell (Kembong, January 25, 1980).

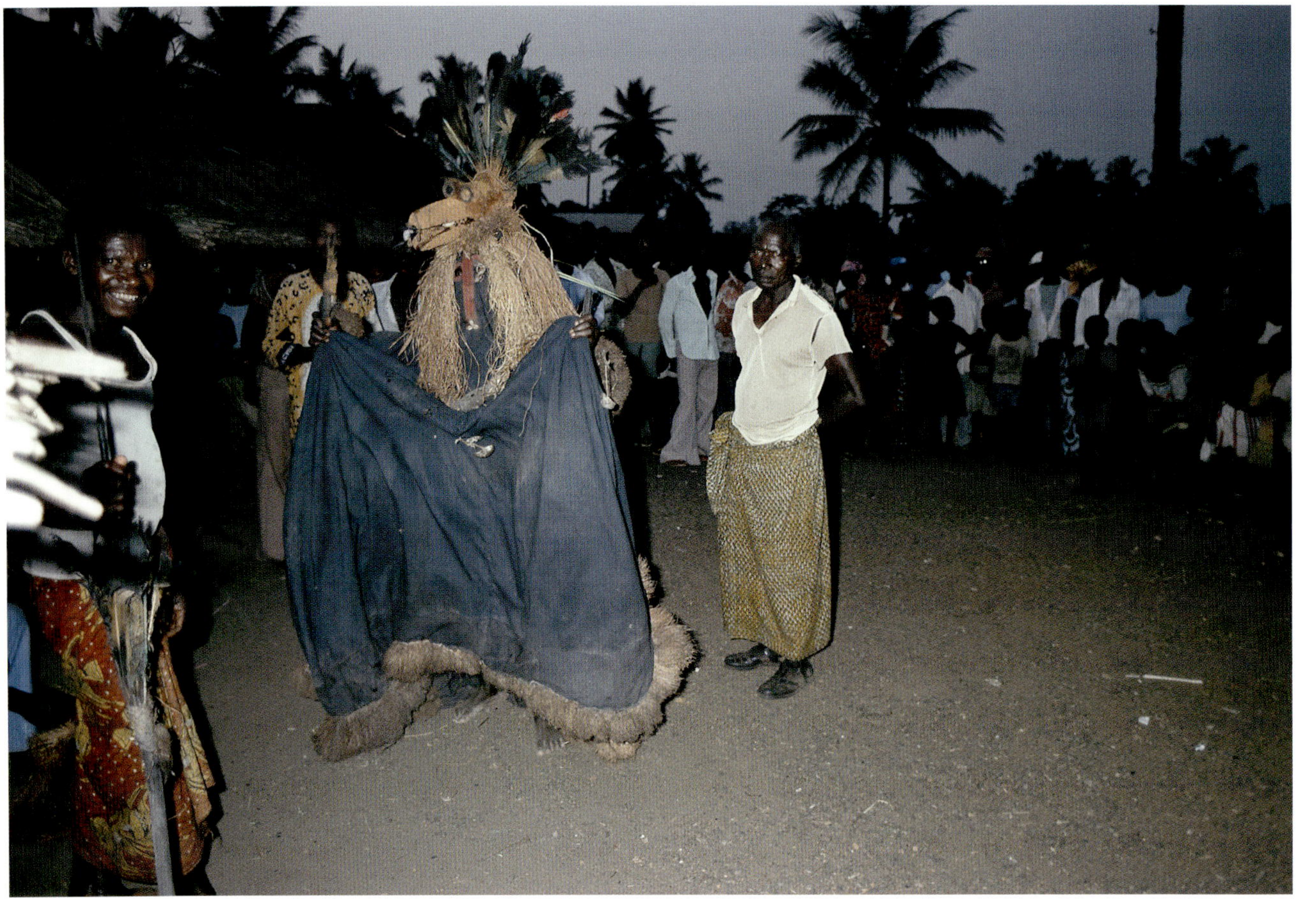

Fig. 190 *Obasinjom* in action (Kembong, January 25, 1980).

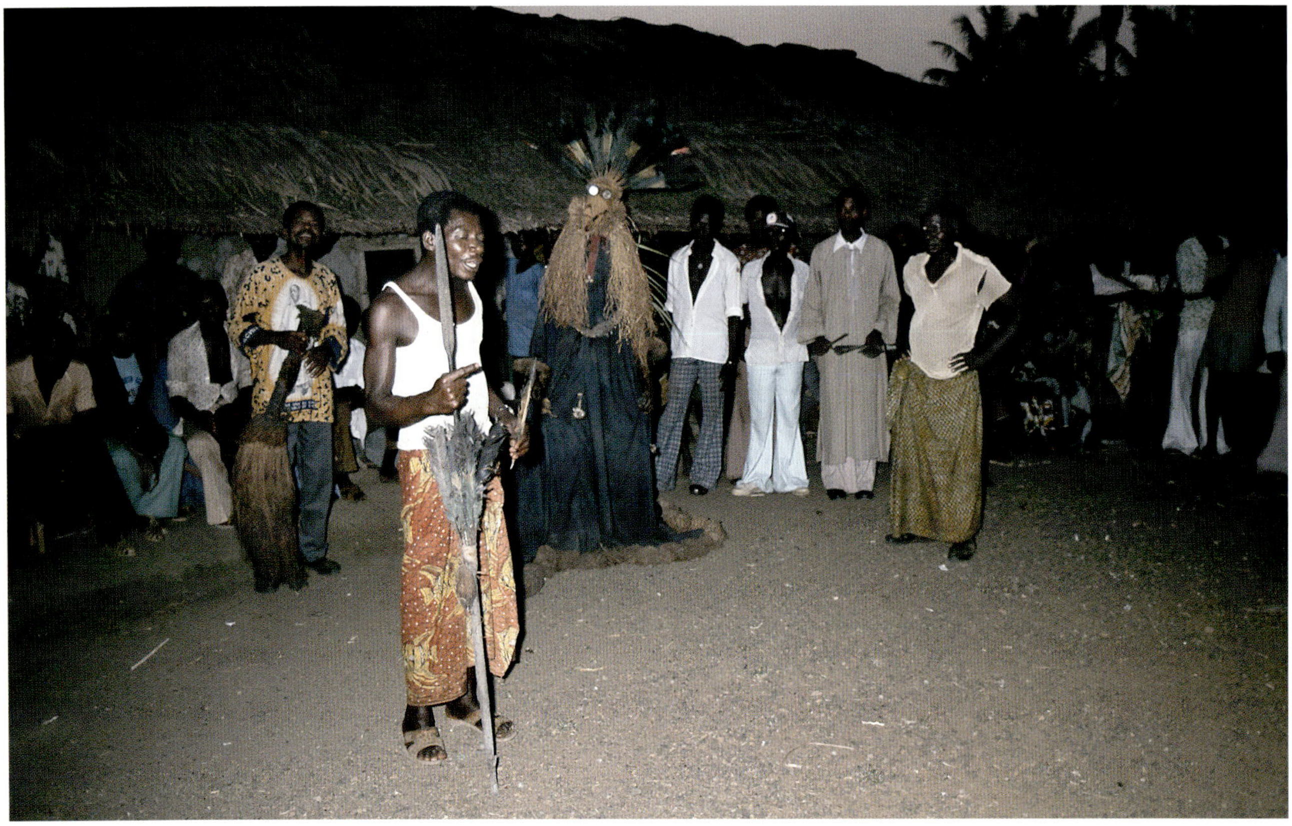

Fig. 191 *Obasinjom* and the interpreter with the staff, *osam Njom* (Kembong, January 25, 1980).

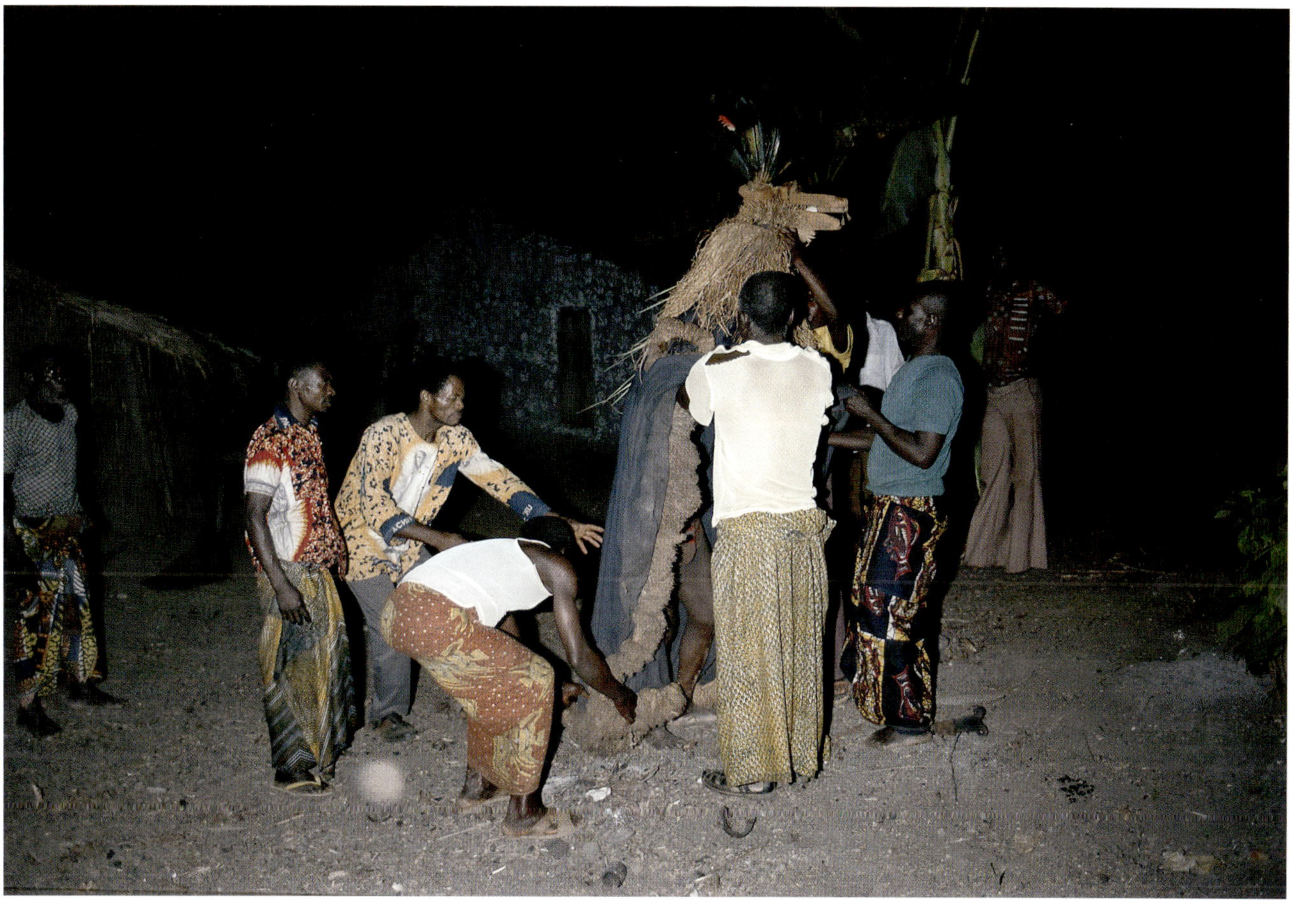

Fig. 192 Members assist the mantlebearer, who is still in a trance, to depart from the mask (Kembong, January 25, 1980).

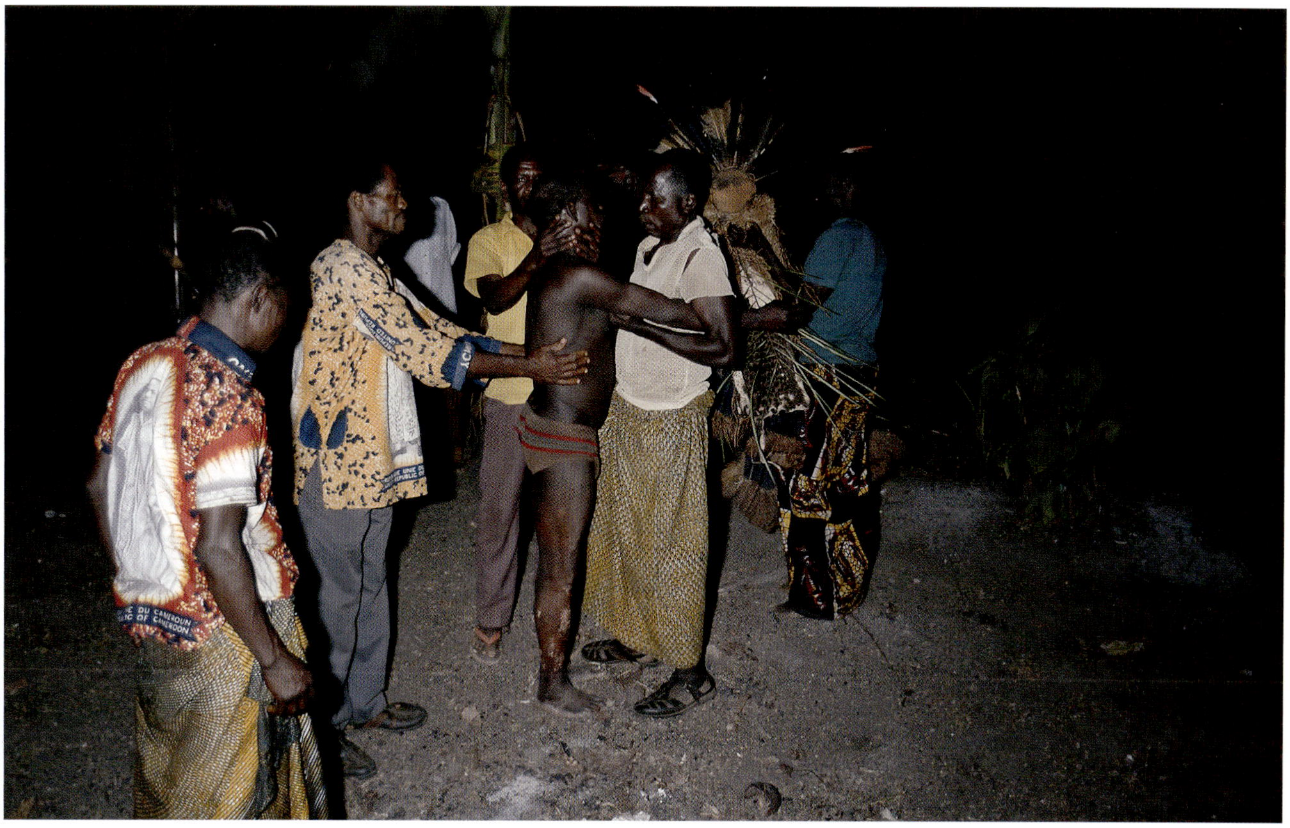

Fig. 193 The members shake the mantlebearer back to consciousness (Kembong, January 25, 1980).

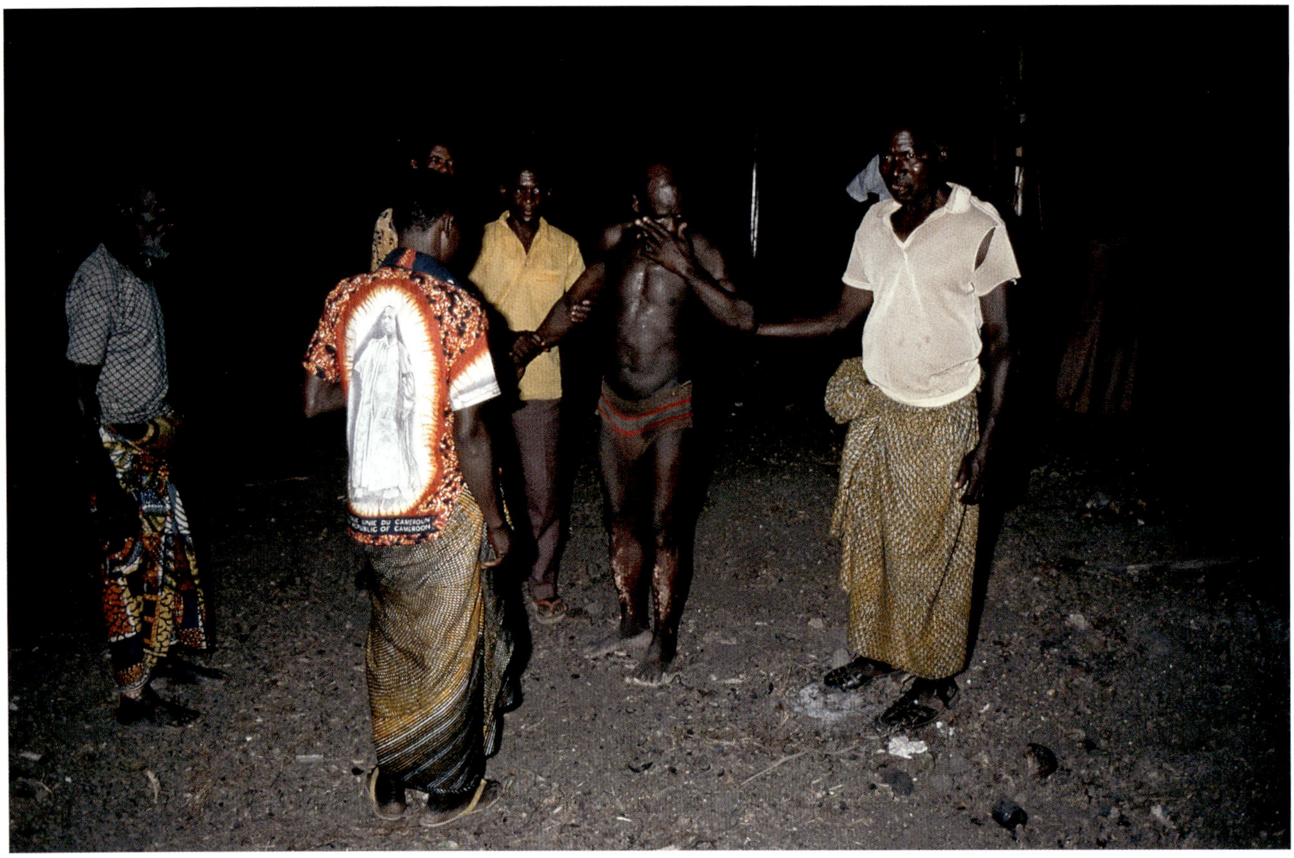

Fig. 194 The mantlebearer is still affected by his performance (Kembong, January 25, 1980).

The mask quietly addressed the interpreter, who translated for the spectators (fig. 191). Now *Obasinjom* answered the questions of petitioners; ordinarily it would not appear unless there were several cases to be heard. The mask might next dictate general rules of behaviour, including a warning against breaking laws. *Obasinjom* might also issue the command to shoot at a certain spot on the ground, where it had detected witches. Finally, the mask might address a bystander, publicly exposing him or her as a witch: "I give seven days for you to set your victim free, to make him to recover." This is notable, because among the Ejagham, anyone who unjustly accuses another person of being a witch is severely punished. Only once has someone rejected *Obasinjom*'s accusation; however, when the person followed the mask's command to spit on the mantle, he fell dead on the spot. Performances last about an hour, ending when the mask "dies". Members of *Obasinjom* freed the mantlebearer, who was still in a trance, from the mantle (fig. 192). Medicine was rubbed upon his forehead and chest, while a particularly strong man, clenching him tightly from behind, shook the mantlebearer's head and shoulders, restoring him to consciousness (fig. 193). The mantlebearer staggered aside, apparently still dizzy (fig. 194; cp. figs. 177–180).

Everyone knew the man who emerged from under the mantle. It was believed that he acted upon *Obasinjom*'s command, as an instrument of the medicine. He was not responsible for anything that had happened during the performance. In fact, the mantlebearer had no recollection of the performance, as he later told me. He was exhausted for several hours. The leader, Tanyiashu, concluded the performance with a prayer to the ancestors: "*Ata*, we have drunk, we come to the end. The whole of Kembong stands here. If someone has come to try you, teach him or her that you are more powerful. *Ata* Nkongho, you handed over your *Obasinjom* to me. We were many, but only eight are left. Take care of us and the entire community. We have drunk and we conclude the performance." Those present chorused in answer, "Yes". *Obasinjom* can take the initiative itself, when it sees calamity or danger approaching. At that moment *Obasinjom* itself can call one of its mantlebearers. The person called falls into a trance and puts on the mask garment.

When *Obasinjom* is engaged by a distant locality to destroy witches and other threatening forces, in some cases its magic drum, *ekpile Njom*, is deposited there a few days prior to the mask's appearance. *Ekpile Njom*

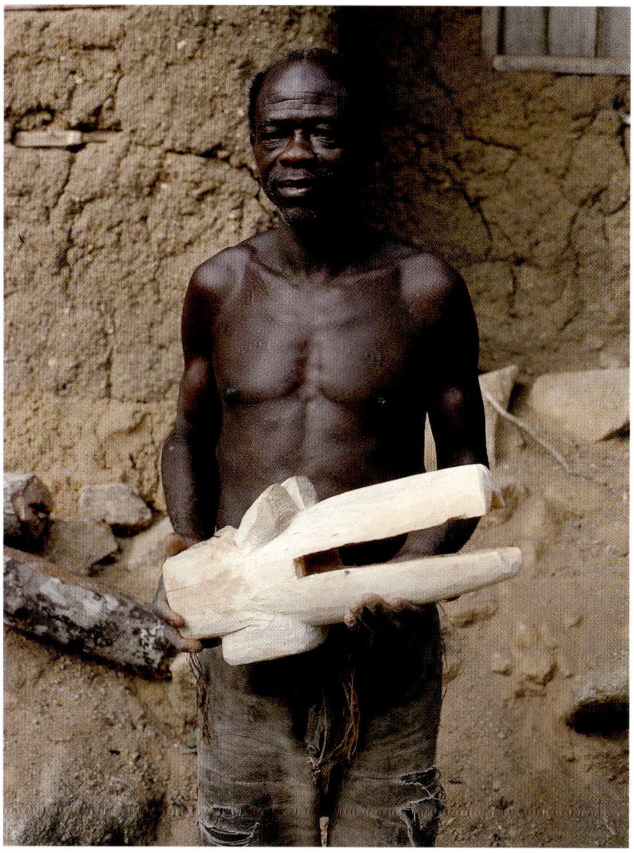

Fig. 195 Johnson Ateko, one of the mantlebearers of *Obasinjom*, holding a newly carved headpiece in the form of a crocodile (Kembong, February 15, 1980).

contains a mixture of medicines, which are found on the head of the mask. It has the power to block the roads leading to the locality, so that the offenders will have no chance of escaping *Obasinjom*. In addition, *ekpile Njom* supplies the mask with important information that aids in its pursuit of the offenders. Only the members of *atemambi*, the "heart of *Obasinjom*", know this medicine.

Ordinarily the performances of *Obasinjom* take place in the mask's own locality. As described in detail, the purpose of this action is to ward off and to pursue inimical and dangerous powers. There are certain characteristic warnings, threats, suspicions and accusations that are typical of *Obasinjom*'s actions, through which *Obasinjom* seeks to restore peace and quiet to the community and to make it secure. Actions of the mask for reasons other than performances are relatively seldom. One such unusual event occurred on April 22, 2004, when *Obasinjom* set out to a farm some three kilometres north of Upper Kembong to find "bad medicine", through which – as everyone was convinced – two people had already been killed. I wondered whether *Obasinjom* would be able to accomplish this task convincingly for all (figs. 196–206).

In this case the source of all the problems with which the locality had long been concerned were conflicts over an inheritance. Upon the death of a man, one of his three wives felt herself cheated by the way in which the inheritance was regulated. This led to serious conflicts within the family. They escalated when the two children, who had already reached adulthood, of one of the two other women died in close succession. The Traditional Council in Kembong was notified, and ultimately three well-known diviners confirmed what had long been suspected: namely, the wife who was dissatisfied with the inheritance had killed both children, in particular, through bad medicine, which had been concealed on the farm of her mother. In order to prevent further misdeeds, *Obasinjom* was finally called to find the bad medicine and destroy it.

On this day of such great import for the entire community, the members of *Obasinjom* had already assembled in the house of the big man before eight o'clock in the morning. The mask garment and accompanying equipment had been placed in a metal box, which, however, had no cover. Thus, the mask garment was visible for everyone (fig. 196). Before the box was carried by one of the younger members (upon his head) to the cocoa farm (fig. 197), the big man turned repeatedly and notably often to the mask and addressed it as follows: "I am splashing this alligator pepper on your head to give you strength and power to see and to talk and to remove the thing. Whether the thing is hidden in the water, in the sky or anywhere else, bring it up to us. Father, I am sending you to war. If the one does not die, the other one must die." – "Father, you are the leader, who leads us to all places. Lead us to the bush, where we are now going. Hold us hand by hand, while we are going to the bush. If somebody pushes you – you also push him down." – "Father, take alligator pepper and eat it. Anybody who wants to argue with us or is against us that we should not do our work, you should attack the person accordingly." – "Everything has an end. People all over have come to end this matter today. Here before you is the X family. They have come and ask you to do your work. Follow them and bring us victory."

The cocoa farm, which through the envy and greed of a woman was said to have been changed into an "evil forest", was actually a dense forest of trees and underbrush. It was quite dark, hard to see and – as soon became obvious – covered quite a large area. The mask garment was spread out in the presence of some 30 to 40 people, among them numerous women. Then the big man began to activate the mask in the usual way, by fulfilling its demands for alligator pepper, whisky and

***Obasinjom* is engaged to find and destroy bad medicine on a farm (Kembong, April 22, 2004) (figs. 196–206).**

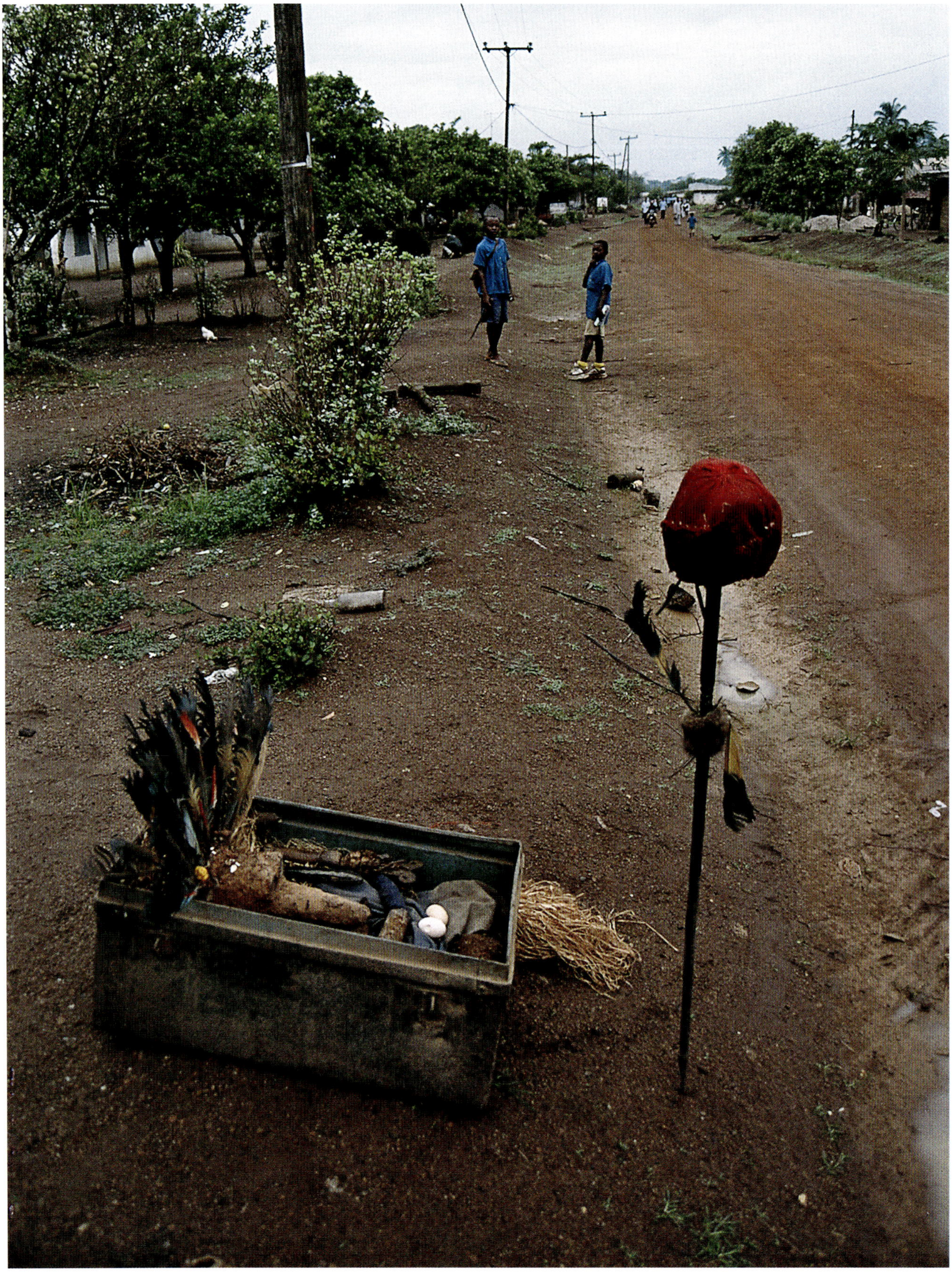

Fig. 196 Equipment for *Obasinjom* in a metal box on the main street in Kembong (Kembong, April 22, 2004).

an egg, and by repeatedly referring to its duties and calling for it to be successful and victorious (figs. 198–199). In view of the extraordinary tasks on that day a cock was sacrificed as well (fig. 200). One of the elders killed the cock by wringing the animal's neck until the head separated from the body. He let the blood flow over the mask headpiece. Then the mask bearer appeared. He was in a trance, with glassy staring eyes and trembling outstretched hands. A few minutes before I had seen how he had departed from the people present and in the accompaniment of another man had taken a few puffs at a cigarette. The big man placed a red cap, which belongs to the mask equipment, upon the head of the mask bearer[24] and spoke: "Father go gently. Remove the shoes and come forward and take the gown." Quick as lightning the mask bearer grabbed the lower part of the garment, held it up high and drew it over his body (figs. 201–202). A few minutes passed before the mask, with the help of a few *Obasinjom* members, was fully dressed and ready for action.

With a few quick steps the mask separated from the group and constantly looked in all directions, as if orienting itself. Again and again it swept *besom Njom* across the ground and then held its ear to the ground, and all the persons present knew that the mask was calling for information. The interpreter, *osame Njom*, who occasionally spoke to the mask, was always near it. The mask moved forwards slowly, looking to the left and right with some uncertainty (figs. 203–204). Some twenty minutes had gone by, when *Obasinjom* suddenly stormed up the slope at such a pace that the men and women could hardly follow it. After about 300 m it stopped abruptly. Its movements with the head and arms became more and more rapid. Now the mask conveyed a nervous and hectic impression, as if something was irritating it and making it insecure, and this affected the whole group as well. At that moment one of the *Obasinjom* members distributed the most important medicine, *nchip Njom*, which each person rubbed on their bodies as a protection against hostile influences (fig. 205). Obviously the mask was close to its objective. After several minutes of further searching and hunting, during which the interpreter spoke with the mask noticeably often, it suddenly pointed with *besom Njom* at a place beneath a tree. Upon the directions of the interpreter one of the men began to dig a hole in the ground at that place with his cutlass. And, indeed, at a depth of c. 50 cm he found a bottle (fig. 206). The bad medicine had been discovered. In order to render it harmless, the remaining *nchip Njom* medicine was poured over it. With that the danger and

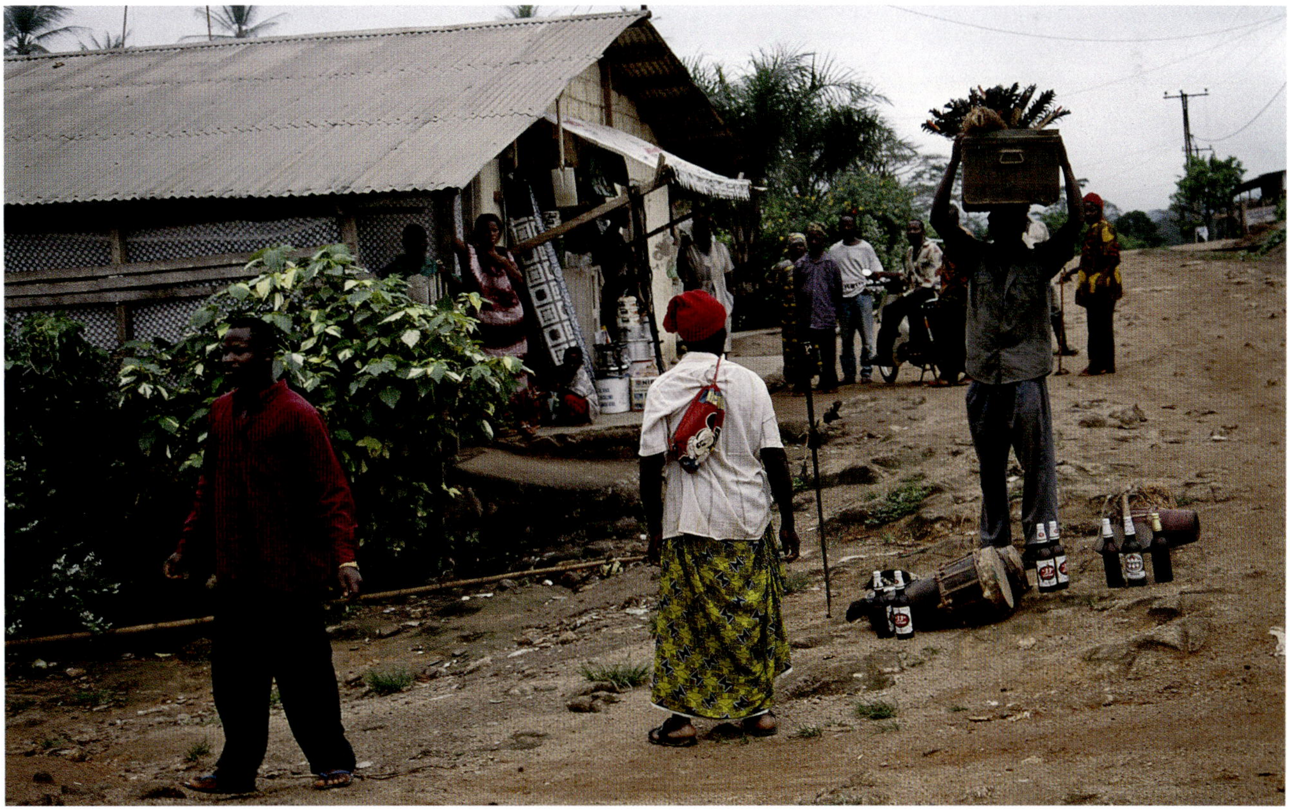

Fig. 197 A young member of *Obasinjom* carries the metal box to the farm (Kembong, April 22, 2004).

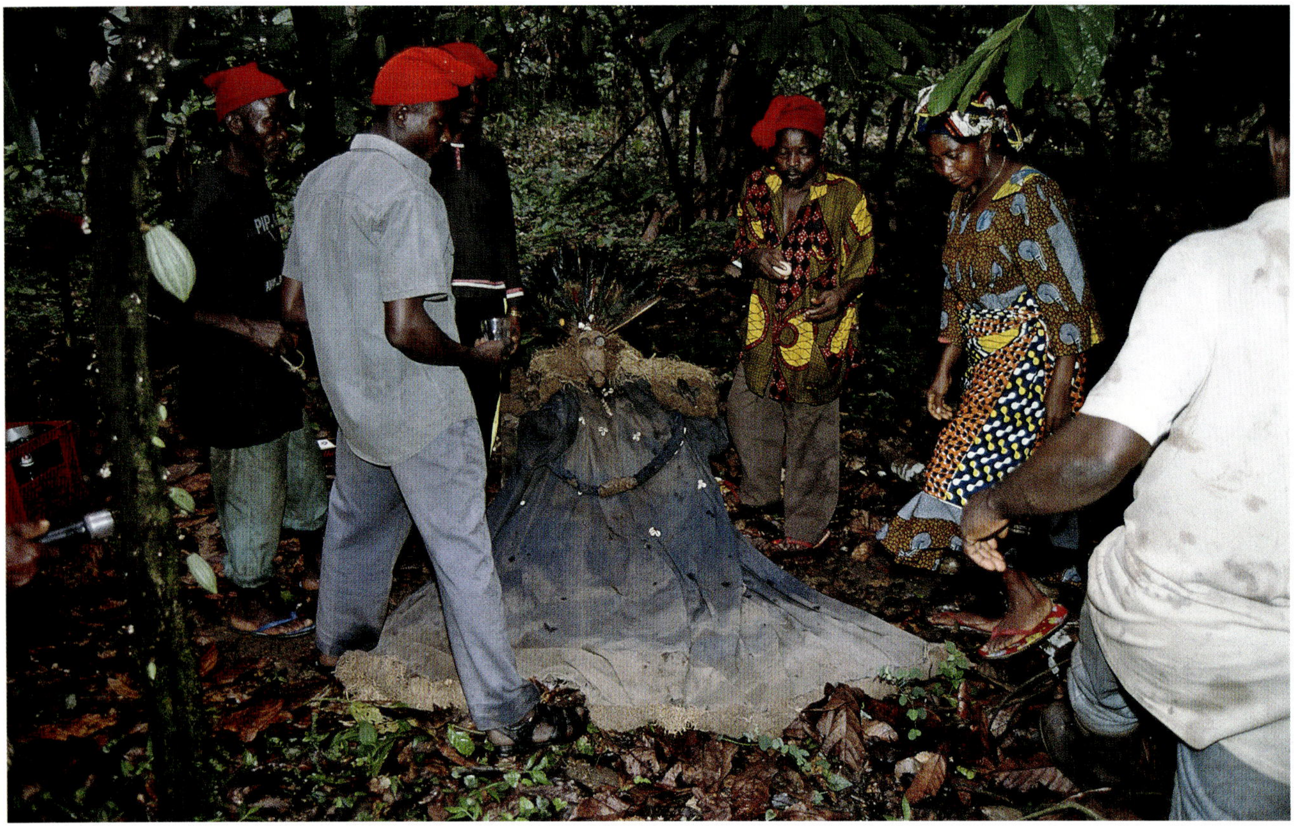

Fig. 198 The mask garment and equipment are spread on the ground and activated, even in the presence of a woman (Kembong, April 22, 2004).

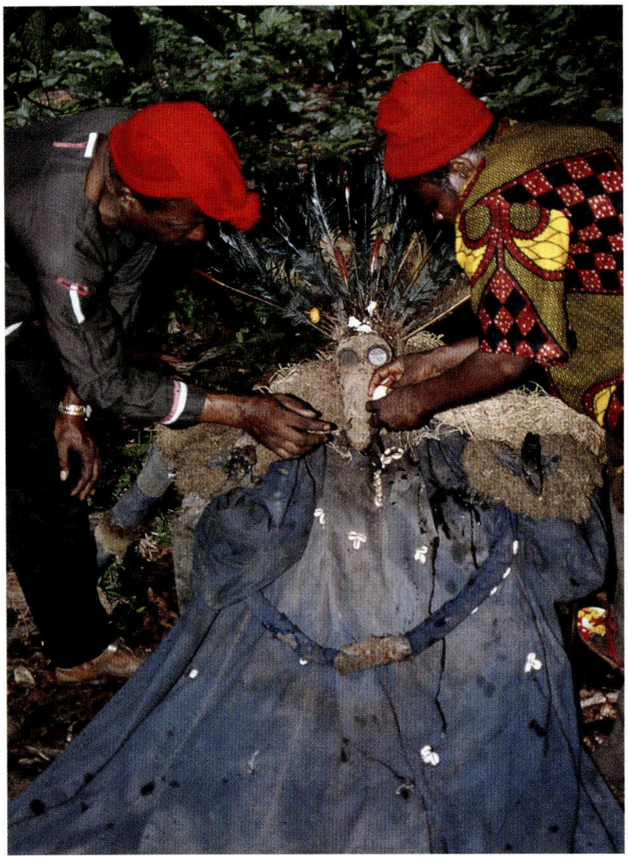

Fig. 199 In offering, alligator pepper is spit upon the headdress and whisky poured into its mouth; finally an egg is offered and its shell placed in the mouth (Kembong, April 22, 2004).

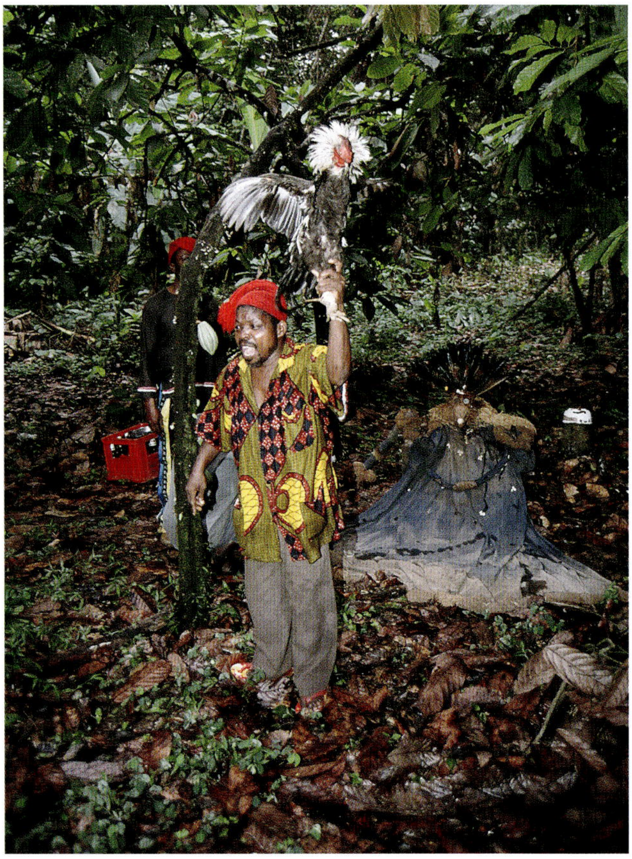

Fig. 200 A cock is sacrificed by the leader of *Obasinjom*, Adolf Ojong Agbor (Kembong, April 22, 2004).

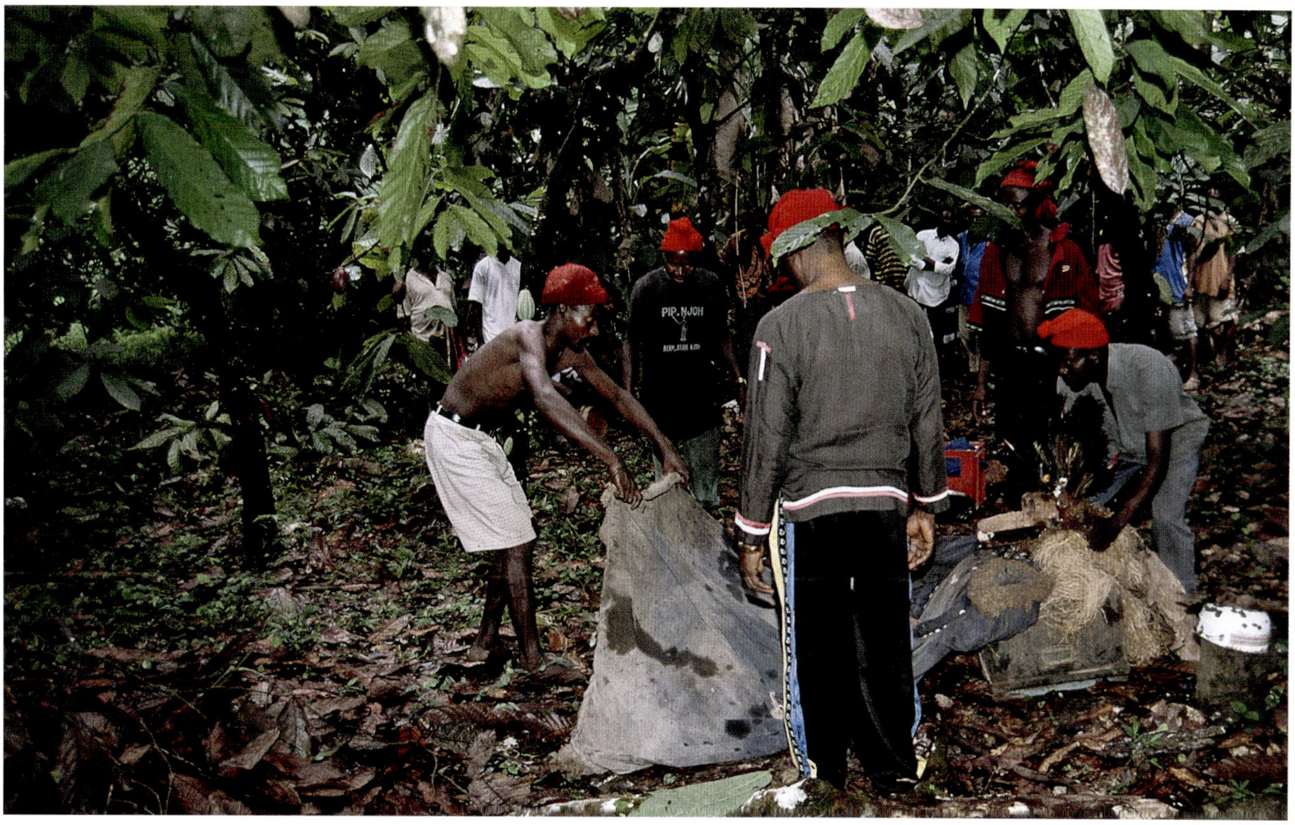

Fig. 201 The mantlebearer wearing a red cap appears in a trance and grasps the mask garment (Kembong, April 22, 2004).

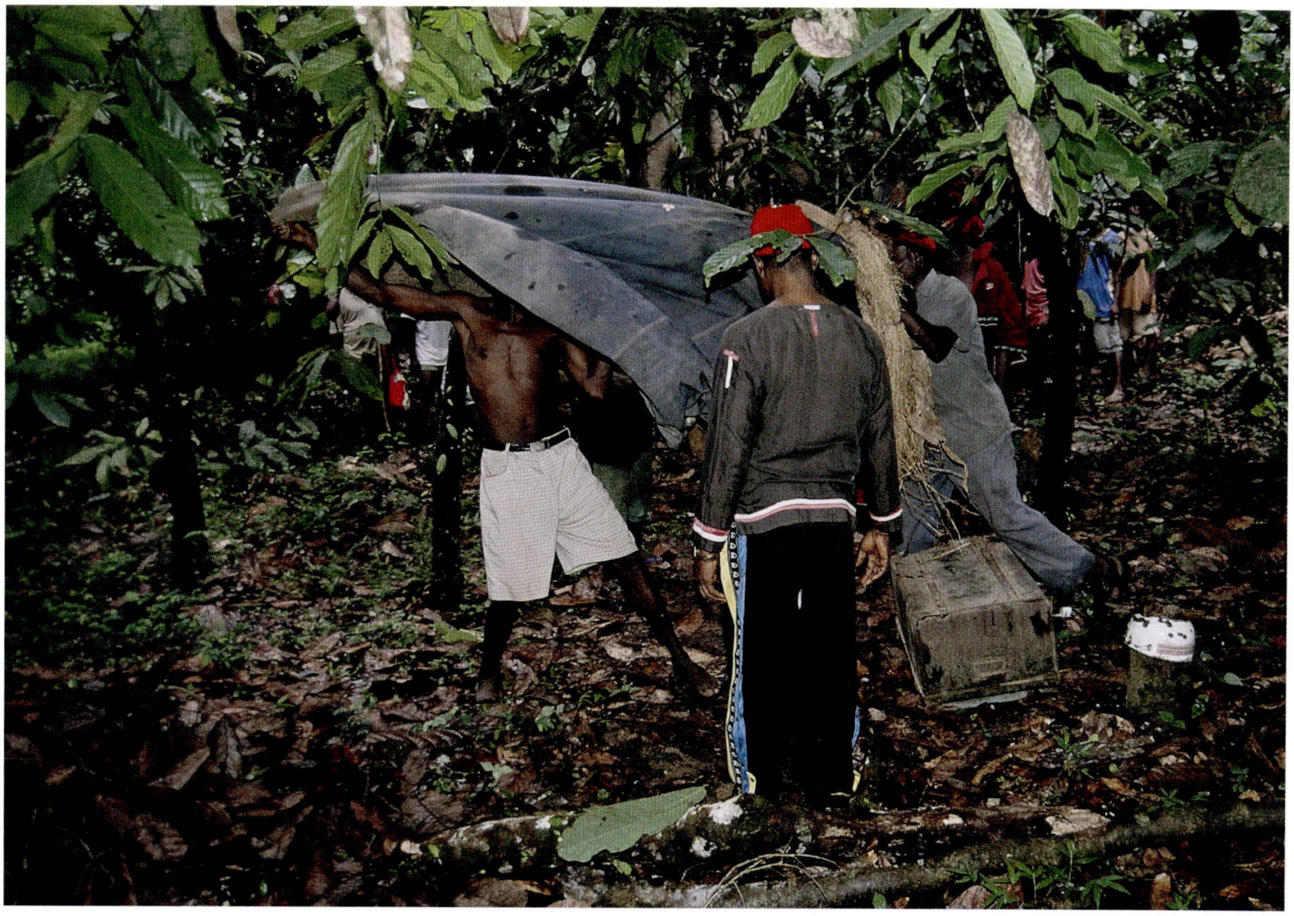

Fig. 202 In a split second the mantlebearer pulls the garment over his body (Kembong, April 22, 2004).

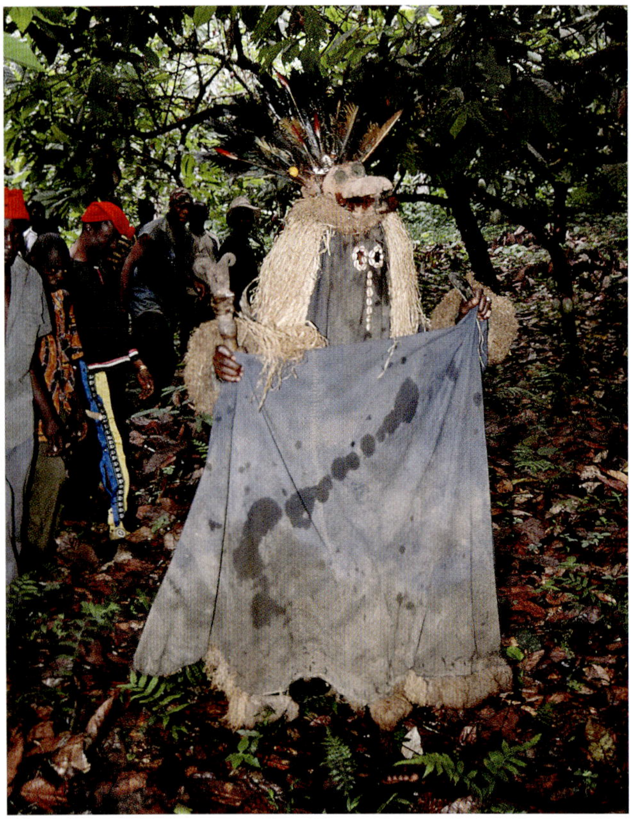

Fig. 203 *Obasinjom* in action on the farm (Kembong, April 22, 2004).

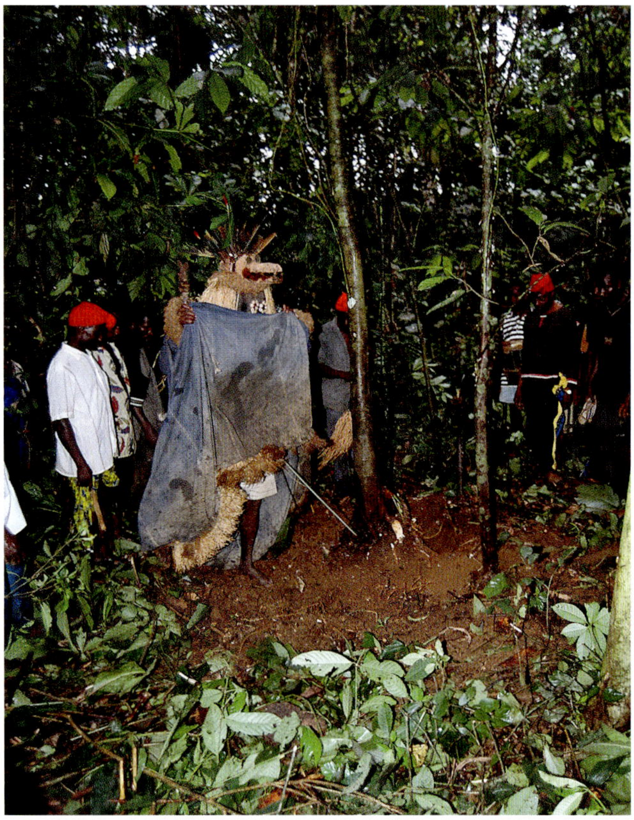

Fig. 204 *Obasinjom* in search of the bad medicine (Kembong, April 22, 2004).

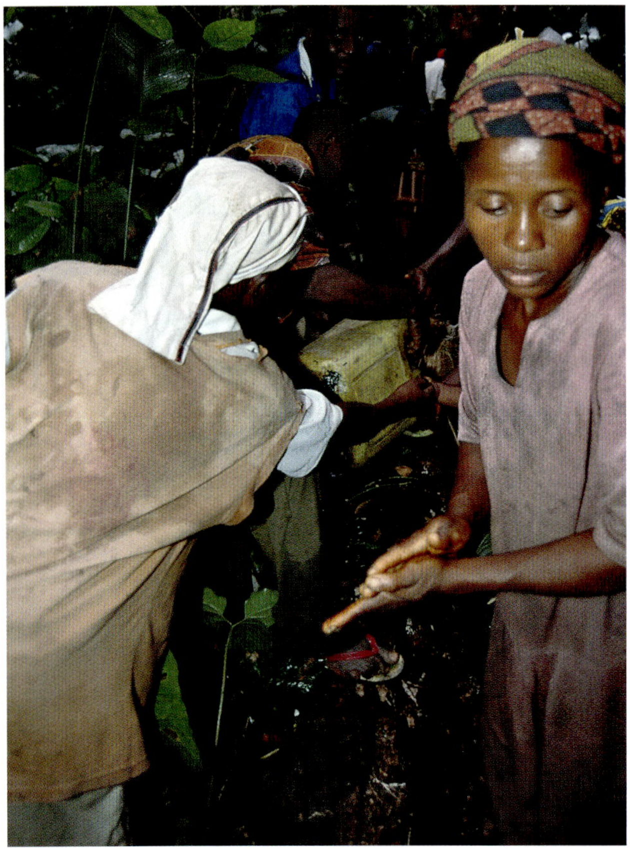

Fig. 205 The persons present rub the medicine *nchip Njom* upon themselves as a protection against hostile forces (Kembong, April 22, 2004).

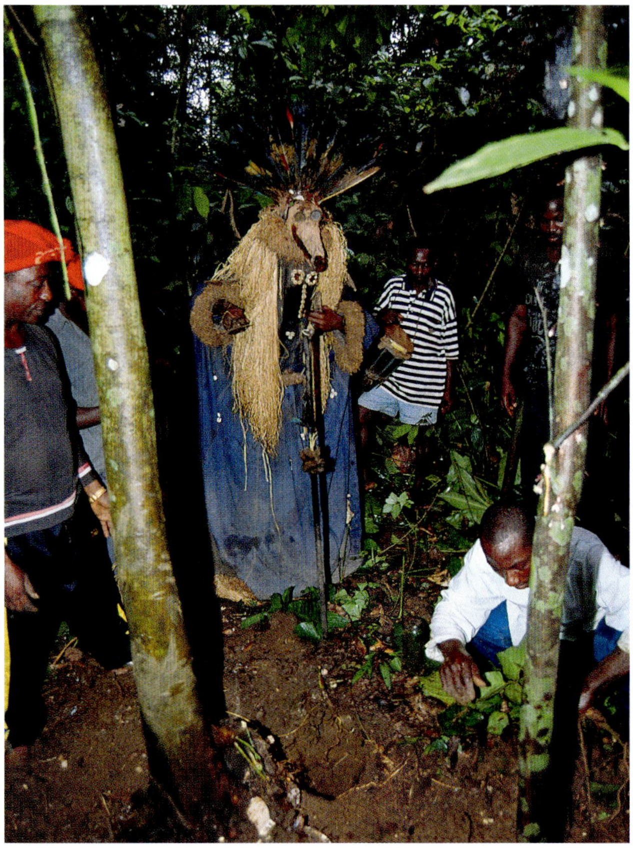

Fig. 206 *Obasinjom* discovers the place where a bottle containing bad medicine is buried in the ground. The mask itself holds the staff *osam Njom* to fight hostile forces (Kembong, April 22, 2004).

calamity which had long oppressed the family were banned at once. All persons present were correspondingly relieved and glad, but also amazed and dumbfounded. For although one could expect wonders from *Obasinjom*, everyone was nevertheless surprised and speechless that the mask was successful in finding the buried bottle with bad medicine in that expansive and impenetrable forest.

In a triumphal march the bottle was taken to Kembong. All those who had participated in the march to the farm took part in the feast that was held that afternoon in the house of the big man of *Obasinjom*. The day before the obligatory payments from the family involved in the conflict had been made: one goat, one cock, one bunch of plantains, one cup of salt, one cup of pepper, one cube of Maggi (dried bouillon), 40 litres of palm wine, two crates of beer and two bottles of whisky. At the end of the meal the big man of *Obasinjom* admonished the members of the family. They would suffer severely in future, if they were not prepared to live in peace and cooperation with one another. Then he ended the assembly with a prayer to God and the ancestors: "I thank God and the ancestors for the successful journey to the bush and back home. Those who look on *Obasinjom* with bad eyes should be perished with the left hand, while those wishing good success should continue to rise with blessings from God Almighty and the ancestors." According to tradition he made an offering of palm wine to them.

It was the general opinion that with the operation on the cocoa farm, *Obasinjom* had put an end to a long period of misery. No matter how it was able to discover the bottle with bad medicine, once again *Obasinjom* proved that it is unsurpassed and the champion of all medicines. Before the head of the family involved went on his return trip to the coast, where he had already resided for a long time, he called together all of the men and women in his family once more. He informed them to forget about the past and to look to the future: "what has passed is past."

Among the other activities of *Obasinjom,* one more medicine ritual should be mentioned here. It is used to counter the occurrence of serious illnesses, especially smallpox, into the community. In the presence of the mask, which also dictates what is to be done, medicine is buried at both entrances to the village: "We have buried *njom* here now. Anybody from anywhere or from amongst us, who wants to bring any illness into the community, let *Obasinjom* destroy him and also the power of the illness." This ritual was last conducted by *Obasinjom* of Lower Kembong in 2002.

5.5.5 *Obasinjom* as *njom*

Although *Obasinjom* is primarily known as a mask, it is basically a medicine, *a njom*, and the rituals connected with activating and pacifying it are similar to those of other medicines. If a client wants to invoke *Obasinjom* against witches but without activating the mask, he has to take *besom Njom* in the right hand and tell the medicine himself what to do. For example, he says: "The witch that is disturbing my child. If she does not stop disturbing it, let *Obasinjom* enter into her family and destroy all the family members. If she forces my child to die, let her give seven heads from her own family and destroy even the whole family. If the witch leaves her hand from her victim, she should, however, be saved. But if not then destroy her."

Should *Obasinjom* catch a thief, the fees consist of one "animal", one cock and palm wine. A meal is prepared, and then an egg is sacrificed, its contents poured down the throat of the mask and the shells stuck to the inside of the mouth. If an additional cock is killed, its blood is allowed to flow over the mask, and a prayer in the following sense is said. "*Obasinjom*, Mr. X, who sent you to war against the thief some days ago, has come back to tell you that he has received the things for which he sent you to war and that you should not go to war against the thief any longer. This is your food that the thief brought, so do not go against that man any longer."

Fees for unrepentant persons caught by *Obasinjom* are higher: one goat, one cock, one "animal", plantains, one bottle of palm oil and 30 litres of palm wine. The actual ceremony takes place in the *ebaah Njom* and may be attended by the patient or his deputy. While the blood of the goat flows over the mask, a prayer is offered: "*Obasinjom*, here is your meat. Here are your plantains and your cock. I have come to tell you that Mr. X, who was caught by you, accepts his guilt. He has done as you wanted. Let him be well, and cease going to war against him and his family members." The cock is also sacrificed, and the colour of the testicles is inspected to see whether *Obasinjom* has accepted the offerings. For the return trip to the leader's house, the mask usually avails itself of a mantlebearer. When the ceremony is over, the therapy can begin. This, too, is determined by *Obasinjom*, who names the member of the society who will conduct the treatment, and prescribes the necessary medicinal herbs. These herbs may only be used for the specified treatment, at the express command of *Obasinjom.*

Sacrifices are extensive when a witch has been caught: "*Ata*, I have come to give you food. The man you have caught has brought all the requirements that are necessary. You shall not kill him. Set him free and give him back to us." Like the medicines *(ajom)* discussed in the last chapters, *Obasinjom* forgives a witch only once. Should the witch commit another offence, the witch is lost and her family will be in danger of death. Appeasement of the medicine then requires substantial fees.

Once created, *Obasinjom* cannot die. It sleeps occasionally, but wakes up again and demands food. Whenever it is not needed for a longer period of time, the leader assures *Obasinjom* that it is by no means forgotten. He spits upon the mask with medicine and sacrifices an egg and a cock: "*Ata*, this is your food. Do not think that we have neglected you. Keep watch over your children and over the whole society." A special ceremony is necessary when the wooden headpiece of the mask is renewed and the old parts buried (fig. 195): "Your mask was old, and now we have made a new one. We give this new one the same powers as the old one. See well, hear well, speak nothing but the truth, and act in time. Bring us new herbs, fight witchcraft, attack wicked people, but do not kill them, so that when they are discovered and confess, they shall be healed. Be the nightwatch of the entire community. In everything you do, may you be victorious."

The direct translation of the name *Obasinjom* is "God of medicine"; there is, however, no special deity of medicine. All of the powers that *Obasinjom* has derive from God and the ancestors in the same way as the other *ajom*, the magic medicines. In answer to my question concerning the "spirits", who supposedly lead and direct the mask during its performances, came the prompt reply: "The spirits of *Obasinjom* are our forefathers."[25] And indeed, all prayers pertaining to *Obasinjom* are directed to God and the ancestors just as with the other magic medicines (*ajom*). According to my informants' interpretation, *Obasinjom,* however, is not just one *njom* among others, but "God of medicine", meaning that it is the strongest of all medicines.

5.5.6 Origin and expansion of *Obasinjom*

Obasinjom is widespread in parts of western Cameroon and eastern Nigeria, where it is the custom to use it in the pursuit of witches and criminals.[26] Substantial information concerning the origin of this important mask is provided by Talbot.[27] According to him at the beginning of the 20th century there were three masks in Oban, southeastern Nigeria (where Talbot was assigned as District Officer starting in 1907): *Akpambe*,[28] *Ekuri Ibokk*,[29] and *Mfuor*. All three were used primarily to ward off dangerous powers and, in view of their dark blue garment and wooden headdress in the form of a crocodile's head, can be seen as forerunners of *Obasinjom*.[30] This applies in particular to *Akpambe*, about whose emergence Talbot reported extensively: "Early in 1909 the cult of *Akpambe* invaded the District and rapidly gained such a reputation that lodges were established in almost every town. The cult was started about a year earlier by a man named Obassi Abong, who was taught the necessary rites by his mother, a celebrated *juju* woman of Okuri in the Cameroons, where its first shrine still exists."[31] This context was confirmed to a certain extent by a new study by R. A. Ojage. His investigations established that *Obasinjom* first appeared in Mbinda, a neighbouring locality of Okuri.[32] From there *Akpambe* began its triumphal progression, ultimately becoming the best-known mask in southeastern Nigeria and southwestern Cameroon.

In Kembong little could be learned about the history of *Obasinjom*. For example, no one had ever heard that *Obasinjom* had been created by a woman. However, it was known that the mask had come from outside the area and that its acquisition had been connected with a difficult and dangerous situation, which confronted Kembong when it was established through the joining of sixteen hamlets. This period of time was marked by an abundance of witches. Many people were killed by witches, oftentimes in their preferred animal form as leopards. Consequently, when word reached the people of Upper Kembong about an extremely powerful and successful mask and medicine, they resolved to acquire it for themselves. According to the information that I received in Kembong, it was Tabot Besong Nyang from Mbiofong who purchased the mask at the price of seven slaves in Ekonoman-Ojongarrey, a small rural village about fifty kilometres southwest of Kembong. His son Tanyiashu, my chief informant and the leader of *Obasinjom* during my research in 1980, said that he himself was about twenty-five years old (presumably between 1910 and 1912) when he, as part of the delegation from Upper Kembong, was sent to Ekonoman-Ojongarrey to be initiated into the secrets of the mask and to bring it back to Kembong.[33] This date is confirmed to a certain degree by a report of K. Stolz, a missionary of the Basler Mission, according to which Akpambe had reached Banyang in 1912.[34]

This information is of even greater significance when considering that Ekonoman-Ojongarrey, the supposed source of Kembong's *Obasinjom*, is only 16 kilometres southeast of Okuri and that the mask's acquisition date (between 1910 and 1912) corresponds with Talbot's findings. Furthermore, Mansfeld, whose *Urwald Do-*

kumente covers the period from 1904 to 1907, does not mention *Akpambe*, which of course he could not do if Talbot's date of 1909 is correct. This mask was soon confiscated by German troops and thrown into the Cross River. It is said that the mask later emerged from the water and returned to Upper Kembong. After several years, Lower Kembong acquired the same mask as well.

Today it is still general knowledge in Kembong that the former name of the mask was *Okpambe* (that is, not *Akpambe* as among the Ejagham in Nigeria). The successes of the mask and the medicine were so singular, so overwhelming and with that so superior to the other medicines (*ajom*) that a new name emerged, *Obasinjom*, which, as mentioned above, expresses its outstanding position: *Obasinjom* was and continues to be the "God of medicine". When and where the name *Akpambe* was replaced by *Obasinjom* is unknown. Likewise, no one knows when the new name became common use in Kembong. According to information from older men, this change occurred presumably in the 1920s, about the same time as the arrival of the first missionaries. As far as I am aware, the name *Obasinjom* was first mentioned in ethnological literature in 1939 by the Swiss missionary J. W. Zürcher.[35]

For the Ejagham, *Obasinjom* is of utmost importance, and so it helped the people of Kembong to overcome the period of terror at the beginning of the 20th century. Yet *Obasinjom* does more than fight evil. Because of its clairvoyance it knows the reasons for illnesses and for infertility in women; it also perceives when God and the ancestors are displeased and prescribes the necessary ceremonies. Finally it reveals to man the healing properties of plants. The gratitude that people feel towards *Obasinjom* is evident in their choice of endearing names for the mask: "the one with graceful movements", "the one who speaks", "the one who never tells lies", "the one who tells and acts", "good man of the village", "caretaker of the village" and "protector of the village".

5.6 Summary and recent developments

As this chapter has demonstrated, *ajom* have played an important role in the struggle for life among the Ejagham, especially since in former times scientific explanations of illness and death were rare, and the individual's life expectancy was short. Ostensibly the potency of *njom* comes from plants, but it is God and the ancestors who activate it and who operate through *njom*. That God is the ultimate source of *njom* was confirmed by my informants and by the prayers at the *sure njom* or "swearing of medicine".[36] This does not exclude their also having a certain mechanical life of their own: *Obasinjom* and *Mfam*, for example, occasionally sleep, but nevertheless remain alert and require constant sacrifice. Their wilful and uncanny character comes to light, when rituals are forgotten and they turn against their owners.

Compared with the powers inherent in the medicine, the objects that serve as its vehicles or containers may seem of less importance. Despite the weight accorded to them by Western observers, their form and material are arbitrary and apparently without direct relation to the potency of the medicine. The vehicles for the medicine are in no way tied alone to figures or other static objects, in the way that the term "fetish" suggests. When medicine manifests itself in the form of a mask, it takes on a dynamic character. In the Cameroon Grasslands medicine can even be located in a person, as – for example - when a king is treated with special medicines during the period of installation, which makes him dangerous so that he cannot be approached by ordinary people.[37]

Despite considerable differences in outward form, the use of medicine – as an antidote to witches and criminals, and in rites of appeasement – is largely the same in all medicine societies. Nevertheless, every society has its own special rules and regulations, and it is generally impossible to find out why this is so. The "swearing of medicine" should, however, not be reduced alone to its juridical functions; it has definite economic consequences. Those for whom *njom* has been activated often have to pay high fees for this assistance, and fees are even greater for those who need to appease it – lest it destroy the victim's whole family. Furthermore, the cost of acquiring these medicines is uncommonly high and can usually be afforded only by the well-to-do. That is why medicines are commonly acquired by several families together or by a whole village. Although induction into the societies and later ascent to higher ranks involve considerable expenses, membership is desirable for a number of reasons. For instance, it allows one to use the medicine free of charge, and it provides the opportunity to take part in the feasts that always include meat dishes, a rarity in daily life. Membership – a matter of prestige – was no doubt a sensible step for every adult male in the past.

Even if *ajom* are the private property of individual families, they serve the interests of the community, as was and is God's intention. The medicine fights all that is evil or criminal, and anyone may appeal to it for assistance – it is a factor of vital importance within the tra-

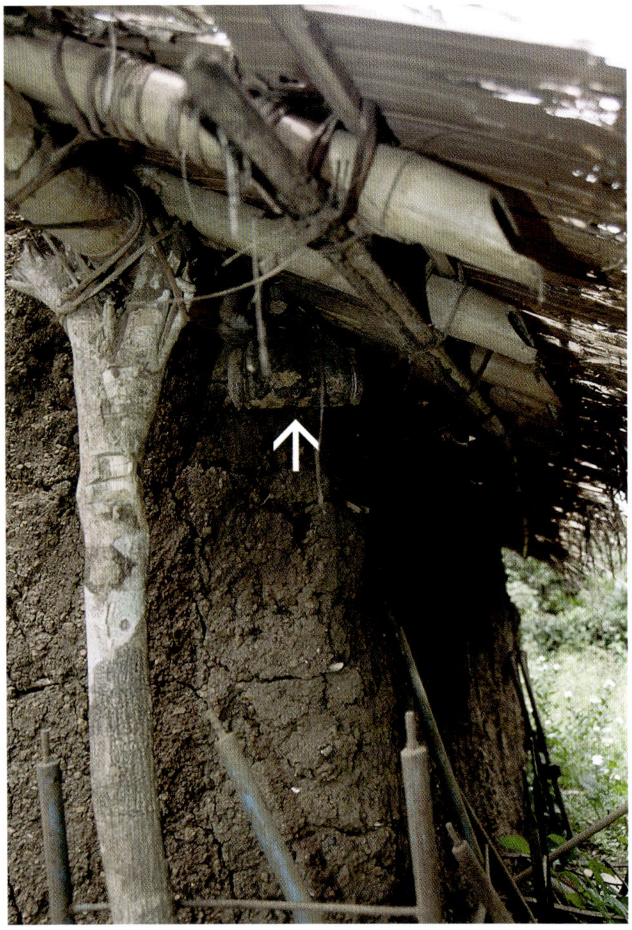

Fig. 207 *Enok Ateng* in its form today: a simple block of wood fastened underneath the roof of a hut (Afap, March 4, 2005).

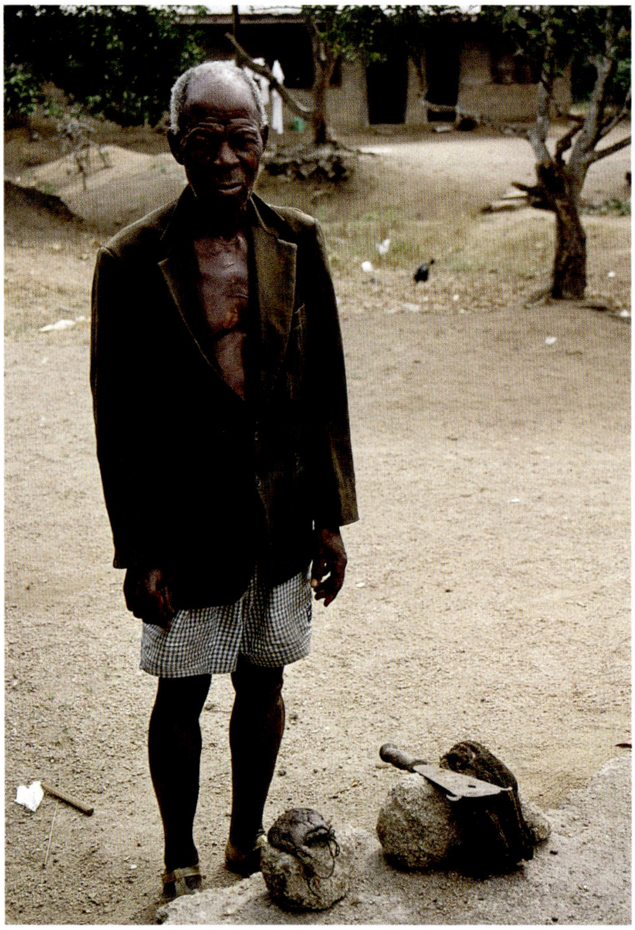

Fig. 208 *Okeboho*, a magic medicine (*njom*) in the form of small raphia bags. Here Akobenem Sampson, owner of *Okeboho* and a *seseku*, stands next to a stone upon which is one example (left); on the stone on the right is the ritual cutlass (Kembong, January 24, 2004).

ditional judicial system. It is, however, impossible to use *njom* against the innocent. Another important social aspect of medicine is that the members themselves are under constant control. Should one of them break the law, they are sure to be punished by their own *njom.*

My informants stressed repeatedly that the antidote to witches in older times had been the ordeal. A suspected witch was brought before the village council, *Etek,* and forced to take poison. If the accused survived the ordeal, they were considered innocent and set free. The person who carelessly made the accusation was severely punished. It was not clear why these ordeals were replaced by the medicine in the course of the 19th century.

When I returned to Kembong in 2004, I was astonished to find that the *ajom*, about which I had learned and studied intensively in 1980, scarcely played a role in the life of the community anymore. Interest in them had dwindled immensely, and upon the deaths of some of the big men and other high-ranking members of medicine societies, there were no replacements for them.[38]

When I met Ayuk Tambla again, he was – as he himself said – a sick old man, who was dependent upon himself alone. He still had neither wife nor children. He still possessed his medicine *Enok Ateng*, but there were few people in need of his help. The last time that he had activated it was about five years before. I was highly surprised to see that *Enok Ateng* no longer was embodied in a human figure, as in 1980, but consisted of an uncarved piece of wood (fig. 207). Ayuk Tambla had sold that magic figure to me in 1980. At that time he intended to have a new figure carved, but – as he "confessed" to me in 2004 – he needed the money elsewhere, and, hence, the "medicine bearer" remained a simple, amorphous block of wood. But, as Ayuk Tambla explained, the important thing is the medicine, not the object. Moreover, he was greatly hindered in his work as a healer through increasing problems with his eyesight.

Similarly, *Mfam* also is of little significance today. After the deaths of Hollford Ndip (1994) and other members, the society was practically dissolved. At present

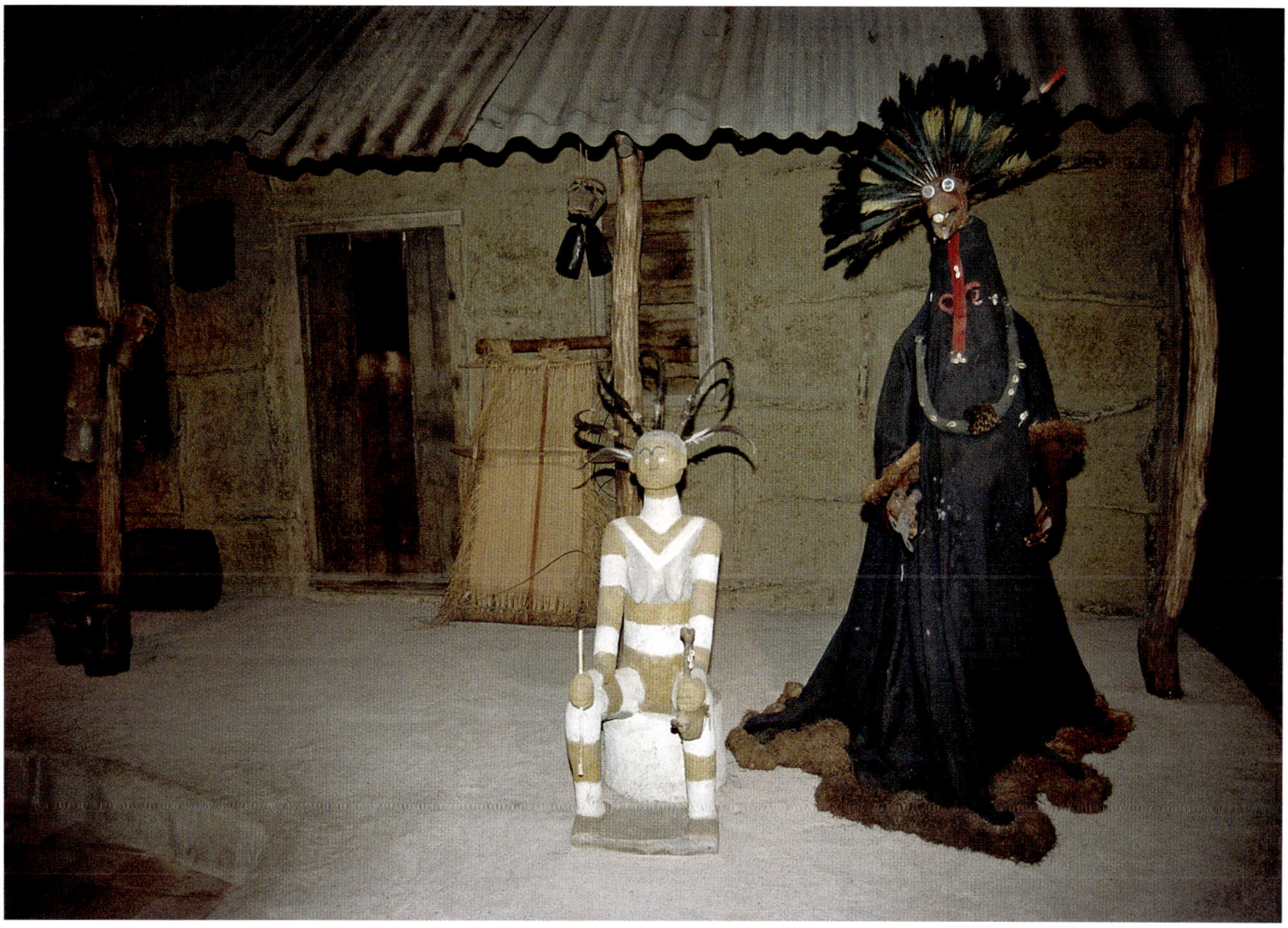

Fig. 209 The mask *Obasinjom* (right) and a commemorative figure of *mgbokandem* on exhibition in the Linden-Museum in Stuttgart, Germany (May 5, 2005).

Mfam is in the sole possession of Macndip Marcel Besong, but there is little occasion for its use.

In contrast to *Enok Ateng* and *Mfam*, which are still in existence despite the little notice taken of them, *Amok* was destroyed forever by its last owner Moses Ojong shortly before his death. On July 9, 2000, when Moses Ojong went with one of his sons into the forest to collect wild mangoes, he was bitten by a snake. As Moses Ojong was unable to walk, his son carried him home on his back. In the face of death Moses Ojong was only concerned at that point about protecting his family from *Amok*. He requested that his son bury the objects of *Amok*, which itself was made of the substance from a termite mound, in a mound that was inhabited by active termites. Everyone knows that that signifies the end of everything under the sun. Thus, nothing was left of *Amok*; it had gone to its death.

Okeboho is also of little significance in the community now. The present chief of the society, Akobenem Sampson, a *seseku*, took over *Okeboho* about twenty years ago. Several members have passed away since then, so that now only four members remain. The medicine itself is rarely requested. In addition, it is considered too dangerous, as once activated it is difficult to "cool down" the medicine. When Akobenem Sampson departs from life (he is already quite old, lame and almost blind), it will probably mean the end of *Okeboho* in Kembong (fig. 208).

Obasinjom, by contrast, the "God of medicine", is still active in Kembong as well as in many other villages of the region. And, as described above, during my stay there in 2004/2005 it still made some spectacular performances. Notwithstanding, the medicine is consulted and the mask employed in ever fewer cases.[39] Although its importance today has greatly diminished as compared to the place and role it occupied and played in Kembong society 25 years ago, I was able to continue my research from 1980 on this important institution and to increase and deepen the knowledge gained before. Oppositely, there was no new information to be obtained about the other *ajom*.

According to the unanimous opinion of most of my informants, there is scarcely any need for *ajom* today. In the case of disputes and other conflicts people turn to the police or the courts. In the meantime many inhabitants have joined Christian congregations and no longer wish to become involved with old practices of cult. For many the efficacy of the *ajom* has become dubious, and whoever is seriously ill goes to the hospital. However, a few people still consult medicine men and diviners. In most cases, they are, as is generally said, "the poor and ignorant of the society".

Footnotes

1 As mentioned above, "swearing of medicine" was also practised in Oku, but it is illegal, for it is associated with great dangers and can even lead to the death of humans. When witches are revealed by diviners, it is the duty of *Kwifon*, the secret society that together with the king formerly constituted the government, to punish the offender (Koloss 2000:306 f.).

2 *Njom* among the Ejagham. In: African Arts 18 (1), 1984, 71–73, 90–93. I am grateful to the editors of African Arts for their permission to make use of and to alter parts of that text in this contribution.

3 The figure of *Enok Ateng* in the Linden-Museum, Stuttgart, has the Inv.-No. F 52328.

4 Partridge 1905:273; Talbot 1912:51, 139; 1926:II:126, 245; Mansfeld 1908:177; Staschewski 1917:25; Jeffreys 1939:99; Ruel 1969: 137 ff. 169 f.; Röschenthaler 1993:153; 2004 (b): 255.

5 I was able to purchase two horns of *Mfam*, which were no longer in use. They are now in the Linden-Museum, Stuttgart (Inv. No. F 52326).

6 Talbot 1912:51, 139.

7 I had the opportunity to acquire two lumps of *Amok* for the Linden-Museum, Stuttgart (Inv. No. F 52329).

8 According to Agbor (2001:5*)* *Amok* was acquired by the Nchemti clan (to whom Kembong also belongs) in 1870 from Babong, who used it in conflicts with the Kebus.

9 References that God or the ancestors revealed the secrets of medicines to human beings in dreams can be found in Mansfeld (1908:210 f.; 1924:26) and Ojage, cit. in Röschenthaler 2004(b):258; see also Koloss 2000:313.

10 The medicine bag of *Okeboho* has the Inv.-No. F 52327.

11 An initial report on *Obasinjom* by the author appeared thereafter in African Arts (Koloss 1985).

12 Nicklin 1977:31.

13 For the ranks in *Obasinjom* of the Banyang, see Ruel 1969: 210 ff. and Röschenthaler 2004(b):265.

14 Sound recordings made during both of these trials are accessible in the Department of Ethnomusicology in the Ethnological Museum, Berlin (Inv. No. VII OA 0407.024 and VII OA 0739.004).

15 A similar method to summon the mantlebearer is found among the Banyang. There specific roots are used, which stand for the mantlebearer: "The roots (inserted within the feathered headdress) symbolize members entitled to wear this gown ... If you are going to dance in the gown, I will remove the root, chew on alligator pepper, take the root and blow on it, repeating your name, and crying *apa toi! apa toi! toi!* mention your name and finish with the word *aba*! This will awaken the spirit and make you become possessed by Basinjom" (Thompson 1974:212).

16 According to Talbot (1912:55 ff., 196 ff.) pipes made of crab claws were blown during many ceremonies in eastern Nigeria. He even designated the crab as the "father of all jujus" (1912: 408).

17 Cp. Röschenthaler 1993:147. Similarly, in the Cameroon Grasslands, where the sphere of the *jujus* is strictly taboo for women, the *Samba* society, a military society especially widespread in the east, is dependent upon the aid of a woman, particularly during the most important medicine rituals. For only a woman is capable of taking over certain duties at that time. Women also have access to the houses of *Samba*, which itself was once founded by a woman, but they are not entrusted with any secrets (Koloss 2000:206).

18 Important information on medicines and symbolism in *Obasinjom* of the Banyang can be found in Thompson (1974:209 ff.).

19 Thompson as well mentions a special knife employed by *Obasinjom* of the Banyang, which is called *isome* and with which "one sees many things" (1974:212, 214).

20 Talbot likewise reports that dogs in eastern Nigeria are considered as animals with "four eyes" (1912:175); cp. Röschenthaler 1993:35.

21 As far as I am aware, in the Cameroon Grasslands eggs have no special meaning in the sphere of cult. However, chickens are important sacrificial animals (Koloss 2000:58). In this context it should be mentioned that *Kheghebchioh*, a mask widespread in the eastern Grasslands whose duty – like *Obasinjom* – is the pursuit and destruction of witches, holds a "garden-egg" (a fruit that resembles an egg) in its mouth, again like *Obasinjom* (Koloss 2000:292 ff.).

22 For the performances of *Obasinjom* among the Banyang, see Ruel 1969:212 f. and Thompson 1974:213 ff.

23 A sound recording made of the performance on January 28, 1980 is accessible in the Department of Ethnomusicology in the Ethnological Museum, Berlin (Inv. No. VII OA 0407.024).

24 Thompson also mentions the red cap of the mask bearer of *Obasinjom* (1974:214).

25 In contrast to that Röschenthaler states: "*Obasinjom* is ... a spirit of the wild, who by means of *njom* can be called to the mask and then begins to speak" (1993:239; cp. p. 192).

26 For the history and dissemination of *Obasinjom*, see the detailed work of Röschenthaler 2004(b). The mask garments and headdresses of *Obasinjom* represent further important historical documents, which were acquired by German museums at a remarkably early time. As early as November 1910 the Museum für Völkerkunde in Dresden received a mask garment of *Obasinjom* (Homberger 1999:286). It is simply designated as "dance costume" in the inventory records; any reference to *Obasinjom* is absent. Allegedly the garment was from the Ekoi in the Ossidinge district in Cameroon. A mask of the same type was acquired by the Überseemuseum in Bremen in 1913. Unfortunately in the records there is merely the reference that the garment came from Cameroon. Equally sparse is the information about the *Obasinjom* masks from the Ekoi in the Cameroon-Nigeria frontier, which were sold by the Umlauff Museum in Hamburg in 1926. One of these masks was purchased by the Museum für Völkerkunde in München (Kecskési 1987:188), the other by the Museum für Völkerkunde in Basel. The mask in Basel was later published by Leo Frobenius with the designation "*juju* dancer" (1954:Pl. 63), without any mention of *Obasinjom*. In his letter of November 26, 1916, to the Museum für Völkerkunde in Basel, Umlauff himself made

mention of "fetish" with reference to the mask. Further *Obasinjom* masks are in the Seattle Art Museum (McClusky 2002: 220 f.) and in Dublin (Thompson 1974:241, fn. 232). In 1980 I was able to acquire an *Obasinjom* mask for the Linden-Museum (Stuttgart) in Kembong (Forkl 1989:71); it has the Inv.-No. F 52317 (a–e). Museums in Nigeria have *Obasinjom* masks in their holdings as well as in Lagos (Thompson 1974:241, fn. 232) and Oron (Nicklin 1977:24, 26, 28). Here I extend my sincere thanks for this information to Silvia Dolz (Dresden), Bernhard Gardi (Basel) and Silke Seybold (Bremen).

27 Talbot 1912:51 ff., 198; 1926:127.

28 Photographs of *Akpambe* can be found in Talbot 1912:198 and Talbot 1923:258. The masks also appeared in murals of the Ejagham (Talbot 1926:III:937). In this reference mention should be made of *Ofiom Inyang* by the Efik: "a masquerade foretelling events of tribal importance" (Anonymous 1957: 162).

29 Cp. the photograph of *Ekuri Ibokk* in Talbot 1912:44.

30 Ruel 1969:210; Thompson 1974:210; Nicklin and Salmons 1984:35; Röschenthaler 2004(b):251, 257 ff.

31 Talbot 1912:51 f.

32 Ojage (1995:19), cited in Röschenthaler 2004(b):257 f.

33 Koloss 1985:63.

34 Stolz, cited in Röschenthaler 2004(b):258. *Obasinjom* was later sold by the Banyang to others: to the Bakwiri (Ardener 1970:149 ff., cp. also Geschiere 1997:149 ff.) and to the Bakossi (Balz 1984:322). It was also said that *Obasinjom* was "already on the doorstep" to the Grasslands (Chilver 1990:244).

35 Zürcher 1939:72.

36 It was P. A. Talbot, who first showed intensive interest in the magic medicines of the Ejagham and also noted the prayers that were said during medicine rituals. They were all directed to God and the ancestors (Talbot 1912:22, 53, 66), occasionally also to the *juju* itself (Talbot 1912:139 f.; cp. Mansfeld 1908: 177). The powers of the medicines were derived from God (Talbot 1932:31), but they were not regarded as everlasting: "...but will fade away after the owner's death if the proper rites are not continued...If a 'medicine', however, is neglected by its owner, it will send sickness or accident to him" (Talbot 1923:21).
Ruel makes some reference to medicines among the Banyang: "These cult-agencies", as he terms the medicines, "of which the most important is *Mfam*, are thought to operate against actions of wrong-doing or deceit within the community..." They "are believed ultimately to owe their efficiency to God ..." (Ruel 1965:15). Ruel devotes as little attention to the medicine rituals as to the prayers spoken in that association. The same applies to Röschenthaler, who views the *ajom* as mechanistic: a *njom* "consists of a certain combination of mineral and organic substances; the secret of the *njom* lies in the way and manner of its production" (Röschenthaler 1993:28).
Interestingly, *njom* is also known in Meta', a kingdom in the western Grasslands, not far from the Cross River region. According to Dillon (1990:69 ff.) there it represents "the speech of the offended party that was believed to cause *ndom* ('bad luck or curse that was manifested in illness, death, poverty, and the infertility of women among other things'). His utterance was described as an *njom* ('statement of correct words'), a term applied to supernaturally powerful speech in many other contexts. This was a complaint in which the person whose rights had been violated described the offense in a truthful way".

37 Koloss 2000:99.

38 Cp. Agbor 2001:35.

39 In order to counter the decline of *Obasinjom* in the entire region (Ejagham, Banyang, Boki and Anyang), the Manyu Obasinjom Association was founded in March 1999: "It aimed to consolidate and coordinate all Obasinjom powers and to save Obasinjom knowledge and the institution as a whole" (Röschenthaler 2004(b):270).

6 Institutions for women

As in many other societies in traditional Africa, in earlier times the position of women of the Central Ejagham was at a great disadvantage and prejudiced as compared to that of men. Women were clearly considered second-class at best and thought to be lacking in intelligence and self-control, whereas men were considered physically, intellectually and morally superior.[1] While women had hardly any right to speech or opinion when important decisions were made, neither in the family sphere nor in the community, they nonetheless bore the major burdens within the traditional division of work. The polygamous family system together with the brideprice were and still remain a sign of their degradation and a means to drive women into the background. At least in earlier times women were more or less fully dependent upon their husbands. This is demonstrated particularly in the case of divorce. Then the children, insofar as they were not young and still nursed by the mother, almost always remained with the husband or father and his family. In such a case the question as to who caused the separation was irrelevant.[2] The children and even the wife were the property of the family of the husband. If the husband died, his widow did not have the right to return to her family. On the contrary, it was quite common that one of the deceased's brothers would take the woman as wife. Although women were and still are greatly underprivileged, nevertheless, in general they enjoy high esteem, especially if they have borne many children. Indeed, everywhere in Africa it was and still is considered a serious offence, when someone behaves improperly towards a woman or insults or even attacks her. Yet, here it should be noted that the position of women is not the same in all African societies.

As has become clear through the descriptions and accounts thus far, the position of women in the traditional society of the Ejagham was and still is definitely more liberal and influential than that of women, for instance, in the Cameroon Grasslands. To summarise the most important points in brief, women of the Ejagham are excluded from the secret societies of men, just as women in the Grasslands. However, unlike women in the Grasslands, Ejagham women are not punished severely by the bad medicine of the men's secret societies, if they by chance encounter secrets of the masks and medicines of these societies. Contrary to women in the Grasslands, who dare not even speak about the dangerous medicines and masks of men, Ejagham women are well informed about the background of the masks. It must also be surprising from the viewpoint of the Grasslands, that women of the Ejagham have the opportunity – at least theoretically – to assume the position as head of the family, if there is no man suited for this office. Probably equally surprising is the fact that among the Ejagham offerings to the ancestors are not carried out exclusively by men, as is the case in the Grasslands, but by women, too. This significance of the female element in Ejagham society is further illustrated by the appearance of certain divine powers. Whereas most of the supreme gods in Africa are considered to be male, among the Ejagham the deity is both male and female: *Ata Obasi* and *Mma Obasi*. Furthermore, the influence of women predominates in the *arem* cult (cp. p. 36).

A further important point is indicative of the female element not only in Ejagham society, but also among other peoples in the Cross River region. It is the fact that there are notably many cases in which medicines and secret societies, which are now exclusively for men, were originally discovered or founded by women and later taken over from them by men – f. e. *Mgbe* and *Obasinjom*[3] There are similar reports and evidence of this background in other parts of Africa,[4] but it seems that they do not compare with the great number of cases known among the Ejagham. Talbot was one of the first to report on this: "The feminine origin of the cult is a secret, unknown save to very few even among natives, and hitherto, I believe, carefully guarded from the knowledge of Europeans. Later we were fortunate enough to discover that nearly all the principal societies were originally feminine cults." He then reaches the conclusion "that in olden days among Ibibio, as until yesterday with the Ekoi, woman, not man, was the dominant sex."[5] Today it is difficult to verify this assertion. However, in the cultural area of southwestern Cameroon and southeastern Nigeria there are still remarkable traditions and institutions that foster women's well-being and further development and also serve for their protection, while at the same time expressing both the respect and esteem that are shown them. Specific institutions exist, which can be seen as expressions of a social and political culture, in which women apparently have greater opportunity for self-determination, self-fulfilment and political as well as

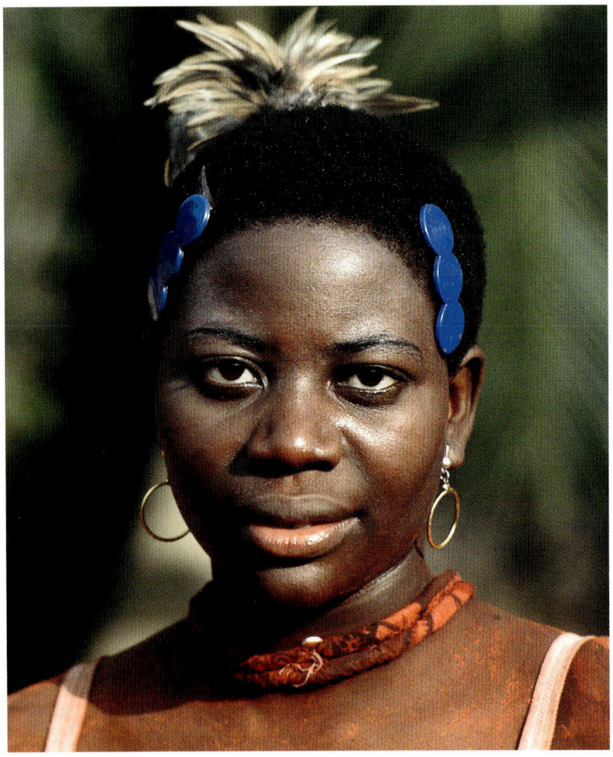

Fig. 210 A *moninkim*, adorned with a necklace and earrings and a cluster of feathers in her hair (Babong, February 21, 1980).

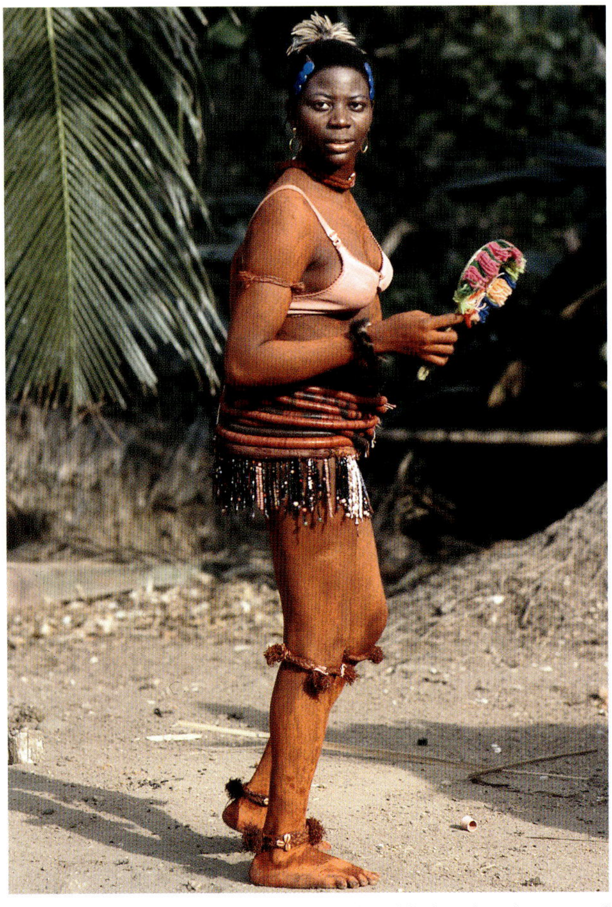

Fig. 211 The same *moninkim*, her body rubbed with red camwood and adorned with many strings of beads. She holds a fan in the right hand (Babong, February 21, 1980).

social influence than in other parts of Africa. In the following examples of such institutions will be described.

6.1 *Aboninkim*, the "children of circumcision"

Special note should be made of the *aboninkim* (sg. *moninkim* or "child of circumcision"), an institution from pre-colonial times, which concerned the transition of a young woman into the status of an adult woman and held remarkably great significance.[6] To my knowledge, however, this institution was totally unknown in the Cameroon Grasslands. In specific, *moninkim* among the Central Ejagham referred to the practice of circumcision on girls and young women; it was also conducted on boys and young men, but without any ritual ceremony. In the case of women, the climax of the procedure was the clitoridectomy itself, "an exercise conceived of as a means of ensuring fidelity of women in marriage".[7] It was carried out after the birth of the first child, as – it was reasoned in Kembong – the bleeding could be best controlled at that time. Scarification was also applied above the cheeks bones. Following this operation the woman or *moninkim* went into seclusion in a "fattening house", where the *aboninkim* were exempted from all work and where they received food in abundance. This was considered very important, "since plump women were generally conceived of as beautiful in traditional Ejagham society".[8] Every day the *moninkim's* body was rubbed with camwood.[9] During the time directly following circumcision, the *moninkim* could not receive any visitors. When the wounds began to heal, she was instructed in all the important aspects of her future role as wife and mother by older and experienced women and learnt by them "... various ways of preserving her husband's love, with a view to ensuring the emergence of peaceful and stable families. Accordingly, she was taught various forms of domestic activities like cooking and child-care, cloth weaving and embroidery. Such feminine past-times like singing and dancing were also vastly taught."[10] The length of time that a woman could spend as *moninkim* depended upon the financial situation of her parents. If they were wealthy, it might last two or more years; less affluent families might afford a few months or even only a few weeks. The period of seclusion concluded with a big festivity, in the course of which the *moninkim* performed the dances that she had learned from the older women (figs. 210–211).

The circumcision or clitoridectomy was officially prohibited by the Cameroon government several years ago and is no longer practised. As a result, it has become difficult to obtain reliable information about this institution.

6.2 *Mawu*

The most important and powerful society of women among the Ejagham is generally *Ekpa Atu*. Its primary responsibility is to defend the rights of women. The society's nocturnal performances, during which women appear in the nude, are much feared everywhere. The dances and rituals that take place during these appearances are strictly forbidden to men.[11] In the Ngunaya area this society for women is called *Mawu*.[12] It already existed there "when people still lived in hamlets", and it is said that the society was originally established by a woman named Wu. As Wu was very old in age, she was called *Mawu*, and this name was apparently transferred to the society as well.

This association represents all women, and from its very inception it acted as a counterbalance to *Mgbe*, the powerful society of men. The moment of her birth itself was considered the initiation of a girl into the society, at least in earlier times: Girls were born into *Mawu*, which indicates that *Mawu* is not a typical "society" with a special initiation, several levels and corresponding fees.

Mawu not only has the power attained through an aggregation of many people, it also possesses a special magic medicine, that is, *njom*, which in Africa is otherwise usually the strict privilege of men. Yet, this particular medicine of *Mawu* is not made of plants and other substances, like those of men's societies, but of the God-given part of their own body: Their strongest medicine are the sexual organs.[13] They are, as it is said in this region, "medicine by itself". Explicitly, not only do women of the Ejagham alone possess such dangerous powers, indeed all women in the world have them. However, the latter – so the belief in Kembong – are not aware of their powers and are thus unable to apply them. The "sleeping mat of the night" (*ekpa atu*), upon which sexual intercourse takes place, is considered equally dangerous as the female sexual organs. It is therefore all the more understandable that its name is

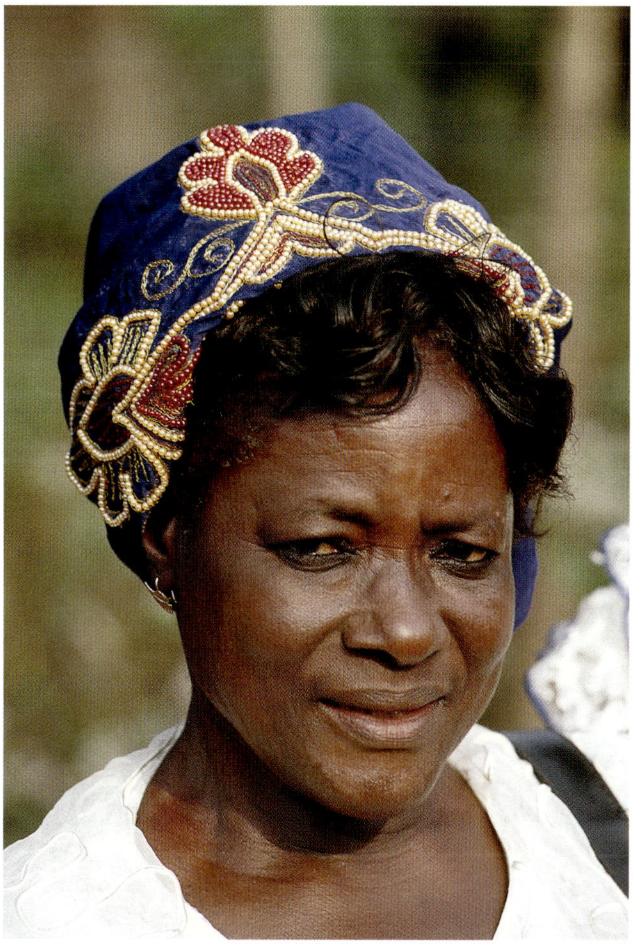

Fig. 212 Manchang Alice, "president" of *Mawu* (Kembong, January 23, 2004).

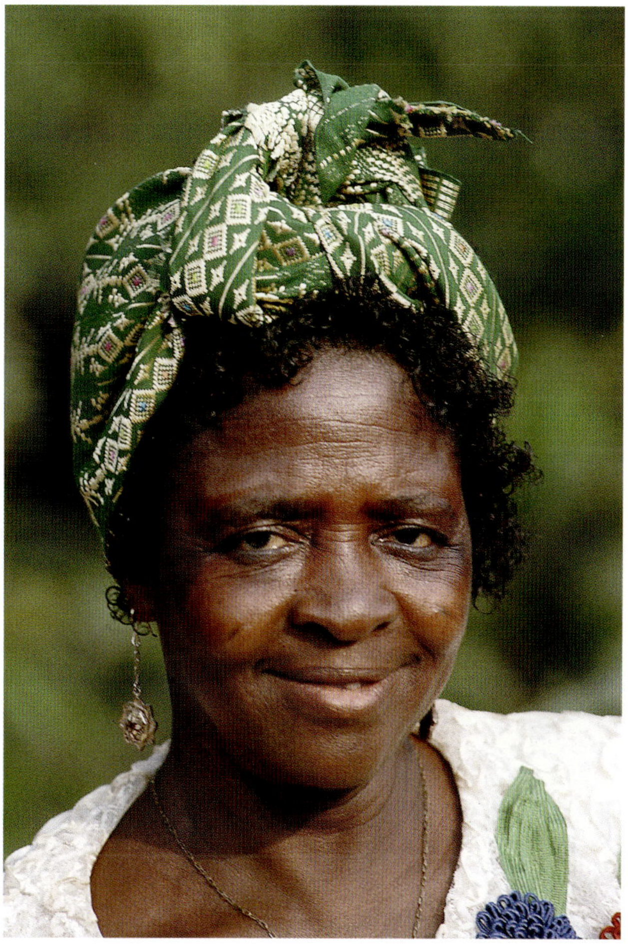

Fig. 213 Batemanyo Pauline, "vice-president" of *Mawu* (Kembong, January 23, 2004).

the same as that of the women's society, *Ekpa Atu*, in the greater area of the Ejagham.

Mawu has a "president" (*nne echi*) and one deputy president (*montui*) (figs. 212–213). If the president should die, her deputy automatically succeeds her. Just as *Etek*, *Mawu* is present for all women in Kembong, and in each quarter women have their own section. The assemblies of *Mawu* (*echeme Mawu*, "come together") are held in the house of the respective "president". They are mostly concerned with resolving conflicts and charging fines for misdemeanours, and thus involve controversial discussions, just as in *Etek* and *Mgbe*, too. When a problem arises, regardless whether the injustice that a woman suffers stems from a man or from another woman, the women of the respective quarter first attempt to solve the difficulty alone. If this is not successful, *Mawu* in the neighbouring quarters is consulted. Should this consultation be unsuccessful as well, the problem is brought before the assembly of *Mawu* of entire Kembong, where a final solution is found. Like *Mgbe*, *Mawu* has the unlimited right to impose fines. They usually comprise payments of palm wine, goats and – as of recent times – money. Also like *Etek* and *Mgbe*, *Mawu* can impose social isolation (cp. p. 76). The sentenced person is excluded from the community – no one may speak or visit him/her – until his/her fine is paid.

The worst punishment for which *Mawu* is feared most is the "swearing of medicine". It is almost always directed against men who have assaulted women. The swearing of medicine takes place at night, during which the women dance naked. As mentioned above, the dances are absolutely taboo for men. Should they view the activities of *Mawu*, they are threatened with impotence, besides other possible maladies. Women who are pregnant or already have a male child are not permitted to participate in the dances. At the end of the dance the women wash their genitals and then proceed to "swear medicine against the offender", i. e. they pour the water used in this cleansing ritual in front of the door of the offender's house. When he leaves the house, he becomes infected. Even today there is still no doubt that the offender concerned will meet with a terrible punishment; he will become impotent or physically or psychically ill, or he might even die. In some cases *Mawu* takes action during the day. The women occupy the house of the offender, they remove their clothes, and after encircling him they scold and threaten him. Following a measure such as this, the offender must reckon with severe consequences. In the case of a serious offence, a woman can take measures alone against the offending man by "swearing medicine" against him – with the cleansing water – in like manner. This often occurs when a man refuses to pay the sum agreed upon for prostitution or when, for example, a man boasts in public of having committed adultery with a woman.

Furthermore, through nocturnal dances *Mawu* is able to pursue witches and other dangerous and hostile forces and to punish them. The society's dances that are performed upon the installation of a new chief also have the purpose of warding off misfortune and evil. In the prayers spoken on this occasion the ancestors are likewise addressed and their blessings entreated. The blessings of the ancestors are also invoked in the dances that take place at the beginning of the year as "thanksgiving to God and the ancestors". One of these dances was performed during the night of January 24–25, 2004. It began with a prayer of the president of *Mawu* to the ancestors: "As the women are out in that form, let whatever they want to do, be cordial and peaceful. They give blessings to the children of the nation, to their husbands and to all their family members. And whatever any of them intends to do, he or she should do it joyfully to the purpose of development. Evildoers should stay quite away from the community. Those with bad medicines and anybody who is involved or seen in actions of atrocity, will be held liable to pay heavy fines to *Mawu*." Then water was poured onto the ground in offering to the ancestors. Seeds and seedlings were planted in this blessed spot to assure a good harvest. Afterwards the dances were performed in every quarter, beginning in Upper Kembong and continuing to Lower Kembong. They were accompanied by the singing of the text of the prayer.

Aside from the vagina, women possess with their breasts (*abe*, sg. *ebe*) yet another magic medicine or *njom*. This is activated in the ritual *asure abe*, meaning "to swear the breasts", when an older or even adult child has refused to show the mother the obligatory respect and obedience or has insulted her in any way. The "swearing of the breasts" can be uttered even in the presence of the offending child: "If you, my child, did not suck my breasts, then what I say against you shall not happen to you. But if you did suck my breasts, and now you have done this to me, then let, what I say against you, affect you. From now whatever you do, goodness and success shall not follow you." A malediction such as this is linked with a special condition. Contrary to the other *ajom*, which can be lessened or recalled at any time, the *asure abe* is irrevocable – it can never be retracted.

Like all traditional institutions, *Mawu* has also undergone new developments, which have made themselves felt in all spheres of life. Thus, in the year 2000 *Mawu* made the decision that dances during which medicine is sworn will not be performed anymore. If a man offends or insults a woman in any manner, he will be brought before a public court: "The dances themselves have been completely abolished." Insofar, the use of the "ethnological presence" in describing the significance and activities of *Mawu* might be misleading.

Societies for women that protect the rights of women are not only found in the egalitarian communities in the Cross River region; they also exist in the kingdoms of the Cameroon Grasslands. In the kingdom of Oku the respective society is called *Fembien*; in other kingdoms it is known by a similar name. As almost all women belong to *Fembien*, death celebrations for deceased women are marked in particular by the performance of *Fembien*. In addition, *Fembien* looks after the interests of women; for example, it organises communal work. Contrary to *Mawu*, *Fembien* does not conduct ceremonies of offering for the well-being of the community nor does it have any medicines. In Oku *Fembien* has, however, a more or less secret musical instrument – a percussion instrument consisting of two stones – which is used out of the sight of men. *Fembien* is respected and even feared. If a man should injure a woman in any way or behave improperly towards her, he must reckon with *Fembien's* disciplinary measures against him – he must fear that the women will destroy his compound with their hoes. In fact, *Fembien* is even considered the "daughter of *Kwifon*", the most powerful of all secret societies in Oku, and belongs, together, with the military societies and certain medicine societies to the "three strong arms" of *Kwifon*.[14]

6.3 *Njom Ekpa*

Special attention should be drawn to *Njom Ekpa*, that women's society which although not represented in Kembong itself, is nevertheless known there through its performances at important death celebrations in the region.[15] The society originally came from the Calabar area and was later adopted by the Ejagham; today it is particularly widespread among the Ekwe (figs. 214–216). As far as I am aware, *Njom Ekpa* reached the Ngunaya area around 1945. It was the women of Mbakang, who at that time acquired *Njom Ekpa* in Inokum (Nigeria). The society *Njom Ekpa* that was acquired by Ajayukndip in 1959 likewise came from Nigeria, from Ojock. Today *Njom Ekpa* is found foremost in the western part of the Ngunaya area: in Akwen, Mbakem, Taboh, Ayukaba, Ebinsi, Mbakang (two lodges), Ajayukndip (two lodges), Ewelle[16] (figs. 217–219) and Mfuni.

In general, not all women in a community are members of *Njom Ekpa*, for initiation into the society as well as into its various ranks requires the payment of fees. In the organisation of the society, *Njom Ekpa* is oriented considerably towards *Mgbe*. The "president" of *Njom Ekpa* is titled with *seseku* or *eyamba*, just as in *Mgbe*, and she likewise has a staff that is used only at ceremonies and as in *Mgbe* is called *monyo*. *Seseku* or *eyamba* is also the person who makes ancestral offerings. The senior members are called *anne eboho*, ("mud-bed people"), just as in *Mgbe*; the "young" members, *abo mfe* ("new children"). Further, the designation for the lodge (*ocha Ekpa*), the grove (*Ekpa eteme*) and the table (*efem Ekpa*) are also reminiscent of *Mgbe*.

The particularly special possession of *Njom Ekpa* is its mask, which, contrary to the masks of men, is worn with the bearer's face exposed (figs. 214–215, 217).[17] The mask headdress consists of a box-like platform that is decorated with mirrors and colourful cloths and upon which several human figurines stand. The central and largest figure usually represents the woman who founded the respective society. The smaller figures stand for the other members. It is quite noteworthy that during the society's performances, the members dance the roles of men; in particular, they imitate positions in *Mgbe* and *Nkanda*. Thus, in addition to a diviner and hunters, members perform as *okina*, *iroko* and *Ema* as well as the men with cutlasses in *Nkanda* (fig. 219). Two other women who wear mirrors always stay near the mask; one in front of the mask, the other behind.

Njom Ekpa is one of the societies of the Ejagham that has no further duties other than admitting new members and performing at the death of deceased members. This also means that the society can be engaged to perform at other events, for example, at death celebrations that are held for non-members. Yet, it is not the duty of *Njom Ekpa* to acknowledge and defend the interests of women in general. That is the charge of *Mawu* alone, which is established in all villages in the Ngunaya area and was "always" present there.

With *Njom Ekpa* the Central Ejagham acquired a mask society that follows another kind of mask tradition, namely that of the southern Nigeria region to the west of Cross River. It is typified by a mask headdress, in which human figures are shown in motion, an element that apparently was not present among the Central Ejagham in earlier times.

Performance of *Njom Ekpa* in Babong (February 21, 1980) (figs. 214–216).

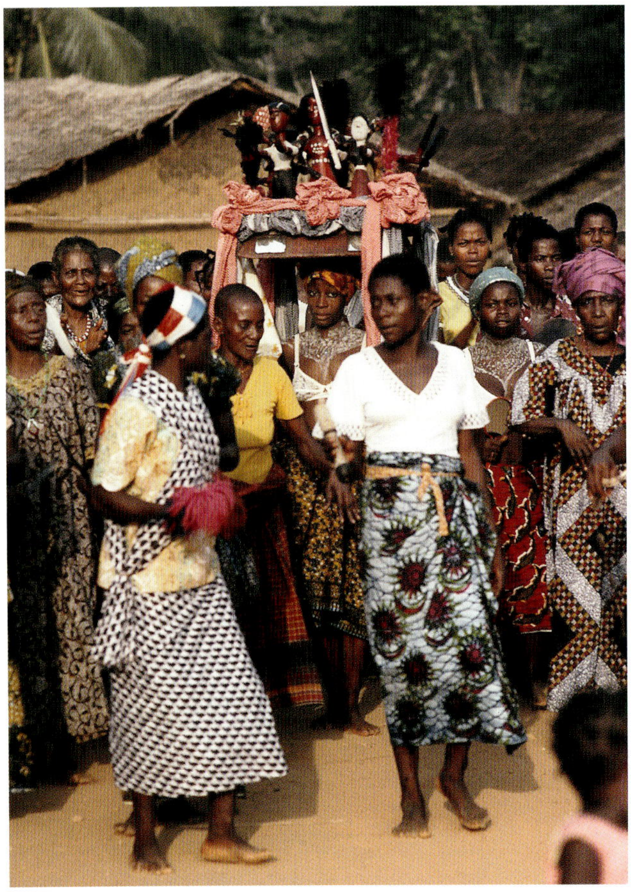

Fig. 214 The mask of *Njom Ekpa* is worn by a woman, whose face is not concealed (Babong, February 21, 1980).

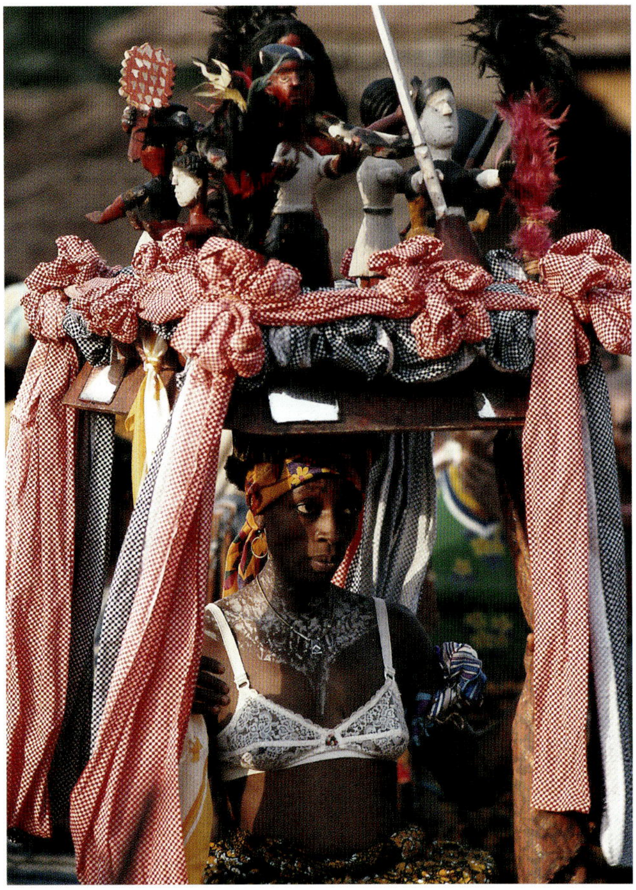

Fig. 215 The mask bearer of *Njom Ekpa* with the headdress (Babong, February 21, 1980).

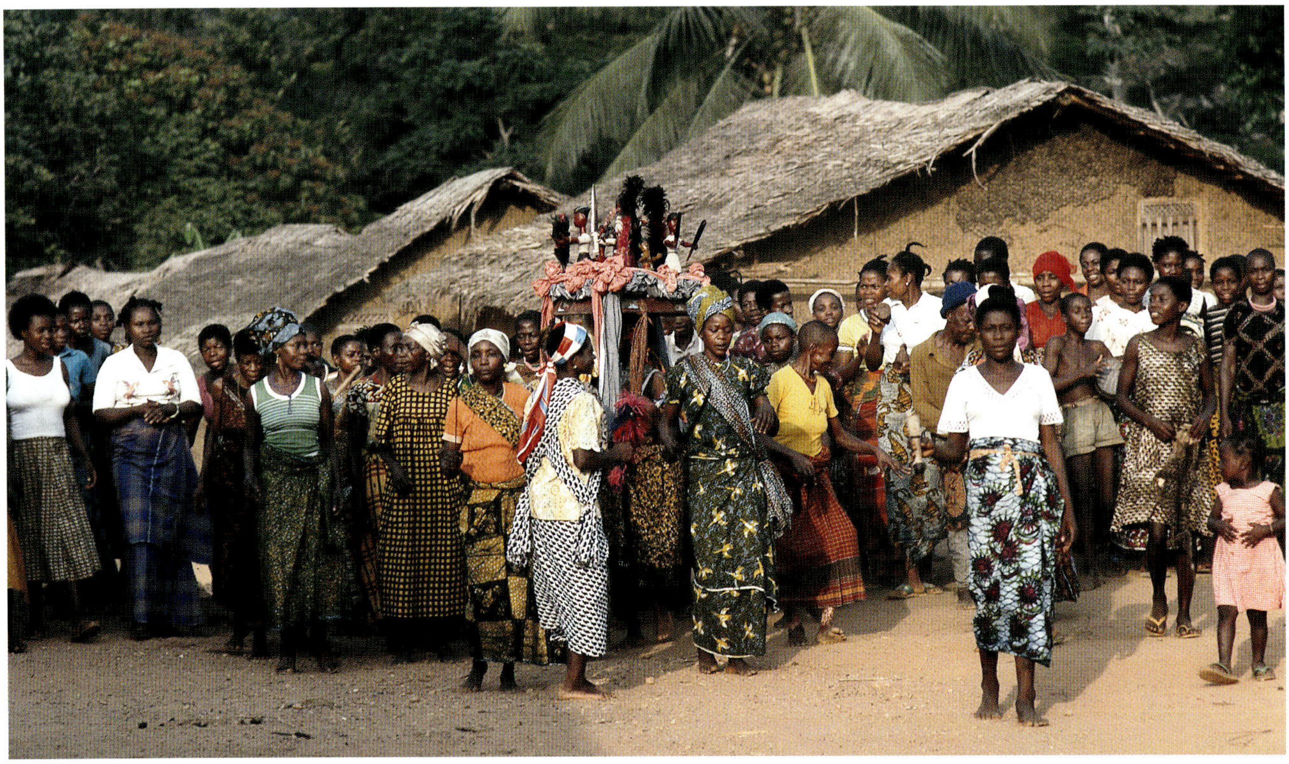

Fig. 216 *Njom Ekpa* with its many members (Babong, February 21, 1980).

Performance of *Njom Ekpa* in Ewelle (March 26, 2005) (figs. 217–219).

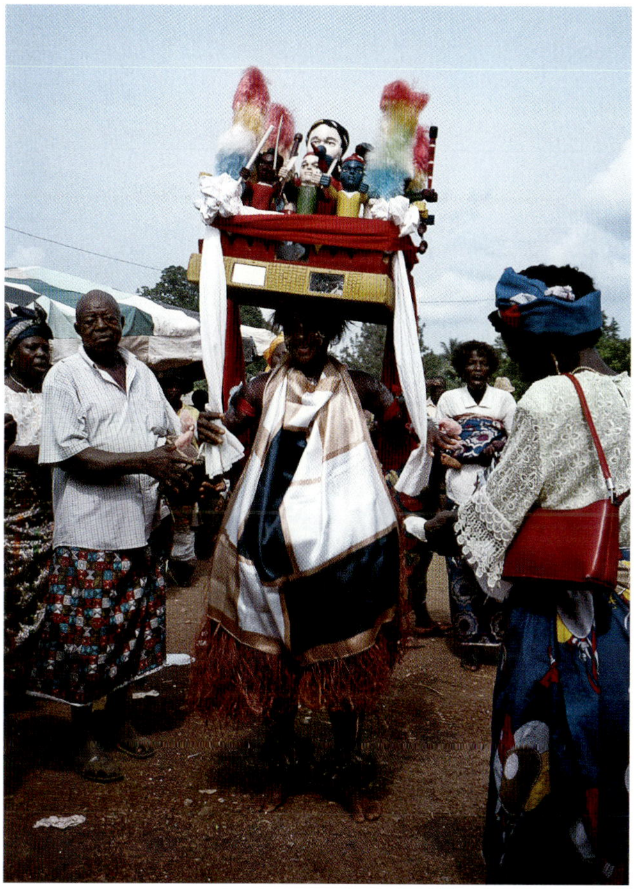

Fig. 217 The mask bearer of *Njom Ekpa* with the headdress; her face is not concealed (Ewelle, March 26, 2005).

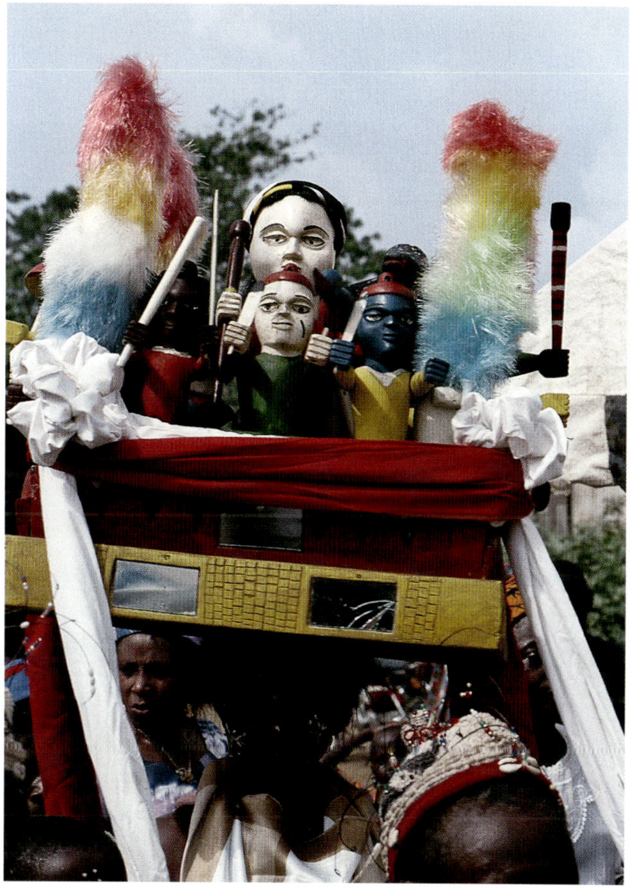

Fig. 218 The box-shaped headdress of *Njom Ekpa* with wooden figures, some with a white face, others with a black face (Ewelle, March 26, 2005).

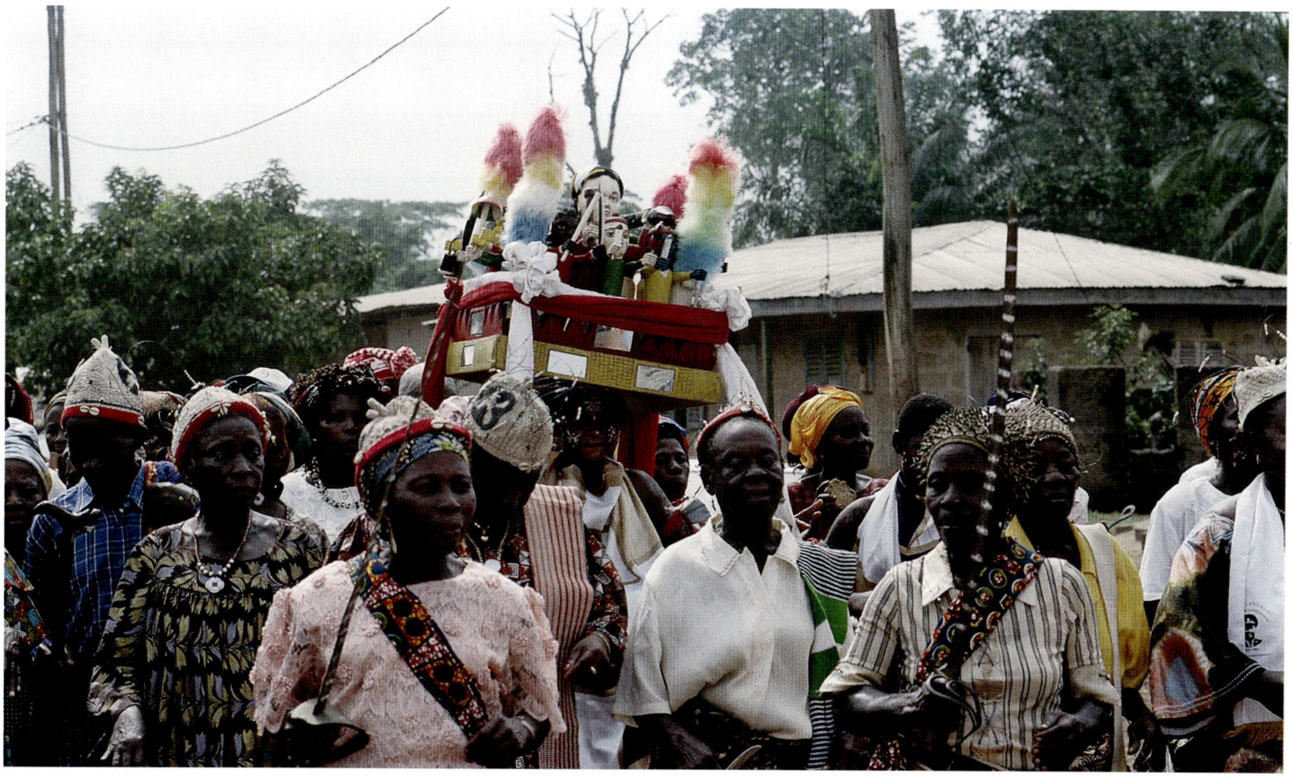

Fig. 219 The mask of *Njom Ekpa*, surrounded by members of the society; two members carry a cutlass like the men of *Nkanda* (Ewelle, March 26, 2005).

6.4 *Ndem*, the society of the elite *agbokarem*

6.4.1 Dignity and importance of the *agbokarem*

Generally *Ndem* counted as the society of the *agbokarem* (sg. *mgbokandem*), who like the *abhoninkim* were obliged to absolve a long period of initiation.[18] *Ndem* had nothing to do with the practice of circumcision, which followed later after the initiation into *Ndem* within the context of *moninkim*. According to tradition, *Ndem* was founded by the Central Ejagham, and later spread as far as the Ekwe and Obang and had even reached the Banyang. According to Mansfeld, at the beginning of the 20th century there were about 200 *agbokarem* in the entire Ngunaya region.[19] However, as will be explained further on, the society no longer exists: "The Keaka people now remember it only by name."[20]

In view of the enormous costs involved only wealthy families could "afford" a *mgbokandem*. Aside from the financial aspect, only the eldest daughter of a woman was eligible for initiation. Moreover, the daughter had to be especially intelligent and beautiful, and she had to be a virgin. Indeed, it was the *agbokarem* who, with regard to intelligence, beauty and above all morality, embodied the highest social ideal through the status and organisation of their association as well as through their own behaviour. Every family was proud, if they succeeded in creating a *mgbokandem*, and a corresponding memorial figure erected after her death was the sign of prosperity and diligence. The brideprice for a *mgbokandem* was disproportionately higher (formerly about seven slaves) than that for an ordinary woman (two to three slaves). The man who was financially able to take a *mgbokandem* as wife also enjoyed repute – she was a sign of his outstanding social position.

The *agbokarem* were highly esteemed and formed with *Ndem* an elite society.[21] Their special signs were scarifications, found variously on the temples, cheekbones, neck, back, arms and legs, and a white feather, which they wore in their hair on festive occasions (fig. 262). They had a special stool and, furthermore, they held the right to carry a staff, just like the big men. At all festivities the *agbokarem* were among the first personalities, to whom palm wine was offered. Conversely, they had to observe a number of taboos, for example, they were not allowed to eat beef and the meat of sheep. However, I was informed that they nevertheless did have the opportunity to partake in some of the forbidden foods, if they were treated with certain medicines beforehand. A man married to a *mgbokandem* was obliged to act towards her with the utmost consideration and respect; he had to fulfil her wishes as far as possible. She was not expected to carry out any greater and strenuous work.

The society of the *agbokarem* is named *Ndem*, and *mgbokandem* is translated correspondingly with "to fall under *Ndem*" or "to become a member of *Ndem*". The *agbokarem* were the only members of *Ndem*; other women were not accepted. *Ndem* (pl. *arem*) is the designation for a "wild spirit", but according to all of my informants the society of the *agbokarem* had nothing to do with supernatural spirits (*arem*).[22] Yet, the state of trance, a characteristic of the *arem*, did play an important role among the *agbokarem*.[23] If a *mgbokandem* were treated with disrespect, she would fall into a trance, and only with the help of another *mbgokandem* could she be revived to consciousness. The person whose censurable behaviour caused the trance had to pay a high fee for reviving the *mgbokandem*. A *mgbokandem* could also fall into a trance, if she saw a centipede (*nyakayong*).

The centre of *Ndem* was – at least since the beginning of the 20th century – Kembong, the largest community in the Ngunaya area. It was also the home of the last and long-term president of *Ndem* (*ntui mfam agbokarem*) Ma Oneki Mbu, until her death on January 17, 1990 (figs. 220–222). Members of the society met occasionally in her house in Okonyenge (Kembong) to discuss general matters. In other words, just as most societies in the Cross River region, *Ndem* did not possess its own meeting house, but it did have a financial reserve to cover the costs for food and drink at such meetings. *Agbokarem* appeared in public foremost on occasions that were associated with the initiation or the death of their members. They were also seen at "ordinary" death celebrations, where in performing their dances – as is always the case with special mask societies (*Nkanda*, *Nchebe*, *Mkpe*, *Njom Ekpa*) – they offered an additional great attraction for visitors and rendered a special meaningfulness to the festivity.[24] Prior to all important activities it commemorated the ancestors. Nonetheless, *Ndem* was a purely secular institution, as Ruel noted with reference to the *agbokarem* among the Banyang: "My informants denied any supernatural aim in the association and asserted its primary purpose as giving status to women."[25]

However highly reputable and esteemed *Ndem* may have been, it was not charged with defending the rights

Figs. 220–222 Ma Oneki Mbu, a *mgbokandem* from Kembong and the last leader of the *agbokarem* (died on January 17, 1990), wearing a feather headdress and bead necklaces around her neck. Her body is rubbed with yellow camwood (Kembong, February 26, 1980). ▸

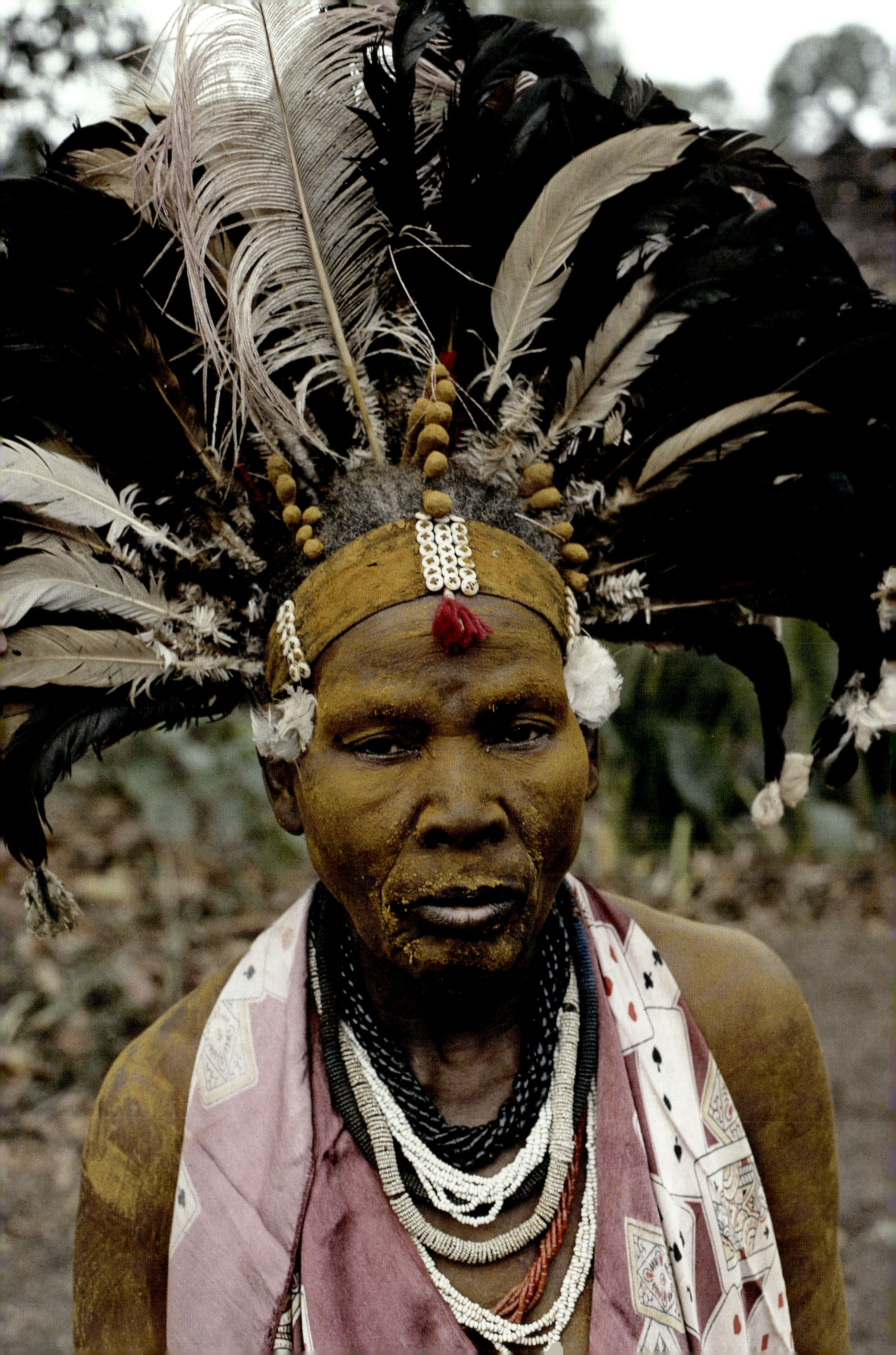

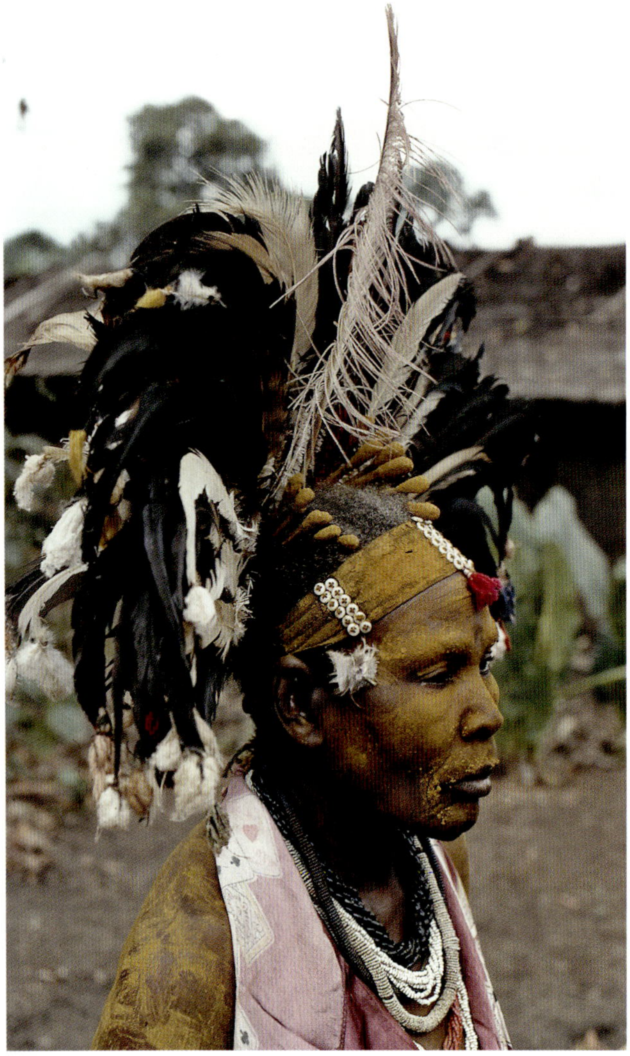

Fig. 221 Close-up of Ma Oneki Mbu (Kembong, February 26, 1980).

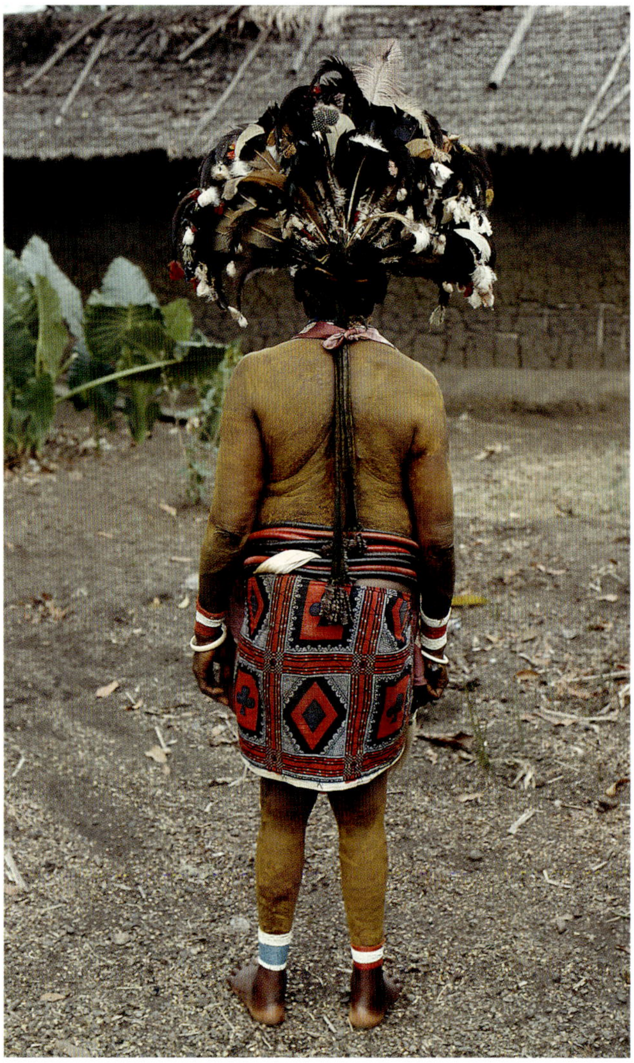

Fig. 222 Ma Oneki Mbu with the colourful skirt and ropes of beads around the waist (Kembong, February 26, 1980).

and interests of women in general nor did it have the facilities to do so. That was the responsibility of *Mawu*. *Ndem* was not a political factor in the strict sense; it could neither make any political decisions nor impose any punishments. However, *Ndem* did hold political power in that it contributed towards integrating the numerous, mostly small groups of settlements in the region, which had the same language and culture, yet never had formed a political unit. And, thus, its special significance lay in fostering identity and furthering peace in the entire region.

Correspondent with the outstanding position of the *agbokarem*, there was – on the one hand – a specific essential condition for acceptance into this elite and exclusive circle, and – on the other – the initiation involved unusually extravagant and intensive rituals and festivities. The preparations for initiation began when the girls were between 12 and 15 years of age, "when the breasts began to develop."[26]

6.4.2 The long period of initiation into *Ndem*

6.4.2.1 *Agbut etene Ndem*, "to set aside *Ndem*"

When a family decided that one of their daughters should be initiated into the circle of *agbokarem*, the father invited an older *mgbokandem* to his house to discuss the preparations and proceedings. The girl was now "set aside" from the normal social life of an ordinary woman and was "reserved" for full membership into the *Ndem* society in the future. First, one feather of the guinea fowl (*enyeng*) and the small carved "stick of *Ndem*" (*beti Ndem*) were stuck into her hair. From this time onwards her hair must not be cut, and she had to continue to maintain her virginity and purity. It was her duty to attend all *Ndem* dances and thereby to watch the various styles of dancing. She had to learn the songs and the general behaviour of the society. There was no time limit between this stage and the next, but usually what she was requested to learn might take between six to nine months. As soon as the elderly members observed that the girl knew the dances and songs and also the secret language (*esoble Ndem*), the father was informed to carry out the next stages of making her a *mgbokandem*. Her teacher, the older *mgbokandem*, was given one jug of palm wine, one "animal" and a bowl of plantains.

6.4.2.2 *Akesu Ndem*, "to wash *Ndem*"

Seven or fourteen days before the initiation started, the father looked for an "animal" to purchase, many plantains and palm wine; he then invited the villagers (*Etek*) to announce that his daughter would soon undergo the initiation of a *mgbokandem*. Thereafter the father invited the older *mgbokandem* to become her teacher once more. She was informed that his daughter would soon enter the house of *Ndem* (*ayi nju Ndem*). The woman was given one "animal", a jug of palm wine and a bowl of plantains (*eboko eghoh*). When the actual initiation proceedings began, the woman was already in the compound in the early morning. The girl bathed in warm water and was then led into a room, where no outsiders saw her again. At this point she had "entered the house of *Ndem*". During this stage, which lasted seven days (usually called *ejah*), she was strictly forbidden to leave the room. If she wanted to go to the latrine, she was carried by somebody on the back and a mat was placed over her head to conceal her head and whole body. Her hair was now long enough so that a few feathers of the peacock (*nkundak*) could be inserted in it. During these seven days she no longer had a name; she lost it the moment she entered the house of *Ndem*.

Early in the morning of the seventh day the officiating *mgbokandem* woman "killed" the girl ritually. She was placed as a dead person (*ayu Ndem*). upon a bed, while the officiating woman went to the bush to collect the necessary herbs. During this time a fence made of fronds from the palm tree was erected in front of the girl's compound. It had to be finished by the time the woman returned with the herbs.[27] Upon the arrival of the officiating *mgbokandem*, a hole was dug at the entrance of the fence and the medicine herbs were buried in it. Fire was kindled on top of the medicines, and more plants were put on the fire including pepper to provoke coughing. The "dead" girl (*ayu Ndem*) was held over the smoking fire seven times. If she coughed, she could never become a *mgbokandem*. If she resisted the choking smoke throughout the seven times she was held over the fire, she was qualified to become a *mgbokandem*.[28] She was taken back into her room to the satisfaction of the officiating woman and her parents and relatives. Then her body was rubbed with medicines by the officiating woman "to bring her back to life" again.

The initiated girl remained in the house of *Ndem* for another period of seven days. From the day on which she had become a *mgbokandem*, she did not eat any food except plantains and meat. Since she had been a "dead" person, she had to be taught how to walk again and she was also given a new name – usually the name of her deceased grandmother. On the fourteenth day one or two curved feathers (*aneng nifut*) were added to her hair. They were similar to those of the tail of a cock. After these feathers had been inserted in her hair, she began to eat *elolo Ndem*. Some medicine was put in a cup together with palm wine and also a long narrow tube; the person in charge of this ritual blew air through the tube into the palm wine. The air caused foam to form, which the young *mgbokandem* took with her palms to eat. It was said that the foam helped to make *mgbokandem* fat and fresh. The process was repeated daily as long as the father of the girl wished, yet not exceeding fourteen days.

6.4.2.3 *Ayi nju Ndem*, "to enter the house of *Ndem*"

On the fourteenth day the girl was presented to the public, an occasion which was called *ake sangha Ndem* ("exposing the new *mgbokandem*"). Relatives and well-wishers gave presents to the new *mgbokandem*. From that day on the young *mgbokandem* returned to normal life, as regards her daily actions. However, she had to observe certain taboos and duties. For example, she was not allowed to be touched by rain and by water in general. Thus, it was forbidden for her to take a bath. Further, she was not allowed to eat the meat of sheep and beef or fufu (*olang*), the main dish in the region. In their stead she lived mainly on plantains. She rubbed her body daily with red palm oil and camwood. The feathers remained on her head all the time, even when in bed, and she never carried a load upon her head. From then on she did not speak the ordinary language, but communicated only with the special, secret language of *agbokarem* and through signs. The period of seclusion was extremely long and could last anywhere from two to seven years. After about three months, always by a waning moon, her body was scarified (*ake gbe nko Ndem*). These body marks served not only as ornamentation and a sign of a special person; special medicine was inserted into the cuts which was meant as a protection for the respective *mgbokandem*. The principal components of this medicine came from cattle, sheep and also millipedes, and for this reason these animals were taboo for *agbokarem*. Seclusion was a time of little contact with the outside world; and when the girl did receive a visitor, this person was obligated to bring gifts. And yet, a *mgbokandem* could marry and bear children during the period of seclusion.

6.4.2.4 *Agbep mfut Ndem*, "inserting the feathers of a peacock"

When the family was ready for the final stage of the long period of seclusion, announcements were made inviting all *agbokarem* of the region to the festivities. On the eve of the day of the ceremony, *agbokarem* assembled at the new *mgbokandem*'s compound. There was great feasting and dancing till morning. In the morning the feathers, which the initiate had worn on her head for many years, were removed. At this time she received only a few feathers. This stage was called *agbep mfut Ndem* ("inserting the feathers of a peacock"). If the family was rich, the guests remained in the compound, enjoying food, drink and dance for seven days. During this time the new *mgbokandem* visited relatives, who accorded her with great honour and respect and also gave her gifts.

On the fourteenth day she was dressed in full as a *mgbokandem*. She held the actual sign of a *mgbokandem*, the bone of an ape, the so-called staff of *Ndem* (*osa Ndem*) in her left hand; in her right hand, a dance fan. Her body was painted with ash and yellow camwood, her face decorated with geometric designs. As a headdress she wore a headband and a very attractive arrangement of long feathers of the chicken, guineafowl and other birds. Bead necklaces were obligatory around the neck, hips and wrists as were ribbons and small cloths. Further accessories included small calabasses, snailshells, bones and the like. Rattles worn on the ankles (*ngya Ndem*) were indispensable for dancing, and a skin with small brass bells (*ngu Ndem*) was worn on the back. Wearing this outfit the *mgbokandem* was set upon a stool (*elo Ndem*), and at that moment the scene greatly resembled the commemorative monument for a *mgbokandem* (see below).

The dances on that day were called *efale Ndem* ("going round in a circle") and were repeated six times. At the last dance the new *mgbokandem* was carried upon the shoulders of her husband's friends to the husband's house. If she was not married, male members of her family carried her to her father's compound.[29] This brought the ceremony to an end. Thereafter the new *mgbokandem* returned to normal life, which means that she did not have to observe most of the taboos that were imposed upon her during the period of seclusion. Thus, she could use the common language of the Ejagham again, and she was permitted to wash herself. As mentioned above, initiation into *Ndem* was not connected with the ritual of circumcision. This was carried out later, and young *agbokarem* underwent this as a *moninkim* just like all women.

6.4.3 Commemorative monuments for the *agbokarem*

The outstanding position that the *agbokarem* attained – usually there were no more than two or three in a settlement – was emphasised in particular through the commemorative figures (*ayem*, sg. *oyem*), which were erected to honour them after their death.[30] These life-sized figures are among the most renowned and remarkable works of art ever produced by the Central Ejagham. They have no religious significance and are not to be seen as ancestral figures. No ceremonies of offering were conducted before them. Their sole purpose was to commemorate an important woman, while at the same time they were also the sign of a successful and esteemed family. The figures depict women in a seated position, which – typical of African art – do not display any movement; the hands rest upon the knees. The figures were not seen as portraits of particular persons. This was also explained to me in 2004 by an old bricklayer from Ayukaba, who was probably the last craftsman capable of creating such figures in the Ngunaya area. He had made a total of 45 figures in his lifetime. Supposedly they were, at least as he emphasised, "all the same", and none of the contractors had ever expressed any special wish concerning the appearance of the figure. The bricklayer himself had never seen most of the *agbokarem* in life, for whom he had made a commemorative figure.

Originally the figures were made of clay and sheltered from rain by a protective roof. Later during the colonial period they gradually came to be made of cement and, thus, remained preserved much longer. The *mgbokandem* figures are the easternmost representatives of the widespread west African clay figures in the form of grave and cult figures.[31] Clay figures of this kind are not found any farther to the east, neither in the Bamenda region nor among the Bamileke.

Upon the death of a *mgbokandem*, the corpse was taken to the parents' compound and placed upon a bier. Attired with the special jewellery of a *mgbokandem*, the deceased was arranged in a seated position. It is this position that is typical of the commemorative monu-

Commemorative figures for *agbokarem* in Ashum (southern Banyang) (March 15, 1975) (figs. 223–227).

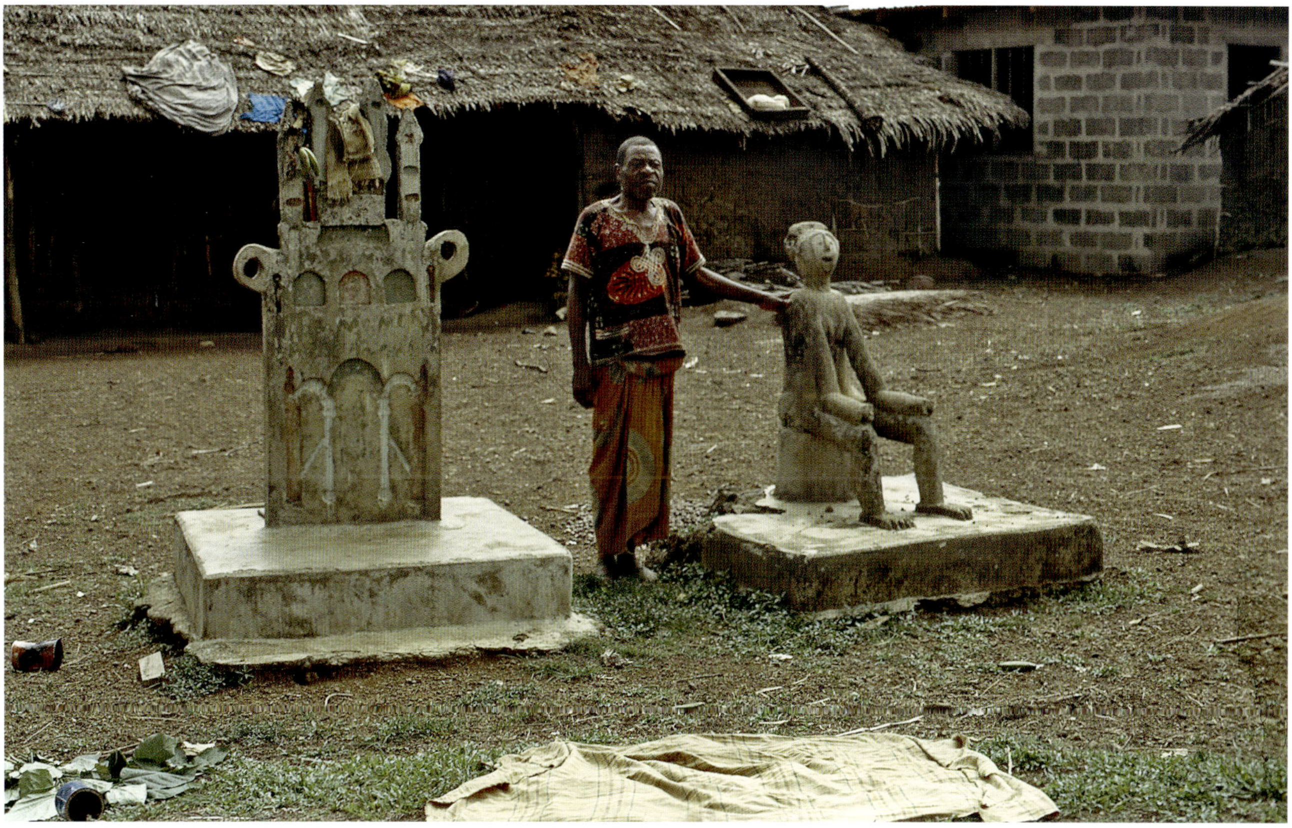

Fig. 223 Commemorative figure for a *mgbokandem*. The board-shaped decorated monument next to it has nothing to do with the *agbokarem* and is a recent development (Ashum, March 15, 1975).

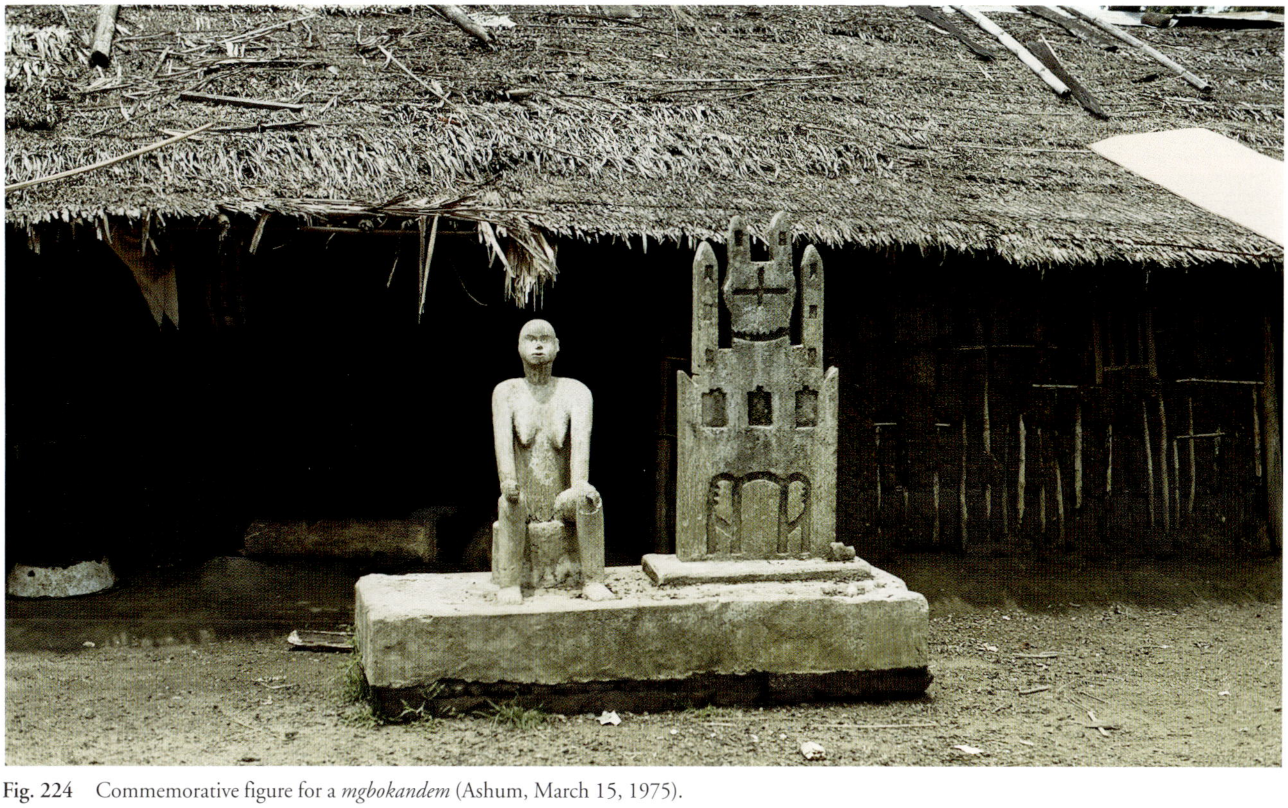

Fig. 224 Commemorative figure for a *mgbokandem* (Ashum, March 15, 1975).

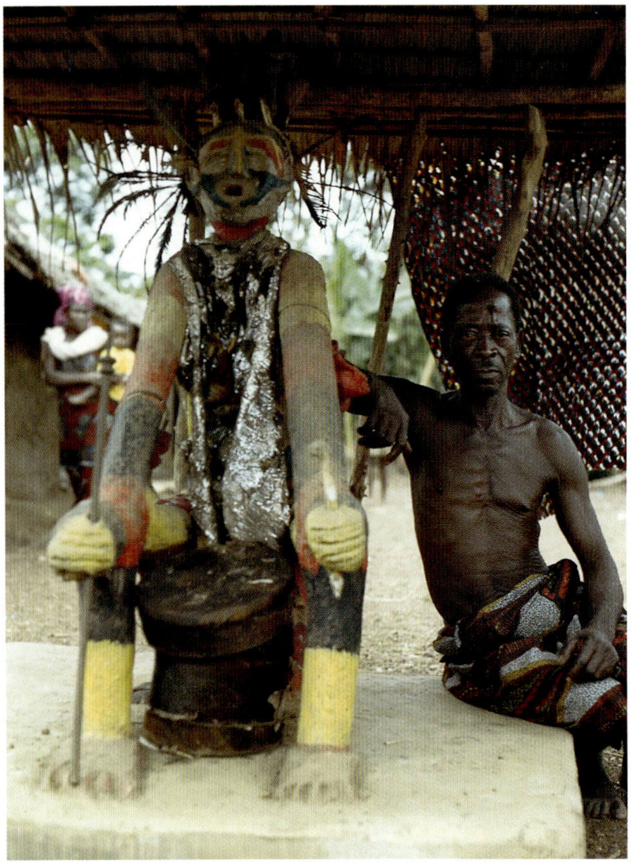

Fig. 225 Newly erected commemorative figure with the jewellery and insignia of the deceased *mgbokandem*; on the right one of her sons (Ashum, March 15, 1975).

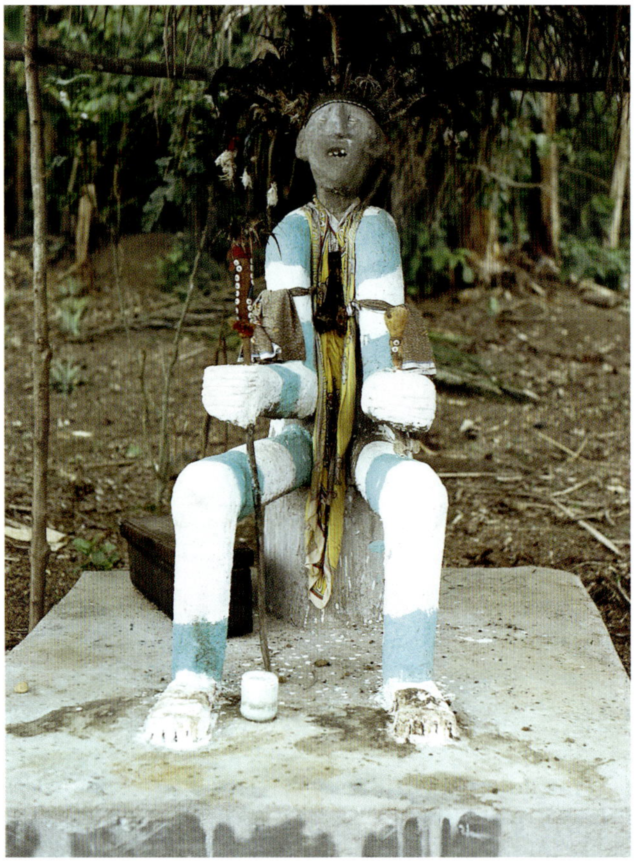

Fig. 226 Newly erected commemorative figure for a *mgbokandem* (Ashum, March 15, 1975).

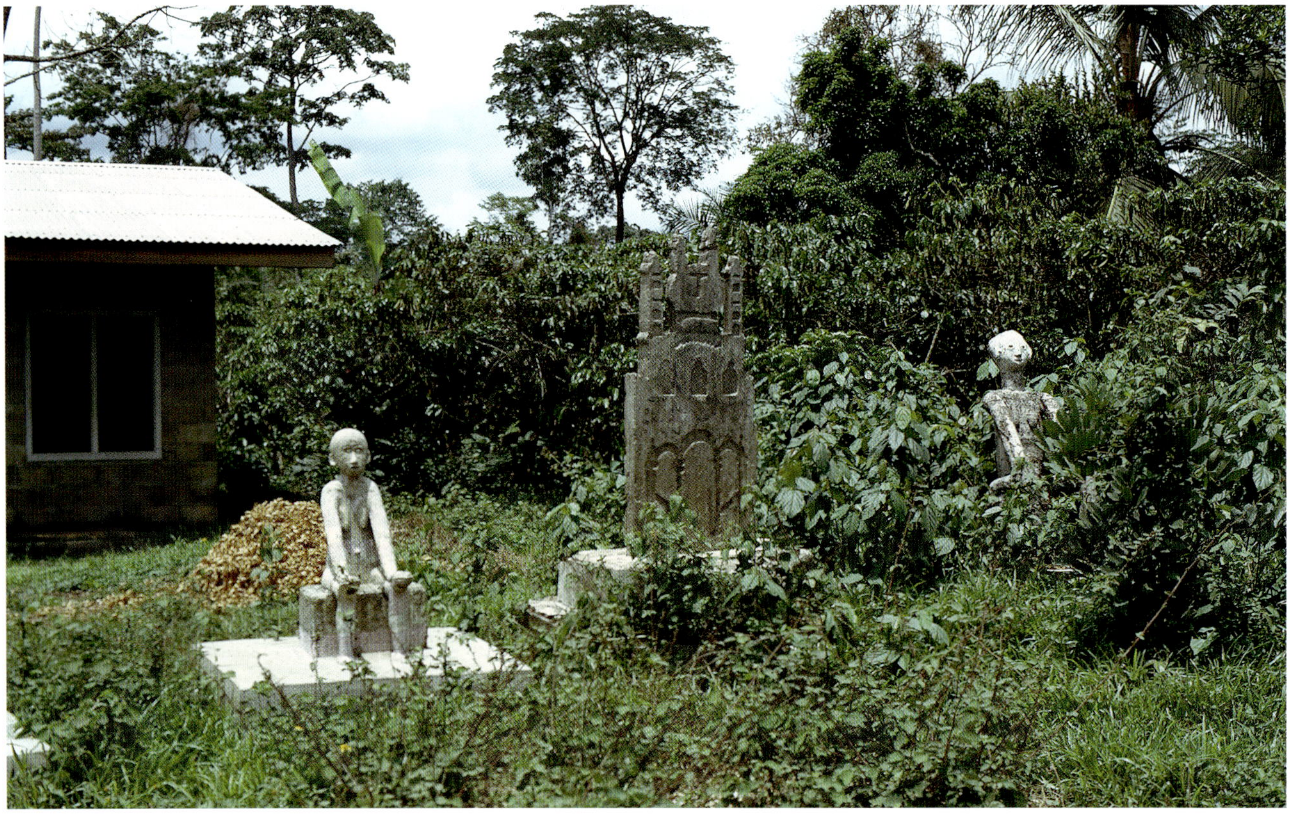

Fig. 227 Two commemorative figures for *agbokarem* (Ashum, March 15, 1975).

Commemorative figures for *agbokarem* in Kembong (January 1980) (figs. 228–234).

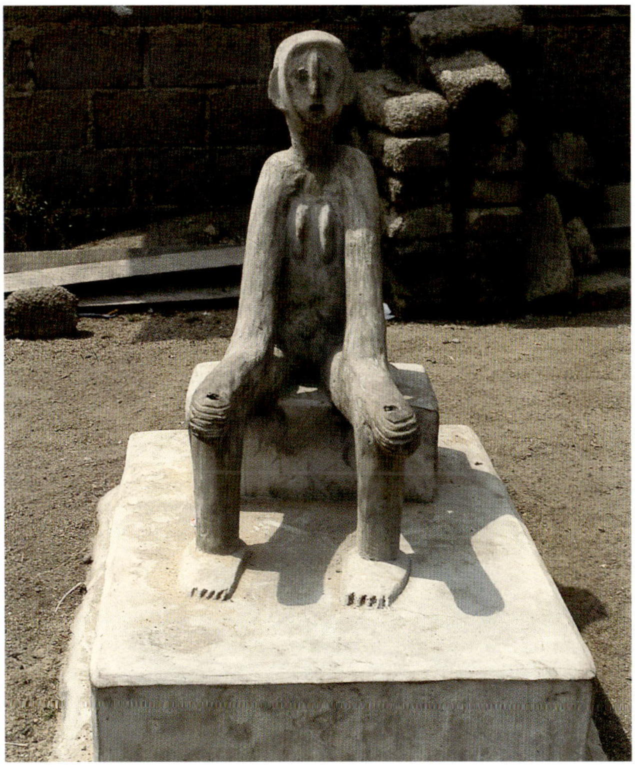

Fig. 228 Commemorative figure for a *mgbokandem* (Kembong, January 30, 1980).

ments. The burial ceremony was marked by the dances of the *agbokarem*, who could come from anywhere in the vicinity. The dances lasted through the night until dawn. Then the corpse – without any jewellery – was buried in the same manner as an ordinary woman.

The production of a commemorative monument usually began soon after the burial and the memorial ceremony (*aboku*) had taken place. That is to say, this occurred if the particular family had the financial means for both the figure and the ceremony. Sometimes there were cases of families who could not afford a commemorative monument for the deceased *mgbokandem*. Craftsmen needed about two weeks' time to make the figure. If the contractor lived at a far distance, the craftsman stayed in this person's compound during the time of work and, of course, was accommodated generously by the host. Work on the figure itself was carried out under the exclusion of the public. No one was allowed to see how such a figure was created; the craftsmen were not ready to reveal their secret methods of production. Whereas the graves of the deceased were and still are generally located behind the houses, in most cases commemorative figures were placed in front of the houses, towards the street, so that they could be easily seen.

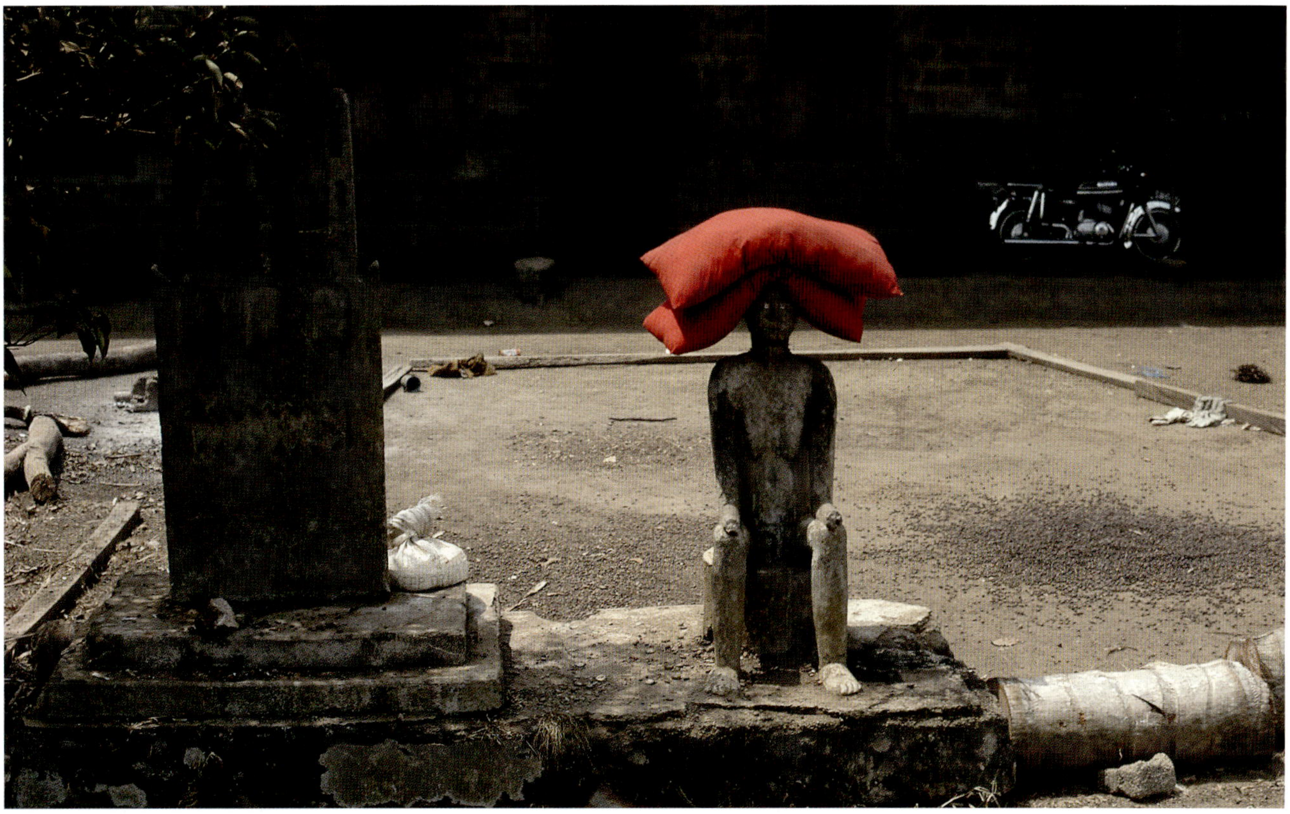

Fig. 229 Commemorative figures were not sacred; sometimes they served quite ordinary purposes, such as here – airing pillows (Kembong, January 31, 1980).

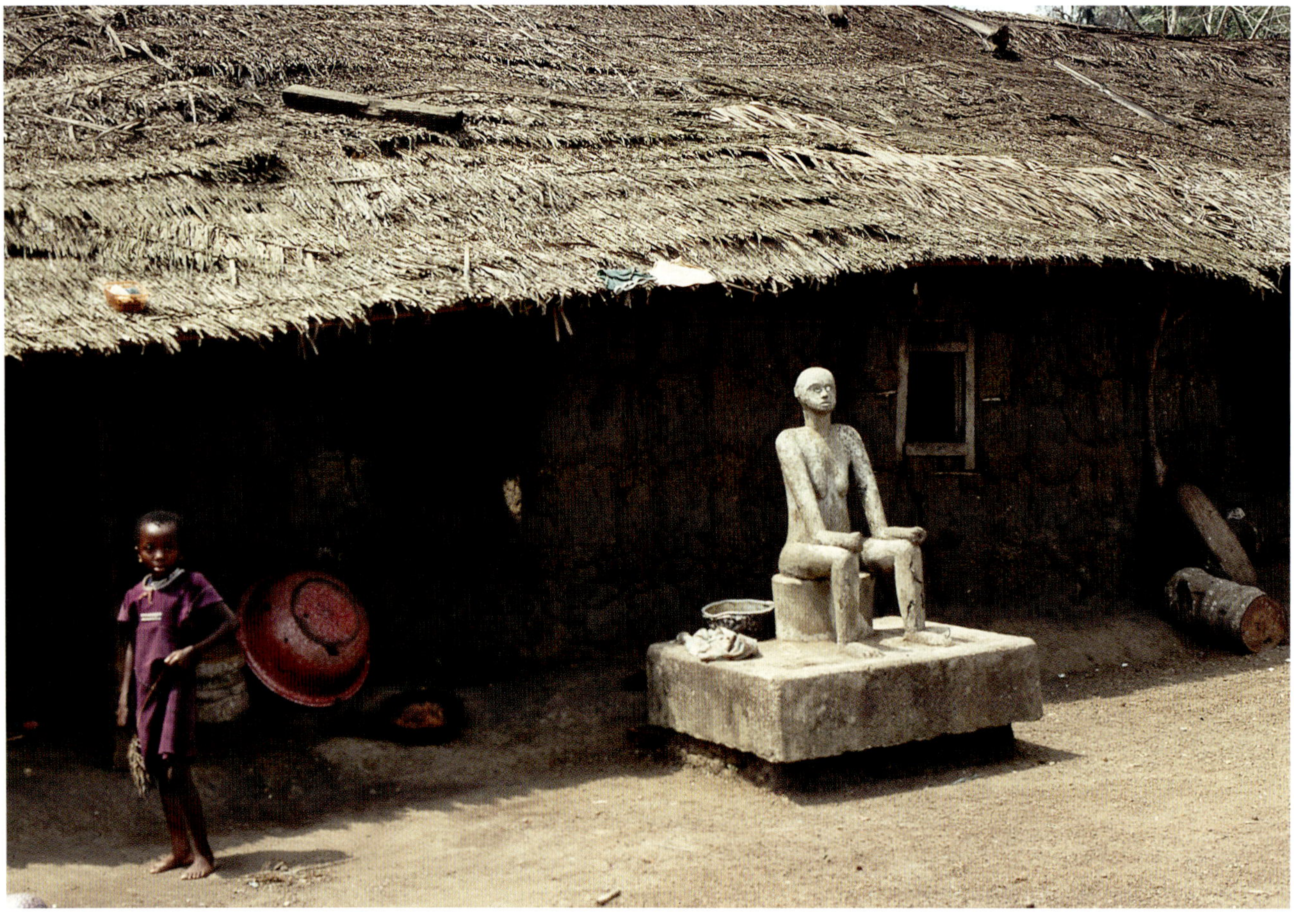

Fig. 230 Commemorative figure for a *mgbokandem* (Kembong, January 31, 1980).

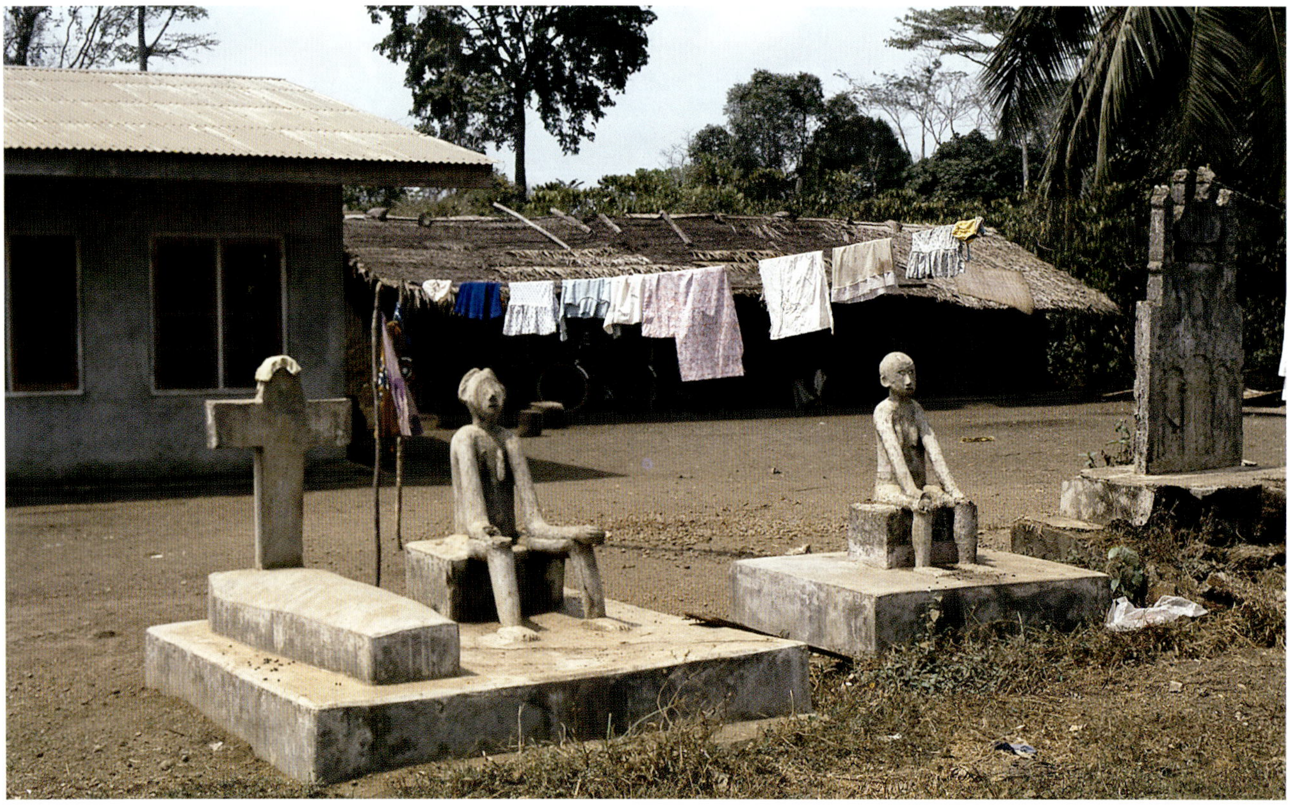

Fig. 231 Two commemorative figures for *agbokarem* next to new grave monuments (Kembong, January 31, 1980).

A newly erected commemorative figure for a *mgbokandem* (Kembong, January 28, 1980) (figs. 232–234).

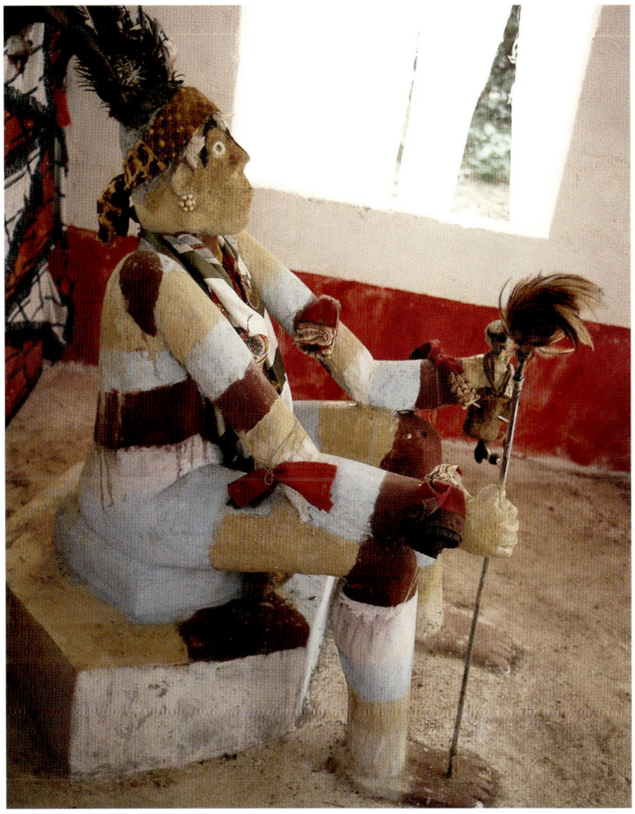

Fig. 232 The figure is adorned with feathers, jewellery and other accessories of the deceased inside a protective shelter (Kembong, January 28, 1980).

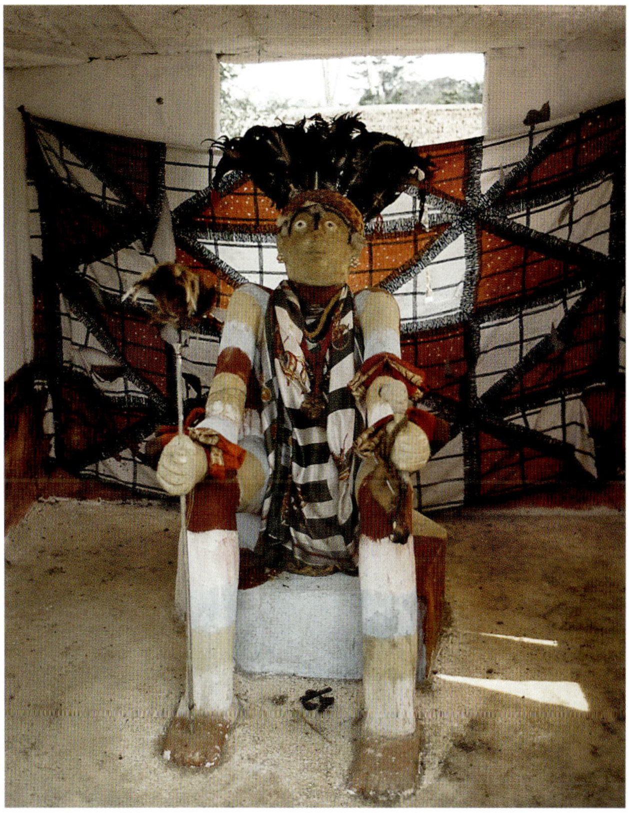

Fig. 233 Frontal view of the newly erected figure (Kembong, January 28, 1980).

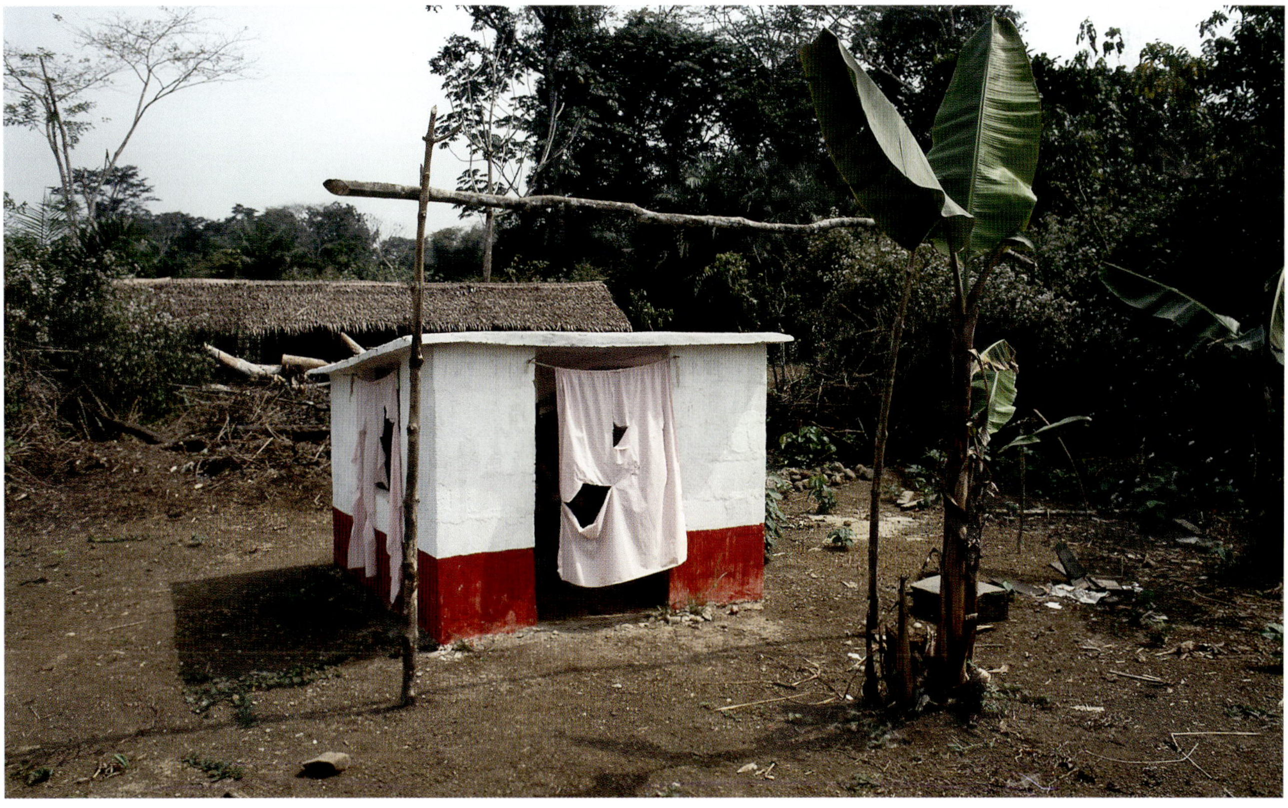

Fig. 234 The shelter as seen from outside (Kembong, January 28, 1980).

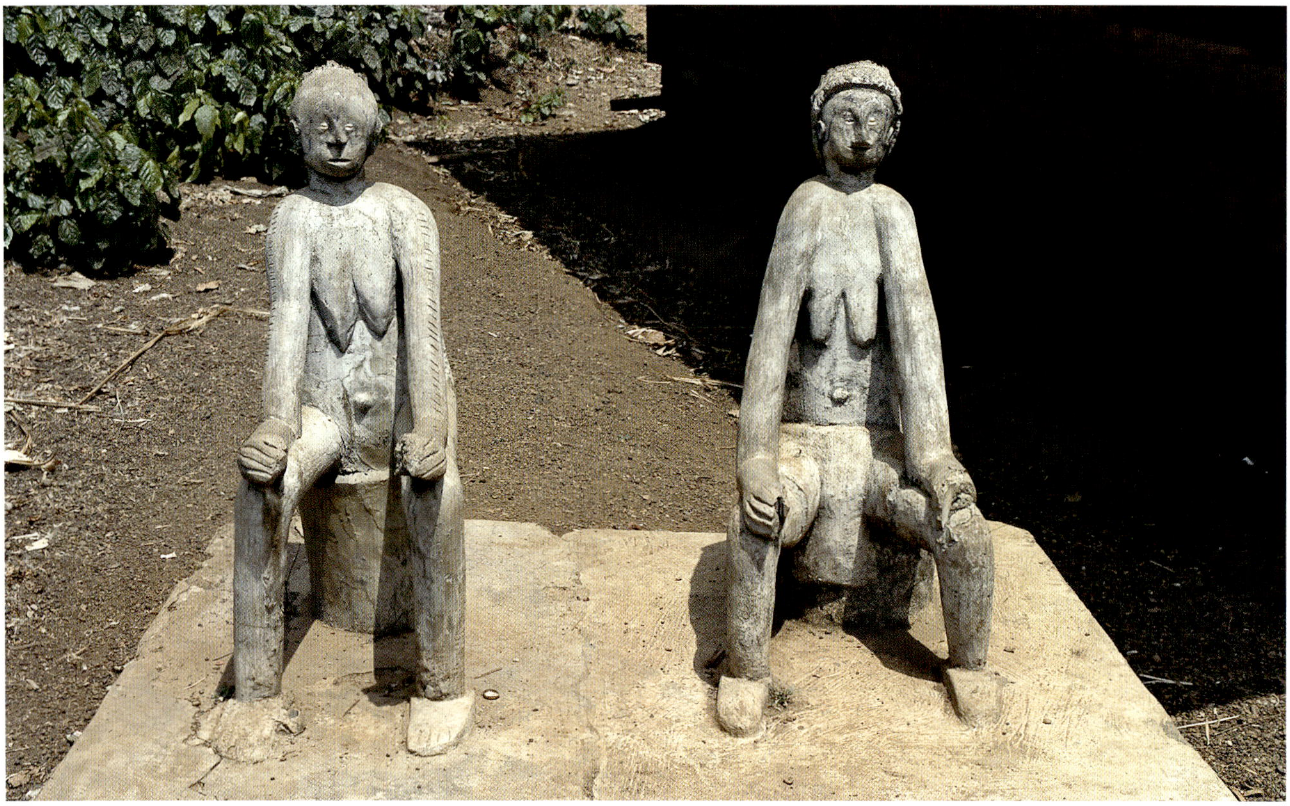

Fig. 235 Two commemorative figures for *agbokarem* in Ajayukndip (February 22, 1980).

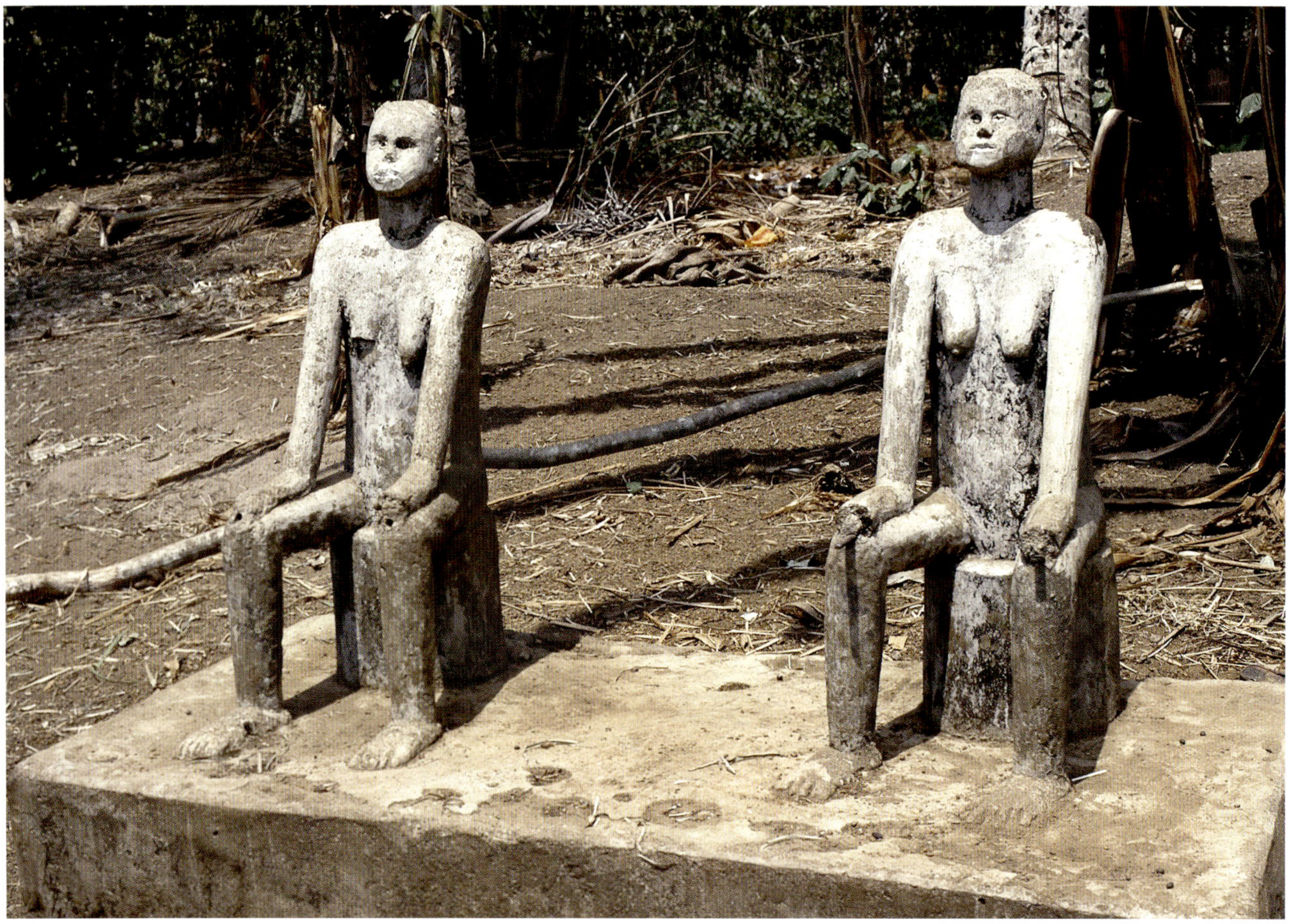

Fig. 236 Two commemorative figures for *agbokarem* in Ajayukndip (February 22, 1980).

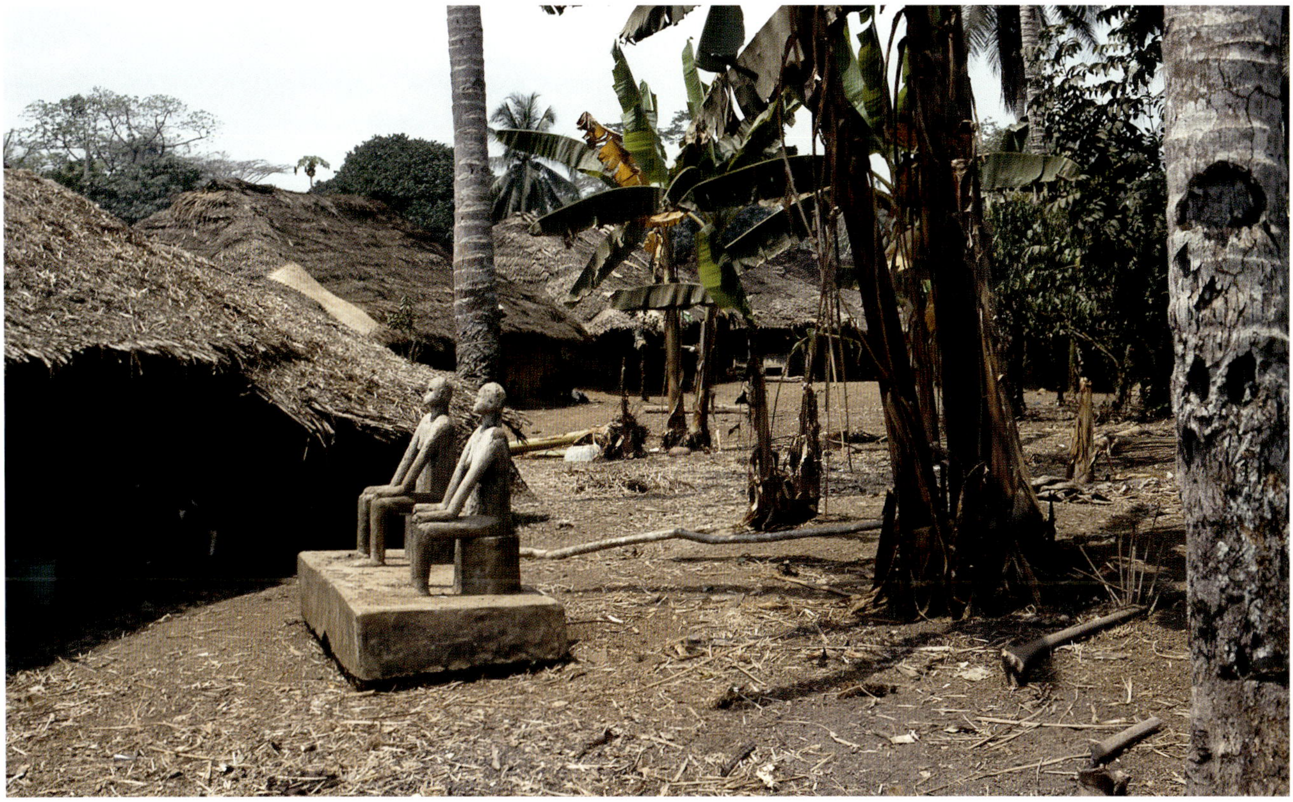

Fig. 237 Two commemorative figures for *agbokarem* in Ajayukndip in their surroundings (February 22, 1980).

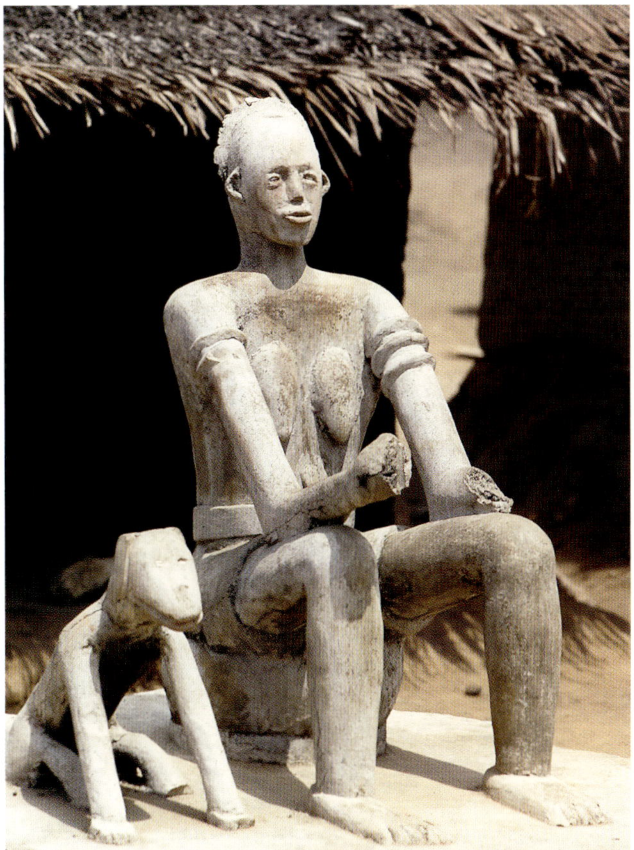

Fig. 238 A *mgbokandem* commemorative figure in Babong with an exceptional feature: the figure of a dog at its side (February 21, 1980).

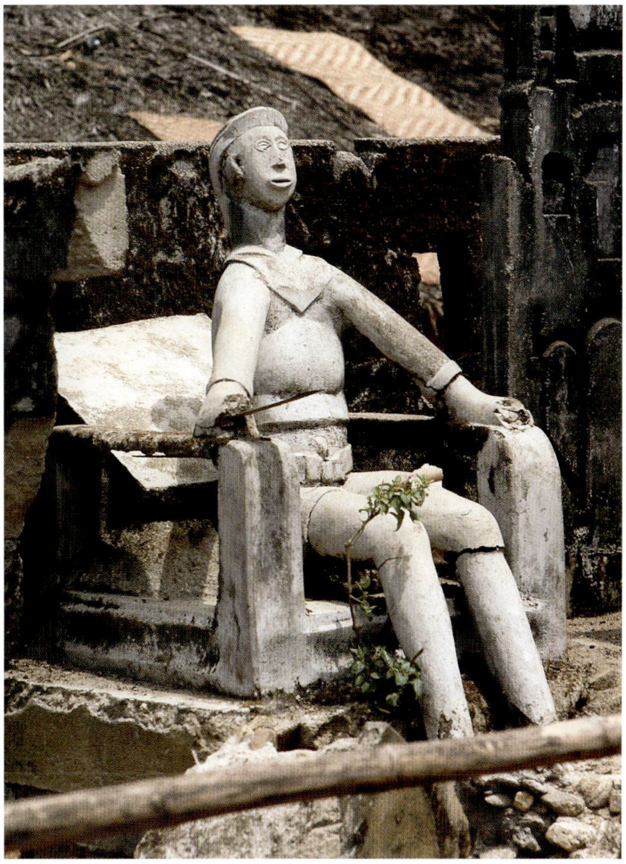

Fig. 239 Commemorative figure for a *mgbokandem* from Babong in an atypical form: it wears clothes and a head covering and is seated upon a modern chair (February 21, 1980).

The public presentation of the figure (*oyem olebe*) followed directly upon completion of work. Now the jewellery of the deceased was placed upon the figure (figs. 225–226, 232–233, 242–243). All of this went on within the context of a big festivity that lasted for several days. Besides other animals, even a cow was slaughtered for the occasion. Such festive occasions were distinctly marked by the performances of the *agbokarem*. In earlier times one could reckon with the appearance of some twenty to thirty *agbokarem*, most of them from the vicinity. They were all accommodated in the compound of the host, which they were not allowed to leave during the festivities. Otherwise, it would have meant that they had only come for a sexual adventure.

The first day of the occasion was the "burial" and – as with a proper burial – this belonged to the *agbokarem*. They danced throughout the entire night until the next evening. This was concluded with an offering to the ancestors (*ajom Ndem*), and it was of the eldest *mgbokandem* who addressed a prayer to the deceased. First an offering of ritual food was made: "Your *Ndem* society has danced for you, and your monument has been made. Do not say that it has not been made. We have come to open the monument. Ma, we have made your monument, so give us luck and not ill-luck. Let your family prosper. Those members of your family who are in white man's countries and those who are at home or in any other part of Africa, let them be blessed in all undertakings." This was followed by a libation with water: "*Ma*, as you have gone ahead and some coming behind – all cannot die at the same time. We need your total support by blessing us." Holding the glass in both hands, the eldest *mgbokandem* poured the water onto the ground: "When an ancestor has eaten, he will drink water. This is your water, I am giving it to you. May your soul rest in perfect peace." This prayer was usually repeated when the offering of palm wine was made. The following day was *aboku*. The feasting and drinking continued, and now other societies had the opportunity to honour the deceased with their dances.

6.4.4 The decline of *Ndem*

Ever since Western influence has called the basis of the old world order into question in the broadest sense, such formerly fundamental and central institutions such as that of the *agbokarem* have lost their meaningfulness and significance. In a social system, in which the social integration of the individual is not as important as in earlier times, and in its stead economic and material goals are given top priority, the extensive financial as well as temporal efforts of this exclusive association were no longer warranted.

The last initiation into *Ndem* took place sometime between 1940 and 1950. During my stay in the Manyu Division in 1980 there were some ten *agbokarem* still living, all of old age. No more initiations could take place, because none of the *agbokarem* were knowledgeable about the medicines that were needed for the rituals. The last commemorative figure was erected in Ewelle in 2002. It was not made by a local artist, but by an Igbo from Nigeria (fig. 243). On the occasion of its presentation to the public only three *agbokarem* were present.
Even in 1980 it was difficult to find sufficient and authentic information about this subject matter, despite the fact that I had the opportunity to speak with nearly all of the *agbokarem* who were still living at that time. The information was contradictory sometimes, especially when complex rituals were concerned. However, the commemorative monuments could still be seen everywhere. They radiated a special peace and dignity and were one of the greatest attractions in every community (figs. 223–239). During my research trip in 1980 I was able to acquire a damaged and no longer "usable" commemorative figure in the village of Ogomoko for the Linden-Museum in Stuttgart (Germany).[32] First the monument was repaired by the bricklayer, Ajbornkongho Ayukndip Dickson, in Kembong. Then the *mgbokandem* Ebob Arrey decorated it with old objects from her family possessions, in accordance with tradition, as all emphasised who saw the monument. The figure has been on display in the permanent exhibition on Africa in the Linden-Museum since 1985 (figs. 209, 240–242).

Today, 25 years later, some commemorative figures still exist in the Manyu Division, but fewer by far and mostly in a neglected, desolate and ruinous condition. Almost all of the figures are damaged, many are without head or arms, and oftentimes they have even toppled over and now lie on the ground next to the base, surrounded by dirt and rubbish (figs. 244–251). Interest in them seems to have disappeared.

Purchase and restoration of a damaged commemorative figure for the Linden-Museum, Stuttgart (Germany) (January 28 and February 3, 1980) (figs. 240–242).

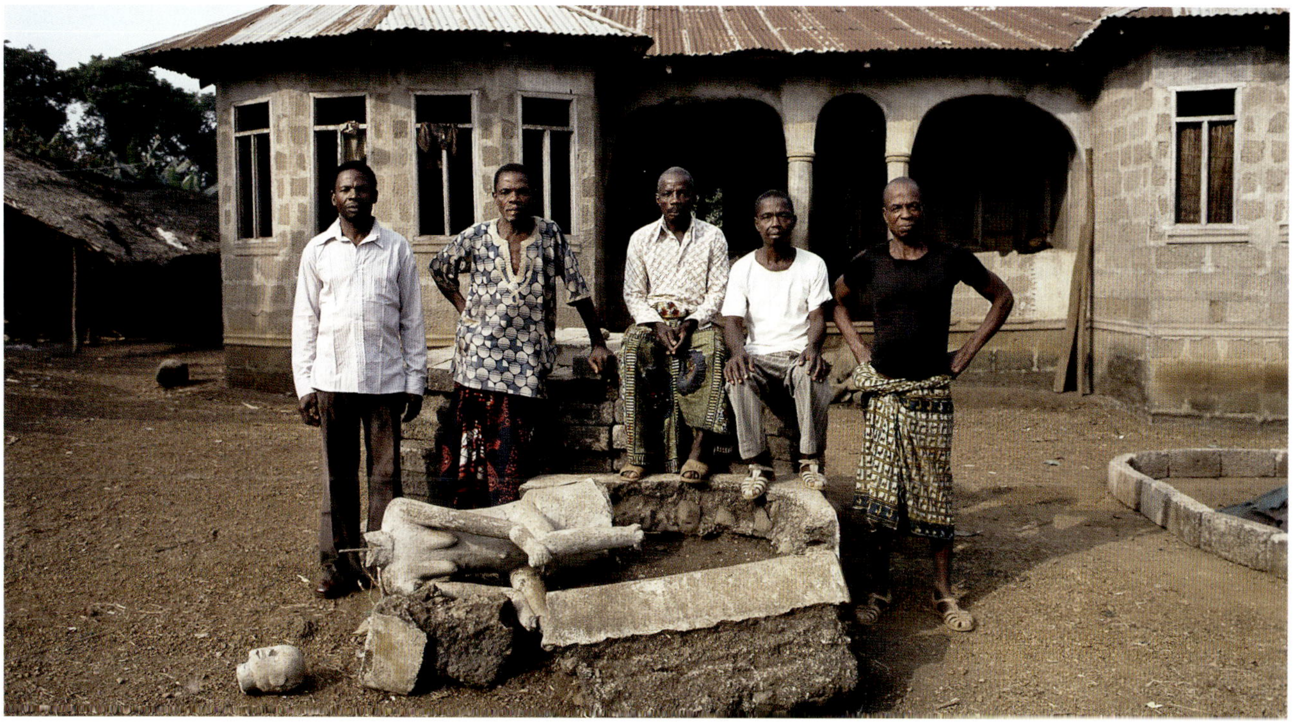

Fig. 240 Older commemorative figure, damaged, toppled over and no longer in use. The figure was acquired in Ogomoko, restored and is now on display in the Linden-Museum in Stuttgart, Germany (cp. fig. 209) (Ogomoko, January 28, 1980).

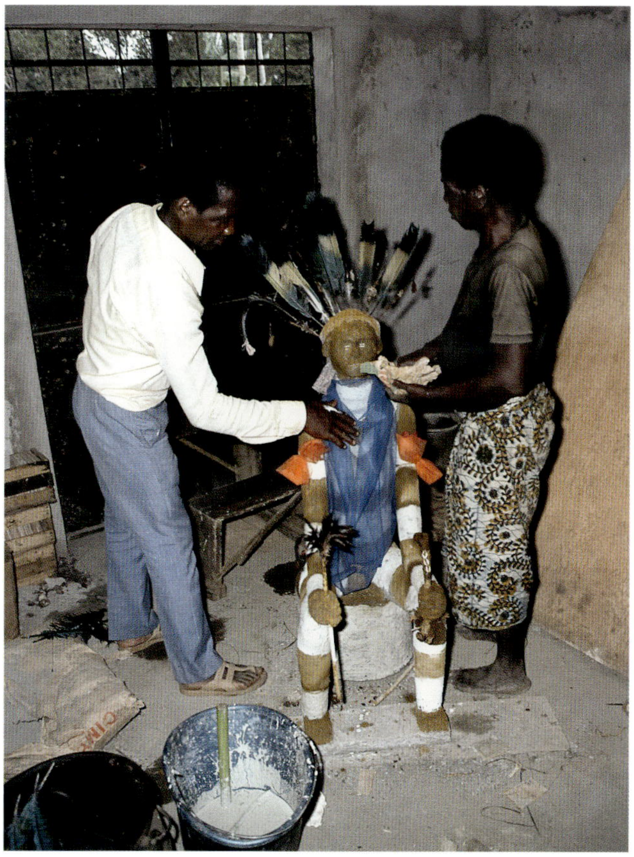

Fig. 241 Restoration of the damaged commemorative figure. Ebob Arrey, the *mgbokandem* (right), and Ajbornkongho Ayukndip Dickson, the bricklayer (left) (Kembong, February 3, 1980).

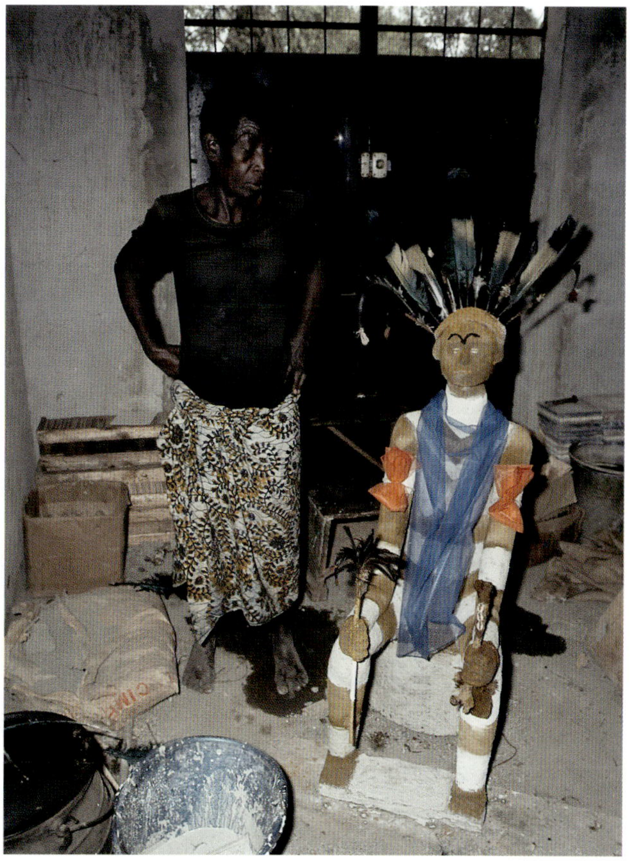

Fig. 242 Ebob Arrey, the *mgbokandem*, next to the restored figure (Kembong, February 3, 1980).

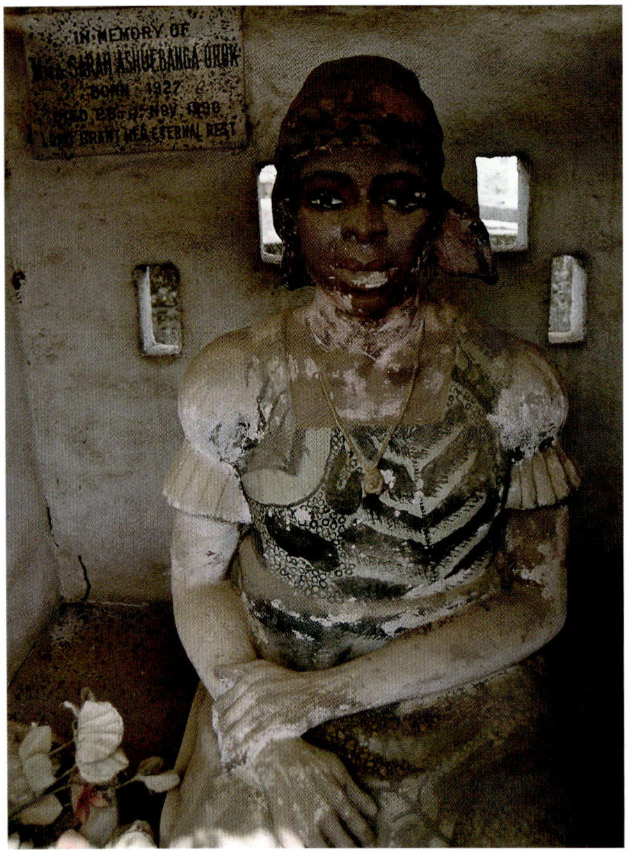

Fig. 243 An unusual commemorative figure that is rather like a portrait and – unlike earlier figures – displays features of the face and body as well as many details of the clothing. It was created by an artist of the Igbo from Nigeria (Ewelle, January 29, 2004).

Commemorative figures for *agbokarem* in their present-day damaged and neglected condition (figs. 244–251).

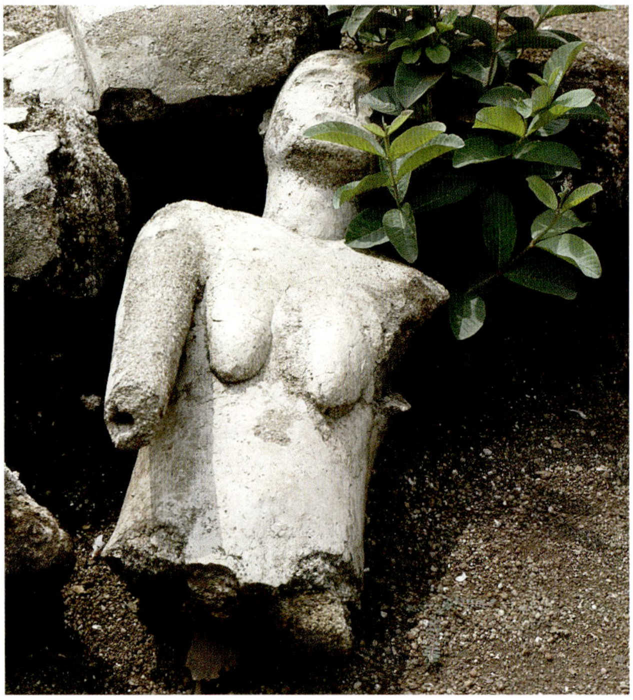

Fig. 244 The torso of a commemorative figure (Kembong, January 21, 2004).

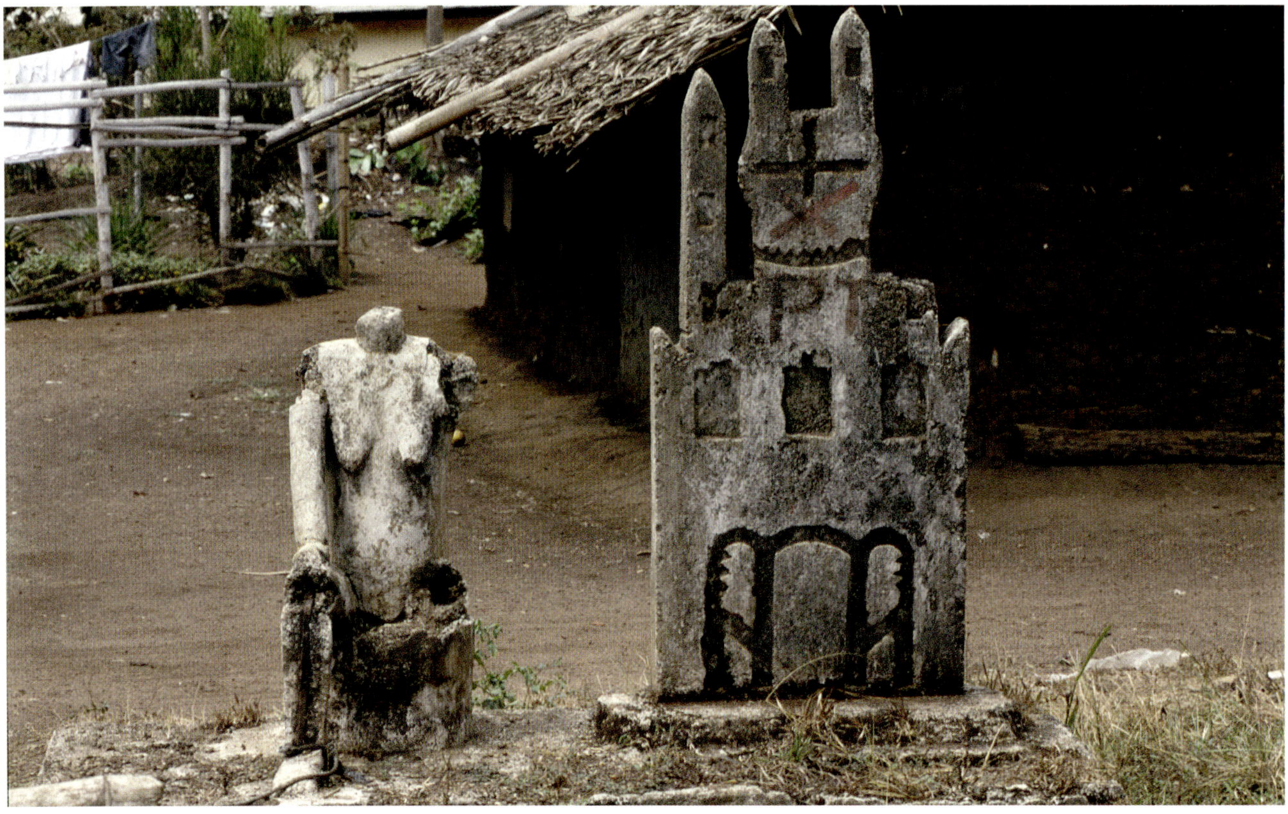

Fig. 245 A headless commemorative figure (Kembong, January 21, 2004).

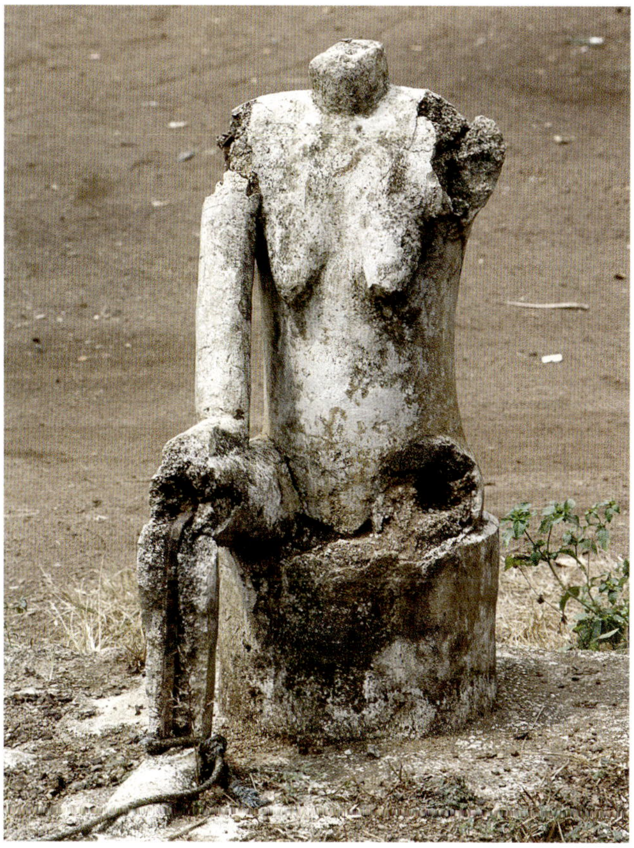

Fig. 246 The remains of a commemorative figure (Kembong, January 21, 2004).

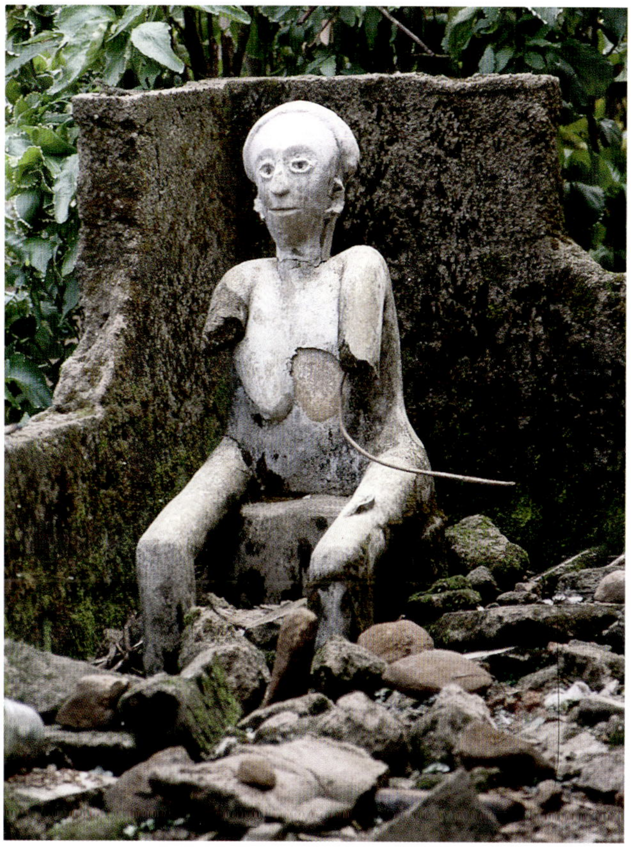

Fig. 247 The remains of a commemorative figure (Afap, April 19, 2004).

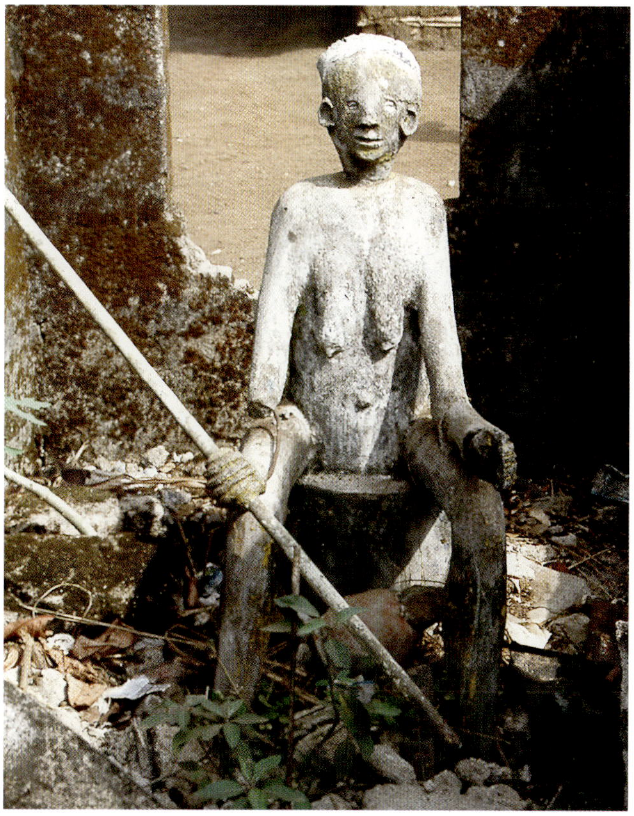

Figs. 248 A relatively well-preserved commemorative figure in its shelter, surrounded by rubbish (Ewelle, January 29, 2004).

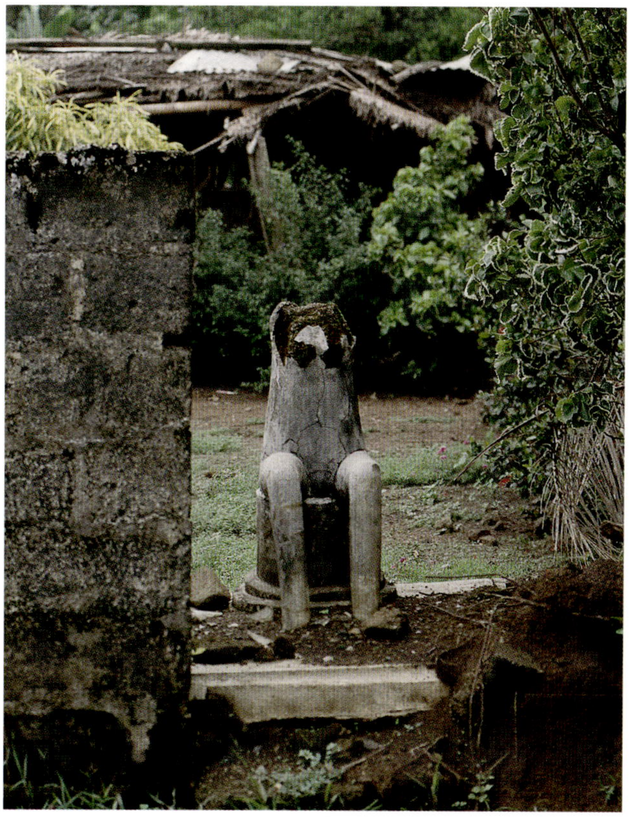

Fig. 249 The remains of a commemorative figure (Ewelle, April 15, 2004).

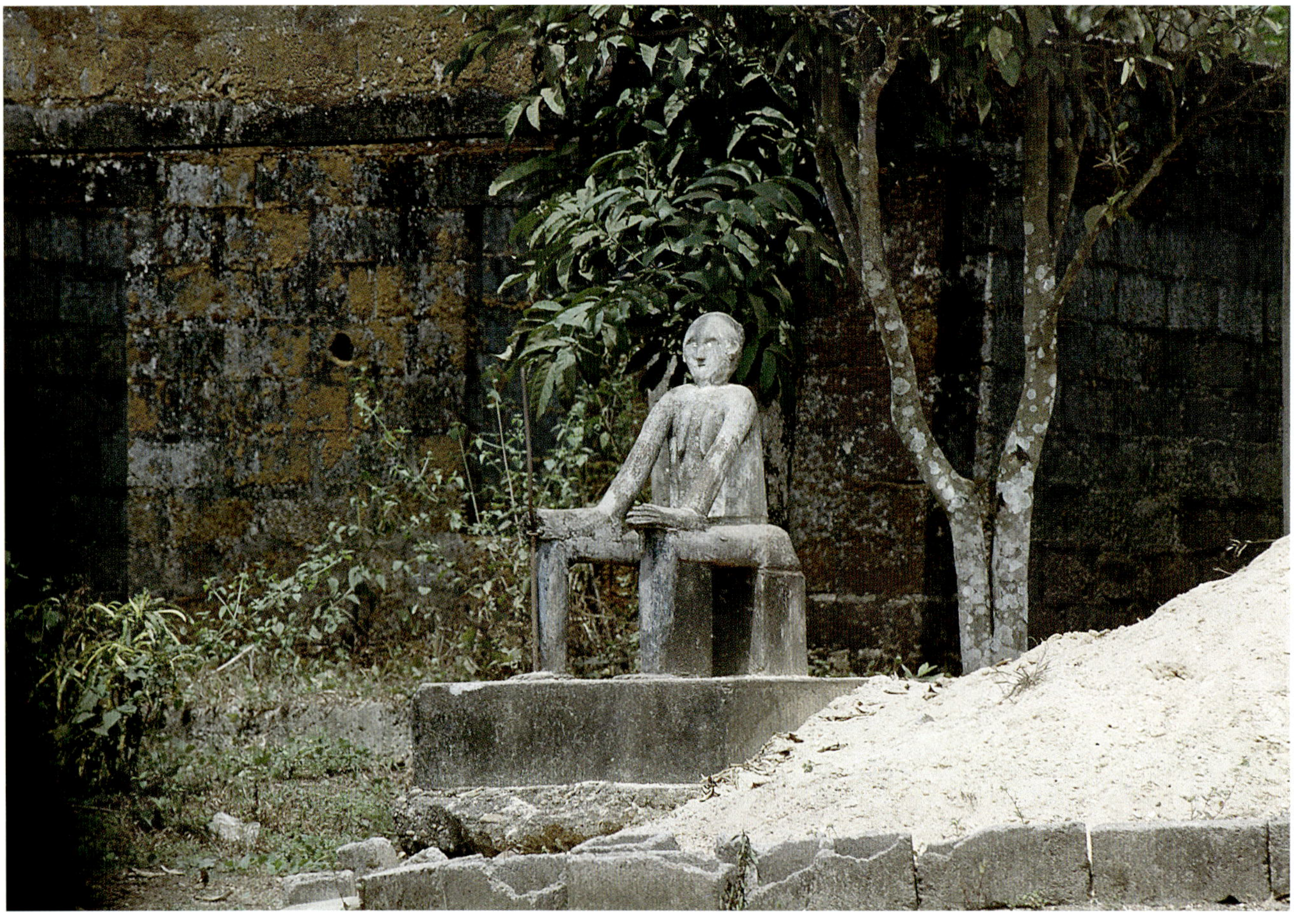

Fig. 250 A well-preserved commemorative figure (Ewelle, January 29, 2004).

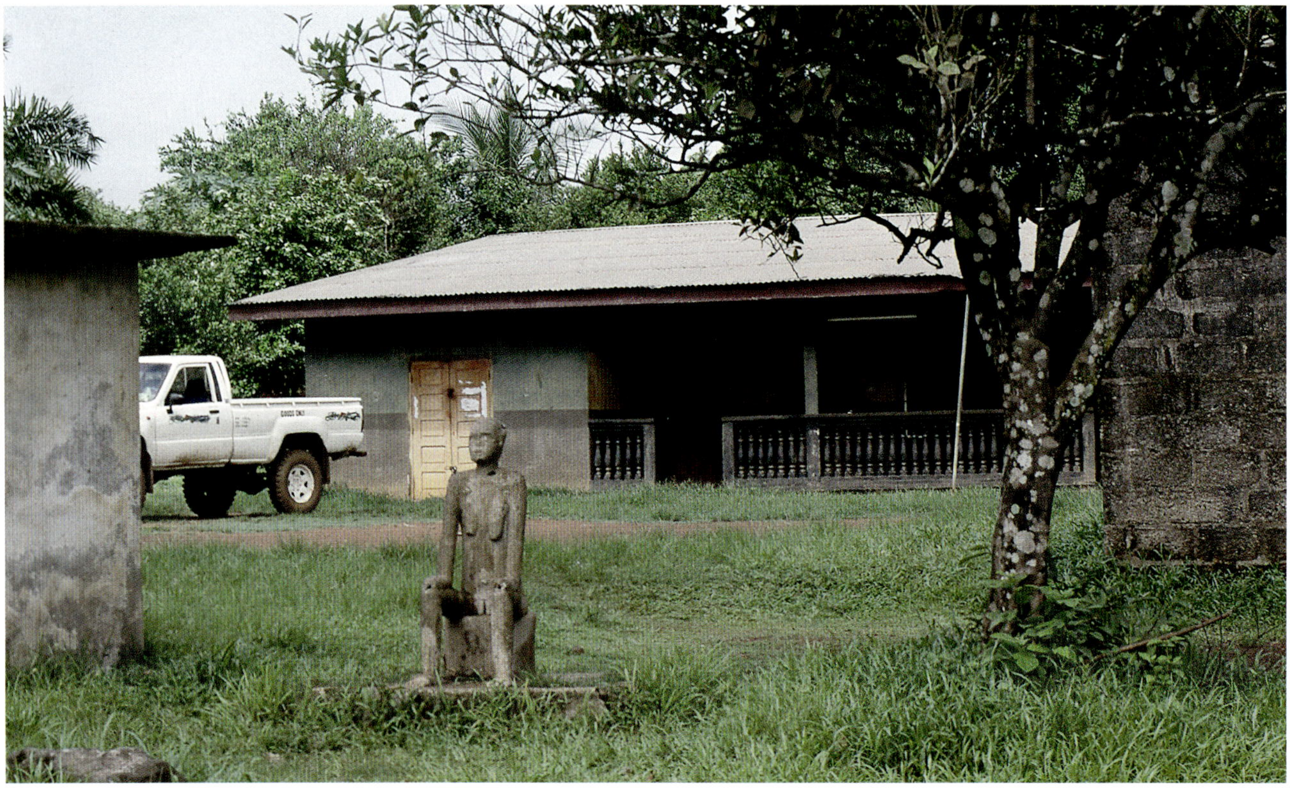

Fig. 251 Commemorative figure for a *mgbokandem* in front of a modern house (Eyang, April 19, 2004).

6.4.5 Bessem Bate from Ewelle, the last of the *agbokarem*

In 2005, only one *mgbokandem* still lives in the entire region, Bessem Bate in Ewelle (figs. 252–261). She concluded her period of seclusion in 1939. Only a few days later she gave birth to her first son, and then she underwent clitorodectomy. In the course of our lengthy conversation, she offered to perform the traditional dance of the *agbokarem*, although alone, which I gladly accepted. The dance took place a few days later, on January 29, 2004, in her compound. She was accompanied by two drummers and the singing of male and female members of her family and neighbours. Dressed and ornamented in the traditional attire, she began with an offering to the ancestors (figs. 252–253). This commenced with a long prayer (fig. 254): "*Ma* Ewube Bate, *Ma* Njock Bate, *Ma* Ewube Ashu Mangang, *Ma* Bessem Egbe, *Ma* Bessem Awu Eta, *Ma* Ebanga Arrey, *Ma* Oyere Eta Egbe, *Ata* Johnson Arrey, Tabe of Bessem Aja, *Ma* Bessem Njock Obi – amongst others who were present at my marriage ceremony. I was to be married at Kembong, where I should have enjoyed a better life than here, but you convinced me to go to Ewelle. Come now and eat this food offered to you by me. Those ancestors I know and those I do not know should all come and eat this food. Do not say that I am giving you this food at noon time. I should have given it to you early in the morning, before you went to the bush. I am doing so, because I promised a white man who is doing cultural research to dance for him the dance of *Ndem*. At first he invited me to Kembong, but I refused, because I wanted him to meet me here in Ewelle, where my father-in-law and my mother-in-law will see me animating. I am giving this food with my left hand. The left hand is for you, the ancestors. Now I am giving the food with my right hand. The right hand is for us, the living. This is your water, ancestors. Drink it after you have eaten. Now I

Dance of Bessem Bate, the last living *mgbokandem*, in Ewelle (January 29, 2004) (figs. 252–260).

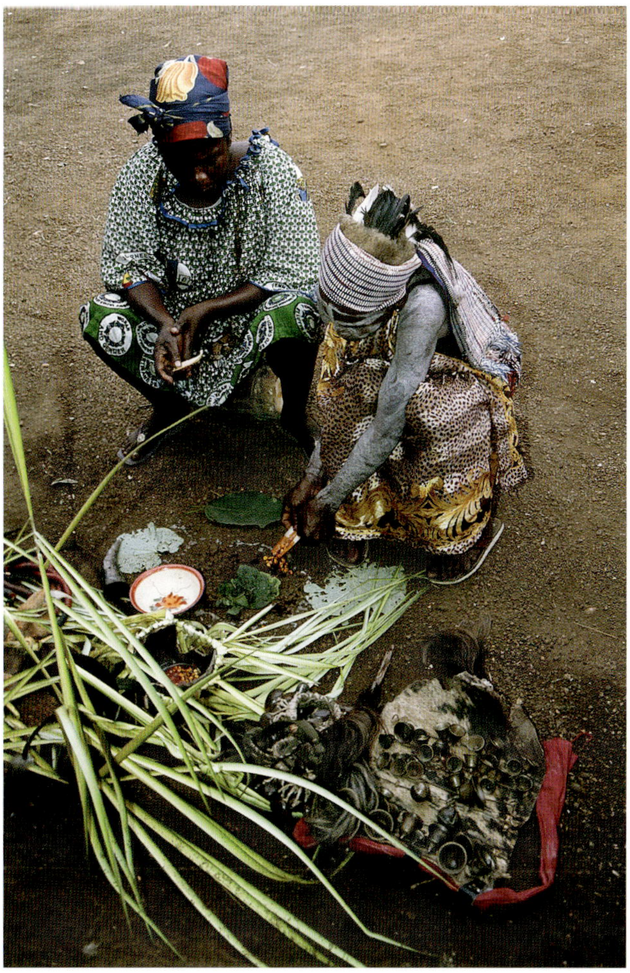

Fig. 252 The dance begins with an offering of food to the ancestors; right foreground: *ngu Ndem*, the skin with small brass bells, worn by Bessem Bate during the dance (Ewelle, January 29, 2004).

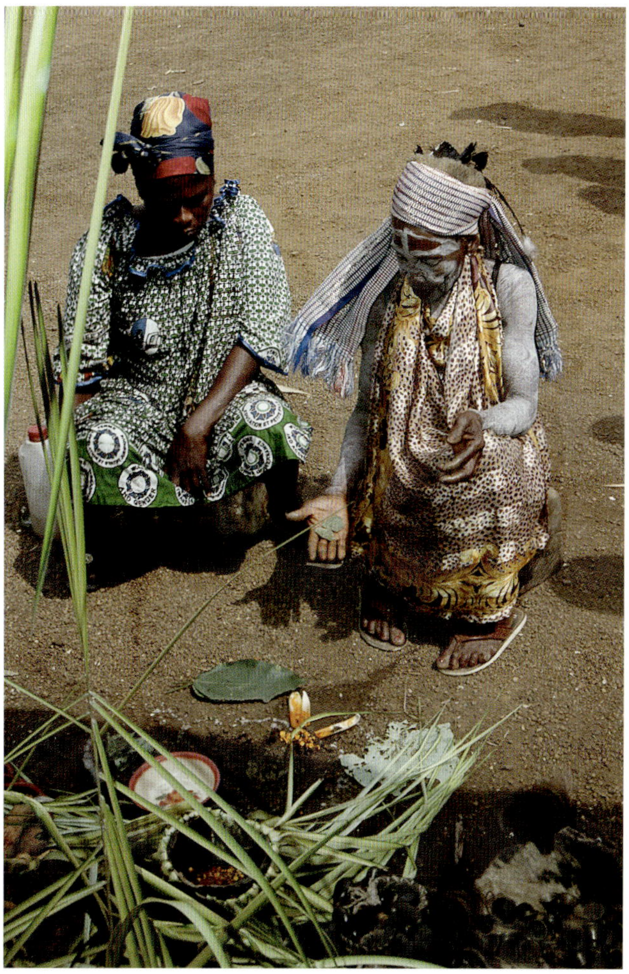

Fig. 253 The offering ends with an oracle with two leaves (*ebanghaah*); the result shows its acceptance by the ancestors (Ewelle, January 29, 2004).

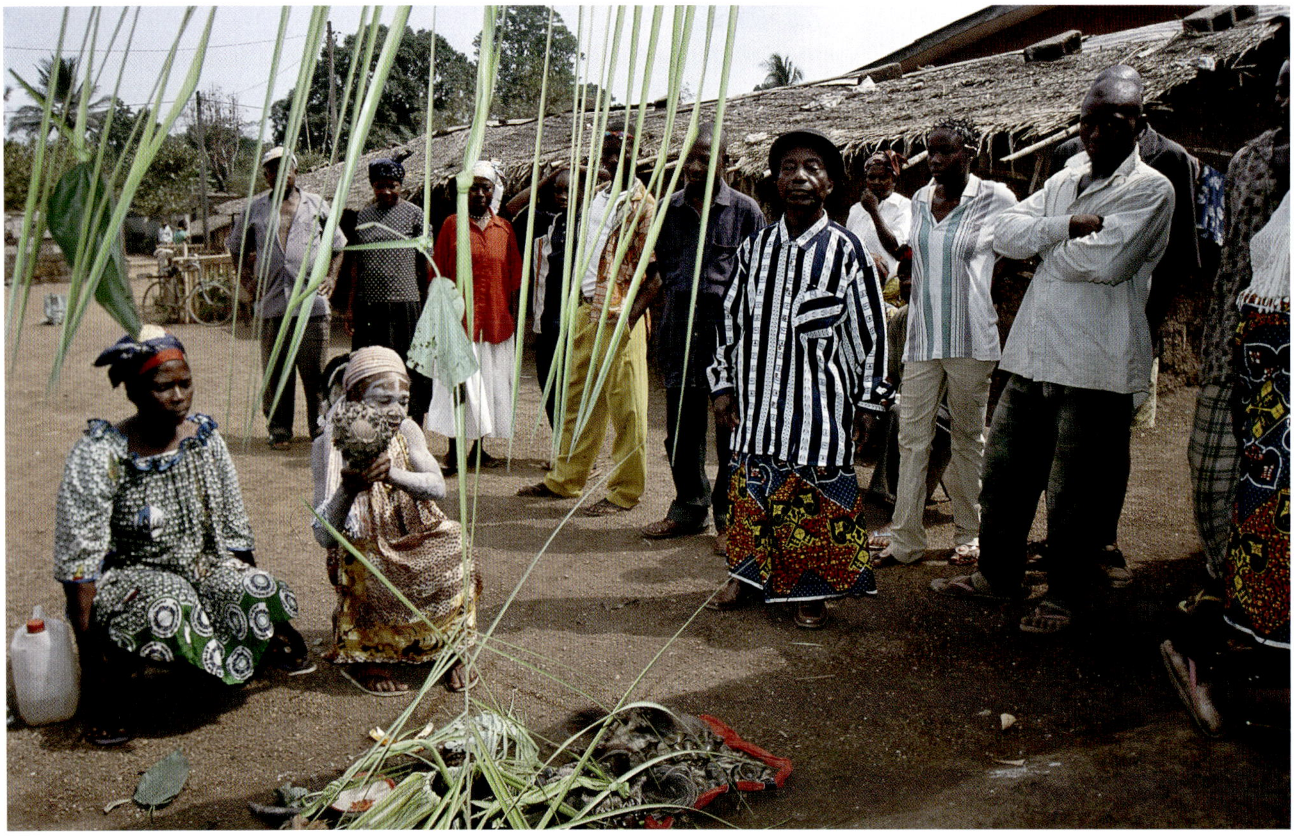

Fig. 254 Bessem Bate making a long prayer to the ancestors (Ewelle, January 29, 2004).

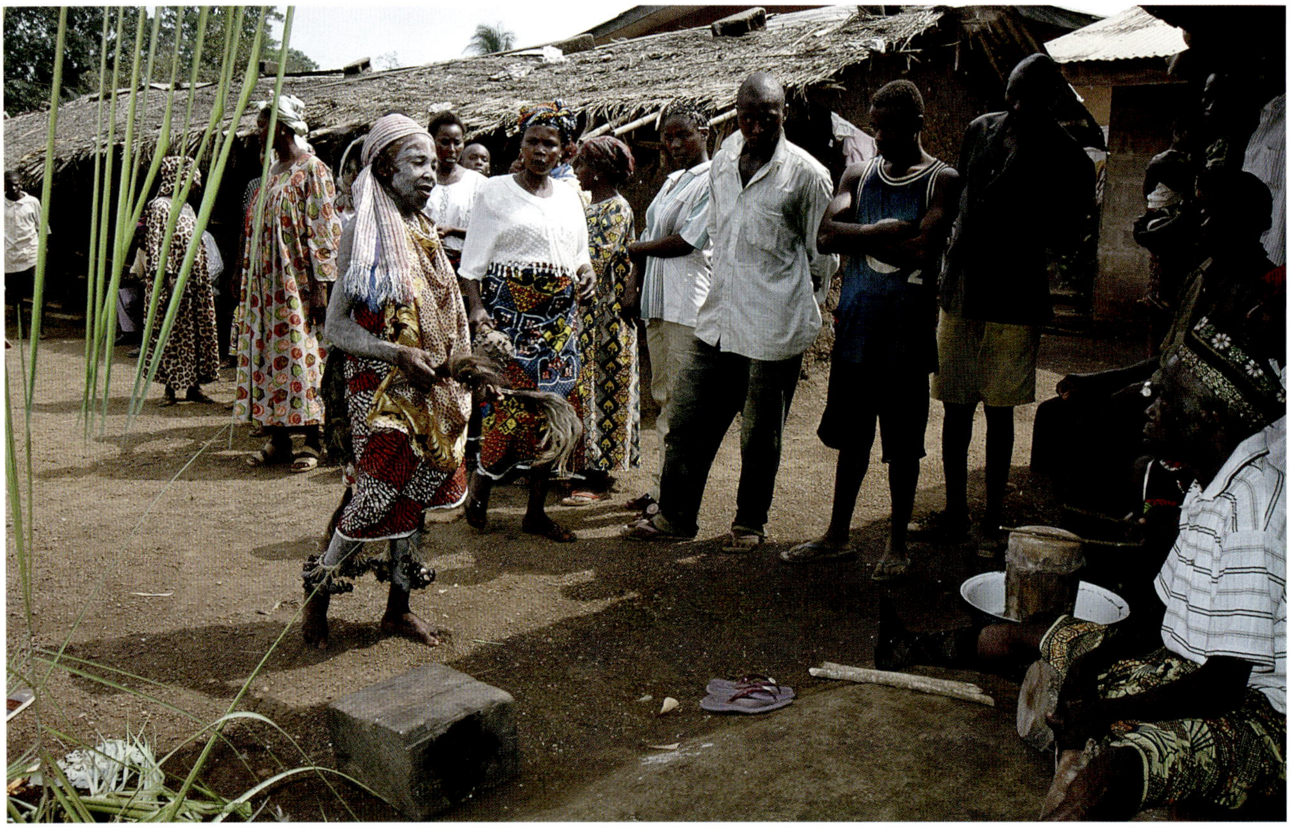

Figs. 255 Dance performance of Bessem Bate, dressed in several clothes, adorned with brass bells on her back and around the ankles, bead necklaces, her face decorated with white colour, and feathers in her hair. She holds a flywhisk in each hand (Ewelle, January 29, 2004).

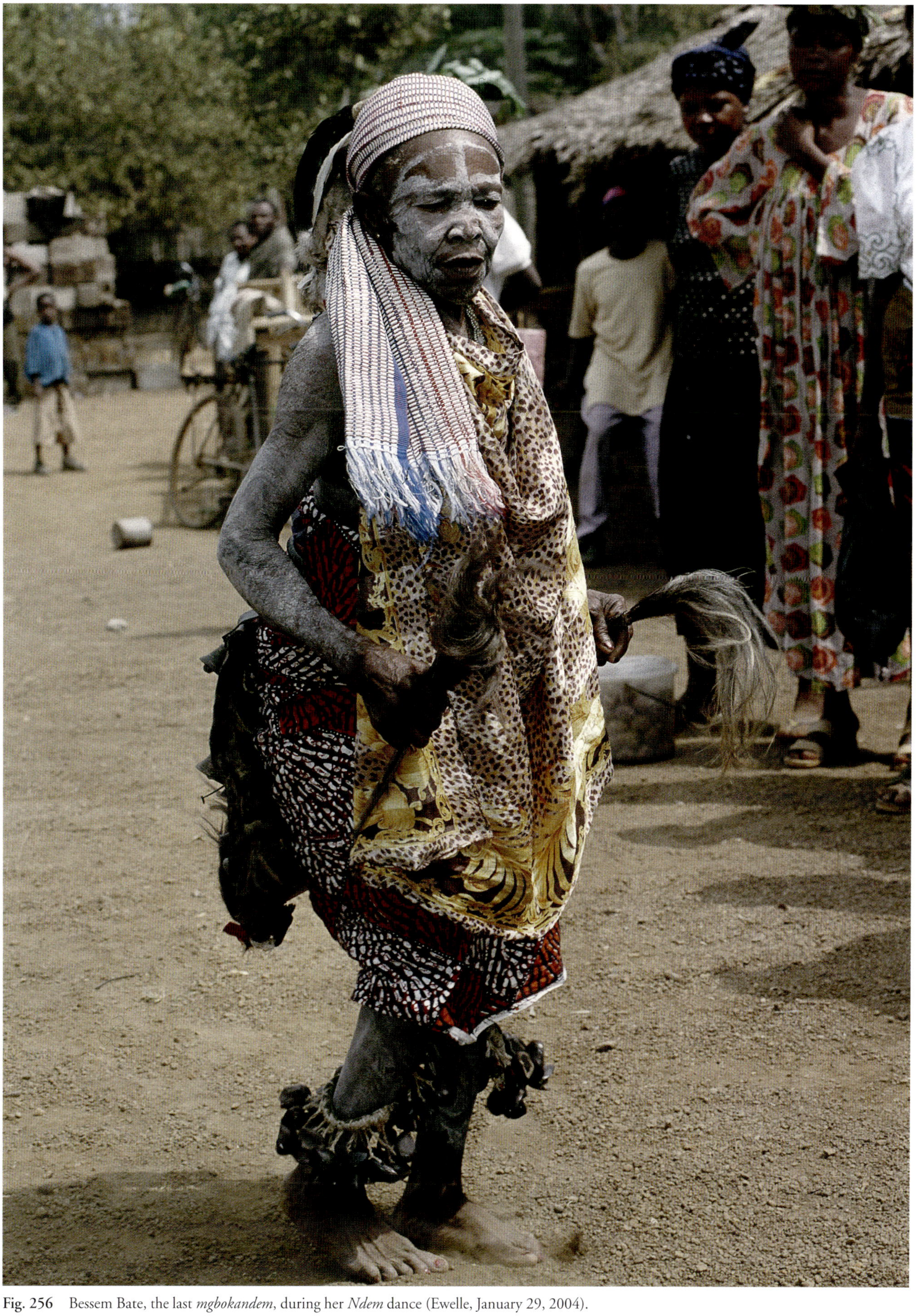

Fig. 256 Bessem Bate, the last *mgbokandem*, during her *Ndem* dance (Ewelle, January 29, 2004).

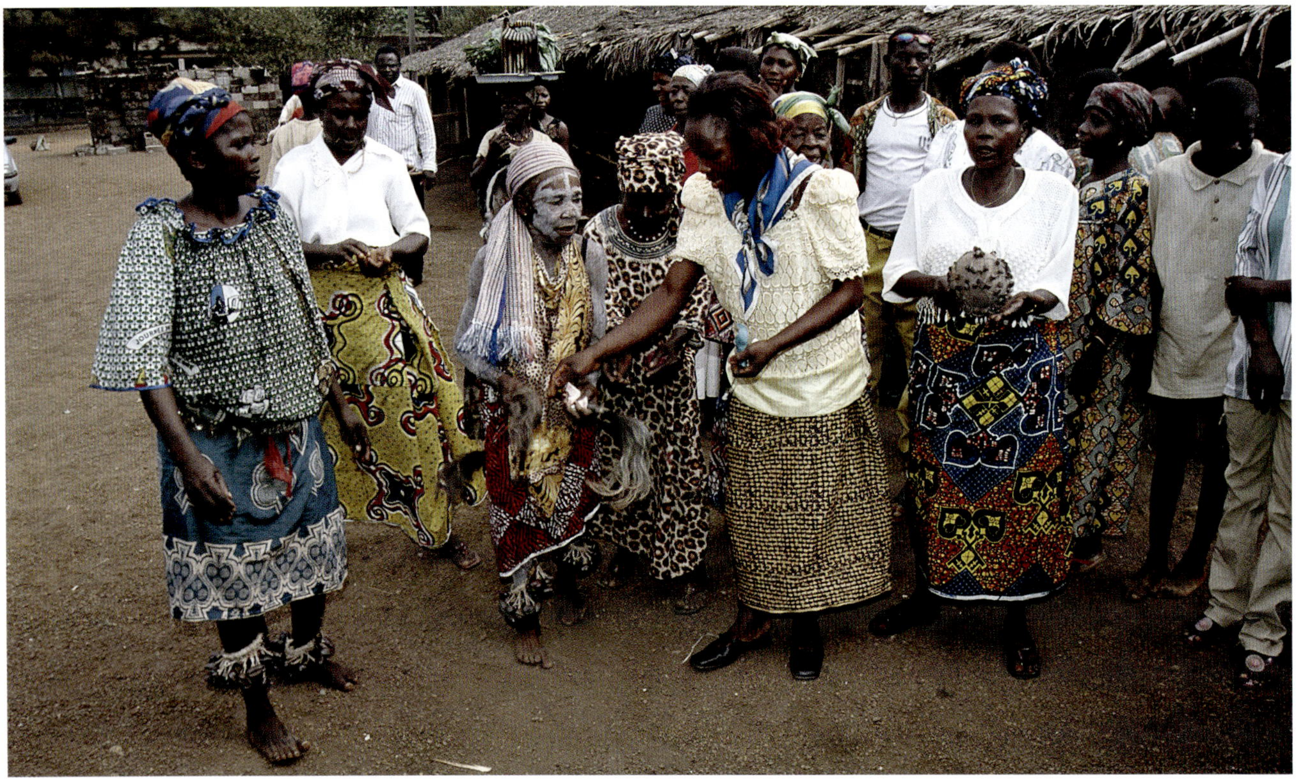

Fig. 257 Bessem Bate doing the *Ndem* dance, together with members of her family and neighbours (Ewelle, January 29, 2004).

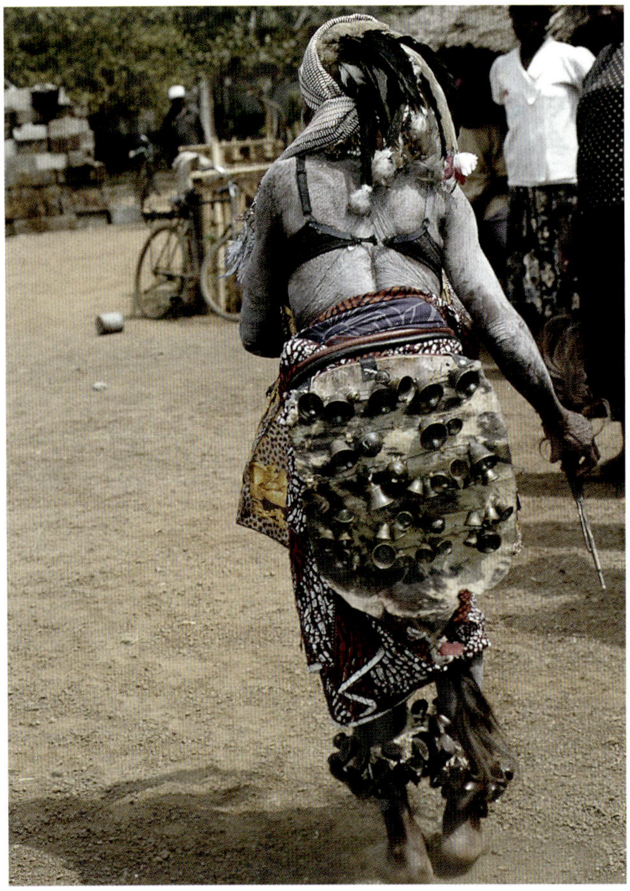

Fig. 258 *Ndem* dance of Bessem Bate; she is wearing *ngu Ndem*, the skin with small brass bells, on her back (Ewelle, January 29, 2004).

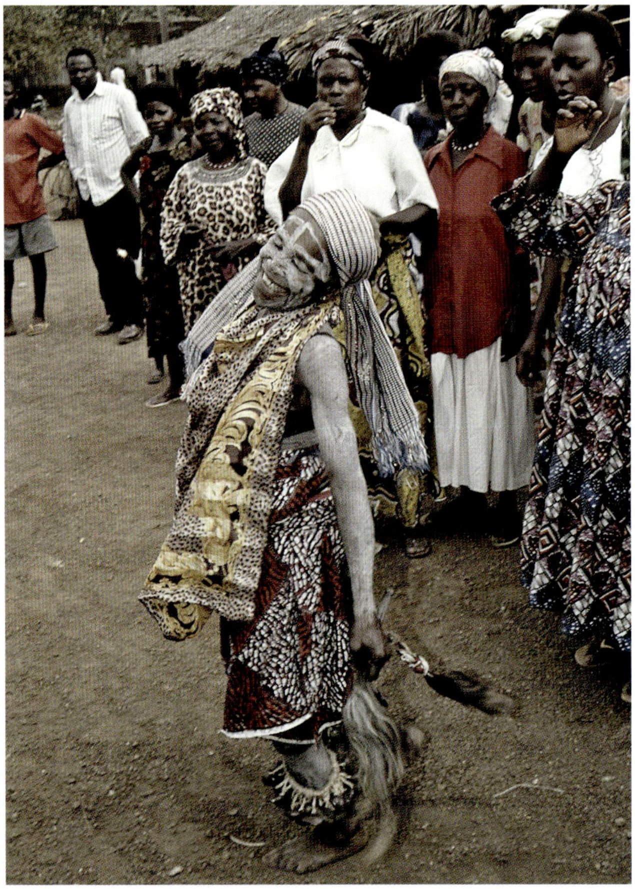

Fig. 259 Bessem Bate's *Ndem* dance (Ewelle, January 29, 2004).

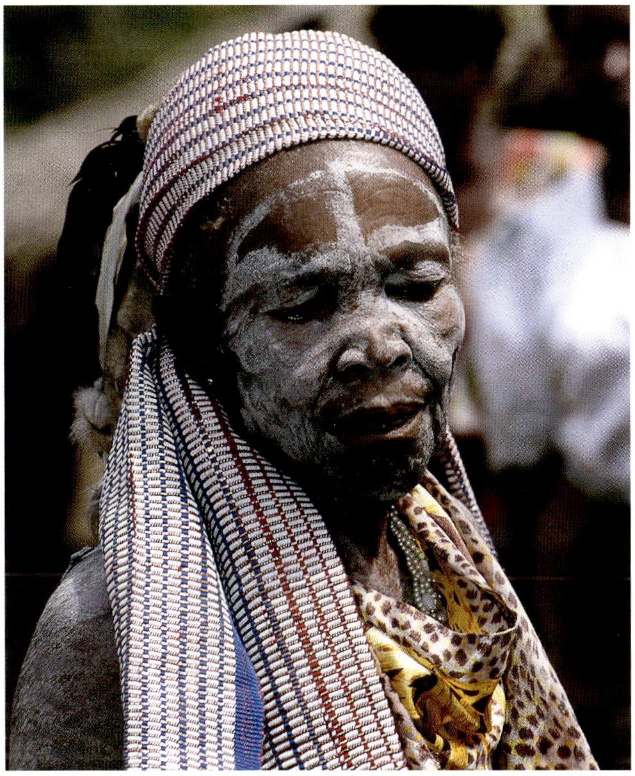

Fig. 260 Dance performance of Bessem Bate; her face is decorated with geometric design (Ewelle, January 29, 2004).

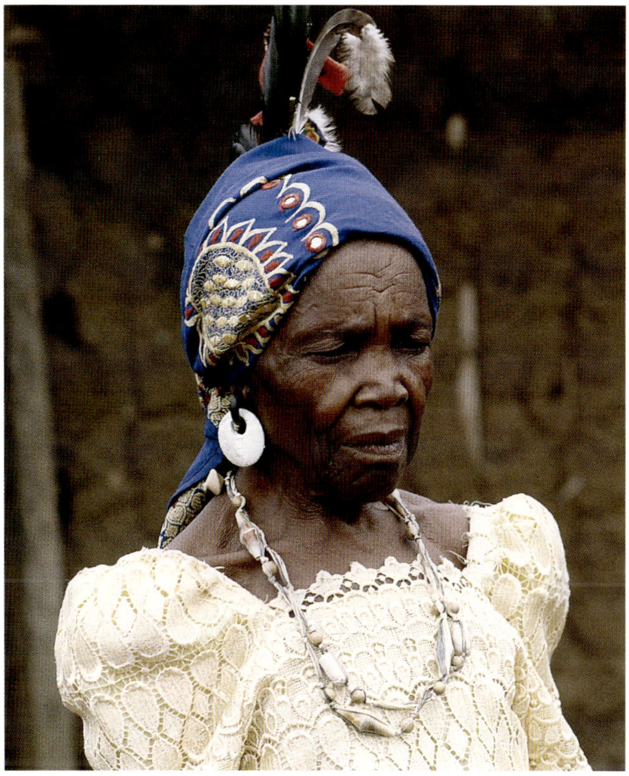

Fig. 261 Bessem Bate at an official occasion. The feathers in her hair are a sign of a *mgbokandem* (Ewelle, April 15, 2004).

am mixing the food with mud. The Ewelle ancestors should now come and bless us, taking note that your wife Bessem Bate is the one calling for your blessings. You know, I am very poor. Let food, clothes and money enter my hands through your blessings. Your children here are often quarrelling with each other. Unite them with peace and love. The blessings are declared good, if *ebanghaah* (i. e. the oracle with two leaves) agrees. If it is not my right hand, send us blessings." The two leaves of the oracle fell upon the ground, one facing upwards, the other downwards. It was the perfect sign; all people present were convinced that the ancestors had accepted the corn, the palm wine and water with satisfaction, and the joy of the people was great. It was said that tradition had become effective, as the white man gave money to the *mgbokandem,* and the other people did the same, too. After the traditional blessing was granted, the *Ndem* dance started at once. (figs. 255–260). [33]

Footnotes

1 The difficult situation of women in traditional as well as modern society is one of the pressing problems, with which churches in Africa and especially in the Cameroon Grasslands have been confronted for the past two decades. An extensive overview of the present state of discussion is offered by Zimmermann 2002.

2 Talbot reports the opposite: "Each wife has complete control over her children, and the latter almost invariably go with her if she leaves her husband" (1912:97). This regulation was almost non-existent among the Central Ejagham and nearly as seldom in the Cameroon Grasslands (Koloss 2000:76).

3 Talbot 1923:164, 170, 199; 1926:III:780; 1932:309. Corresponding information can be found in Anonymous 1957:167; Horton 1963:94 f.; Alagoa 1963:145 f., 150 f.; Balz 1984:257; Ukpong 1989:14; Röschenthaler 1993:240, 244, 248 f.; 1999: 42 ff.

4 Cole 1985:15; Koloss 2000:103 (fn.19).

5 Talbot 1923:162. Extraordinary significance is held by the Yoruba women, which pertains not only to: "… female fertility and fecundity. They claim that women possess the secret of life itself, the knowledge and special power to bring human beings into the world and to remove them...The power of the mothers is equal or superior to that of the gods, for, as a number of informants suggest, the mothers own and control the gods" (Drewal and Drewal 1983:8).

6 The first overview of the initiation rituals for girls and young women of the Ejagham was made by Talbot (1912:106 ff.). Since then many works on this topic have been published, of which the following should be mentioned in particular: Röschenthaler 1993:55 ff.; Onor 1994:88 f.; Umoetuk 1985 (among the Ibibio); Iyalla 1968 (among the Kalabari).

7 Onor 1994:88.

8 Onor 1994:88. "Fattening periods" are known in the Cameroon Grasslands as well. The period of seclusion, which newly installed kings and heads of families must undergo, is similarly designated (Koloss 2000:71 f., 105 f.).

9 In the Cameroon Grasslands red camwood holds great meaningfulness within the ritual sphere. This applies especially to the installation of kings and other dignitaries: "Over a longer period of time, the period of seclusion, the person is washed

several times a day and anointed with camwood, so that he/she will forget his/her earlier life and gradually assume the new position. He or she should change into a new person" (Koloss 2000:59).

10 Onor 1994:89.

11 Quite likely the very first reports about *Ekpa Atu* stem from Talbot. He viewed this association among the Ejagham as "by far the most important" society of the women: "The women dance stark naked the whole night through, and, should any man attempt so much as a glance at these mysteries, his strength will ebb away, and all his vital powers shrivel up forever." (Talbot 1912:225; see also Talbot 1926:III:525, 756, 792). Corresponding information about *Ekpa* in Babong is found by Leib and Romano (1984:94 f.). Likewise important information about *Ekpa Atu* is presented by Röschenthaler (1993:183 ff.; 1998:45 f.; 1999:42 ff.) and also by Onor: "*Ekpa* was an all-female institution which … represented in some sense, the female variant of the men's *Mgbe* … *Ekpa* only occasionally embarked on its outings during the day. Most of its activities took place at night, during which men were constrained to remain indoors throughout the period of its operations. Indeed, any man who proved obstinate by exposing himself to the secrets of *Ekpa*'s activities, ran the risk of becoming impotent for the rest of his life" (Onor 1994:109).
Women's societies of this kind with corresponding masks existed, although with other names, in other tribes, for example among the Efik (Anonymous 1947:150 ff.). Staschewski (1917:46) provided early evidence, according to which there were certain ceremonies among the Banyang, in the course of which women danced naked "while their husbands had to stay in the house". The Bakwiri were familiar with such dances as well, which were likewise strictly taboo for men (Ittmann 1957:169).

12 See also Röschenthaler 2004(a):215, 218.

13 Elderly women of the Yoruba are attributed with similar powers, as indicated by the word *Gẹlẹdẹ*, which is the name of an important masquerade: "*Gẹ̀* means 'to soothe, to placate, to pet or coddle'; *ẹ̀lẹ̀* refers to a woman's private parts, those that symbolize women's secrets and their life-giving powers; and *dẹ̀* connotes 'to soften with care or gentleness'" (Drewal and Drewal 1983:XV).

14 Koloss 2000:262.

15 For detailed information about *Njom Ekpa* see Röschenthaler 1993:139 ff.; 1998:45 f.; 1999:39 f. Photos of *Njom Ekpa* can be found in Röschenthaler 1993 Fig. XII–XIV; 1998:43 ff.; 1999:30 ff. and 2004(b):200.

16 As Röschenthaler reports (2004[b]), Ewelle acquired the society in 1997 from Ajayukndip. The price, including the mask, was 400,000 Francs CFA (about 650 Euros).

17 Masks by which the woman's face is not concealed are also found among the Bangwa (Brain and Pollock 1971:112). They are present in the Grasslands as well, for example, in Nso.

18 Preliminary information about the *agbokarem* among the Central Ejagham and about the commemorative figures dedicated to them is found together with photographs and sketches in Mansfeld (1908:28, 31, 55, 64, 70 f., 149 ff., 163, 184, 216; 1924:18 Fig. 91–95). The "*mbogondem*" women of the Banyang were first mentioned by Staschewski (1917:35, 48 f., 52). For further information about the *agbokarem* see Migeod 1925:65 ff.; Talbot 1926:II:130 ff.; Ittmann 1957:158 f. and Ruel 1969:203 f. Important and extensive information about the *agbokarem* is contributed by Röschenthaler (1993:50 ff., 65, 73 ff., 201 ff.; 1998:41 ff.; 1999:36 ff.).

19 Mansfeld 1924:18.

20 Agbor 2001:31.

21 Röschenthaler reports on a women's association ("Frauenbund") called "*ngobogha-ndem*" (1993:73; see also 1998:41). But in fact the society of the *agbokarem* is, as described above, called *Ndem*.

22 We have to thank Ruel for important information about *Ndem* among the Lower Banyang. He translates *Ndem* with "corpse", "dead person", "ancestor" and "foetus", and concludes, "From its name one might surmise that the association was concerned with fertility or procreation, but this was stoutly denied by both my Upper and Lower Banyang informants: they said that its name came from the fact that on initiation its members were given medicines which made them 'unconscious' (i.e. as an *ndem*) from which they were revived or 'woken up.'" (Ruel 1969:203 fn. 1). Röschenthaler, however, associates the *agbokarem* with the spirits of the wilderness (1993:73 ff.). Talbot (1912:97) also drew attention to similarities between the *agbokarem* and priestesses of the *nimm* cult in Oban.

23 See also Röschenthaler 1999:37.

24 This was already noted by both Staschewski (1917:49) and Talbot (1926:II:133).

25 Ruel 1969:204.

26 For detailed information about the initiation of the *agbokarem* see Röschenthaler (1993:73 ff.).

27 A photograph of a "house of *Ndem*" with such a fence can be viewed in Mansfeld (1908:31). As he noted, this "fence" is connected to the house through chains of liana vines that are three metres in height. They are supposed to represent the "ladder to heaven, upon which the first *Mboandem* woman descended from heaven" and founded the *agbokarem* society (Mansfeld 1924:18).

28 According to Staschewski (1917:48), the Banyang believe that sneezing is seen as the sign of acceptance into the circle of *agbokarem* (see also Talbot 1926:II:130). My informants, on the contrary, did not agree with this statement.

29 This information is confirmed by Talbot (1926:II:133). Apparently it was customary that on special occasions the *agbokarem*, for example when entering the dancing area, were carried upon the shoulders of men. Migeod also (1925:66) reports encountering two *agbokarem*, who were carried on men's shoulders. A drawing depicting a "fattening girl" in Oron upon the shoulders of a young man can be viewed in Udo Ema (1940:386).

30 See photographs of commemorative figures of *agbokarem* in Mansfeld (1908:150 ff.; 1924:77 f.); Migeod 1925:81 and Röschenthaler (1993: XXIV, XXVII–XXIX).

31 Beier 1956 and 1963; Butler 1963; Peek 1976; Cole 1982. See also the figure in the shrine of the Bini god Olokun (Talbot 1926:II:21).

32 The figure has the Inv.-Nr. F 52315.

33 Sound recordings of this dance (January 29, 2004) are preserved in the Department of Ethnomusicology in the Ethnological Museum, Berlin (Inv. No. 0430.003).

7 Conclusion: The concept of an ideal society and the importance of masks

A community that lives in peace and harmony and in unity with its ancestors was the social ideal that prevailed in most of traditional Africa, and the traditional norms and institutions there accorded with this ideal. It was the concept of the Ejagham as well. Developments in the modern world, however, have led to an emancipation from long-observed and respected social ties and promote rather an independent life style, so that this model concept is hardly heeded today. For example, thirty years ago I was fascinated in the Kingdom of Oku by the concord and readiness towards cooperation, which were the basis for daily thoughts, actions and ceremonies within the family in particular and society in general.[1] The same could be said of the Ejagham, for whom peace, unity and harmony once represented the highest social values, too. Today, however, – in the view of my informants, most of whom were elderly men – little effort is made to live according to these traditional ideals in Kembong as well as in other parts of Africa in general.

All traditional political systems in Africa, however much they might have differed individually in structure, were based upon the highest moral principles of equality and justice, and these principles led to a special form of leadership. However different the position of big men among the Ejagham and in the Cameroon Grasslands may seem in comparison, it should be emphasised that both structures were essentially the same, insofar as the leaders in both political systems were dependent upon their people. One particular example are the kings of the Grasslands, who were in no way all-powerful, but were accountable to a secret society variously known as *Kwifon*, *Nwerong*, *Ngumba* or other names, according to the respective region in which the society resided. The most important members of this society were the heads of the numerous extended families, who represented the entire population. These family heads were, in turn, dependent upon their family council. This situation prevailed in both regions, in the Grasslands and among the Ejagham as well as among many other societies in Africa: The actual sovereign was the people.[2]

The ideal of a community that lives in peace and harmony and in unity with its ancestors is implied in a number of sayings in Kembong, as generally among African peoples, for example: "A community is more than a single person.", "One person cannot overcome a community.", "The shoulder cannot be above the head.", "The whisper of the community is louder than the scream or shout of an individual.", "When you cook and give food to the community, it will eat; but when it cooks, you cannot eat all of it."[3]

Not only is the absolute dominance of the community over the individual interests of its members noteworthy, but its personification as well. Ruel gave a convincing description of this in his impressive analysis of the political system of the Banyang: "Rather in the manner of a similar verbal device in English law, this way of personifying or reifying the community serves (at least conceptually) to 'incorporate' it: it is no longer a mere aggregate of individuals but becomes an entity in its own right, with interests and demands independent of those of all its individual members."[4] The power and resoluteness of the respective social institutions, whether *Etek* or *Mgbe*, can at times reach dimensions that are inestimable and awesome. They are manifested above all in the discussions carried on when making important decisions. Consequently, the direction and result of these discourses are often unpredictable; for aside from the matter at hand, the main concern is always to demonstrate and strengthen unity in the community, and at the same time balance it with individual interests.

Among the Central Ejagham and in the Cameroon Grasslands such discussions are carried on in a manner that can be very controversial, and all participants have the basic right to state their own opinion. This applies not only to *Etek* and *Mgbe* of the Central Ejagham with their acephalous political system, but also to *Kwifon* in the Grasslands where the monarchical system with hierarchical differences is prevalent. Yet these differences disappear within the closed context of *Kwifon*, and even the king, who otherwise acts with seemingly unlimited power in public, is only "primus inter pares" there. Both the personal and impersonal character of *Kwifon* becomes apparent, in that the person who takes a stand in a discussion no longer speaks as an individual but solely in the name of *Kwifon*, or indeed even as *Kwifon*.[5]

In order that all interests can be taken into consideration, among the Ejagham as well as in the Grassland kingdoms decisions are not taken through majority accord, but through concession. An attempt is made to find a solution which is acceptable to all people. Once decided, it is rarely possible to revise a decision. At the same time everyone is expected to comply with the decision without contradiction. The authority and power with which decisions are made and enforced are not dependent upon the actual "physical" strength of the respective community; the actions that are carried out in its name are legitimised through the protection of the ancestors. Whoever turns against the community, also contradicts and assails the ancestors. Moreover, should the community come to a decision that violates the law, it must reckon with sanctions from the ancestors.

The fundamental sovereignty of the community is – without question – the decisive feature of the political systems in the rain forest and in the Grasslands. In both regions there is a consciousness that this sovereignty is strong and successful only as long as its members live together in peace and unity, despite all of the problems that might arise. For then they do justice to the laws of the ancestors, which have no other purpose than to provide guidance for a successful and happy life.[6] Like many other societies in traditional Africa, the Ejagham have many proverbs that not only celebrate the principle of unity but also vow to honour it: "To be in one voice" is a metaphor well-known among the Ejagham as well as the Banyang[7] and in the Kingdom of Oku.[8] Further examples of such sayings are: "The right hand washes the left hand, and the left hand washes the right hand"[9] and "One hand alone can never tie a bundle."[10] Numerous images are connected with a community united in harmony, such as "one leg", "one thought", "one heart" etc. One of the most profound experiences during my field work in Oku was my realisation that there a maximum of life force was seen as being totally dependent upon social harmony. Correspondingly, it was said in *Kwifon* that the greatest strength imaginable, the strongest of all medicines, is a community united in peace and harmony.[11]

Associations in the Cameroon Grasslands act in strict secrecy, today as in former times. *Kwifon* societies as well as other circles of special dignitaries are completely separated from non-members. The king is dependent upon those circles, and, moreover, they are the forum for the most important duties of the community: for the political and judicial decisions and for conducting the most meaningful offerings, that is, offerings to the gods of the land and for the royal ancestors. The general public are excluded from these activities. This situation, by contrast, is found among the Ejagham only to a very limited extent. Decisions that affect the whole community are not made in the seclusion of a secret society. Instead, all men have the opportunity to participate in political discussions and controversies in the assembly of *Etek*, which also includes offerings to the ancestors. Compared with the political traditions of the Grasslands, according to which the power of decision lies with the representatives of the numerous extended families, among the Ejagham, on the contrary, the power is always exercised directly by the people, and, thus, political disputes remain transparent and open to view. One exception is that the public is generally excluded from severe criminal cases that are dealt with by *Mgbe*.

Even today a certain consciousness of the ancestors exists among the Ejagham. For many it is still customary to honour the ancestors daily in short prayers and small offerings. Ceremonies of offerings with palm wine and special food as the most important oblations are dedicated to the ancestors at important events. These can be seen as " offerings of food", although here just as in Oku[12] the main concern is not to simply provide the ancestors with food and drink, but far more to demonstrate the belief that the ancestors are not forgotten. This applies especially to important ceremonies. The offerings made to the ancestors at that time are the share to which they are entitled. Simultaneously through these offerings the ancestors' direct presence is ensured and demonstrated. In this way the obligation is fulfilled not only of recognising their presence, but also of showing gratitude for their support to the living. Moreover, following the "eternal" laws of the ancestors means to choose the right path in life, for indeed the ancestors are the leading light of life. If the oracle, which is usually made at ceremonial offerings, shows that the ancestors have accepted the gifts, there is a noticeable relief among the persons present, because this is a sign of the benevolence of the ancestors towards the living. The ancestors are now satisfied. It signifies that the whole family – the living and the dead – is united in harmony. Yet, the bond with the ancestors does not depend on their blessings alone, which aid mankind in mastering life. Equally as important for mankind's existence are the material and cultural achievements that the ancestors once made. Ultimately mankind has to thank the ancestors for life itself.

Medicines and masks are meant to protect people from all hostile and threatening powers and are believed to be very special gifts from the ancestors. And because they are repeatedly discussed in the course of this study, are indeed even one of its major topics, it seems appropriate at this point to give a short summary of the most important aspects of masks and medicines. Thereby attention will be drawn to the prevailing theory in African studies that masks are a depiction of spirits or ancestors.[13] It must be asked to what extent this theory can be applied to the mask traditions among the Central Ejagham and in the Grasslands.

Both medicines and the more prominent masks are associated with special powers and are one of the most important and at the same time most secret possessions of secret societies. They are a manifestation of power and prosperity, and performances of the masks are always extraordinary events. That masks and medicines are not ordinary commonplace things is demonstrated foremost by the special rituals that are necessary to activate them. The secrecy that surrounds them is carefully guarded and kept from outsiders. The Ejagham are generally not as restrictive in their treatment of and behaviour towards medicines and masks in comparison to secret societies in the Grasslands. Even today in the Cameroon Grasslands non-members and non-initiates, above all women, do not dare approach the vicinity of a medicine or mask house; otherwise they must reckon with severe punishment. There medicines and masks are means through which the kings and dignitaries maintain and protect their exclusive and exalted position. By contrast, the Ejagham do not shield medicines and masks from the public to any greater degree; moreover, there are neither special medicine nor mask houses – just as there is no privileged or ruling class forced to defend its privileges.

Whereas the function and handling of magic medicines (*ajom*) are more or less the same, regardless of the variations in material and form of the actual object of medicine, there are considerable differences among the masks in this respect. In principal two types of masks can be distinguished, and this differentiation applies not only to the masks of the Central Ejagham but to the Grasslands as well, indeed as far as I am aware to many other mask traditions in Africa. The typical feature of the first type is that these masks are "dangerous"; they are treated with medicines and are used in certain medicine rituals to protect people. Thus, their appearances are in most cases not connected with dancing. *Obasinjom* and *Angbu* belong to this type of masks in Kembong. The second type of mask is constituted by "dancing" masks, which are neither associated with strong medicines nor used in medicine rituals. The primary purpose of these masks is to perform in dance, foremost at death ceremonies. With their dances they not only entertain the visitors, but provide the deceased with an honourable departure from life. Furthermore, they can also function in maintaining social order.[14] In Kembong masks belonging to this group are *Ebongu* and *Ema* of *Mgbe*, *Nkanda* and *Nchebe*. Even though these masks are not frightening or much feared like the "bad *jujus*" (*Obasinjom*, *Angbu*), they possess authority and are supported by the ancestors as well as the particular secret society to which they belong. Principally, all masks are strictly taboo for non-members. During their appearances the masks are in complete control, and their actions must be accepted without objection.

Masks of the Central Ejagham and in the Grasslands are – and this is my leading theory – autonomous beings in their own right, which were created by the ancestors; they are not representations of any ancestors or of spirits.[15] The Central Ejagham definitely do not possess masks that serve as a means for reincarnation, as is the case among many ethnic groups in southern Nigeria. There, according to tradition, the ancestors use certain festivities as the occasion to visit the living in the form of masks. This belief, as emphasised by my informants, never existed among the Central Ejagham. The differences between the two mask traditions – on the one hand, among the Central Ejagham and in the Grasslands and, on the other, among the above-mentioned ethnic groups in southern Nigeria – will be discussed in the following.

R. Horton provided comprehensive studies and interpretations of the Kalabari masks.[16] The performances of these masks are primarily meant "to bring the gods into the village".[17] It is the duty of *Ekine*, a secret society that is found everywhere among the Kalabari and to which most adult males belong, to organise all mask performances that are associated with ceremonies of offering and invocations. These masks represent various deities, and their representation is considered to be perfect, when the mask bearer becomes possessed by the particular deity and falls into a trance. At the mask performances different characters and figures in society are represented, likewise mythical and historical events, yet basically it is the point of the performances to make the particular community aware of and to understand itself: "All in all, the themes of Kalabari masquerades cover a great diversity of social experience, ostensibly drawn from the world of the water spirits, but recognizably reflecting the life of Kalabari town and village."[18] No advantages are expected from the spirits at these performances; the main concern is social contemplation and the viewers' enjoyment: "We are here for laughing, drinking and, for the play."[19]

Similar mask traditions, in which spirits and especially ancestors are portrayed by masks, are encountered among numerous other peoples in southern Nigeria, for instance, among the Ibibio,[20] Igbo, Idoma, Igala[21] and Yoruba. The most renowned example of these are probably the *Egungun* masks of the Yoruba, which are "regarded as physical representations of ancestral spirits".[22] Just like the masks of the Kalabari, the *Egungun* masks portray a number of different characters, and they relate to mythical and historical traditions. Like the Kalabari masks, their principal aim is to bring the population closer to reality. Corresponding to this, M.T. Drewal notes: "*Egungun* performances reshape perceptions of the world and give concrete form to ontological concepts. Ritual specialists bring that which is normally inaccessible, unseen, or imagined, into the phenomenal world where it can be observed and contemplated."[23] The actual centre of interest is understanding and examining social conditions and questioning their legitimacy in the sense of the laws handed down from the ancestors: "Just as the masks themselves refer backward in time, to ancestral spirits, to a presumed past, they simultaneously renegotiate the present."[24] The spectacle of the masks "honors the spirits of the ancestors";[25] it entertains the people, while at the same time it serves for social control. According to J.A. Adedeji, *Egungun* was established by Sàngó, Alafin of Oyo, presumably in the 14th century.[26] He maintains that this founding was the beginning of the theatre-culture of the Yoruba, which developed later into performances of more or less professional theatre troops "to satisfy the people's desire for entertainment and diversion."[27] Nonetheless, the question arises as to whether all masks of this region represent spirits and ancestors. Hence, H. J. Drewal noted that among the Yoruba, "only some masqueraders, but by no means all, are literally 'for the ancestors'".[28] There are similar reports pertaining to this question with reference to other peoples.[29]

The importance accorded to the dramaturgical aspects of masks in southern Nigeria obviously went hand-in-hand with similar developments in artwork, insofar as they were likewise associated with social themes and problems. In the religious sculpture of traditional Africa human beings are usually depicted in a static position. The images do not show any movement nor do they depict a specific incident. When several persons are shown together, they do not signify a group, in which the individuals act jointly. Instead, they are an enumeration rather than a group picture in the strict art historical sense.[30] In contrast to this traditional concept, the art of southern Nigeria is typified by a remarkable number of objects representing humans in movement and even a great number of scenic representations. Included among these objects are not only cult figures such as the clay images in the Mbari houses of the Igbo,[31] but also a multitude of mundane articles, whose ornamentation displays actual daily scenes, such as house posts, panels, doors, stools, bowls and especially mask headdresses.[32] In particular the oftentimes over-dimensional and heavy headdresses are well-known among the Yoruba[33] and Igbo[34]. Perched above the actual head of the mask are several – at times even a great number – of human figures that are often shown together in a scene, involved in an incident. The easternmost representatives of such mask headdresses are those of the *Njom Ekpa* among the Ejagham, as mentioned above (cp. p. 193 ff.).

To return to my own areas of research once again, it can be stated that mask traditions in the form described above are unknown among the Central Ejagham and in the Cameroon Grasslands. In none of these cultural regions, however diverse their social and religious traditions may be in essence, do masks represent spirits or ancestors nor do the performances of masks deal with mythical or historical themes. Furthermore, mask performances are definitely not associated with social criticism or contemplation.[35]

Besides, "dangerous" masks appear only when they are needed within their particular purpose, such as the pursuit and destruction of witches. In the Grasslands such masks are also obligated to appear at commemorative ceremonies for deceased members. The "dancing" masks are expected, above all, to perform "beautiful" dances, entertain the spectators and thereby render a sense of meaningfulness to the festivities. Mask societies in the Grasslands belong to the various extended families and possess masks in the form of humans as well as animals, amongst these: "leader", "wife", "big man" and "old man", or "elephant", "buffalo", "ram", "bird", "bat" etc.[36] Although the masks differ distinctly in appearance, they are not assigned a specific role according to the particular mask headdress. All masks move or dance in the same way, with the exception of the leading masks. For example, the "big man" dances just like the "bird" or the "ram". As far as I know, theatrical elements, like those that typify mask traditions in southern Nigeria, do not exist among the Central Ejagham and in the Grasslands.

The most important elements of their world-view are, nonetheless, the same. As with most African peoples, for the Ejagham it is the ancestors to whom the living should be grateful for life and for all cultural endowments and whose laws have only one purpose: to foster a community that lives in harmony. It is the observance of their laws that guarantees a life full of meaning and success. Since a community united in peace and cooperation represents the highest social value of the Ejagham, efforts to achieve wealth and esteem are of course approved and even encouraged. However, every form of hierarchical thought and action is all the more foreign and unacceptable – indeed, that is the distinguishing characteristic of the political and social culture of the Ejagham: "Everybody is a chief by himself. You make yourself what you are."

Footnotes

1 Koloss 2000:58, 446 ff.
2 Koloss 2000:447 f.
3 The Banyang have similar sayings (Ruel 1969:135 f.).
4 Ruel 1969:193.
5 Koloss 2000:101, 133.
6 Koloss 2000:27, 451.
7 Ruel 1969:65, 185.
8 Koloss 2000:452.
9 Agbor 2001:III.
10 Ruel 1969:136; Koloss 2000:447.
11 Koloss 2000:453.
12 Koloss 2000:401, 452.
13 Cole 1985:19 ff.; Kasfir 1988:6 f.; Herreman 1993:14 ff.; Kecskési and Vajda 1997: 24 ff.
14 Even though the medicines of the mask societies, which belong to the various extended families, are not as strong and potent as the medicines of *Kwifon*, military societies and medicine societies, they serve to protect the respective family, even the community (Koloss 2000:223). Normally it is the "running mask" of the respective mask society that is used to sustain social control in different ways. It oversees community work, is present at public announcements, carries out punishments and formerly checked houses for any fire hazards during the dry season. As representative of the whole secret society it appears at the burial for deceased members (Koloss 2000:236).
15 *Kwifon* (with its masks *Mabuh* and *Nkock*) as well as *Samba*, *Ngang*, *Kheghebchio* and *Nontang*, just to mention some of the most important secret societies and masks found in the eastern Grasslands, are in no way connected with spirits and ghosts. All of the necessary rituals for activating medicines and masks are directed towards the ancestors alone – as is the case among the Ejagham. In addition, masks of the Grasslands display a remarkable multiformity. Especially among the mask societies that belong to extended families, there are masks with human and animal attributes, masks with wooden headdresses and those with a feathered head-covering. Aside from these, there are masks that consist of a garment and simply a dense net that covers the face. It is hardly imaginable that there could be a corresponding multiplicity of spirits and ghosts that might compare with this extraordinary diversity of masks (Koloss 2000:99 f., 114 ff., 191 ff., 223 ff., 279 ff.). An overview of mask traditions in the Cameroon Grasslands is provided in Koloss 2008: 86 ff.
16 Horton 1960 and 1963.
17 Horton 1960:20.
18 Horton 1963:97.
19 Horton 1963:102.
20 Messenger 1973:119 f.; Ukpong 1989:16; Akpan 1994.
21 Kasfir 1984:163.
22 Drewal, M.T. 1992:90.
23 Drewal, M.T. 1992:90.
24 Drewal, M.T. 1992:94.
25 Drewal, M.T. 1992:90.
26 Adedeji 1972:255.
27 Adedeji 1972:257. Nzekwu (1960:141) pointed out the "non-religious, 'purely aesthetic' values" of traditional mask performances in southeastern Nigeria: "People like the Kalabari recognised that masquerading, as ballet and drama, had an intrinsic value quite apart from its worth as a means of coercing the Gods." In the question of a theatrical tradition in all of Nigeria, Ogunbiyi (1981:3) stated very clearly: "What is, however, not speculative ... is the existence, in many Nigerian societies, of a robust theatrical tradition. The primitive root of that tradition must be sought in the numerous religious rituals and festivals that exist in many Nigerian communities."
28 Drewal, H. J. 1978:18.
29 (Kalabari) Alagoa 1963:150; (Ibo) Boston 1960:58; (Mbembe) Harris 1984:63.
30 Koloss 2000:23.
31 Cole 1982.
32 Fagg 1963; Fagg and Pemberton 1982.
33 Fagg 1963:Fig. 81, 85; Wardwell 1989:183, 195 ff.
34 Cole and Aniakor 1984:124, 129 f., 132, 141 ff., Pl. 25, 35, 36.
35 From that point of view one can only wonder at a study recently published by N. Argenti (2006), who tries to demonstrate, giving the *Kwifon* mask from Oku as an example, that mask dances "have their origin in the experience of the slave trade" (2006:53). The author takes *Mabuh* for the "running mask" of *Felingang*, a group of masks that *Kwifon* in Oku is in charge of besides the traditional masks *Mabuh* and *Nkock*. Moreover, in his analysis the alleged running mask develops into a "driver", who, according to Argenti, formerly belonged to slave caravans and later, in colonial times, to those caravans "often led by German officers with the rank of Captain, and that they were guarded by drivers armed with clubs and whips watching out for those attempting to escape into the bush" (2006:62). To my knowledge there is not the slightest proof for such an interpretation of *Mabuh,* which can in principle be found among all *Kwifon* societies in the Grasslands; especially in Oku there was hardly any evidence relating to the time of the slave hunts. Nobody can tell when and under what circumstances masquerades developed or were adopted. Interestingly, *Felingang* does not even possess a running mask. True, among the *Felingang* masks there is one also regarded as *Mabuh* – but it does not represent the "real" *Mabuh* that fills everyone with fear (Koloss 2000:256 ff.). Apart from that, the "real" *Mabuh* is not a "dancing" mask and consequently never appears in connection with *Felingang*. Nor do the leading masks of *Felingang* dance with "Fulani-style swords" (2006:55). Although those speculations are far beyond the scope of generally accepted historical and ethnological evidence, Argenti (2006:63) himself considers them as a "Copernican model". (Cp. Koloss 2008:110, fn. 21).
36 Koloss 2000:236 ff.

Glossary

The glossary covers general terms pertaining to objects and subject matters in daily life. Proper names of individuals, families, communities, secret societies, deities and their ceremonies can be found in the index.

Singular	Plural	Explanation/Translation
abang	bebang	horn
abang Mfam		"the horns of Mfam"; first stage of Mfam
aboku	aboku	"washing hands after death"; the feasting day of a death celebration
abo Mgbe		young members of Mgbe
abonche		plural of monche
aboninkim		plural of moninkim
abo Njom		young members of Obasinjom
abo Obon		young members of Obon
abu arem		plural of mbu arem
abuebu		plural of mbuebu
agbep mfut Ndem		"inserting the feathers of a peacock"; the last stage of initiation into Ndem
agbokarem		plural of mgbokandem
agbut etene Ndem		"to set aside Ndem"; the first stage of initiation into Ndem
ajom		plural of njom
ajom	ajum	a sacrifice for the ancestors
akachak		woven rattles
ake gbe nko Ndem		making bodymarks on a new mgbokandem
ake kale eri mba Obasi		"giving food to God"; a ceremony of offering to God at the beginning of the planting season
akeku akale		"gift for the ancestors"; a sacrifice for the ancestors
akeku efohe		"fanning the ancestors"; a sacrifice for the ancestors
akeku efoko		"appeasing the ancestors"; a sacrifice for the ancestors
akeku ejoho		"placation of the ancestors"; a sacrifice for the ancestors
akeku ka nsi		ancestors in the earth
ake sangha Ndem		exposing the new mgbokandem
akesu Ndem		"to wash Ndem"; a stage of initiation into Ndem
akum		plural of okum
amenge ezum		"he knows something"; name of an oracle instrument
Amok		"to push away", a magic medicine (njom) in the form of lumps of clay (no longer existent)
Angbu		a secret society
angwa ribo		"jumping cat"; nickname for Ebongu and Ema, the masks of Mgbe
anne akangkang		men armed with cutlasses in the procession of Nkanda
anne atemambi		plural of nne atemambi
anne eboho		plural of nne eboho
arem		plural of ndem
asu Mgbe		"washing the living and the dead"; a ritual of Mgbe at burial ceremonies
asure abe		"to swear the breasts"; a medicine ritual of Mawu, the society of the women
Ata		"father"; title for an old honoured man
Ata Obasi		Father God

Singular	Plural	Explanation/Translation
Ata Obasi ka oso		Father God above (in heaven)
atemambi		"heart" of Obasinjom; the members of this rank control the medicines and make all decisions concerning the society
atui amfa Obon		the level of the two chiefs of Obon
atunyak		"the night has fallen"; refers to strong members in Obasinjom
aye nne amenge ejun		"making a person know something"; name of an oracle instrument
ayi nju Ndem		"to enter the house of Ndem"; the long period of seclusion during the initiation of the new members into Ndem
ayu Ndem		the "dead" (ritually killed) initiant of Ndem
bebang	abang	Horn
bechi Obon		leaders of Obon
bekeneku	nkenekun	money contributed by family members for a death celebration
bekundi		a rank in Mgbe and taboo-sign of Mgbe
bese	nse	duiker, dwarf antelope
besom Njom	asom Njom	a big knife with a flat end, which is empowered with medicines, held in the right hand by the mask of Obasinjom
beti Ndem		"stick of Ndem", a small carved piece of wood stuck into the hair of a new initiant into Ndem
boseseku		plural of seseku
dikaba	bodikaba	a title in Mgbe; the person who divides and shares food or drink in any lodge of Mgbe
ebaah Angbu	bebaah Angbu	grove ("evil forest") of Angbu
ebaah Njom	bebaah Njom	grove ("evil forest") of Obasinjom
ebanghaah	mbanghaah	oracle with two leaves to find out the wishes of ancestors
ebanghaah Njom	bebanghaah Njom	the head or chief of Obasinjom
ebe	abe	female breast
ebhe	bebhe	a condition that requires a sacrifice or purificatiofor seven days, or else it is a curse
ebiolak	abiolak	knitted red cap
ebla	abla	medicine for healing, "good medicine"
eboho	boho	mud-bed
eboko eghoh	beboko eghoh	bowl of plantains
ebone		special food offered to the ancestors (made of fried dry corn mixed with palm oil)
Ebongu	Bebongu	mask and dance in Mgbe
ebore		red palm oil
ebu	bebu	divination, oracle
ebu Njom	bebu Njom	mask carrier of Obasinjom
echakara ngomba		a man with a special staff in the procession of Nkanda
echem atu		"meeting in the night"; meeting of witches
echeme Mawu		"come together"; meeting of Mawu women
echi Mgbe	achi Mgbe	the core members of a Mgbe lodge
echi ndebenju	achi arebeoju	head of a family
echi Njom	achi Njom	headdress of the mask of Obasinjom and designation for a core member of Obasinjom

Singular	Plural	Explanation/Translation
efale Ndem	befale Ndem	"going round in a circle"; a dance of Ndem
efe	befe	mirror
efem	befem	table
efem Mgbe	befem Mgbe	ritual table of Mgbe, upon which certain signs, symbols, instruments and objects of Mgbe are displayed for a deceased member in the lodge during death ceremonies
efe Njom		strong medicine on the back of the headpiece of Obasinjom
efi nyam		"bush-baby"; a small animal of prey
efune Njom		a special piece of wood with strong medicine worn by the mask of Obasinjom in its left hand
efune Mgbe		medicine leaves, held by Ebongu/Ema, the masks of Mgbe, in the left hand
egbelle olak	mgbelle olak	a special cap of Mgbe members, usually those who have reached the rank of eteme Mgbe
Egbo		the name in Pidgin-English for Ngbe/Ekpe, the most important secret society in the Cross River region
ejah		seven days, a week
ekachak	akachak	plaited rattles
ekasi Nkanda		a man carrying a hoop in the procession of Nkanda
ekeneyamojeh		pipe made of the claws of a crab
ekokonne	bekokoanne	elderly man, old person
ckong	bekong	a succulent plant used in burial ceremonies by Mgbe lodges, that originate from Echoko
ekot Angbu	nkot Angbu	grove ("evil forest") of Angbu
ekot Mgbe	nkot Mgbe	grove ("evil forest") of Mgbe
Ekpa Atu		"sleeping mat of the night"; a women's society among the Central Ejagham
ekpang Nkanda		a man wearing a basket on his head in the procession of Nkanda
Ekpe		the most important secret society of the Efik (called Mgbe among the Central Ejagham)
ekpile	mpkile	larger drum
ekpile Njom		magic drum of Obasinjom
eku ebi	beku ebi	bad death
ekume atu		"sitting in the night"; meeting of witches
ekye	bekye	crab
ekye nyam ojeh		"crab, the meat of witches"; a whistle made from a claw of the crab, used in Obasinjom performance
elo Ndem	belo Ndem	stool of a mgbokandem
elolo Ndem		ritual food consumed during initiation into Ndem
Ema	Bema	mask and dance of Mgbe
emangha Obasi	bemangha Obasi	illness from God
engeh Njom		test of Obasinjom: young men are tested if they are qualified to be a mantlebearer
Enok Ateng		"fighting alone"; a magic medicine (njom) from Afap in the form of a small wooden human figure
enyeng	benyeng	guinea fowl
epwangha Nkanda	bepwangha Nkanda	an oblong basket of Nkanda (made of cane ropes)
eri mba Obasi ya akeku /	beri mba Obasi ya akeku /	food to God and ancestors (in the form of a sacrifice)
esene Njom		lower part of the garment of Obasinjom
esoble Ndem		secret language of Ndem
etaah	betaah	a meal as the last stage of aboku

Singular	Plural	Explanation/Translation
etaah nji eyatek	betaah mbu eyatek	"food which is outside"; sacrifice of food to the ancestors (as last stage of aboku)
etaah nji ojyanju	betaah mbu ojyanju	"food inside the house"; food for the living (as last stage of aboku)
etakoko nne	betakok andeh	old person
eteh Mgbe	ateh Mgbe	stone of Mgbe
Etek	Ntek	a settlement (quarter, village, town, etc.) and also the assembly of a community, in which all important decisions are made
etek akeku		the land of the dead people
eteme Mgbe	beteme Mgbe	grove ("evil forest") of Mgbe
eteme Nkanda		"grove of Nkanda"; the stage of full membership of Nkanda
eti Njom		magic tree of Obasinjom
etobe ntui	betobe ntui	vice-chief, assistant president
etokobi atu	betokobi atu	the "night dance"
etokobi efe	betokobi efe	a part of etokobi ("night dance") during the day
eturu Njom	beturu Njom	a wind instrument of Obasinjom made of wood and blown like a trumpet; therefore usually referred to as "trumpet"
ewonghonne	awonghoanne or ngonghoanne / young people, youths	
eyamba	beyamba	another designation for the seseku, chief of Mgbe
eyok	beyok	big slit-drum
eyume Mgbe		"the voice of Mgbe"; a rank in Mgbe
iroko	beroko	messenger, announcer of Nkanda
juju		drawn from the French word 'joujou' and adopted in Pidgin-English; stands for the whole complex of magic medicine, designates also an individual mask and a whole secret society
ken nkeku		to bury a corpse
Kwifon		the most important secret society in the kingdoms of the Cameroon Grasslands with the king and the heads of the extended families as most important members. Kwifon in cooperation with the king formed the government in pre-colonial times
mammy wata		water nymph, mostly in coastal areas
Mawu		society of the women
mbenghe	obenghe	heart
mbenghe Njom		"heart of Obasinjom"; a band made of thick textile which contains all medicines of Obasinjom and which is worn by its mask round the neck
mbom	abom	towel or piece of cloth, a sign of a seseku which he wears over his left shoulder
mbu arem	abu arem	"priest" or "priestess"of the spirits, diviner
mbuebu	abuebu	diviner
mbung	abung	fool
mengú	djĕngu	female spirits (similar to mammy wata) on the Cameroon coast

Singular	Plural	Explanation/Translation
Mfam		"community"; a magic medicine (njom) in the form of two bushcow horns
mfa Nkanda		"fork of Nkanda"; a man with a special staff in the procession of Nkanda
mgbaahetek	agbaahetek	notable, wise, strong man
Mgbe		the most important secret society of the Central Ejagham
mgbokandem	agbokarem	a member of the women's society Ndem (no longer existent)
Mkpe		a mask covered with skin; appears during Mgbe and night dances
mma	boma	"mother"; title for an old honoured woman
mma Njom	boma Njom	the wife of Obasinjom
Mma Obasi		Mother God
mo mfe	abo mfe	"new children", the first rank in Njom Ekpa
monche	abonche	child (plural: young people)
moninkim	aboninkim	"child of circumcision"; status of a young woman who has been circumcised
mo Njom	abo Njom	"child of Njom"; young member of Obasinjom
monkem	amonkem	young cripple
montui	aboatui	sub-chief, quarterhead
monyo	bomonyo	ceremonial staff of a seseku
naob elemembhi		oil palm tree
nbeneben	abeneben	dancer
Nchebe		a mask covered with skin; appears during Mgbe and "night dances"
nchip Njom		the strongest medicine of Obasinjom
Nchockandah		mask dance of children ages 5 to 12 during aboku
nchokot Obon		a secret musical instrument of Obon
nchotekuble	achotekuble	speaker, spokesman
ndebenju	arebeoju	family, kinsmen
ndeck ebu	areck ebu	"rope of ebu"; oracle artefact
Ndem		women's society of the agbokarem (no longer existent)
ndem	arem	spirit
ndum nne	arum anne	great, noble, important man ("big man")
nekhi (or etakoko) nne	bakhi (or betakok) andeh	old person, elder, chief
Ngbe		the most important secret society of the Ejagham and Banyang (called Mgbe by the Central Ejagham)
ngilako		a thick leaf of underbrush used by Mgbe in burial eremonies
ngok Njom	agok Njom	garment of Obasinjom
Ngunaya		"main land of the river"; homeland of the Central Ejagham
ngu Ndem		a skin with small brass bells worn on the back of a mgbokandem
ngya Ndem		foot rattles of Ndem
ngyime		language
nja Ndem		rattles of a mgbokandem worn on the ankles
nje	aje	witch
Njemaya		"back of the river"; the area of the Ekwe, i. e. west of the Munaya River
njoho Nkanda		the chief of Nkanda, "the man who performs the sacrifice"
njom	ajom	"bad" medicine, medicine society
Njom		designates medicine societies, especially Obasinjom

Singular	Plural	Explanation/Translation
Njom egeh		"medicine-try"; the process of searching for potential mask carriers of Obasinjom
Njom Ekpa		a secret society of the women which possesses a mask
nju	oju	house
nkakamem	akakamem	sharer of wine
nkan	okan	age-group
Nkanda		secret society, often, however, a separate section of Mgbe
nkankang	okankang	iron double bell
nkeku	akeku	dead person, ancestor, ghost, devil
nkekwet	akekwet	widow or widower
nkem	akem	cripple; name of the small slit-drum of Angbu
nkepansi	akepansi	devil
nkundak	okundak	peacock
nkwen okum	akwen okum	mask dancer or bearer of a mask
nkwui	okwui	tortoise; in Mgbe used as a musical instrument
nne atemambi	anne atemambi	"a man of atemambi"; a full member of Obasinjom
nne eboho	anne eboho	"man sitting on the mud-bed"; a leader of a secret society
nne echi	anne bechi	"head of people", chief
nne echi ka quarter	anne bechi ka quarter	quarterhead
nnenkwui ndebenju	bakwui ndebenju	family head, elderly person of a family
nnenkwuinne	bakwuianne	old man or elderly person
nse Amok		"father of Amok"; the largest medicine container of Amok
nse nju	ase or base oju	father, head of a house or a family
nsibiri		"bad feelings and intentions"; name of a section in Mgbe and also the name of the secret sign language in Mgbe
nsibiri Nkanda		the first stage of Nkanda
nsu ayong		"washer of blood"; one who performs the cleansing ceremony after a murder
ntufam emong		chief or king in Ikom and Ogoja regions (Nigeria)
ntui mfam	atui afam	chief, head of a community
ntui mfam okarara		"white man's chief"; chief, installed formerly by the colonial authorities
ntui oyim	atui oyim	"chief of wickedness"; the person who was formerly in charge of slaying the victims during night dances
nya	oya	animal
nyakayong	onyakayong	millipede, "one who makes blood black" (a witch)
Nyampkwe		another name for Mgbe
Obasinjom		"God of Medicine"; a magic medicine (njom) in the form of a mask
Obasi Nsi		God of the earth
Obon		a secret society of men
ocha Mgbe Mgbe	acha Mgbe	the lodge of Mgbe (parlour of a seseku) and assembly of
ocha Njom		assembly of Obasinjom
ochantui	abhaatui	house of the chief, "palace", where cases are tried
ofegh		white-wash, chalk, white earth
ofu akeken nkeku	afu akeken akeku	day of burying the corpse
oghork		yellow camwood
ojahne Angbu		autopsy performed by Angbu

Singular	Plural	Explanation/Translation
oje ba kpang		a special ritual of Obasinjom in which the medicine nchip Njom is made
oje Njom		"Obasinjom's witch"; concoction of medicinal leaves and herbs ound at the back of Obasinjom's head
okahah Mgbe		"to answer Mgbe"; a rank in Mgbe, where the members can enter the lodge with shoes and drink while sitting down
okat Mgbe		"curtain of Mgbe"; a rank in Mgbe
Okeboho		a magic medicine (njom) in the form of small bags woven of raffia fiber
okina or okinaribo		messenger of Mgbe
okongo	akongo	a section of Mgbe that appears only at night
Okpambe		the old name of Obasinjom among the Central Ejagham
okum	akum	(secret) society
okume eboho		"sitting on the bed"; the rank of the big men in secret societies
olang		fufu, made of cocoyams or cassava
oneng nfut	aneng nfut	curved feathers
orongho Mgbe	arongho Mgbe	"board of Mgbe" in the form of a square-woven mat hung on the wall of the sitting room of a seseku
osam Njom	asam Njom	staff of Obasinjom, also the designation for the interpreter of Obasinjom
osa Ndem	nsa Ndem	staff of a mgbokandem
osangito	abosangito	one who performs an ugly job, scavenger of any secret society, mask bearer of Angbu society
osongaribo	asongaribo	title in Mgbe; deputy of the seseku
osuamet		"washing the eyes"; a medicine ritual in the initiation in secret societies
oyem	ayem	grave, monument, pit
oyem olebe		presentation of a new commemorative figure for a deceased mgbokandem
oyot	ayot	blessing, healing
oyotnsi	ayotnsi	blessing of the ancestors
oyot obasi	ayot obasi	blessing from God
seseku	boseseku	highest title in Mgbe that qualifies one to own a lodge
sure njom		to swear or activate a magic medicine (njom)

Bibliography

Abalogu, U. N., 1978: Ekpe society in Arochukwu and Bende. In: Nigeria Magazine. Nos. 126–127: 78–97.

Adedeji, Joel A., 1972: The origin and form of the Yoruba masque theatre. In: Cahiers d'Etudes Africaines. 12: 254–276.

Agbor, Ayukonchong Williams, 2001: The influence of German rule in Keaka country 1884–1916. B. Th.-Thesis. Presbyterian Theological Seminary, Kumba (Cameroon).

Akpan, Joseph J., 1994: Ekpo society masks of the Ibibio. In: African Arts. 27 (4): 48–53, 94–95.

Alagoa, E. J., 1963: Delta masquerades. In: Nigeria Magazine. No. 93: 145–155.

Anonymous, 1956: Calabar. In: Nigeria. 52: 70–98.

Anonymous, 1957: Efik dances. In: Nigeria. 53: 150–169.

Ardener, Edwin, 1970: Witchcraft, economics, and the continuity of belief. In: Mary Douglas (ed.), Confessions and accusations. London: 141–160.

Ardener, Edwin, Shirley Ardener and W. A. Warmington, 1960: Plantation and village in the Cameroons. London.

Argenti, Nicolas, 2006: Remembering the future: slavery, youth and masking in the Cameroon Grassfields. In: Social Anthropology. 14: 49–69.

Balz, Heinrich, 1984: Where the faith has to live. Studies in Bakossi society and religion. Part I: Living together. Berlin.

Bastian, Adolf, 1884: Der Fetisch an der Küste Guinea's. Berlin.

Beier, Ulli, 1956: Ibibio monuments. In: Nigeria Magazine. 51: 318–336.

id., 1963: African mud sculpture. London.

Blier, Suzanne Preston, 1980: Africa's Cross River. Art of the Nigerian-Cameroon border redefined. New York. L. Kahan Gallery.

Boston, John Shipway, 1960: Some northern Ibo masquerades. In: Journal of the Royal Anthropological Institute. London. 90: 54–65.

Brain, Robert and Adam Pollock, 1971: Bangwa funerary sculpture. London.

Butler, V. F., 1963: Cement funeral sculpture in Eastern Nigeria. In: Nigeria Magazine. No. 77: 117–124.

Campbell, Kenneth F., 1983: Nsibidi update. In: Arts d'Afrique Noire. 47: 33–46.

Chem-Langhëë, B. and E. S. D. Fomin, 1995: Slavery and slave trade among the Banyang in the nineteenth and early twentieth centuries. In: Paideuma. 41: 191–206.

Chilver, Elizabeth M., 1990: Thaumaturgy in contemporary traditional religion: The case of Nso' in mid-century. In: Journal of Religion in Africa. 20 (3): 226–247.

Cole, Herbert M., 1982: Mbari. Art and life among the Owerri Igbo. Bloomington.

id., 1985: Introduction: The mask, masking, and masquerade arts in Africa. In: Herbert M. Cole (ed.), I am not myself: The art of African masquerade. Los Angeles: 15–27.

id. et al., 1970: African arts of transformation. Santa Barbara.

id. and Chike C. Aniakor, 1984: Igbo arts. Community and cosmos. Los Angeles

Crowder, Michael, 1962: The story of Nigeria. London.

id., 1977: West Africa. An introduction to its history. London.

De Wolff, P. P.. 1981: Die afrikanischen Sprachfamilien. I. Niger-Kordofanisch. In: Bernd Heine et al. (eds.), Die Sprachen Afrikas. Hamburg: 45–76.

Dike, P. Chike, 1987: Art, symbol and authority among the Aro of South-East Nigeria. In: Nigeria Magazine. No. 55: 30–35 .

Dillon, Richard G., 1990: Ranking and resistance. A precolonial Cameroonian polity in regional perspective. Stanford, California.

Drewal, Henry John, 1978: The arts of Egungun among Yoruba peoples. In: African Arts. 11 (3): 18–19, 97.

Drewal, Henry John and Margaret Thompson Drewal, 1983: Gelede. Art and female power among the Yoruba. Bloomington.

Drewal, Margaret Thompson, 1992: Yoruba ritual. Bloomington and Indianapolis.

Ekpo, Ikwo A., 1978: Ekpe costume of the Cross River. In: African Arts. 12 (1): 72–75, 108.

Evans-Pritchard, Edward E., 1977: Nuer-Religion. Oxford.

Eyo, Ekpo, 1981: Description of a headdress from the Ekoi. In: Susan Vogel (ed.), For spirits and gods. New York: 167.

Fagg, William, 1963: Nigerian images. New York.
id., 1964: Africa. 100 Tribes – 100 Masterpieces. Berlin.

Fagg, William and John Pemberton, 1982: Yoruba sculpture of West Africa. New York.

Forkl, Hermann, 1989: Linden-Museum Stuttgart. Abteilungsführer Afrika. Stuttgart.

Fowler, Ian and David Zeitlyn (eds.), 1996: African crossroads: Intersections between history and anthropology in Cameroon. Oxford.

Frobenius, Leo, 1898: Die Masken und Geheimbünde Afrikas. Halle.
id., 1954: Kulturgeschichte Afrikas. Zürich.

Geschiere, Peter, 1993: Chiefs and colonial rule in Cameroon: Inventing chieftaincy, French and British style. In: Africa. 63: 151–175.
id., 1997: The modernity of witchcraft. Politics and the occult in postcolonial Africa. Charlottesville and London.

Hackett, Rosalind I. J., 1989: Religion in Calabar. The religious life and history of a Nigerian town. Berlin, New York.
id., 1996: Art and religion in Africa. London, New York.

Harris, Rosemary, 1984: Mbembe men's associations. In: African Arts. 18 (1): 61–63, 96.

Herreman, Frank, 1993: Face of the spirits. In: Frank Herreman and Constantijn Petridis (eds.), Face of the spirits. Masks from the Zaire basin. Antwerpen: 11–20.

Homberger, Lorenz, 1999: Trance-Wahrsager. In: Museum Rietberg Zürich (ed.), Orakel. Der Blick in die Zukunft. Zürich: 273–297.

Horton, Robin, 1960: The gods as guests. An aspect of Kalabari religious life. Lagos.
id., 1963: The Kalabari Ekine society: a borderland of religion and art. In: Africa. 33: 94–114.
id., 1971: From fishing village to city-state. A social history of New Calabar. In: Mary Douglas and Phyllis M. Kaberry (eds.), Man in Africa. New York: 38–60.
id., 1993: Patterns of thought in Africa and the West. Cambridge U. P.

Hutchinson, Thomas J., 1858: Impressions of Western Africa. London.

Hutter, Franz, 1902: Wanderungen und Forschungen im Nord-Hinterland von Kamerun. Braunschweig.

Ittmann, Johannes, 1954/1955: Bemerkungen zu den Altersklassen der Douala und ihrer Nachbarn. In: Afrika und Übersee. 39: 83–88.
id., 1957: Der kultische Geheimbund *djĕngú* an der Kameruner Küste. In: Anthropos. 52: 135–176.

Iyalla, B. S., 1968: Womanhood in the Kalabari. In: Nigeria Magazine. No. 98: 216–224.

Jeffreys, M. D. W., 1939: Some notes on the Ekoi. In: Journal of the Royal Anthropological Institute. London. 69: 95–108.
id.,1949: The bull-roarer among the Ibo. In: African Studies. 8: 23–34.

Jones, G. I., 1956: The political organisation of Old Calabar. In: Daryll Forde (ed.), Efik traders of Old Calabar. London, New York, Toronto: 116–160.
id., 1963: The trading states of the Oil Rivers. London, Ibadan, Accra.

Kasfir, Sidney Littlefield, 1984: Masks from the towns of the dead: The Igbo – Idoma borderland. In: Herbert M. Cole and Chike C. Aniakor (eds.), Igbo arts. Community and cosmos. Los Angeles: 163–165.
id., 1988: Introduction: Masquerading as a cultural system. In: Sidney L. Kasfir (ed.), West African masks and cultural systems. Tervuren: 1–16.

Kecskési, Maria, 1987: African masterpieces and selected works from Munich: The Staatliches Museum für Völkerkunde. New York.

Kecskési, Maria und László Vajda, 1997: "Ich bin nicht ich selbst". Maske und Maskenwesen in Afrika. In: Iris Hahner-Herzog, Maria Kecskési und László Vajda, Das zweite Gesicht. Afrikanische Masken aus der Sammlung Barbier-Mueller, Genf. München, New York: 11–36.

Koloss, Hans-Joachim, 1984: Njom among the Ejagham. In: African Arts. 18 (1): 71–73, 90–93.
id., 1985: Obasinjom among the Ejagham. In: African Arts. 18 (2): 62–65, 98–101, 103.
id., 1986: Zaubermedizinen in West-Kamerun. In: Joseph F. Thiel (ed.), Was sind Fetische? Frankfurt am Main: 233–279.
id., 1992: Review of: Dillon, Richard G., Ranking and resistance. A precolonial Cameroonian polity in regional perspective. Stanford 1990. In: Tribus. 41: 199–201.
id., 2000: World-view and society in Oku (Cameroon). Berlin.
id. (ed.), (2002): Africa. Art and culture. Masterpieces of African art. Ethnological Museum Berlin.
id.. 2008: Court art and masks in the kingdoms of the North West Province of Cameroon. In: Lorenz Homberger (ed.), Cameroon. Art and kings. Zürich: 67–109.

Langheld, W., 1909: Über die Stammesorganisationen in Kamerun. In: Koloniale Rundschau. Berlin: 542–545.
Latham, A. J. H., 1973: Old Calabar. 1600–1891. Oxford.
Leib, Elliott and Renee Romano, 1984: Reign of the leopard: Ngbe ritual. In: African Arts. 18 (1): 48–57, 542–545.
Lifschitz, Edward, 1988: Hearing is believing: Acoustic aspects of masking in Africa. In: Sidney L. Kasfir (ed.), West African masks and cultural systems. Tervuren: 221–229.

Mansfeld, Alfred, 1908: Urwald-Dokumente. Vier Jahre unter den Cross-Flussnegern Kameruns. Berlin.
id., 1924: Westafrika. Urwald- und Steppenbilder. Berlin.
Matiba, Jean Ikelle, 1966: Adler und Lilie in Kamerun. Ein Lebensbericht. Herrenalb, Schwarzwald.
McClusky, Pamela, 2002: Art from Africa. Long steps never broke a back. Seattle.
MacGaffey,Wyatt, 1986: Religion and society in Central Africa. The BaKongo of Lower Zaire. Chicago, London.
id., 1991: Art and healing of the BaKongo: commented by themselves. Stockholm.
Meek, C.K., 1937: Law and authority in a Nigerian tribe. London, New York, Toronto.
Messenger, John C., 1973: The carver in Anang society. In: Warren L. d'Azevedo (ed.), The traditional artist in African societies. Bloomington and London: 101–127.
Migeod, Frederick William Hugh, 1925: Through British Cameroons. London.
Müller (Oberst), 1904: Der Anjang-Feldzug. In: Deutsches Kolonialblatt. 15: 698–701.

Nair, Kannan K., 1972: Politics and society in South Eastern Nigeria. 1841–1906. A study of power, diplomacy and commerce in Old Calabar. London.
Ngoh, Victor Julius, 1996: History of Cameroon since 1800. Limbe.
Nicklin, Keith, 1974: Nigerian skin-covered masks. In: African Arts. 7 (3): 8–15, 67–68, 92.
id., 1977: Guide to the National Museum Oron. Lagos.
id., 1979: Skin-covered masks of Cameroon. In: African Arts. 12 (2): 54–59, 91–92.
id., 1980: Annang Ibibio raphia weaving. In: Dale Idiens and K. G. Ponting (eds.), Textiles of Africa. Bath: 142–162.
id., 1983: No condition is permanent: Cultural dialogue in the Cross River Region. In: The Nigerian Field. 48: 66–79.
id., 1984: Cross River Studies. In: African Arts. 18 (1): 24–27, 96.
id., 1991: An Ejagham emblem of the Ekpe society. In: Tribal Art Bulletin: Barbier-Mueller Museum, Geneva. 1991: 3–18.
id., 1995: Emblem of the leopard spirit society. In: Tom Phillips (ed.), African Art of a Continent. Munich, New York: 372–373.
Nicklin, Keith and Jill Salmons, 1984: Cross River art styles. In: African Arts. 18 (1): 28–43, 93–94.
N'Idu, Ado 1959: Ekpe-Cross River cult. In: West African Review. 30 (No. 384): 747–749.
Northrup, David, 1978: Trade without rulers. Precolonial economic development in South-Eastern Nigeria. Oxford.
Nzekwu, Onuora, 1960: Masquerade. In: Nigeria Magazine. A special independence issue: 134–144.

Ogunbiyi, Yemi, 1981: Drama and theatre in Nigeria: A critical source book. Lagos.
Olderogge, Dmitrij, 1969: Afrikanische Kunst. Aus den Afrika-Sammlungen des Museums für Anthropologie und Ethnographie, Leningrad. (Fotografien von Werner Forman). Hanau/Main.
Onor, Sandy Ojang, 1994: The Ejagham nation in the Cross River Region of Nigeria. Ibadan.
Ottenberg, Simon, 1975: Masked rituals of Afikpo. The context of an African art. Seattle and London.
Ottenberg, Simon and Linda Knudsen, 1985: Leopard society masquerades: symbolism and diffusion. In: African Arts. 18 (2): 37–44, 93–95, 103–104.

Parkinson, John, 1907: A note on the Efik and Ekoi tribes of the Eastern Province of Southern Nigeria, W.C.A. In: Journal of the Royal Anthropological Institute. London. 37: 261–267.
Partridge, Charles, 1905: Cross River natives. Being some notes on the primitive pagans of Obubura Hill District, Southern Nigeria.
Peek, Philip M., 1976: Isoko sacred mud sculpture. In: African Arts. 9 (4): 34–39, 91.
Poynor, Robin, 2001: Cross River, Cameroon Grasslands, and Gabon. In: Monica Blackmun Visonà et al. (eds.). A history of Art in Africa. New York: 331–365.

Röschenthaler, Ute, 1993: Die Kunst der Frauen. Zur Komplementarität von Nacktheit und Maskierung bei den Ejagham im Südwesten Kameruns. Berlin.
id., 1998: Honoring Ejagham women. In: African Arts. 31 (2): 38–49, 92–93.
id., 1999: Frauenbünde der Ejagham im Cross River Gebiet. In: Anne Helfensteller (ed.), Afrikanische Frauen. Frauen und Frauendarstellungen in

Kunst und Kultur Schwarzafrikas. Naturkunde-Museum Coburg: 26–50.
id., 2000: Lokalität und Siedlungsgeschichte im Cross River-Gebiet. In: Zeitschrift für Ethnologie. 125: 189–214.
id., 2004 (a): Neuheit, Bricolage oder Plagiat? Zur Entstehung neuer Tanzbünde im Cross River-Gebiet (im Südwesten Kameruns und Südosten Nigerias). In: Paideuma. 50: 193–223.
id., 2004 (b): Transacting Obasinjom: The dissemination of a cult agency in the Cross River area. In: Africa. 74: 241–276.
Rosevar, D. R., 1984: Cross River tombstones. In: African Arts. 18 (1): 44–47, 94.
Rubin, William (ed.), 1984: 'Primitivism' in 20th century art. New York.
Ruel, Malcolm, 1962: Banyang settlements. In: Man. 62: 99–103, 115–119.
id., 1965: Witchcraft, morality and doubt. In: Odu. 2: 3–27.
id., 1969: Leopard and leaders. Constitutional politics among a Cross River people.
London etc.
Rutherfoord, J. W.C., 1926: An Assessment-Report of the Keaka speaking area in the Mamfe Division of the Cameroons Province, from notes of Mr. J. W. C. Rutherfoord, Divisional Officer, edited by Mr. H. O. Anderson, Assistant District Officer. (Buea National Archives No. Af 27, Original File No. 115/1927).

Salmons, Jill, 1977: Mammy Wata. In: African Arts. 10 (3): 8–15, 87–88.
Schädler, Karl-Ferdinand, 1975: Afrikanische Kunst. München.
id., 1982: Ekoi. München.
Sigrist, Christian, 1978: Gesellschaften ohne Staat und die Entdeckungen der social anthropology. In: Fritz Kramer and Christian Sigrist (eds.), Gesellschaften ohne Staat. Band 1: Gleichheit und Gegenseitigkeit. Frankfurt am Main: 28–44.
Staschewski, F., 1917: Die Banjangi. Berlin.

Talbot, P. Amaury, 1912: In the shadow of the bush. London.
id., 1923: Life in Southern Nigeria. London.
id., 1926: The peoples of Southern Nigeria. A scetch of their history, ethnology and languages with an abstract of the 1921 census. 4 vols. London.
id., 1932: Tribes of the Niger delta. Their religions and customs. London.
Thompson, Robert Farris, 1974: African art in motion. Washington.
id., 1983: Flash of the spirit. African and African-American art and philosophy. New York.
Thormählen, Y., 1885: Mitteilungen über Land und Leute in Kamerun. In: Mitteilungen der Geographischen Gesellschaft in Hamburg 1884: 328–334.
Tunis, Angelika, 1985: Der Crossriver in Kamerun 1904–1909. Ein Beitrag zur Juju-Frage. In: Baessler-Archiv. 33: 497–519.

Udo Ema. A. J., 1938: The Ekpe society. In: Nigeria Magazine. No.16: 314–316.
id., 1940: Fattening girls in Oron, Calabar Province. In: Nigeria Magazine. No. 21: 386–389.
Ukpong, Edet Akpan, 1989: Government precolonial Ibibio-land: the role of secret societies. In: Nigeria Magazine. No. 57: 14–27.
Umoetuk, Okom U., 1985: Body art in Ibibio culture. In: Nigeria Magazine. No. 53: 40–56.

Waddell, Hope Masterton, 1863: Twenty-nine years in the West Indies and Central Africa: A review of missionary work and adventure. 1829–1858. London.
Wardwell, Allen (ed.), 1989: Yoruba. Nine centuries of African art and thought. New York.
Weston, Bonnie E., 1984: Northeastern Region. In: Herbert M. Cole and Chike C. Aniakor (eds.), Igbo arts. Community and cosmos. Los Angeles: 145– 161.
Wirz, Albert, 1972: Vom Sklavenhandel zum kolonialen Handel. Wirtschaftsräume und Wirtschaftsformen in Kamerun vor 1914. Zürich und Freiburg i. Br.

Zimmermann, Armin, 2002: The conditions of traditional and modern life for women in Cameroon. In: Armin Zimmermann (ed.), Voices from Kumba. Theological reflections for Cameroon, Africa and the world. Celebrating 50 years Presbyterian Theological Seminary, Kumba: 70–95.
Zintgraff, Eugen, 1895: Nord-Kamerun. Berlin.
Zürcher, J. W., 1939: Tanzmaske des Obaschinyom. In: Der Heidenbote. Monatsblatt der Evangelischen Missionsgesellschaft in Basel. 112 (5): 72.
Zwernemann, Jürgen, 1972: Eine außergewöhnliche Aufsatzmaske von den Bangwa, West-Kamerun. In: Tribus. 21: 69–75.

Index